Handbook of the Spinal Cord

VOLUMES 2 and 3: Anatomy and Physiology

HANDBOOK OF THE SPINAL CORD

series editor
Robert A. Davidoff

Professor and Vice Chairman, Department of Neurology
Professor, Department of Pharmacology
University of Miami School of Medicine
and Chief, Neurophysiology Research Laboratory
Veterans Administration Medical Center
Miami, Florida

Volume 1 Pharmacology

Volumes 2 and 3 Anatomy and Physiology

Volumes 4 and 5 Clinical Disorders: Injury and Diseases

Handbook of the Spinal Cord

VOLUMES 2 and 3: Anatomy and Physiology

edited by Robert A. Davidoff

*University of Miami School of Medicine
and Veterans Administration Medical Center
Miami, Florida*

MARCEL DEKKER, INC.   New York and Basel

Library of Congress Cataloging in Publication Data
(Revised for volumes 2 & 3)
Main entry under title:

Handbook of the spinal cord.

Includes bibliographical references and indexes.
Contents: v.1. Pharmacology --v. 2-3. Anatomy and
physiology.
1. Spinal cord--Handbooks, manuals, etc.
2. Spinal cord--Diseases--Handbooks, manuals, etc.
I. Davidoff, Robert A., [date].   [DNLM: 1. Spinal
cord. WL 400 H236]
QP371.H36 1983   612'.83   82-23674
ISBN 0-8247-1708-2 (v. 1)
ISBN 0-8247-7091-9 (v. 2 & 3)

MARCEL DEKKER, INC.
270 Madison Avenue, New York, New York 10016

Current printing (last digit):
10 9 8 7 6 5 4 3 2 1

PRINTED IN THE UNITED STATES OF AMERICA

INTRODUCTION TO THE SERIES

In recent years the spinal cord has been the subject of intense study by clinicians, physiologists, pharmacologists, and biochemists. The literature in this area is already formidable, and its exponentially accelerating volume provides abundant testimony to major advances that have already occurred and portends an increased and rapid growth in the future. It appears, then, that this is an opportune time to appraise and review, summarize and integrate, the current status of endeavors in this field.

The present series of volumes offers such an appraisal: a broad and comprehensive survey of the state of our knowledge about the spinal cord. It is my hope that the *Handbook* will be of value in the laboratory, in the clinic, and in the classroom to every student interested in the spinal cord, whether he or she be a beginner, an established investigator, a seasoned clinician, or a dedicated teacher.

The *Handbook* has been developed in three sections. Volume 1 deals with the pharmacology of the spinal cord with emphasis on the identification and action of neurotransmitters at specific spinal synapses. Volumes 2 and 3 review the anatomy, ultrastructure, and physiology of the cord. The last two volumes assess a variety of clinical problems affecting the cord with special attention given to pathophysiological mechanisms.

The design of the *Handbook* derives largely from my own enthusiasms and interests. These, in turn, reflect my clinical and laboratory training. To Morris B. Bender I owe a great obligation for teaching which emphasized minute examination of the patient so as to obtain clues to the physiological basis of normal function. He taught me to search for facts rather than for complicated and untestable theories. From Robert Werman and M.H. Aprison I received invaluable research training which emphasized the idea that advances arising from collaborative efforts between physiologists and chemists must be based on a firm understanding of anatomy. I also wish to acknowledge my inestimable debt to my wife Judith for her critical and logical approach to scholarship and for her aid in this and in all my other endeavors.

Robert A. Davidoff, M.D.

PREFACE

The purpose of these two volumes is to present a comprehensive description of our current knowledge of the structure and function of the spinal cord. Although an attempt has been made to cover the breadth and depth of the subject, a major focus has been placed on cellular mechanisms because this is the area of knowledge in which the greatest amount of progress has been made in the past several decades.

As indicated in the first volume of this series, much of the material is subject to varying interpretation and for this reason the divisions of topics among the various chapters are sometimes not very sharp. Some points were considered important enough to be covered from different, and sometimes from similar, points of view. Even though many areas remain controversial, advances in our understanding of the operations and morphology of the spinal cord have been so cast that they have led to a considerable revision of previously accepted ideas and concepts. A review of the material covered in these two volumes indicates that the spinal cord is a comprehensible structure and that a thorough conception of it may soon be possible. In addition, a common thread ties these two volumes to the first one in this series, for it is impossible to describe the spinal cord without realizing that structure and function must be correlated with, and are inseparable from, the pharmacological aspects of chemical synaptic transmission.

It is hoped that students, basic scientists, and clinicians will find in these volumes an accessible body of current concepts and data relevant to the spinal cord. As such, they should serve as an impetus for further research and study.

Robert A. Davidoff, M.D.

CONTRIBUTORS

Chandler McC. Brooks, D.Sc. Distinguished Professor Emeritus, Department of Physiology, Downstate Medical Center, State University of New York, Brooklyn, New York

Peter L. Carlen, M.D., F.R.C.P.(C.) Associate Professor, Department of Medicine (Neurology) and Physiology, Playfair Neuroscience Unit, Addiction Research Foundation Clinical Institute, University of Toronto, Toronto, Ontario, Canada

Ronald G. Clark, Ph.D. Associate Professor, Department of Anatomy and Cell Biology, University of Miami School of Medicine, Miami, Florida

Wayne E. Crill, M.D. Professor and Chairman, Department of Physiology and Biophysics, University of Washington School of Medicine, Seattle, Washington

Robert A. Davidoff, M.D. Professor and Vice Chairman, Department of Neurology, and Professor, Department of Pharmacology, University of Miami School of Medicine; and Chief, Neurophysiology Research Laboratory, Veterans Administration Medical Center, Miami, Florida

Dominique Durand, Ph.D.* Scientist, Playfair Neuroscience Unit, Addiction Research Foundation Clinical Institute, University of Toronto, Toronto, Ontario, Canada

Robert E. W. Fyffe, Ph.D.† Research Fellow and Visiting Assistant Professor, Departments of Anatomy and Physiology, School of Medicine, University of North Carolina at Chapel Hill, Chapel Hill, North Carolina

Present affiliation: Case Western Reserve University, Cleveland, Ohio

†*Present affiliation*: John Curtin School of Medical Research, Australian National University, Canberra, Australia

vii

Barth A. Green, M.D., F.A.C.S. Associate Professor, Department of Neurological Surgery, University of Miami School of Medicine, Miami, Florida

John C. Hackman, Ph.D. Assistant Professor, Departments of Neurology and Pharmacology, University of Miami School of Medicine; and Research Physiologist, Veterans Administration Medical Center, Miami, Florida

Ziaul Hasan, Ph.D. Assistant Professor, Department of Physiology, College of Medicine, University of Arizona Health Sciences Center, Tucson, Arizona

Nariyuki Hayashi, M.D.* Research Assistant Professor, Department of Neurological Surgery, University of Miami School of Medicine, Miami, Florida

Kiyomi Koizumi, M.D., Ph.D. Professor, Department of Physiology, Downstate Medical Center, State University of New York, Brooklyn, New York

Donald M. Lewis, Ph.D., M.B., B.Chir. Reader, Department of Physiology, The Medical School, University of Bristol, Bristol, England

David A. McCrea, Ph.D.[†] Assistant Professor, Playfair Neuroscience Unit, Addiction Research Foundation Clinical Institute, University of Toronto, Toronto, Ontario, Canada

John B. Munson, Ph.D. Professor, Departments of Neuroscience and Neurological Surgery, University of Florida College of Medicine, Gainesville, Florida

Ottavio Pompeiano, M.D. Professor, Department of Physiology, Institute of Human Physiology, University of Pisa, Pisa, Italy

Donald D. Price, Ph.D. Associate Professor, Department of Anesthesiology, Medical College of Virginia, Virginia Commonwealth University, Richmond, Virginia

Miklós Réthelyi, M.D. Associate Professor, Second Department of Anatomy, Semmelweis University Medical School, Budapest, Hungary

William Z. Rymer, M.D., Ph.D. Associate Professor, Departments of Physiology and Rehabilitation Medicine, Northwestern University Medical School, Chicago, Illinois

Arnold B. Scheibel, M.D. Professor, Departments of Anatomy and Psychiatry, and Brain Research Institute, UCLA School of Medicine, Los Angeles, California

Present affiliation: Nihon University Medical School, Tokyo, Japan

†*Present affiliation*: University of Manitoba, Winnipeg, Manitoba, Canada

Peter C. Schwindt, Ph.D. Associate Professor, Departments of Physiology and Biophysics, and Medicine (Neurology), University of Washington School of Medicine; and Veterans Administration Medical Center, Seattle, Washington

Paul S. G. Stein, Ph.D. Associate Professor, Department of Biology, Washington University, St. Louis, Missouri

Douglas G. Stuart, Ph.D. Professor, Department of Physiology, College of Medicine, University of Arizona Health Sciences Center, Tucson, Arizona

George W. Sypert, M.D. Professor, Departments of Neurological Surgery and Neuroscience, University of Florida College of Medicine; and Veterans Administration Medical Center, Gainesville, Florida

Richard P. Veraa, B.M.E. Director of Research Division, National Spinal Cord Injury Association, Lauderhill, Florida

Charles J. Vierck, Jr., Ph.D. Professor, Department of Neuroscience and Center for Neurobiological Sciences, University of Florida College of Medicine, Gainesville, Florida

CONTENTS

CONTENTS OF VOLUME 1: Pharmacology

Handbook of the Spinal Cord

VOLUMES 2 and 3: Anatomy and Physiology

1
ANATOMY OF THE MAMMALIAN CORD

Ronald G. Clark   *University of Miami School of Medicine, Miami, Florida*

I. INTRODUCTION

The spinal cord (medulla spinalis) is the elongated, cylindrical portion of the central nervous system that extends from the medulla oblongata to the upper lumbar vertebrae (Fig. 1). It resides within the cranial two thirds of the vertebral canal, enveloped by the meninges, bathed in cerebrospinal fluid, and attached by ligaments to the vertebrae. Thirty-one pairs of spinal nerves are connected with the cord and have the following distribution: eight cervical, twelve thoracic, five lumbar, five sacral, and one coccygeal. Each pair is formed by a series of dorsal and ventral routlets which merge together in the intervertebral foramina.

Neuronal cell bodies for all sensory input to the cord are located in the dorsal root ganglia within the intervertebral foramina. The sensory axons traverse the dorsal roots to reach the spinal cord. Cell bodies for the motoneurons are located in the gray matter of the spinal cord. Both somatic and visceral motor axons exit through the ventral roots to join the peripheral nerves.

The visceral motor output from the cord is the preganglionic component of the autonomic nervous system, which includes sympathetic and parasympathetic subdivisions. Axons from the first thoracic through the second lumbar cord levels give rise to the sympathetic (thoracolumbar) subdivision, while those from

1

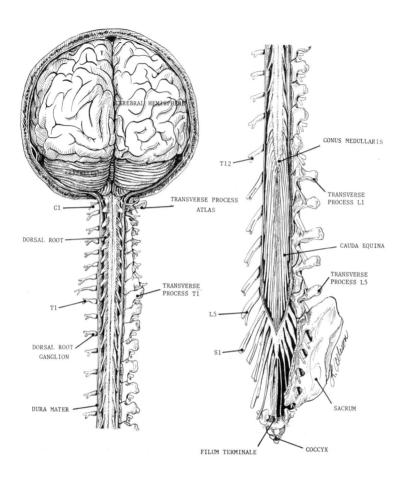

Figure 1 Posterior view of the human central nervous system. The posterior portions of all vertebrae have been removed so that the spinal cord and its relationships to the vertebral canal can be observed. To preserve detail at a greater magnification the diagram is divided into two parts.

the second through the fourth sacral levels contribute to the parasympathetic system. Other preganglionic parasympathetic axons arise from cranial nerves; thus the synonym craniosacral, denoting their combined cranial and sacral origin. The preganglionic axons course peripherally into the body cavities to synapse upon postganglionic neuronal cell bodies of the various autonomic ganglia. Finally the postganglionic neurons innervate glandular, smooth muscle, and cardiac tissue throughout the body.

The spinal cord proper consist of peripheral white matter surrounding central gray matter. Ascending and descending pathways reside in the white matter along with axons that make intersegmental connections. The gray matter is in the shape of an "H" or "butterfly," consisting of paired anterior and posterior horns connected by an intermediate band of gray matter. Neuronal cell bodies are located in the gray matter. They give rise to the ascending pathways, inter- and intrasegmental connections, and the entire motor output of the cord.

The following discussion refers to man except where indicated otherwise.

II. EXTERNAL TOPOGRAPHY AND RELATIONSHIPS WITH THE VERTEBRAL COLUMN

A. Anatomic Terminology

The anatomic terminology employed to describe various structures and pathways of the spinal cord is confusing. The reason for this is that the terms used for quadruped animals are not always applicable to the erect primate. This is particularly true of the terms "dorsal," "posterior," "ventral," and "anterior." For example, in rats it is correct to use the terms dorsal horn and ventral horn, whereas in man the same structures should be called the posterior horn and anterior horn, respectively, because of the cord's anatomic position in the upright posture. Technically, when referring to cord structures in man, the term "dorsal" would actually correspond to "superior" and "ventral" would equate with "inferior"—terms which are infrequently used when discussing the cord. Nevertheless, the terms dorsal and ventral are so ingrained that most authorities use dorsal and posterior, and ventral and anterior interchangeably. Even the absolute purist would find it difficult to use the term "posterior root ganglion" instead of "dorsal root ganglion."

The term "myelin" is based upon a misnomer: It is dervied from "myelos," the Greek word for marrow, which is equivalent to the Latin term "medulla" meaning marrow, or inner portion of an organ, in contrast to the outer portion, or cortex. While it is appropriate to use the term medulla in describing bone marrow, as in medullary cavity of bone, it is incorrectly used in such terms as myelin and myelinization or medullation of axons. The myelin sheath is a cortical not a marrow structure. The term was first used to describe the subcortical white matter of the cerebrum, which in essence is the "medullary substance" of the brain. Subsequent investigators applied the term to the myelin sheath.

B. Relative Cord Length

During the first three months of fetal development the spinal cord extends the entire length of the vertebral canal (1). Subsequently, the vertebral column grows at a faster rate than the spinal cord, and by the time of birth the cord extends to the inferior border of the second lumbar vertebra. In the late teens the spinal cord attains its adult position and terminates at the level of the intervertebral disc between the first and second lumbar vertebrae (Fig. 2). This position, however, can vary from the twelfth thoracic to the third lumbar vertebrae (1).

C. Spinal Cord Shape

The spinal cord does not form a true cylinder. Its transverse width is greater than its dorsoventral dimension, and there are two enlargements at the cervical and lumbar levels which are related to the innervation of the extremities (Fig. 3). Caudally, the cord tapers abruptly to become the conus medullaris, which is attached by the filum terminale, a meningeal structure, to the fundus of the dural sac at the level of the second sacral vertebra (Fig. 2). The length of the spinal cord is approximately 45 cm in men, and varies from 41 to 43 cm in women. The length of the entire vertebral column is 70 cm (1).

D. Spinal Nerves

A spinal cord segment consists of a portion of the spinal cord proper and all of its rootlets that join to form the associated pair of spinal nerves. The number of rootlets that form a spinal nerve varies from one level of the cord to the next, as does the length of the cord segments. Cervical segments average 13 mm, midthoracic segments 26 mm, lumbar segments 15 mm, and sacral segments 5 mm in length (1).

Because of the disparity in length between the spinal cord and vertebral column, the nerve rootlets from lumbar and sacral segments have a much longer distance to travel prior to reaching their respective foramina of exit. Whereas cervical and upper thoracic rootlets are situated nearly at right angles to the cord, lower thoracic, lumbar, and sacral rootlets enter and leave the cord at increasingly more oblique angles. This discrepancy is so pronounced in the caudal third of the vertebral canal that the rootlets run parallel to one another in nearly a superior to inferior direction, thus forming the cauda equina (Figs. 1 and 2).

E. Enlargements

1. Cervical Enlargement

The cervical enlargement corresponds to the innervation of the upper extremities and extends from the third cervical to the second thoracic cord levels (Fig. 3). It is 13 mm in width and 9 mm in dorsoventral diameter (1). The cervical plexus arises from the first to fourth cervical segments, and the brachial plexus arises from the fifth cervical to the first thoracic segments. The cervical enlargement extends from the third cervical to the second thoracic vertebrae.

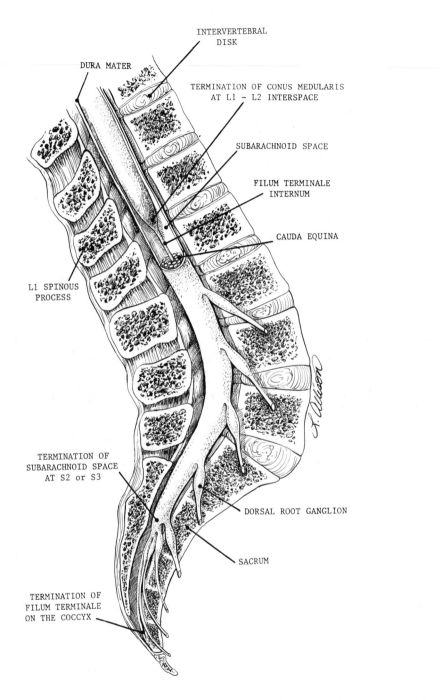

INTERVERTEBRAL
DISK

DURA MATER

TERMINATION OF CONUS MEDULARIS
AT L1 – L2 INTERSPACE

SUBARACHNOID SPACE

FILUM TERMINALE
INTERNUM

CAUDA EQUINA

L1 SPINOUS
PROCESS

TERMINATION OF
SUBARACHNOID SPACE
AT S2 or S3

DORSAL ROOT GANGLION

SACRUM

TERMINATION OF
FILUM TERMINALE
ON THE COCCYX

Figure 2 Diagrammatic representation of the lower portion of the vertebral column and spinal cord in sagittal view.

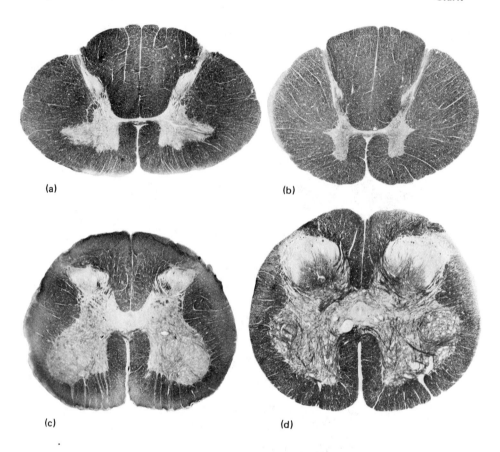

(a)   (b)

(c)   (d)

Figure 3 Transverse sections of the human spinal cord. The Weil stain utilized in treating the tissue imparts a very dark color to the myelin, leaving the gray matter light in appearance. (a) Cervical enlargement. (b) Thoracic cord. (c) Lumbar region of the lumbosacral enlargement. (d) Sacral region of the lumbosacral enlargement. Compare the configurations of gray and white matter at the various levels. The diameter of the cord is greatest at the cervical enlargement due to a larger number of axons in the white matter. This follows from the fact that the long descending and ascending pathways to all cord levels are present in the cervical cord while only those related to lower levels are found in the lumbosacral enlargement. Conversely, note that the relative amount of gray matter is greater in the lumbosacral enlargement than in the cervical enlargement. The greater muscle bulk of the lower extremities requires a larger number of neuronal cell bodies for supply and feedback than is necessary for the upper extremities. Published through the courtesy of Harper & Row. The author is indebted to Dr. Terence Williams for providing these photomicrographs.

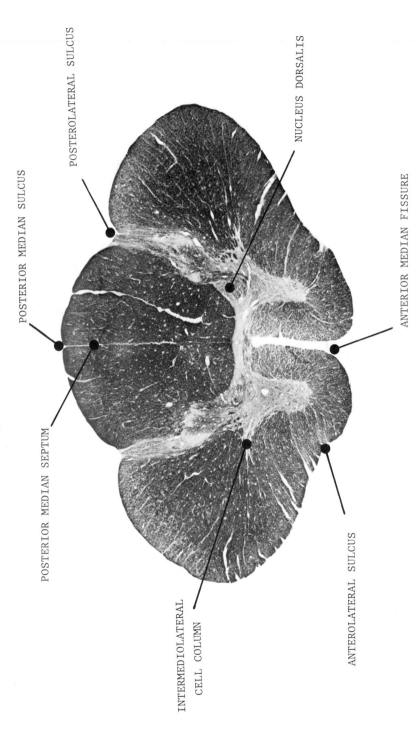

POSTERIOR MEDIAN SULCUS

POSTEROLATERAL SULCUS

POSTERIOR MEDIAN SEPTUM

INTERMEDIOLATERAL
CELL COLUMN

NUCLEUS DORSALIS

ANTERIOR MEDIAN FISSURE

ANTEROLATERAL SULCUS

Figure 4 Photomicrograph of a cross section of the human thoracic spinal cord (T6 level). Weil stain for myelin. ×15. The anterolateral and posterolateral sulci are much more pronounced at thoracic levels than at cervical and lumbosacral levels where they are quite superficial.

2. Lumbar Enlargement

The lumbar enlargement corresponds to the innervation of the lower extremities and extends from the first lumbar to the third sacral cord levels (Fig. 3). Slightly smaller than the cervical enlargement, it is 12 mm in width and 9 mm in dorso-ventral diameter (1). The lumbar plexus arises from the first to the fourth lumbar segments, and the sacral plexus from the fourth lumbar to the second sacral segments. The pudendal plexus arises from the third to fifth sacral levels. The lumbar enlargement extends from the ninth to the twelfth thoracic vertebra.

F. Fissures and Sulci

Several indentations extend the length of the spinal cord surface. The deepest of these is the anterior median fissure, which has an average depth of 3 mm and penetrates the ventral surface of the cord to the level of the anterior white commissure (Fig. 4). Branches of the anterior spinal artery are located in this fissure. There is a very shallow posterior median sulcus, anterior to which is located the posterior median septum, a thin glial tissue structure extending 4 to 6 mm and nearly to the central canal (Fig. 4). From the upper thoracic to the cervical cord, the posterointermediate sulcus overlies the posterointermediate septum, a structure that separates the fasciculus gracilis medially from the fasciculus cuneatus laterally.

Two indistinct sulci are related to the nerve rootlets. The posterolateral sulcus is present in the dorsal root entry zone, while the anterolateral sulcus is located in the ventral root exit zone (Fig. 4).

III. BLOOD VESSELS

A. Arterial Supply

The spinal cord receives its major arterial blood supply from the medullary (radicular) arteries, which are derivatives of the embryonic segmental vessels. The anterior spinal and the posterior spinal arteries also contribute to the spinal cord's blood supply but to a lesser degree.

1. Medullary Arteries

Medullary arteries arise consecutively as spinal branches of the posterior inferior cerebellar, vertebral, deep cervical, intercostal, and lumbar arteries. They enter the spinal canal by passing through the intervertebral foramina, in which location they are referred to as lateral spinal arteries, and then bifurcate to follow the dorsal and ventral nerve roots, becoming the anterior and posterior medullary arteries (also called the anterior and posterior radicular arteries). The term "radicle" means nerve root; consequently, the name radicular arteries should be applied to those vessels supplying only the nerve roots. The medullary arteries follow the nerve roots to the cord and then bifurcate into ascending and descending branches, forming numerous anastomoses with the posterior and anterior spinal arteries.

There is tremendous variation in the number and arrangement of the medullary arteries. Embryologically, there are 31 pairs of medullary arteries accompanying the 31 pairs of spinal nerves. In the adult, neither the number nor the symmetry persists. Usually, there are six to 10 on each side, each of which forms an anterior and posterior medullary artery. Frequently, one of the anterior medullary arteries in the lower thoracic or upper lumbar region is larger than the rest and is referred to as the great anterior medullary artery (arteria radicularis magna of Adamkiewicz).

2. Anterior Spinal Artery

On the anterior surface of the medulla oblongata each vertebral artery gives rise to a descending branch. The artery and branch join to form the anterior spinal artery that passes down the entire length of the spinal cord in or near the anterior median fissure (Fig. 5). It is misleading to think of this vessel as being totally dependent upon the input from the vertebral artery because numerous segmental anastomoses from the medullary (radicular) arteries exist throughout its course. There are large variations in the size of the anterior spinal artery from one level of the spinal cord to the next, and it frequently splits into more than one vessel. It is responsible, however, for the blood supply of much of the entire anterior two thirds of the spinal cord, including all of the anterior horn and most of the intermediate gray matter.

3. Posterior Spinal Arteries

The posterior spinal artery arises either as a branch of the vertebral artery or the posterior inferior cerebellar artery on the posterolateral surface of the medulla oblongata. It originates as a paired structure, one on each side, and descends just lateral to the entry of the dorsal roots (Fig. 5). Shortly after its origin, the posterior spinal artery typically splits into two anastomotic channels, one medial and the other lateral, to the entering dorsal roots. Similar to the anterior spinal artery, the posterior spinal artery has numerous anastomoses with the segmental medullary arteries, and there are great variations in size through its descending course. Along with vessels that enter the cord from the pia mater, the posterior spinal arteries supply the posterior third of the cord and overlap to some extent with the anterior spinal artery to supply the intermediate gray area.

Circumferentially, there are numerous anastomoses between the major channels, which are commonly referred to as pial plexuses. The pial vessels enter the peripheral substance of the spinal cord and are most important in supplying blood to the lateral and posterior aspects of the cord.

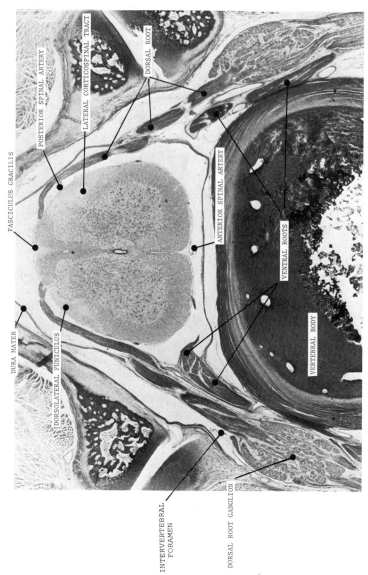

Figure 5 Photomicrograph of a cervical cord cross section (C5 level) from a 10-day-old beagle dog. Luxol fast blue stain for myelin counterstained with cresyl violet for neuronal cell bodies. × 23. At this age myelinization is incomplete in the fasciculus gracilis, lateral corticospinal tract, and dorsolateral funiculus. At cervical levels the dorsal root ganglia are located quite ventrally in the intervertebral foramina. At increasingly more caudal levels the ganglia assume a more dorsal position closer to the later aspect of the spinal cord.

B. Blood-Brain Barrier

It is important to note that like most vessels within the central nervous system (exceptions to this include: arteries of the choroid plexus, median eminence, subfornical organ, subcommissural organ, and area postrema), the endothelial cells of intrinsic spinal cord arteries are connected by tight junctions (2-5). This is unlike the situation in the rest of the body where fenestrated or "leaky" junctions are the rule. Tight junctions prevent certain drugs and other substances from readily entering the brain, a physiologic mechanism referred to as the blood-brain barrier.

C. Venous Drainage

In general, veins and arteries do not accompany one another in the central nervous system. Veins exiting from the spinal cord typically form rich plexuses in the pia-arachnoid layer which usually are deep to the arterial plexuses. Characteristically, six major but highly variable channels can be observed, with the anterior median vein being best defined. It lies within the anterior median fissure and drains most of the anterior portion of the cord. Other less distinct channels are located near the dorsal and ventral root zones and the posterior median sulcus. Of these, the posterior median vein is the most conspicuous and it drains most of the posterior and lateral regions of the cord.

A series of anterior and posterior medullary or radicular veins drain the superficial veins within the pia-arachnoid layer. They do not accompany the medullary arteries, and they are more numerous, with as many as 36 to 60 being present. The medullary veins drain into dense longitudinal vertebral plexuses located posteriorly and anteriorly in the epidural space. These plexuses, referred to as the internal epidural plexuses, are connected together by anastomotic channels. Blood then drains through the intervertebral and sacral foramina to empty into the external vertebral venous plexuses.

IV. MENINGES

Three connective tissue layers, the meninges, envelop the spinal cord and consist of, from without to within: the dura mater, the arachnoid mater, and the pia mater (Figs. 6 and 7). Whereas in lower vertebrates the dura mater arises from mesenchyme and the pia and arachnoid are of neural crest origin, all three layers are of mesenchymal origin in man (6). Neural crest cells, however, apparently contribute to the formation of the pia mater in man (6).

A. Dura Mater

The dura mater is a very tough, opaque membrane consisting of interlacing bundles of collagen with some elastic tissue lined by an endothelium. Although

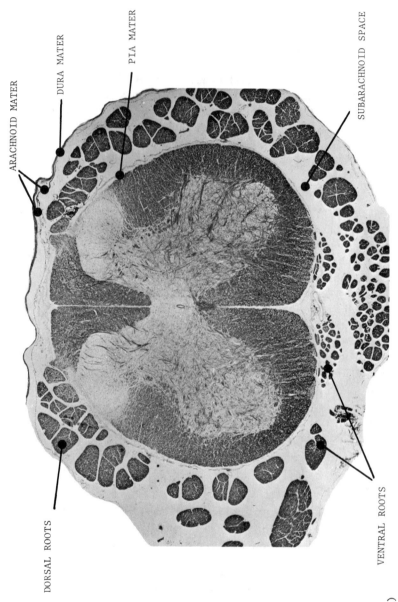

ARACHNOID MATER

DURA MATER

PIA MATER

SUBARACHNOID SPACE

DORSAL ROOTS

VENTRAL ROOTS

(a)

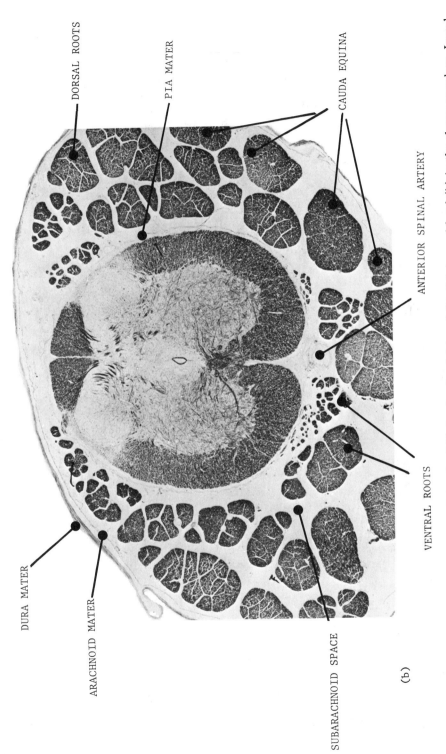

DORSAL ROOTS

PIA MATER

CAUDA EQUINA

ANTERIOR SPINAL ARTERY

VENTRAL ROOTS

DURA MATER

ARACHNOID MATER

SUBARACHNOID SPACE

(b)

Figure 6 Photomicrograph of cross sections from the fifth lumbar level (a) and the third sacral level (b) in the rhesus monkey. Luxol fast blue counterstained with cresyl violet. × 11.

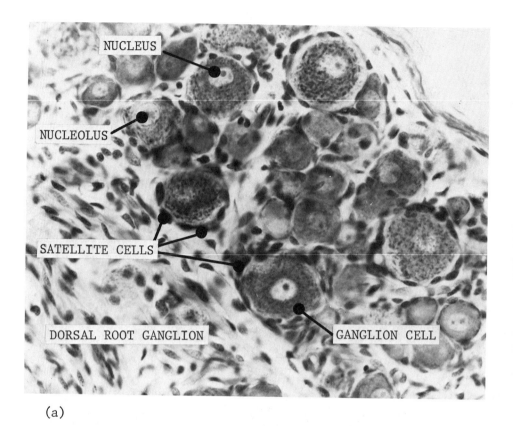

(a)

Figure 7 Photomicrographs of dorsal root (a) and sympathetic chain (b) ganglia. Cresyl violet stain. × 550. The unipolar cell bodies in the dorsal root ganglion are much larger and more spherical than the multipolar neuronal cell bodies in the sympathetic ganglion. The nuclei in sympathetic ganglia tend to be more eccentrically located than those in dorsal root ganglia. Most nuclei have a single, prominent nucleolus. Satellite cells are common to both ganglia.

primarily avascular, blood vessels, lymphatics, and nerve fibers have been reported to occur toward the middle of the dura (7). The dura mater of the spinal cord is continuous with the inner layer of the cranial dura. Whereas the outer layer of the cranial dura subserves as the periosteum of the skull, the bony wall of the vertebral canal has its own periosteum. An epidural space, containing fatty and loose connective tissue and the epidural venous plexuses, separates the

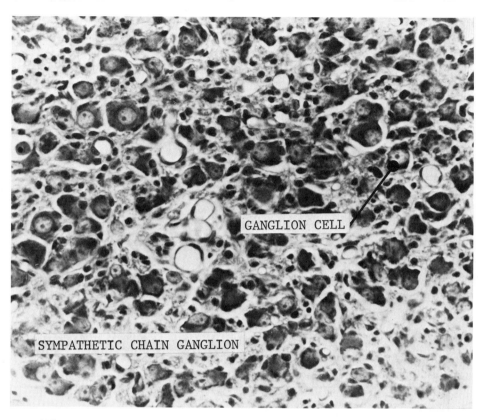

GANGLION CELL

SYMPATHETIC CHAIN GANGLION

(b)

dura from the periosteum of the vertebrae. The dura is in close approximation to the outer surface of the arachnoid matter, such that under normal circumstances the subdural space is almost nonexistent. This space does, however, contain a small amount of fluid resembling lymph. The dura ends at the lower border of the second sacral vertebra.

B. Pia-Arachnoid Mater

The arachnoid mater consists of connective tissue cells several layers thick. With numerous organelles and pinocytotic vesicles present (7), the cells are obviously active in protein transport and synthesis and in fluid uptake. A meshwork of fine trabeculae interconnect the arachnoid with the underlying pia mater.

The connective tissue cells on the inner aspect of the pia overlie a basement membrane which resides on the surface of the spinal cord. The pia-arachnoid, or leptomeninges, is rich in macrophages and blood vessels.

C. Cerebrospinal Fluid

The cerebrospinal fluid flows through the ventricles of the brain and the subarachnoid spaces and cisternae surrounding the entire central nervous system. It is clear, colorless fluid with a specific gravity of approximately 1005, which is nearly protein and cell free (8). It contains less glucose than plasma. In man the total volume of cerebrospinal fluid is approximately 140 ml, with 30 ml in the ventricles and 110 ml in the subarachnoid space. The pressure of the cerebrospinal fluid, as measured by lumbar puncture in the recumbent position, is 100–200 mm H_2O. The pressure is 200 mm H_2O higher than this when measured in the sitting position.

The cerebrospinal fluid is formed to a large extent by the active secretion of the epithelial cells of the choroid plexuses within the ventricular cavities. The nervous system lacks lymphatics; consequently, the interstitial and perivascular fluids drain directly into the ventricles, the central canal of the spinal cord, and the subarachnoid spaces, all contributing substantially to the formation of the cerebrospinal fluid. It is produced at the rate of 0.2 ml/min. Absorption of cerebrospinal fluid occurs through the arachnoid villi into the dural sinuses of the brain, into spinal veins, and perhaps into lymphatics of the vertebral column.

Since the spinal cord terminates between the first and second lumbar vertebrae and the subarachnoid space extends to the second sacral level, cerebrospinal fluid can be removed from the lower lumbar area by needle without fear of cord injury. This same space can be used for the injection of radiopaque substances to enhance the diagnostic capabilities for x-ray and computerized axial tomographic scan evaluations of the spinal cord. This procedure is referred to as positive contrast myelography.

V. GANGLIA

A. Dorsal Root Ganglia

The dorsal root ganglia (spinal ganglia) reside outside the spinal canal and are located within the intervertebral foramina (Figs. 3, 5, and 7). Specifically, they occupy the distal portion of the dorsal roots near their junction with the ventral roots. The ganglia are derived from the neural crest under the influence cᶠ the neurotrophic protein, nerve growth factor (9), and contain the nerve cell bodies of nearly all somatic and visceral sensory input from the body to the spinal cord. The unipolar ganglion cells vary in diameter from 11 μm to 100 μm. Ganglion cells innervating neighboring peripheral receptive fields tend to cluster close together, reflecting a fundamental principle–that of the somatotopic neuronal organization which is maintained throughout the nervous system (10). This neuronal population is part of the peripheral nervous system; consequently, neither glial cells nor meningeal tissues are present.

Each dorsal root ganglion is encapsulated by fairly dense connective tissue that is continuous with the epineurium and perineurium of the related peripheral nerves. It should be noted that peripheral nerves have several connective tissue coverings. The epineurium, or outermost layer, is the most dense and tough, and invests the entire nerve. Within the nerve bundles of longitudinally running axons are separated into fascicles, each of which is invested by another dense connective tissue sheath, the perineurium. This latter envelope is not limiting because axons can leave one fasciculus to enter another. Finally, individual axons are enwrapped by the delicate connective tissue layer, the endoneurium.

Each ganglion cell is invested by a row of satellite cells (Fig. 7) (also called amphicytes) which also are derived from the neural crest and appear to have a function similar to Schwann cells. Indeed, they are probably modified Schwann cells. A basal lamina is present covering the satellite cells, followed by a thin connective tissue layer that is continuous with the endoneurium of the related peripheral nerves. The radicular arteries typically follow the connective tissue investments to terminate in capillary plexuses in the endoneurium.

It has been traditionally accepted that ganglion cells usually have a single myelinated process which bifurcates into a peripheral branch and a central branch. In many instances, prior to bifurcating, the initial segment is highly coiled and is referred to as the glomerular segment. The peripheral branch may course to a peripheral receptor or terminate as an unmyelinated nerve ending in a variety of structures, including the skin, subcutaneous tissue, muscle, and periosteum. The central branch enters the central nervous system to synapse with another neuron.

Recent quantitative data present a more complex picture. According to the classic view, there should be equal numbers of sensory axons in the dorsal root, dorsal root ganglion cells, and sensory axons in the proximal portion of the peripheral nerve. This, however, is not the case. In the rat sacral area there are more than twice the number of dorsal root and proximal peripheral nerve axons than there are ganglion cells (11). This evidence suggests branching in both the central and peripheral axonal processes of the dorsal root ganglion cells. These investigators feel that this may permit a single ganglion cell to receive stimuli from receptive fields in two separate locations.

Structurally and functionally, the peripheral and central processes of ganglion cells are axons, the dendritic component of the neuron being located in its most peripheral portion in the receptor region. The nerve impulse is normally transmitted along the peripheral to the central process without entering the cell body. Schwann cells continue along the centrally directed axons of the dorsal root until it reaches the vicinity of the cord where oligodendrocytes take over the responsibility of maintaining the myelin sheath. This transition does not occur as a sharp boundary, but rather changes gradually.

It is of interest to note than when their peripheral processes are transected, the ganglion cells undergo chromatolysis, but that this fails to occur when the central processes are severed. This may result from the fact that more of the substances synthesized in the nerve cell body are transported into the peripheral than into the central process.

B. Autonomic Ganglia

Preganglionic neuronal cell bodies of the spinal cord are located in the lateral aspect of the intermediate gray matter. Their axons exit the cord through the ventral roots and then pass through the white ramus communicans. Preganglionic sympathetic neurons synapse either in the sympathetic chain ganglia or in the prevertebral ganglia (e.g., celiac ganglion). Preganglionic parasympathetic axons, on the other hand, travel all the way to the viscera to be innervated, and synapse in either of two plexuses. One is the myenteric plexus, or plexus of Auerbach, that is located between the longitudinal and circular smooth muscle layers of the organs. The other is the submucosal plexus, or plexus of Meissner, that resides in the submucosal lining of the viscera.

Connective tissue and satellite cell investments in the sympathetic ganglia are quite similar to those described for the dorsal root ganglia. In general, the neuronal cell bodies are smaller in diameter and their nuclei tend to be more eccentrically located than those of the dorsal root ganglia (Fig. 7). There are major differences, however, that distinguish autonomic ganglia from dorsal root ganglia. Neurons in autonomic ganglia are multipolar and receive synapses. A single preganglionic sympathetic axon may synapse upon as many as 20 to more than 100 postganglionic cell bodies in a sympathetic chain ganglion. The presence of interneurons is another major difference. At least two populations of interneurons are known to exist, small intense fluorescent cells and chromaffin cells. Both types of cells are catecholaminergic neurons.

VI. PERIPHERAL AXONAL STRUCTURES

A. Splanchnic Nerves

The splanchnic nerves carry preganglionic sympathetic axons that originate in the intermediolateral cell column from the first thoracic through the second lumbar vertebrae to synapse in the prevertebral ganglia. They also contain visceral axons whose cell bodies are located in the dorsal root ganglia.

The pelvic splanchnic nerves convey preganglionic parasympathetic neurons that arise from the intermediate gray matter of the second through the fourth sacral levels.

B. Sympathetic Trunk

Quantitative data from the rat cervical sympathetic trunk indicates that 84% of the axons are preganglionic, 11% are postganglionic, and 5% are sensory, resulting in a preganglionic/postganglionic ratio of approximately 4:1 (12).

C. Rami Communicantes

The rami communicantes attach the sympathetic chain to the proximal portion of peripheral nerves. At each level there are two rami, the lateral white ramus communicans and the medial gray ramus communicans. They both contain preganglionic, postganglionic, and visceral sensory axons.

1. White Ramus Communicans

Previously it was thought that the white ramus communicans contained only myelinated preganglionic and sensory axons. Recently, utilizing experimental surgical techniques with subsequent electron microscopic examination of tissues, this was proved to be an oversimplification (13,14). In the cat thoracic region there are 3200 unmyelinated and 1600 myelinated axons. Approximately 85% of the myelinated axonal population consists of preganglionic sympathetics, and the remainder is thought to be visceral sensory input. Of the unmyelinated axons, 30% are preganglionic sympathetic fibers and 60% appear to be postganglionic sympathetics, leaving only 10% as visceral sensory axons.

2. Gray Ramus Communicans

Previously it was thought that the gray ramus communicans contained only unmyelinated postganglionic axons. This also has proved to be an oversimplification (13,14). In the cat thoracic region there are 4 to 5 myelinated sensory axons, 20 to 25 unmyelinated sensory axons, 3000 to 5000 unmyelinated postganglionic sympathetic axons, and 25 myelinated postganglionic axons.

D. Dorsal Roots

Each dorsal root fans out into several rootlets which enter the cord in a row along the posterolateral sulcus. Approximately 40% of the dorsal root consists of the small unmyelinated C-fibers. As each dorsal rootlet enters the cord, it is characteristically divided into medial and lateral segments based upon structural differences (Figs. 1 and 5). The lateral portion in primates, including man, contains very small myelinated and unmyelinated axons which terminate primarily in laminae I and II of the posterior horn (15). A few of the fibers also synapse in laminae III and V (16). In contrast, large myelinated axons enter the medial division to bifurcate into ascending and descending branches which

ultimately project in an arc posteriorly over the posterior horn and then anteriorly down along the medial aspect of the horn to terminate primarily in
laminae III and below (17).

E. Ventral Roots

Each ventral root results from the coalescence of several rootlets which exit the
cord in the anterolateral sulcus (Fig. 4). Immediately distal to the dorsal root
ganglion the ventral root joins the dorsal root in the intervertebral foramen to
form the spinal nerve (Fig. 5).

Traditionally, only myelinated motor axons were considered to be present
in the ventral roots. It is now known that sensory fibers are present, and furthermore, electron microscopic studies reveal that approximately 30% of the ventral
root fibers are unmyelinated (18,19). While one half of these unmyelinated axons
are known to be preganglionic autonomics, many of the remainder are sensory
and arise from both visceral and somatic structures. It is thought that the
majority of the sensory axons are related to pain input. A few myelinated
sensory fibers have also been demonstrated in the ventral roots.

VII. INTERNAL STRUCTURE OF THE SPINAL CORD

A. White Matter

Unlike the cerebrum and cerebellum, white matter is peripheral to gray matter in
the spinal cord. It is white in the fresh state because of the presence of myelin;
however, there are more unmyelinated than myelinated axons (20). In the rat
sacral cord there are approximately 177,000 myelinated and 263,000 unmyelinated axons in the white matter. Surprisingly, more than one half of the myelinated axons are confined to the dorsal part of the lateral funiculus. This region
includes part of the lateral corticospinal tract, part of the dorsal spinocerebellar
tract, and an area referred to as the dorsolateral funiculus (Fig. 8).

Blood vessels and neuroglia are also constituents of the white matter. The
neuroglia includes oligodendrocytes, astrocytes, and microglia. The pia mater
follows the vessels for a short distance into the white matter and then is replaced
by astrocytic processes which are tightly adherent to the vessels. Collagen,
except in blood vessels and the pia mater, is absent from spinal cord tissue,
accounting for its friable consistency.

Neither neuronal cell bodies nor dendrites are normally present in the white
matter. Some of the sparsely situated, large neuronal cell bodies that rim the
circumference of the substantia gelatinosa protrude into the neighboring white
matter, and occasionally isolated large neuronal cell bodies are observed in the
white matter lateral to the dorsal horn.

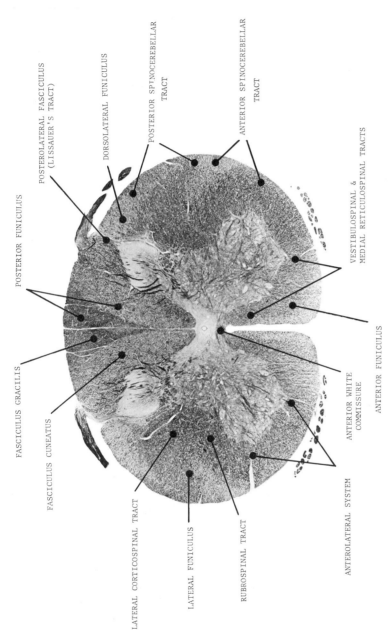

Figure 8 Photomicrograph of a cervical enlargement (C5 level) cross section from a rhesus monkey depicting the major funiculi of white matter and the primary ascending and descending pathways. Weil stain. × 22. Note the difference in appearance between the fasciculus gracilis and fasciculus cuneatus. The axons in the fasciculus gracilis are smaller in diameter than those of the fasciculus cuneatus because the large-caliber fibers ascending from the lumbosacral levels leave this system to join the dorsolateral funiculus.

POSTEROLATERAL FASCICULUS
(LISSAUER'S TRACT)

DORSOLATERAL FUNICULUS

POSTERIOR SPINOCEREBELLAR
TRACT

ANTERIOR SPINOCEREBELLAR
TRACT

VESTIBULOSPINAL &
MEDIAL RETICULOSPINAL TRACTS

POSTERIOR FUNICULUS

FASCICULUS GRACILIS

FASCICULUS CUNEATUS

ANTERIOR WHITE
COMMISSURE

ANTERIOR FUNICULUS

LATERAL CORTICOSPINAL TRACT

LATERAL FUNICULUS

RUBROSPINAL TRACT

ANTEROLATERAL SYSTEM

In each half of the cord the white matter is subdivided into three major regions, referred to as funiculi (Fig. 8). The posterior funiculus is located between the posterior median septum medially and the posterior horn and dorsal root entry zone laterally. The lateral funiculus, in turn, is subtended by the posterior horn and dorsal root entry zone and the anterior horn and ventral root exit zone. The anterior funiculus is bounded laterally by the anterior horn and ventral root exit zone and medially by the anterior median fissure.

Three other regions require explanation. Immediately adjacent to and completely surrounding the gray matter is a region of the white matter referred to as the propriospinal system, or bundle. Myelinated and unmyelinated axons interconnecting gray matter at one level with that of another ascend and descend in this system. Another area, the posterolateral fasciculus, or Lissauer's tract, is located at the juncture between the posterior and lateral funiculi in the dorsal root entry zone. Approximately one third of the axons in this fasciculus are part of the propriospinal system, whereas the remainder are primary sensory axons entering from the dorsal roots (21). Finally, immediately posterior to the anterior median fissure and anterior to the central canal is a small region of decussating fibers called the anterior white commissure.

The diameter of the cervical enlargement is greater than that of the lumbosacral enlargement. This is due to the greater amount of white matter present at the cervical level (Fig. 3). All descending and ascending pathways to both the upper and lower extremities are present at cervical levels, whereas only those related to lower extremities are present in lumbosacral levels.

B. Gray Matter

Although one speaks of spinal cord segments or levels, the gray matter exists as a laminated, neuronal cell body continuum, extending the length of the cord without interruption. Viewed in cross section, the gray matter is shaped roughly in the form of the letter "H," and is subdivided into paired posterior and anterior horns (or columns) interconnected by a central band of intermediate gray substance (Fig. 8). Neuronal cell bodies and dentritic processes are intermixed with axons, blood vessels, and neuroglia. The predominance of the former imparts a gray color to the tissue in the fresh state.

The shape and size of the horns varies from one region to the next; for example, the anterior horns are quite wide in the cervical and lumbar enlargements and much narrower in upper cervical and thoracic levels (Figs. 4 and 9). The reason for this, of course, is that a greater neuronal cell population is required to supply the muscle mass of the extremities than is necessary for the innervation of the neck and truncal musculature. A lateral cell projection of the intermediate gray matter is present in thoracic and, to a lesser extent, in upper lumbar levels but not at other cord levels (Fig. 4). It contains the cell bodies of the preganglionic sympathetic neurons.

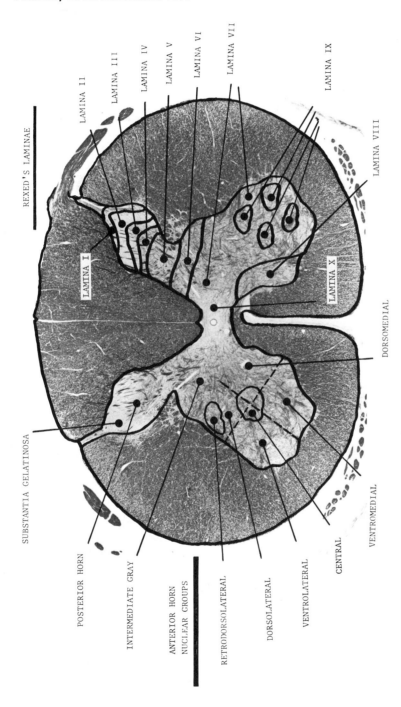

Figure 9 Photomicrograph of the cervical enlargement (C5 level) cross section from a rhesus monkey. On the left side the major nuclear groups are outlined while the right side depicts Rexed's laminae. Weil stain. ×25.

Wide variation exists in neuronal structure and size in the gray matter. Cells possessing long axons which pass out of the gray matter and either into the ventral roots or into the white matter pathways are referred to as Golgi type I neurons. Cells with short axons, on the other hand, which tend to be confined to intra- and intersegmental connections, are called Golgi type II neurons. Interneurons are the primary example of the latter type. All neurons are multipolar and their cell bodies vary in size from 15 to 135 μm in diameter, but small ones (15-25 μm) predominate. Most of the large cells are alpha motoneurons that innervate striated muscle, whereas the small ones serve either as interneurons or as gamma motoneurons that innervate intrafusal muscles fibers of muscle spindles. Other intermediate- to large-sized neurons give rise to ascending pathways.

Two classification systems are utilized to categorize the various regions of spinal cord gray matter. The most precise is based upon cytoarchitectonic studies which reveal the nerve cell bodies to be longitudinally organized into more or less continuous layers or laminae [after Rexed (22,23)]. Although originally described in the cat, this system has proved to be applicable with minor variations to nearly all mammalian species. The second system is based upon the tendency for nerve cell bodies to cluster into functional nuclear configurations.

1. Rexed's Laminae

Rexed described 10 regions (Fig. 9) based upon Nissl stained preparations that extended, in general, as columns throughout the length of the cat spinal cord. Similar laminar patterns have been demonstrated in all species studied, including man and other primates (15-17,22-24).

a. Laminae I through VI. Laminae I through VI are located in sequential, horizontal layers in the posterior (dorsal) horn (column). Lamina I (marginal layer), the outermost layer, is a very narrow band that caps the posterior horn immediately peripheral to the substantia gelatinosa and internal to the posterolateral fasciculus of Lissauer. Internal to this layer is lamina II, which is considered to be the region occupied by the substantia gelatinosa (of Rolando) (24). Continuing anteriorly, or ventrally, laminae III and IV are in the apex of the posterior horn and are generally regarded as the location of the nucleus proprius, or dorsal funicular gray matter. The next layer, lamina V is in the region considered to be the neck of the posterior horn. Finally, lamina VI is in the base of the posterior horn and is most conspicuous at the regions of the enlargements.

b. Lamina VII. Lamina VII is comparable for the most part to the intermediate gray matter. It includes the nucleus dorsalis of Clarke, and the intermediomedial and intermediolateral cell columns. Lamina VII also has a ventral component that extends into the anterior horn between laminae VIII and IX.

c. Laminae VIII through X. Lamina VIII is confined to the medial aspect of the anterior horn at the levels of the enlargements, but extends through much of the base of the anterior horn in the thoracic levels. It gives rise to many commissural fibers that pass to the opposite side of the spinal cord. Lamina IX consists of cell clusters in the anterior horn and contains the alpha and gamma motoneurons and interneurons. Finally, lamina X is a small region with few neuronal cell bodies located in the intermediate gray matter adjacent to the central canal.

2. Nuclear Configurations

While a collection of neuronal cell bodies in the peripheral nervous system is referred to as a ganglion, within the central nervous system it is called a nucleus. Usually, the neurons within a given nucleus subserve a similiar function. Typically, each nucleus contains both interneurons and neurons which give rise to longer projection systems. Some nuclei are quite conspicuous and well circumscribed, whereas others are more diffuse and not so readily delineated. In general, the spinal cord nuclei are distributed in longitudinal columns, some of which persist throughout the length of the cord, while others are more restricted in their extent.

a. Anterior horn (column). The anterior horn contains three columns of nerve cells, including lateral, medial, and central regions (Fig. 10).

Lateral nuclear group. Because its neurons supply the musculature of the extremities, the lateral nuclear group is present only at the levels of the enlargements. It is further subdivided into ventrolateral, dorsolateral, and retrodorsolateral subdivisions. The retrodorsal component innervates the musculature of the hand and foot, which suggests the somatotopic organization of the lateral column; namely, the more dorsal the location of the nerve cell body, the more distal the musculature innervated by it.

Medial nuclear group. The medial nuclear group is present throughout most of the length of the cord. It is primarily responsible for the innervation of truncal and proximal limb musculature. In thoracic and upper lumbar levels it is subdivided into ventromedial and dorsomedial components. Rostral and caudal to these levels, only the ventromedial component is present, except at the first cervical level where only the dorsomedial component is found.

Central nuclear group. The central nuclear group is the most limited and least consistent of the anterior horn nuclear columns. Only two of its nuclear groups are well understood and both of these groups are in the cervical cord. The phrenic nucleus innervates the diaphragm and it is located in the central region from the third to the seventh cervical levels. The accessory nucleus is located from the first to the sixth cervical levels in the central and ventral aspect of the anterior horn. It gives rise to the spinal portion of the accessory nerve.

b. Posterior horn (column). Three nuclear columns extend the length of the cord, including the marginal zone, the substantia gelatinosa, and the dorsal

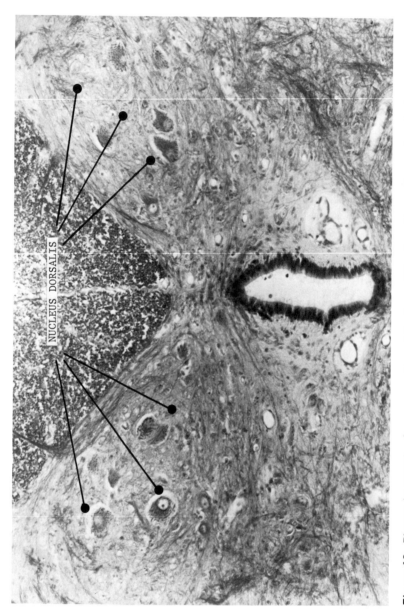

Figure 10 Photomicrograph of a cross section of the base of the dorsal horns from a beagle dog thoracic cord (T12 level). Luxol fast blue counterstained with cresyl violet. × 220. The nucleus dorsalis (Clarke's nucleus) is spherical with large neuronal cell bodies located on the medial aspect of the base of the dorsal horn.

NUCLEUS DORSALIS

funicular gray matter, or nucleus proprius. The marginal zone is a narrow band immediately peripheral and posterior to the substantia gelatinosa. It is comparable to Rexed's lamina I. The substantia gelatinosa (of Rolando) also is present at all cord levels and is considered to be Rexed's lamina II. The dorsal funicular gray matter, or nucleus proprius, is immediately anterior to the substantia gelatinosa and is considered to reside in Rexed's laminae III and IV. It too is present the length of the cord.

    c. Intermediate gray matter. The intermediate gray matter is located in Rexed's lamina VII, and contains the nucleus dorsalis of Clarke and preganglionic autonomic cell bodies (Figs. 4 and 10). The nucleus dorsalis is located on the medial aspect of the base of the posterior horn; it contains interneurons and gives rise to spinocerebellar axons. While it extends the length of the thoracic cord through the second lumbar vertebra, the nucleus dorsalis is largest at the lower thoracic and upper lumbar segments.

    The intermediate gray matter of the thoracic and upper lumbar levels is subdivided into intermediomedial and intermediolateral cell columns. Both contain preganglionic sympathetic neuronal cell bodies. The intermediolateral division is responsible for the lateral column projection which is most conspicuous in thoracic levels. The intermediate gray substance from the second through the fourth sacral segments contains preganglionic parasympathetic cell bodies; however, it lacks a lateral projection and is not subdivided into medial and lateral components.

C. Ascending Pathways

Information from the spinal cord projects along multiple ascending pathways in the white matter to reach supraspinal structures. They are congregated primarily in the posterior funiculus, anterolateral system, and entire lateral margin of the lateral funiculus, including the area referred to as the posterolateral (dorsolateral) funiculus (Fig. 8). Major targets of these systems include: (1) the nuclei gracilis and cuneatus (referred to collectively as the posterior or dorsal column nuclei), (2) the thalamus, (3) the reticular formation, (4) the tectum of the midbrain, (5) the cerebellum, (6) the inferior olivary nuclei, and (7) the vestibular nuclei. The reader is referred to the publications by Wiesendanger and Miles (25) and Brodal (26) for a comprehensive review of ascending pathways.

1. Posterior Column Pathways

The posterior or dorsal column pathways include the tracts that ascend through the posterior funiculi of the spinal cord; namely, the fasciculi gracilis and cuneatus (Fig. 8). Admittedly, the terminology with respect to this system is inconsistent and one must be cautious to differentiate between the term posterior column, meaning posterior horn, and, in this instance, posterior column, meaning posterior funiculus. The majority of axons arise ipsilaterally from the larger myelinated fibers entering from the medial division of the dorsal roots. Thus, the cell bodies of origin are the dorsal root ganglion cells. Approximately 15% of the axons, however, consist of secondary neurons arising from laminae III and IV of the ipsilateral posterior horn. Furthermore, a small proportion of the primary afferent fibers terminate in the posterior horn at various levels. For completion, it must be realized that a small proportion of descending axons reside in the posterior funiculus. Whereas some are intersegmental in origin, others arise from the nuclei gracilis and cuneatus and terminate primarily in lamina V of the posterior horn (an area containing neurons receptive to noxious stimuli).

Proceeding from caudal to rostral, incoming axons add laterally to those axons already present in the posterior funiculus; consequently, the somatotopic organization at the cervical cord is such that sacral representation is most medial and cervical representation most lateral. This arrangement is not absolute in that there is some sorting of fibers as they ascend. Axons that enter from the sixth thoracic level and above give rise to the fasciculus cuneatus, while those from the seventh thoracic and below contribute to the formation of the fasciculus gracilis.

The majority of primary axons in these pathways terminate in the ipsilateral nuclei gracilis and cuneatus (Figs. 11, 12, and 13). Most of the second-order neurons on the other hand do not synapse in these nuclei, but rather cross over to join the contralateral medial lemniscus. Still other second-order neurons course ipsilaterally via the posterior external arcuate system to reach the cerebellum. Most of the axons originating in the nuclei gracilis and cuneatus decussate in the medulla oblongata to form the ascending medial lemniscus and then synapse in the ventral posterolateral nucleus and posterior nuclear complex of the thalamus.

Functional and clinical considerations regarding the posterior column pathways have been revised dramatically over the past few years. At thoracic and cervical levels fasciculus cuneatus is much more heavily endowed with large myelinated axons than is the fasciculus gracilis. This results from the fact that the primary afferents from muscle and joint receptors of the forelimb travel in the fasciculus cuneatus, but similar fibers from the hindlimbs leave the fasciculus gracilis in lower lumbar levels and ascend through other systems (such as the posterior aspect of the lateral funiculus). This particular hindlimb projection terminates in subnucleus Z, which is located immediately rostral to the nucleus gracilis. Posterior column lesions, therefore, should effect more of a pronounced deficit with respect to the upper than the lower extremities. Ataxia, then, would not be an anticipated clinical finding as traditionally conceived.

It now appears that the posterior column pathways are not particularly important with respect to vibratory and joint sensations. In fact, large experimental lesions of this system produce relatively mild deficits. What is emerging, however, is the concept that these pathways are involved in highly complex, discriminative

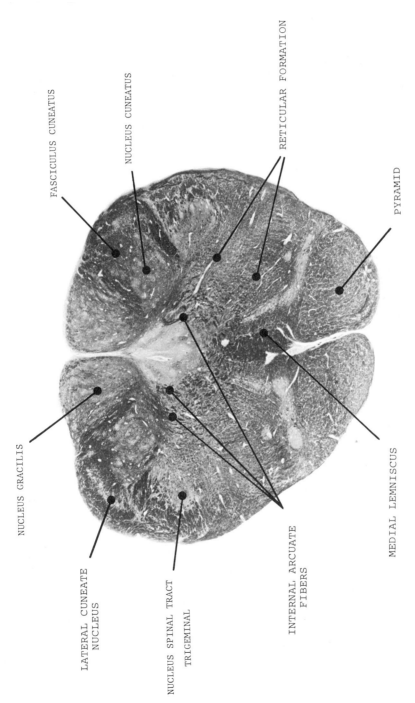

Figure 11 Caudal aspect of the human medulla oblongata, cross section. Weil stain. × 10. The internal arcuate fibers are axons that arise from cell bodies in the nuclei gracilis and cuneatus. The fibers decussate to give rise to the medial lemniscus. This is referred to as the sensory decussation.

FASCICULUS CUNEATUS

NUCLEUS CUNEATUS

RETICULAR FORMATION

PYRAMID

NUCLEUS GRACILIS

LATERAL CUNEATE NUCLEUS

NUCLEUS SPINAL TRACT TRIGEMINAL

INTERNAL ARCUATE FIBERS

MEDIAL LEMNISCUS

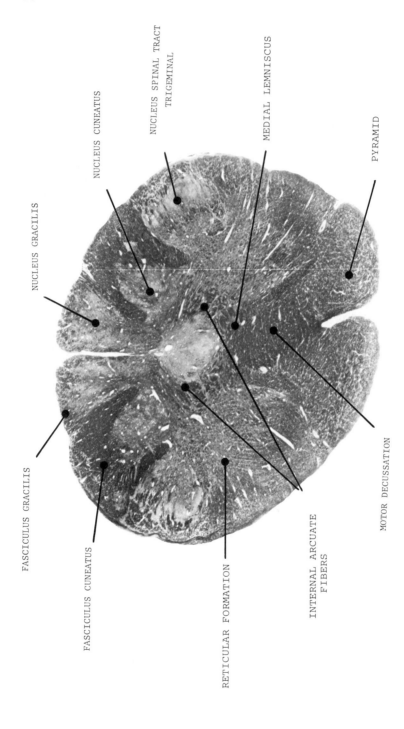

NUCLEUS SPINAL TRACT
TRIGEMINAL

NUCLEUS CUNEATUS

MEDIAL LEMNISCUS

PYRAMID

NUCLEUS GRACILIS

FASCICULUS GRACILIS

FASCICULUS CUNEATUS

RETICULAR FORMATION

INTERNAL ARCUATE
FIBERS

MOTOR DECUSSATION

Figure 12 Caudal aspect of the human medulla oblongata, cross section, at the level of the motor decussation. This section is at a level caudal to that of Figure 11. Weil stain. × 12.

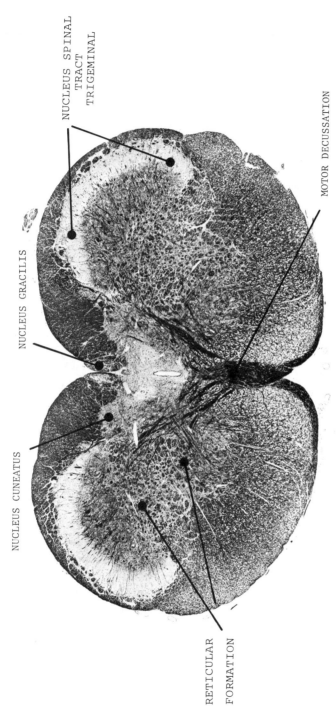

NUCLEUS SPINAL TRACT TRIGEMINAL

MOTOR DECUSSATION

NUCLEUS GRACILIS

NUCLEUS CUNEATUS

RETICULAR FORMATION

Figure 13 Caudal aspect of the rabbit medulla oblongata, cross section, at the level of motor decussation. Luxol fast blue stain. × 20.

tasks, such as judging the magnitude of cutaneous pressure, maintaining the finger grip on an object held in hand, discerning the distance between two applied stimuli, determining the direction of skin movement, and writing.

2. The Anterolateral System

The anterolateral system is located in the white matter peripheral to the anterior (ventral) horn and includes portions of both the lateral and anterior funiculi (Fig. 13). It contains spinothalamic, spinoreticular, and spinotectal projections. No longer is it justified, either functionally or structurally, to subdivide further into anterior and lateral spinothalamic components. The system conveys pain, temperature, touch, and pressure information.

The anterolateral system is not compactly organized, but rather, it is somewhat diffusely structured and intermingles with other ascending pathways. Nevertheless, there is a general somatotopic tendency such that axons arising from lower segments (such as sacral) are located in a more posterolateral position, and those from higher levels (such as cervical) are more anteromedial in location.

a. The spinothalamic system. All cord levels contribute to the formation of the spinothalamic tract. It is a relatively small component of the anterolateral system and arises primarily from the contralateral side of laminae I, V, VII, and VIII. Some fibers also arise from laminae II through IV and VI. It is of interest to note that in the monkey while the majority of axons at the cervical level originate from laminae I and V, those in the lumbar region arise from laminae VII and VIII. A prominent uncrossed bundle of fibers in the spinothalamic tract that arises primarily from laminae VII and VIII of the second cervical segment has been reported in the rat, cat, and monkey.

Spinothalamic neurons synapse in several areas of the thalamus. Many terminate bilaterally in the posterior thalamic nuclear complex and the intralaminar nuclei. Some fibers also project to the ventral posterior intermediate nucleus. While in the cat no fibers terminate in the ventral posterolateral nucleus, in the monkey there is a contralateral projection to this nucleus.

In man the spinothalamic tract is considered to convey temperature sensation; however, this has not been demonstrated experimentally in primates. Recently data in the cat suggest that axons carrying temperature input ascend in several systems, including the posterior column pathways. Similarly, several systems in addition to the spinothalamic tract convey pain information. These include the spinocervicothalamic tract, spinoreticular tract, spinotectal tract, and intersegmental, polysynaptic systems.

Clinically, the anterolateral system is transected to relieve abdominal or pelvic pain in patients terminally ill with cancer, a procedure referred to as a cordotomy. The surgical incision is made on the contralateral side, at least one segment above the level of the pain. Initially, there is nearly a total loss of pain.

After a period of weeks or months some of the pain may recur as a result of either uncrossed pathways or pain mediated by other ascending systems.

b. Spinoreticular tracts. A large number of the axons in the anterolateral system terminate both ipsilaterally and contralaterally in the reticular formation (27). Many are collaterals of the spinothalamic tract. Spinoreticular fibers synapse in nearly all regions of the reticular formation, with a heavy input to the lateral reticular nucleus, the raphe nuclei, and neighboring medial regions. The latter contain the nucleus reticularis gigantocellularis of the medulla, the nuclei reticularis caudalis and oralis of the pons, and the nucleus subcoeruleus. Spinoreticular information can reach the level of the thalamus by a polysynaptic system, spinoreticulothalamic connections. In the monkey a spinoreticular tract has also been demonstrated in the anterior funiculus. The spinoreticular pathways respond to a wide variety of sensory stimulation.

c. Spinotectal tract. In the rat the spinotectal tract arises at all cord levels, travels with the anterolateral system, and terminates in the deep layers of the contralateral superior colliculus. In the cat this system arises from cervical levels only. Little is known of this pathway in primates. There is a projection from the spinal cord to the periaqueductal gray matter of the midbrain. This system arises from cell bodies of laminae I through IV of the posterior horn and terminates upon opiate receptor cells in the periaqueductal gray matter.

3. Spinocervicothalamic System

The lateral cervical nucleus is a narrow, lateral projection located immediately ventral to the base of the dorsal horn in the cat. The nucleus is present in the monkey and has been reported in approximately 50% of human cords studied. Possibly, the cell bodies are incorporated into the base of the posterior horn when the lateral projection is lacking.

Afferent fibers to the lateral cervical nucleus arise at all cord levels from the ipsilateral dorsal horn, primarily from lamina IV. The axons travel in the most dorsal aspect of the lateral funiculus, immediately dorsal to the dorsal spinocerebellar tract (28). Most frequently, this pathway is referred to as the dorsolateral funiculus (Figs. 5 and 8), a term which is misleading and easily confused with the dorsolateral fasciculus (Lissauer's tract). The dorsolateral funiculus, then, would contain the spinocervical component of the spinocervicothalamic system. The fibers synapse in the lateral cervical nucleus, which, in turn, projects its axons through the contralateral medial lemniscus to the ventral posterolateral nucleus of the thalamus. The fibers in the medial lemniscus represent the cervicothalamic component of the entire system (29-32). Some fibers also terminate in the posterior nuclear complex of the thalamus.

This system responds to a variety of sensory stimuli conveyed over very heavily myelinated to unmyelinated fibers, primarily from cutaneous receptors.

Touch, pressure, and pain information, therefore, travels over this system to the thalamus.

4. Spinocerebellar Systems

Several pathways convey information from the spinal cord to the cerebellum (33). The posterior and anterior spinocerebellar tracts (Fig. 8) project sensation related primarily to the lower extremities, while the rostral spinocerebellar and cuneocerebellar tracts subserve similar functions for the upper extremities.

   a. Posterior spinocerebellar tract. The posterior or dorsal spinocerebellar tract resides in the posterior and lateral aspect of the lateral funiculus, and arises from the ipsilateral nucleus dorsalis, Clarke's nucleus, of lamina VII (Figs. 4, 8, and 10). Though present from the first thoracic through the second lumbar vertebrae, the nucleus dorsalis is largest in the lower thoracic and upper lumbar segments. The pathway projects through the inferior cerebellar peduncle to terminate in the vermis and paravermal region of the cerebellum in the hindlimb regions.

   Functionally, the posterior spinocerebellar tract conveys information from muscle spindles, Golgi tendon organs, joints, and touch and pressure receptors of the lower extremity.

   b. Anterior spinocerebellar tract. The anterior or ventral spinocerebellar tract is located anterior to the posterior spinocerebellar tract in the anterior and lateral aspect of the lateral funiculus. It arises from the contralateral laminae V through VII, primarily from lamina VII, of the lumbrosacral segments. Many of the cells of origin are in the most peripheral aspect of the anterior horn in the dorsolateral region. The anterior spinocerebellar tract ascends through the brain stem to the level of the pons, where it enters the superior cerebellar peduncle to enter the vermal and paravermal region of the cerebellum bilaterally.

   Functionally, the anterior spinocerebellar tract receives information from the same types of receptors that contribute to the posterior spinocerebellar tract. The anterior spinocerebellar tract, as a result of numerous polysynaptic inputs, relays information regarding the status of muscle groups and the entire extremity. The posterior spinocerebellar tract on the other hand, with smaller receptive fields, tends to impart information regarding individual muscles.

   c. Cuneocerebellar tract. The cuneocerebellar tract is the upper extremity equivalent of the posterior spinocerebellar tract in the lower extremity. It arises ipsilaterally from the lateral (external or accessory) cuneate nucleus (Fig. 11), passes through the inferior cerebellar peduncle, and terminates in the vermal and paravermal region of the cerebellum (34). The lateral cuneate nucleus is comparable in function to the nucleus dorsalis. Sensory input to this nucleus arises from axons of the dorsal root ganglia from the fourth thoracic through the first cervical levels. Information from muscle spindles, Golgi tendon organs, joints, and touch and pressure receptors of the upper trunk, upper extremity, and neck projects into this system.

d. Rostral spinocerebellar tract. The rostral spinocerebellar tract is the upper extremity equivalent of the anterior spinocerebellar tract in the lower extremity. Although the location of the cell bodies of origin is not firmly established, it appears as though the ipsilateral laminae VII give rise to some of the axons in this pathway. The fibers enter the cerebellum through both the inferior and superior cerebellar peduncles to terminate in the vermis and paravermal regions.

5. Spinovestibular Tracts

A small number of fibers arising from the spinal cord terminate in all of the vestibular nuclei except the superior vestibular nucleus. These fibers may arise as collaterals of the posterior spinocerebellar tract. Information is then relayed, in turn, to the cerebellum by vestibulocerebellar connections.

6. Spino-Olivary Tract

A ventral spino-olivary pathway ascends in the ventral funiculus to synapse in the medial and dorsal accessory olivary nuclei (in the cat, rabbit, hedgehog, pig, and opossum). These same olivary nuclei receive an input from the nuclei gracilis and cuneatus.

D. Descending Pathways

The anterior (ventral) horn cells or motoneurons are the "bottleneck" of the spinal cord through which all motor output must be funneled. They are multipolar and include both the large alpha motoneurons that supply skeletal musculature and the small gamma motoneurons that innervate the muscle spindles. With the exception of monosynaptic input from some primary afferents and a small percentage of the corticospinal tract, all systems influence the anterior horn cells through interneurons. Many descending pathways interact to regulate the anterior horn cells.

Because of the large number of descending tracts and the complexity of their terminations, it is useful to subdivide the pathways into functionally related systems. The somatotopic organization of the motoneurons in the anterior horn guides this endeavor. Motoneurons in the most medial aspect innervate neck and truncal musculature, while those in the lateral region supply the musculature of the extremity. With this in mind, the following generalizations can be made.

Since the lateral corticospinal and rubrospinal tracts descend in the lateral funiculus and innervate the more lateral aspect of the anterior horn (Fig. 8), they are primarily concerned with the regulation of the musculature of the extremity, particularly the most distal portions, including the hands and feet. On the other hand, the vestibulospinal tracts and medial reticulospinal tract travel in the anterior funiculus and synapse in the more medial regions of the anterior horn (Fig. 8). They have more of an influence on the musculature of the trunk and proximal extremity.

Descending systems which terminate primarily in the cervical cord, such as the tectospinal, interstitiospinal, and cerebellospinal tracts, are primarily concerned with upper extremity, head, and neck movements. Pathways that originate in the areas rich in endogenous endorphins and enkephalins, such as the raphe nuclei of the medulla and pons and the periaqueductal gray matter, tend to project to those areas of the posterior horn involved in nociceptive function. Other tracts are more difficult to characterize because of diverse connections. The catecholaminergic systems, for example, influence sensory, motor, and autonomic systems.

The reader is referred to the following publications by Brodal (26) and Kuypers and Martin (35) for a comprehensive review of the descending pathways.

1. Corticospinal System

By definition, the corticospinal tract originates in the cerebral cortex and terminates in the spinal cord. Although the term pyramidal tract is used as a synonym for this pathway, it is not entirely accurate. The pyramidal tract would include any pathway passing through the pyramid of the medulla oblongata. It is true that the majority of axons in the pyramid belong to the corticospinal system, but corticobulbar tracts and other more poorly defined pathways are also present.

Considerable variation exists in mammalian species regarding the connections, loations, and extent of the corticospinal system.

a. Cell bodies of origin. All of the axons in the corticospinal system arise from the frontal and parietal lobes of the cerebral cortex. Specifically, cell bodies of origin are located in the premotor cortex (area 6), primary motor cortex (area 4), supplementary motor zone (superior and medial aspects of areas 4 and 6), primary somatosensory cortex (areas 1, 2, and 3), and parietal association areas (areas 5 and 7). In the monkey approximately 29% of the axons in the pyramidal tract arise from area 6, 31% from area 4, and 40% from the parietal lobe.

b. Axonal numbers and diameters. Results of studies from a number of mammals indicate that the total number of axons in a pyramid is proportional to body and brain weight. Significantly, the corticospinal tract contains four times as many axons in animals in which the pathway extends the entire length of the cord, compared to those species in which it terminates either at cervical or thoracic levels.

In man there are approximately 1,000,000 axons in each pyramid. Only 3% of the fibers are 10–22 μm in diameter. These fibers are thought to arise from the large Betz cells in lamina V of the primary motor cortex (area 4). The largest Betz cells give rise to the largest and longest axons, which innervate the lumbosacral region of the cord. In the cat there are approximately 80,000 axons in each pyramid. Only 2% of these are 6 μm or greater in diameter, and, similar to man, they arise from the large pyramidal cells in lamina V of area 4.

The majority (90%) of axons in the pyramid are small, varying in diameter from 1 to 4 μm. Thus, the corticospinal system is a relatively slowly conducting pathway.

c. Pyramidal decussation. In many mammals, including man, the majority of axons in the corticospinal tract decussate in the caudal aspect of the medulla oblongata and then continue as the lateral corticospinal tract in the spinal cord. Typically, some fibers do not cross in the medulla, but continue into the cord in the anterior funiculus, and then cross in the anterior white commissure. This pathway is referred to as the anterior (ventral) corticospinal tract. Still another small group of axons remains uncrossed in the medulla and joins the lateral corticospinal tract to terminate ipsilaterally with respect to the cell bodies of origin.

The term pyramidal decussation (motor decussation) is applied to the crossing fibers of the corticospinal system in the medulla oblongata (Figs. 12 and 13). Some animals, such as the klitdassi, hedgehog, and mole, lack this decussation. It has also been reported to be sometimes lacking in man.

d. Course in the spinal cord. Most of the axons in the corticospinal system cross in the medulla and then continue in the lateral funiculus of the spinal cord as the lateral corticospinal tract (Fig. 8). This pathway extends the entire length of the cord, innervating each level. The anterior corticospinal tract on the other hand terminates in cervical and thoracic segments and does not project into lumbosacral regions.

In some species the major cord projection of the corticospinal tract does not reside in the lateral funiculus. For instance, in many marsupials and rodents most of the crossed fibers descend in the ventral aspect of the dorsal funiculus. This is also true of the tree shrew. In the armadillo crossed corticospinal fibers descend through both the ventral and lateral funiculi.

e. Termination. Kuypers (35) categorizes the mammalian corticospinal system according to a gradient progressing from a primitive to a highly evolved form. In the more primitive species it terminates in rostral cord segments in the dorsal horn. As the system evolves and becomes more complex, it terminates at increasingly more caudal levels of the cord and progressively more ventral regions of the gray matter. Thus, in intermediate stages the corticospinal system would terminate in both the intermediate gray matter and dorsal horn through thoracic levels, and in the most advanced form it would synapse in the ventral horn as well as in the intermediate gray matter and dorsal horn through lumbosacral levels. Only in primates would a direct, monosynaptic connection with motoneurons be found.

Mammals exhibiting the most primitive corticospinal system include: the armadillo, elephant, goat, rabbit, sloth, and tree shrew. The pathway terminates in cervical or rostral thoracic levels, primarily in the dorsal horn in laminae IV through VI. Whereas many marsupials fit into this category, others have corticospinal tracts that extend through caudal thoracic levels, terminating not only in the dorsal horn but also in lamina VII of the intermediate gray matter and ventral horn. In this more primitive system the cerebral cortical influence upon lumbosacral levels must depend on polysynaptic connections.

The second or next highest level of corticospinal tract evolution includes nearly all other mammals except monkeys, apes, and man. This form involves a crossed corticospinal tract that extends the length of the cord and terminates primarily in the dorsal horn and intermediate gray matter (laminae IV through VII). While in some of these animals (such as the dog) the ventral corticospinal tract terminates in part in lamina VIII bilaterally, neither the ventral nor lateral corticospinal tracts synapse upon motoneurons in lamina IX.

The third highest level of corticospinal system development includes those species in which the tract terminates not only in the dorsal horn and intermediate gray matter, but also in lamina VIII and in the dorsolateral aspect of lamina IX of the ventral horn. Consequently, in these species there exists a direct corticospinal connection with the neuronal cell population regulating the distal musculature of the extremities for fine motor control of the digits. Even the distribution to lamina VII is different in these mammals compared to lower forms in that the medial portions are also innervated. In lower forms the tract projects primarily to the lateral aspect of lamina VII. The majority of monkeys and some of the prosimians are included in this category. Also, as might be anticipated by their manual dexterity, two carnivores, the raccoon and kinkajou, are members of this group.

In the fourth or highest level of corticospinal system evolution the tract terminates in the posterior horn, intermediate gray matter, and anterior horn, including the ventromedial and ventrolateral as well as the dorsolateral aspects of lamina IX. Consequently, there are direct cortical connections, not only to motoneurons innervating the musculature of the distal extremity, but also to those regulating the musculature of the proximal extremity and trunk. Fewer fibers terminate in the posterior horn than in lower forms. The great apes and man are included in this category. It must be emphasized that even in man only 2-3%of the axons terminate directly upon the alpha and gamma motoneurons. On the contrary, most axons innervate interneurons in all of the laminae of termination.

f. Function. The function of the corticospinal system appears to be two-fold. First, there is the obvious influence on the motor output directly by the corticospinal tracts, and indirectly by corticorubrospinal and corticoreticulospinal pathways. With respect to motor control, the corticospinal system tends to have a facilitatory action upon anterior horn cells which innervate flexor muscles, and an inhibitory influence on those that innervate extensor musculature. This applies to both alpha and gamma motoneurons.

The second function of the system relates to sensory phenomena. Collaterals of descending corticospinal fibers synapse in three major regions with sensory functions. These include the posterior horn, the posterior column nuclei (gracilis and cuneatus), and the reticular formation. All of these sites are important in projecting sensory input that ultimately reaches the thalamus and the cerebral cortex. Feedback loops are thus established whereby motor output can influence sensory input.

It should be noted that, in general, corticospinal fibers terminating in the posterior horn and intermediate gray matter are of the smallest diameter and arise from the parietal cortex. In contrast, axons terminating in the ventral horn are larger and originate from frontal cortex motor areas. Consequently, given the phylogenetic history of this system, the tract originally pertained more to sensory functions, and then as it evolved it added motor control while retaining sensory regulation.

2. Rubrospinal Tract

Most of our knowledge regarding the rubrospinal tract is derived from experimental studies in the chimpanzee, monkey, cat, and lower forms. Little is known of this pathway in man but it apparently exists and is assumed to be similar to that of the chimpanzee and monkey.

The red nucleus is a large, spherical nuclear complex located in the tegmentum of the midbrain. It is subdivided into small-cell (parvicellular) and large-cell (magnocellular) components. In primates the large-cell component is most caudal. The nucleus receives its name because of a rich blood supply that imparts a red color in the fresh state. The red nucleus gives rise to a pathway, the rubrospinal tract, that crosses immediately anterior to the red nuclei in the ventral tegmental decussation of the midbrain.

The rubrospinal tract is located in the lateral funiculus of the spinal cord just anterior to the lateral corticospinal tract (Fig. 8). It travels the entire length of the cord and terminates primarily in laminae V through VII, overlapping to a large extent with the distribution of the lateral corticospinal tract input; however, there are no inputs to lamina IX.

The rubrospinal tract, like the corticospinal system, gives off many collaterals to a number of structures, including: the cerebellum, motor and sensory cranial nerve nuclei, lateral reticular nucleus, inferior olive, lateral cuneate nucleus, and posterior column nuclei (gracilis and cuneatus).

The red nucleus, although richly innervated by both the cerebellum and the cerebral cortex, receives a greater input from the cerebellum. Both the dentate and the interpositus nuclei project axons to the red nucleus through the superior cerebellar peduncle (brachium conjunctivum). The cerebral cortex projects axons to the ipsilateral red nucleus. Whereas most fibers arise from the motor areas of the frontal cortex, some originate from the somatosensory cortex of the parietal lobe. Apparently, the supplementary motor zone projects bilaterally to the red nuclei.

Functionally, the rubrospinal pathway acts to a large extent in concert with the corticospinal tract. It is facilitatory to the flexor musculature of the extremities. together, the tracts provide the capacity for the limbs to make independent movements, especially in the distal regions. The corticospinal tract alone has the intrinsic circuitry to orchestrate independent movements of the digits as a consequence of the monosynaptic input to lamina IX.

3. Reticulospinal Tracts

The medial two thirds of the brain stem reticular formation in the pons and medulla oblongata gives rise to descending reticulospinal pathways. In the medulla the nucleus reticularis gigantocellularis is the main nuclear group contributing to this system, while in the pons the nucleus reticularis pontis caudalis and the caudal part of the nucleus reticularis pontis oralis both contribute.

The pontine reticular formation gives rise to the ipsilateral pontine reticulospinal tract, sometimes referred to as the medial reticulospinal tract. This tract extends the length of the cord in the anterior funiculus and terminates primarily in lamina VIII and in the adjacent portion of lamina VII.

The medullary reticular formation gives rise to the crossed and uncrossed medullary reticulospinal tract, sometimes referred to as the lateral reticulospinal tract. This tract extends the length of the cord, located primarily in the anterior aspect of the lateral funiculus near the anterior horn; however, some of the fibers descend in the anterior funiculus, and still others are reported to descend in the posterior aspect of the lateral funiculus (referred to by most investigators as the dorsolateral funiculus). The medullary reticulospinal tract terminates primarily in lamina VII but some fibers terminate in laminae VIII and IX.

The pontine and medullary reticulospinal tracts appear to differ in function, as might be anticipated by their different terminations. The pontine system tends to monosynaptically activate motoneurons to the neck, back, and extremities. In contrast, the medullary pathway, though poorly understood, seems to be polysynaptically inhibitory to these areas.

In contrast to the corticospinal, rubrospinal, and vestibulospinal systems, the reticulospinal pathways are not well organized somatotopically. They tend to make more numerous collateral connections in the cord. For instance, a large portion of reticulospinal fibers terminating in cervical levels send collaterals to thoracic and lumbosacral regions. This occurs with the other descending pathways but to a much lesser degree. In addition, the reticular nuclei receive a bilateral input from the cerebral cortex. Little is known of these pathways in man.

4. Vestibulospinal Tracts

The vestibular nuclei give rise to two vestibulospinal tracts.

The lateral vestibulospinal tract arises ipsilaterally from the lateral vestibular nucleus and descends the length of the cord to terminate in lamina VIII and the anterior and central parts of lamina VII. In cervical areas the pathway is located in the vicinity of the anterolateral system. As it descends, the pathway enters the anterior funiculus in thoracic and lumbosacral regions.

Less is known regarding the medial vestibulospinal tract. It arises bilaterally from the medial vestibular nuclei and joins the medial longitudinal fasciculus to pass into the anterior funiculus of the cord. It descends no lower than midthoracic levels, terminating in laminae VIII and VII.

The lateral vestibulospinal tract experimentally increases extensor muscle tone inhibiting flexor tone. The effect is monosynaptic to hindlimbs but polysynaptic to forelimbs. Apparently, the medial vestibulospinal tract regulates forelimb and neck movements in response to cerebellar and direct vestibular input, but little is known regarding the mechanisms. While there is abundant cerebellar input to the vestibular nuclei, few if any fibers from the cerebral cortex innervate the nuclear complex.

5. Noradrenergic Projections

Catecholaminergic cells located primarily in the pons project axons to various regions of the spinal cord. The cells of origin are located primarily in the nucleus coeruleus and nucleus subcoeruleus/medial parabrachial nuclear complex. These nuclei are positioned near the lateral margins of the fourth ventricle. The parabrachial nuclear complex is located just lateral to the locus coeruleus, and includes nuclei on either side of the brachium conjunctivum (superior cerebellar peduncle).

Other nuclei in the pons contribute to these descending noradrenergic pathways. One is the nucleus of Kolliker-Fuse that is located in the lateral portion of the tegmentum of the pons. The other area is positioned immediately dorsolateral to the superior olive and the facial nucleus, also in the tegmentum of the pons.

The noradrenergic projections influence sensory, motor, and autonomic systems in the spinal cord and the brain stem.

The nucleus coeruleus has an extensive bilateral innervation of somatosensory and motor cranial nerve nuclei. In addition, it sends axons to several parasympathetic centers, including: the Edinger-Westphal nucleus of the oculomotor nerve, dorsal motor nucleus of the vagus nerve, and preganglionic parasympathetic nerve cell bodies of the sacral cord. Most of the fibers that descend to the cord pass in the ipsilateral posterior aspect of the lateral funiculus (dorsolateral funiculus) and terminate in laminae VII and IX. Some fibers also synapse in laminae I, IIa, and IV through VI.

The nucleus subcoeruleus/medial parabrachial complex projects fibers to similar laminae of the posterior and anterior horns but differs in its autonomic input. This system is primarily concerned with sympathetic function and projects to preganglionic cell bodies in the intermediolateral column of the thoracic and upper lumbar regions.

The noradrenergic system has a powerful control over autonomic function of the brain stem and cord. It is strongly involved with the regulation of respiratory and cardiovascular functions, as well as micturition and affective behavior. The latter phenomenon probably is a result of the input from the amygdaloid nuclear complex and midbrain central gray matter. Because of its input to the posterior horn, the noradrenergic system is thought to be involved in the perception of pain.

The noradrenergic pathways are also involved in rather complex motor activity, but the nature of this control is not well understood. Noradrenergic fibers exert a direct facilitatory influence on alpha and gamma motoneurons. They seem to enhance the responsiveness of motoneurons in preparation for various reflexes.

6. Serotonergic Systems

Serotonergic neurons that project to the cord arise primarily from nuclei in the medulla oblongata, including those in the medullary raphe and adjacent ventral medullary reticular formation. It is of interest that several neurotransmitters are known to coexist in these cells, with two or more being present. Such transmitters include serotonin, enkephalins, thyrotrophin-releasing hormone, and substance P. Similar to the noradrenergic fibers, they descend in the posterior aspect of the lateral funiculus (dorsolateral funiculus), and extend to all ipsilateral levels of the cord. Their termination in the posterior and anterior horns also coincides to a large degree in laminae I, IIa, VII, and IX.

The serotonergic neurons have a direct facilitatory influence on motoneurons and in conjunction with the noradrenergic fibers enhance the responsiveness of these cells.

7. Cerebellospinal Connections

Direct connections from the cerebellum to the spinal cord are known to exist. They arise from the contralateral fastigial and interpositus nuclei and descend in the cord in the vicinity of the anterolateral system in the lateral and anterior funiculi. These fibers terminate in upper cervical levels in laminae VII and IX.

Although they must be involved in the regulation of neck movement, little is known of their function.

8. Tectospinal Tract

The tectospinal tract arises in the deep layers of the superior colliculus, crosses in the dorsal tegmental decussation of the midbrain, travels ventral to the medial longitudinal fasciculus, and enters the anterior funiculus of the spinal cord. The pathway innervates cervical levels only.

The superior colliculus receives visual information from the cerebral cortex and somatosensory input from ascending pathways. It also receives projections from the cerebellum and vestibular nuclei. Through the tectospinal and interstitiospinal pathways it regulates head and neck movement in response to visual, vestibular, and cerebellar input. The tectospinal system is facilitatory to contralateral extensor motoneurons of the neck.

9. Interstitiospinal Tract

The interstitial nucleus of Cajal is located near the periaqueductal gray matter but ventral to the medial longitudinal fasciculus in the midbrain. It gives rise to the interstitiospinal tract, which passes primarily ipsilaterally in the medial longitudinal fasciculus to enter the anterior funiculus of the spinal cord. This tract extends the entire length of the spinal cord and terminates in lamina VIII and adjacent lamina VII, with no fibers entering lamina IX. Its function is probably similar to the tectospinal tract for head and neck movement, but because of its extent it can influence musculature rotation of the trunk.

REFERENCES

1. Cayaffa, J. (1981). Anatomy and vascular supply of the spinal cord. In *Radiology of Spinal Cord Injury*, L. Calenoff (Ed.), C. V. Mosby, St. Louis, pp. 3–22.
2. Brightman, M. (1965). The distribution within the brain of ferritin injected into cerebrospinal fluid compartments. I. Ependymal Distribution. *J. Cell Biol. 26*:99–123.
3. Brightman, M. (1965). The distribution within the brain of ferritin injected into cerebrospinal fluid compartments. *Am. J. Anat. 117*:193–219.
4. Brightman, M. (1967). Intracerebral movement of proteins injected into blood and cerebrospinal fluid. *Anat. Rec. 147*:219.
5. Brightman, M., Klatzo, I., Olsson, Y., and Reese, T. (1970). The blood-brain barrier to proteins under normal and pathological conditions. *J. Neurol. Sci. 10*:215–239.
6. Leikola, A. (1976). The neural crest: Migrating cells in embryonic development. *Folia Morphol. 24*:155–172.

7. Waggener, J., and Beggs, J. (1967). The membranous coverings of neural Tissues: An electron microscopy study. *J. Neuropathol. Exp. Neurol. 26*: 412-426.

8. Fishman, R. (1980). Cerebrospinal fluid. In *Diseases of the Nervous System*. Saunders Co., Philadelphia, pp. 19-54, 168-251.

9. Levi-Montalcini, R., and Hamburger, V. (1951). Selective growth-stimulation effects of mouse sarcoma on the sensory and sympathetic nervous system of the chick embryo. *J. Exp. Zool. 116*:321-362.

10. Jones, E., and Cowan, W. (1983). The nervous tissue. In *Histology: Cell and Tissue Biology*, 5th ed., Leon Weiss (Ed.), Elsevier, New York, pp. 283-370.

11. Langford, L., and Coggeshall, R. (1981). Branching of sensory axons in the peripheral nerve of the rat. *J. Comp. Neurol. 203*:745-750.

12. Brooks-Fournier, R., and Coggeshall, R. (1981). The ratio of preganglionic to postganglionic cells in the sympathetic nervous system of the rat. *J. Comp. Neurol, 197*:207-260.

13. Coggeshall, R., Hancock, M., and Applebaum, M. (1976). Categories of axons in mammalian rami communicantes. *J. Comp. Neurol. 167*:105-123.

14. Coggeshall, R., and Galbraith, S. (1978). Categories of axons in mammalian rami communicantes. *J. Comp. Neurol. 181*:349-359.

15. Knyihar-Csillik, E., Csillik, B., and Rakic, P. (1982). Ultrastructure of normal and degenerating glomerular terminals of dorsal root axons in the substantia gelatinosa of the rhesus monkey. *J. Comp. Neurol. 210*:357-375.

16. Réthelyi, M., Trevino, D., and Perl, E. (1979). Distribution of primary afferent fibers with the sacrococcygeal dorsal horn: An autoradiographic study. *J. Comp. Neurol. 195*:603-622.

17. Ralston, H. (1979). The fine structure of laminae I, II and III of the macaque spinal cord. *J. Comp. Neurol. 184*:619-642.

18. Coggeshall, R., Coulter, J., and Willis, W. (1974). Unmyelinated axons in the ventral roots of the cat lumbosacral enlargement. *J. Comp. Neurol. 153*:39-58.

19. Coggeshall, R., Applebaum, M., Fazen, M., Stubbs, T., and Sykes, M. (1975). Unmyelinated axons in human ventral roots, a possible explanation for the failure of dorsal rhizotomy to relieve pain. *Brain 98*:157-166.

20. Chung, K., and Coggeshall, R. (1983). The fine structure of laminae, I, II and III of the macaque spinal cord. *J. Comp. Neurol. 214*:72-78.

21. Chung, K., and Coggeshall, R. (1982). Quantitation of propriospinal fibers in the tract of lissauer of the rat. *J. Comp. Neurol. 211*:418-426.

22. Rexed, B. (1952). The cytoarchitectonic organization of the spinal cord in the cat. *J. Comp. Neurol. 96*:415-495.

23. Rexed, B. (1954). A cytoarchitectonic atlas of the spinal cord in the cat. *J. Comp. Neurol. 100*:297-379.

24. Ralston, H., and Ralson, D. (1982). The distribution of dorsal root axons to laminae IV, V, and VI of the macaque spinal cord: A quantitative electron microscopic study. *J. Comp. Neurol. 22*:435-448.

25. Wiesendanger, M., and Miles, T. (1982). Ascending pathway of low-threshold muscle afferents to the cerebral cortex and its possible role in motor control. *Physiol. Rev. 62*:1234-1270.

26. Brodal, A. (1981). *Neurological Anatomy*, Oxford University Press, Oxford, England.
27. Kevetter, G. A., Haber, L. H., Yezierski, R. P., Chung, J. M., Martin, R. F., and Willis, W. D. (1982). Cells of origin of the spinoreticular tract in the monkey. *J. Comp. Neurol. 207*:61–74.
28. Craig, A. (1978). Spinal and medullary input to the lateral cervical nucleus. *J. Comp. Neurol. 181*:729–743.
29. Craig, A., and Burton, H. (1979). The lateral cervical nucleus in the cat: Anatomic organization of cervicothalamic neurons. *J. Comp. Neurol. 185*: 329–346.
30. Craig, A., and Tapper, D. (1978). Lateral cervical nucleus in the cat: Functional organization and characteristics. *J. Neurophysiol. 41*:1511–1534.
31. Morin, F. (1955). Central connections of a cervical nucleus (nucleus cervicalis lateralis of the cat). *J. Comp. Neurol. 103*:17–32.
32. Taub, A., and Bishop, P. (1965). The spinocervical tract: Dorsal column linkage, conduction velocity, primary afferent spectrum. *Exp. Neurol. 13*: 1–21.
33. Grant, G., Wiksten, B., Berkley, K., and Aldskogius, H. (1982). The location of cerebellar-projecting neurons within the lumbosacral spinal cord in the cat. An anatomical study with HRP and retrograde chromatolysis. *J. Comp. Neurol. 204*:336–348.
34. Rustioni, A. (1977). Spinal Neurons project to the dorsal column nuclei of rhesus monkeys. *Science 196*:656–658.
35. Kuypers, H., and Martin, G. (Eds.) (1982). Anatomy of descending pathways to the spinal cord. In *Progress in Brain Research*, vol. *57*, Elsevier Biomedical Press, New York.

2
ORGANIZATION
OF THE SPINAL CORD

Arnold B. Scheibel *UCLA School of Medicine, Los Angeles, California*

I. INTRODUCTION

No other portion of the central nervous system reflects with such clarity its ontogenetic and phylogenetic origins as does the spinal cord. Preserved within a tubular structure running the length of the trunk lies much of the drama of several hundred million years of vertebrate development. Structure and, undoubtedly, function become more complex beyond the foramen magnum, but it is uniquely in the spinal cord that one can sense the derivative relationship between the segmented invertebrate with its ganglionic chain and the continuous neural tube of all subsequent vertebrate forms. We can only hypothesize how the transition occurred, assuming that its evolution was gradual and not the product of some prodigious genetic leap that compressed tens of millions of years of evolution into a few generations! Picture an "educated," wormlike form, behaviorally a creature of its neural ganglia which lie individual and isolated, perhaps at the head end, thorax, and abdomen, communicating with each other by axonal bundles or connectives. As the demands for information processing increase, these ganglia find themselves hard-pressed to fill the need. Further growth of the individual ganglion is limited—or perhaps impossible—since at this evolutionary juncture, nature has not yet discovered the trick of introducing a microvascular plexus into the substance of working neural tissue. Perhaps as a result, cells begin to creep along the connectives, progressively narrowing the gaps between populations of functioning nerve cell bodies. Thus, by degrees, a continuous tube of neurons, each closely associated with their connecting axons, can be imagined to develop.

Whether or not such changes were indeed the prolegomena to the structure we know today, harbingers of spinal-cordlike systems are to be found in some invertebrates. In the hemichordate. Enteropneusta, part of the nervous system arises as a medullary tube from the dorsal body ectoderm; and in tunicates of the genus *Appendicularia* there is a dorsal cordlike structure from which emerge pairs of nerve roots, suggestive of vertebrate organization (1,2).

Ontogeny is mirrored in the from-within-outward pattern of the vestigial central canal that is lined with ependymal neuroglia, neuron-rich gray matter, and surrounding white matter; a remarkably accurate elaboration of the primitive neural tube and its germinal layer surrounded concentrically by mantle and marginal zones. It is in fact the elaboration of this basic pattern which provides the substance for this chapter and, in turn, the background for all structural, functional, and chemical considerations that will follow.

II. ORGANIZATIONAL OVERVIEW

The internal structure of the spinal cord varies from level to level, but the basic pattern remains constant. It is essentially a virtually bilaterally symmetric tube consisting of an inner arc of neurons and their processes surrounded by an outer shell of axons (white matter); the latter representing not only the efferent projections of the cells of the inner core (spinal gray matter) but also the afferent projections from all peripheral and suprasegmental areas which play upon the spinal neuronal matrix. [I add the disclaimer, "virtually," because of the increasing evidence for asymmetry as a very common phenomenon, not only in the cerebral cortex (3) but at varying levels of the forebrain and upper brain stem.] Both gray and white matter are supported by an interstitial neuroglia framework, and both are richly supplied by a microvascular stroma made up of loops and arcades generated by larger radicles penetrating from anterior and posterior spinal arteries and from smaller radicular components entering over each rootlet. The denser vascularization of the spinal gray matter is appropriate to the higher level of metabolic demand in the neuropil (Fig. 1).

In coronal sections, the gray matter generates its familiar H-shaped outline that is formed by elaboration of the primitive mantle layer into dorsal and ventral horns on each side, joined by the horizontal, bridgelike spinal gray commissure. The dorsal horn, arising as it does from the *alar plate*, is sensory in function; the ventral horn, a *basal plate* derivative, is at least in part motor in functional role. The intermediate region connecting the dorsal and ventral fields is composed entirely of *interneurons*, some of which project upon supraspinal

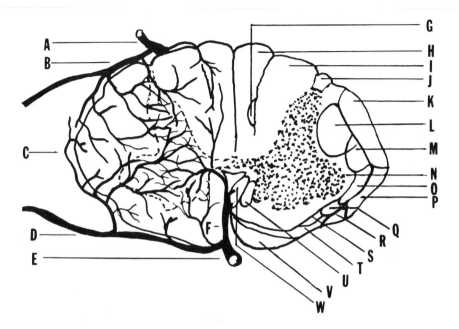

Figure 1 Cross-section through cervical level of spinal cord showing arterial supply on left, tracts on right. A, posterior spinal artery; B, posterior radicular artery; C, arterial vasocorona; D, anterior radicular artery; E, anterior spinal artery; F, sulcal artery; G, fasciculus interfascicularis; H, fasciculus gracilis; I, fasciculus cuneatus; J, dorsolateral fasciculus of Lissauer; K, posterior spino-cerebellar tract; L, lateral corticospinal tract; M, rubrospinal tract; N, fasciculus proprius; O, lateral spinothalamic tract; P, anterior spinocerebellar tract; Q, spinotectal tract; R, spino-olivary tract; S, anterior spinothalamic tract; T, vestibulospinal tract; U, medial longitudinal fasciculus; V and W, portions of uncrossed (anterior) corticospinal tract.

targets (i.e., spinothalamic cells and the nucleus of Clarke's column), while others, and probably the majority, are true *propriospinal* neurons dedicated to intersegmental and polysegmental loops within the spinal cord.

Cord structure varies somewhat with the level studied, and its internal configuration, especially in terms of profiles of the gray matter, reflects the input-output arrangements peculiar to that level. Thus, the ventral horns of the cervical and lumbosacral enlargements are particularly prominent owing to the increased numbers of motoneurons supplying the musculature of the upper and lower extremities. Similarly, the intermediolateral horns achieve prominence at thoracic levels because of concentrations of sympathetic effector neurons of the visceral nervous system. It has been suggested also that the unusually large rounded profile of the dorsal horn at sacral levels is due to the strength and bio-logic urgency of sensory stimulation from the genitalia and perineum.

III. WHITE MATTER

The white matter can be described in terms of segments of two half circles or arcs extending clockwise from the dorsal medial septum at 12:00 through the ventral medial fissure at 6:00, and back to the dorsal medial septum. At least 100 years of study with techniques of increasing refinement have resulted in a highly accurate characterization of tract position, fiber content, pattern of axonal termination, and function. Here, we shall content ourselves with an over-view of presently recognized ascending and descending systems, with some addi-tional comments about several of the functionally more important systems (Fig. 1).

A. The Dorsal Columns

Occupying the zone between dorsal medial septum and the medial edge of the dorsal horn, the dorsal columns are sensory in nature, being made up largely, though not exclusively, of the rostral continuation of large medial division spinal sensory root fibers subserving epicritic modalities such as touch-pressure and kinesthesia. Fibers of this system show high degrees of locus and mode speci-ficity (4), contributing as they do to spatial sensation (two-point discrimination), temporal modulation of tactile sensibility (flutter-vibration), and joint position. In addition, many group 1a muscle spindle afferents ascend for varying distances in the dorsal column before terminating in the dorsal nucleus of Clarke or, in the case of upper thoracic inputs, the accessory cuneate nucleus (5), prior to their projection to the cerebellum. Limited numbers of these rapidly conducting ele-ments also may project directly upon cortical pyramidal cells of area 4, provid-ing short-latency feedback guidance during ongoing motor activity.

Ascending fibers from lower levels shift medially and posteriorly as they ascend, under the pressure of additions from succeeding levels. The result is an approximately laminar arrangement of fibers, with those of sacral origin being most medial. In the upper thoracic and cervical levels the dorsal column is divided by a posterior intermediate septum into a medial-lying fasciculus gracilis and a lateral-lying fasciculus cuneatus. The latter, lying lateral to the septum, carries the long ascending branches of the upper five or six thoracic and all cervical dorsal roots.

A large proportion of dorsal column fibers are of limited length and never leave the cord. Descending components of dorsal root origin include: (1) the fasciculus interfascicularis (comma tract of Schultze), lying in the middle of the posterior funiculus at cervical and thoracic levels; (2) the septomarginal fasciculus at cervical and thoracic levels; (2) the septomarginal fasciculus (oval area of Flechsig), situated near the middle of the posterior septum at lumbar levels; and (3) its caudal continuation at sacral levels, the triangle of Gombault-Philippe. Fibers of propriospinal origin also are represented, primarily at the ventromedial apex of the posterior column as the cornu-commissural bundle of Marie (6).

A wide range of fiber sizes are represented in this column, as in other spinal fillets, and a few figures may be of interest. According to Hwang, Hinsman, and Roesel (7), one fasciculus gracilis in the cat contains 25,284 fibers at a mid-cervical level. Fiber diameters range from 4 μm to 15 μm, with 97% being below 8 μm in diameter, and the majority of these being in the 2-5 μm range.

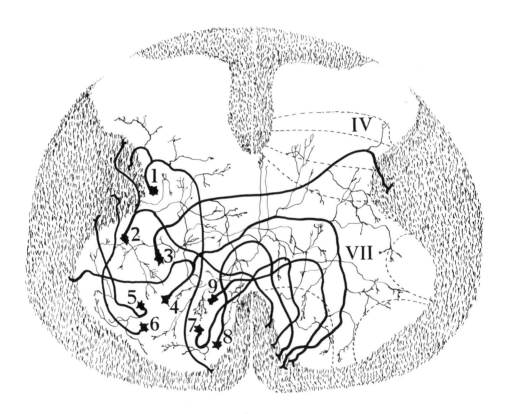

Figure 2 Somewhat schematized drawing of cross section of kitten spinal cord through a lower lumbar segment showing the intrasegmental portion of the axonal trajectories of nine interneurons (1-9). The major axonal projection is darkened to differentiate it from its local collaterals. Two laminae (IV and VII) are shown on the right. Rapid Golgi modification. $\times$ 70. (From Ref. 68.)

B. The Lateral Columns

The arc of white matter extending from the dorsal horn and the dorsal root entry zone to the area of the ventral root exit zone constitutes the lateral white matter, which is made up of a number of discrete fiber systems, both ascending and descending. Most medial, and shaped to the outline of the gray matter, is the propriospinal system, containing axons of the spinal internuncial cells (Fig. 2). These axon systems are complexly branched and may run for from one or two to six or eight segments before developing terminal synapses (Fig. 3). The frequent collateral systems that reenter the gray matter at every level are substrate to the varied and powerful polysegmental spinal reflexes out of which almost all spinal mediated activity is constructed. Along the peripheral border from posterior to anterior are dorsal and ventral spinocerebellar tracts that transmit information from muscle spindles and Golgi tendon organs to the cerebellum

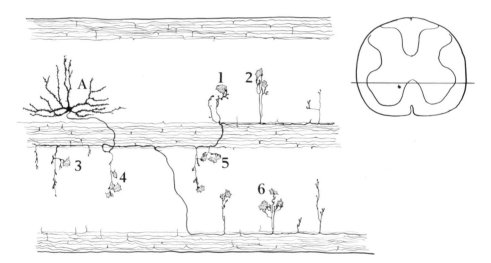

Figure 3 Somewhat schematized drawing of a horizontal section through the base of the anterior horn of kitten spinal cord showing part of the rostral-caudal trajectory of an interneuron whose location is marked in the cross section inset diagram. Neuron A sends it axon into the contralateral ventral white matter where it bifurcates into rostral and caudal running branches. A secondary branch crosses to the contralateral lateral fasciculus. Collaterals from these major axon stems reenter the gray matter at right angles, apparently effecting contact with ipsilateral mononeurons (1,2), contralateral motoneurons (4,6), contralateral interneurons (3,5). Only the relatively small number of axosomatic contacts are shown here, and this represents only a fraction of the axonal course of this interneuron. Rapid Golgi modification. × 72 (From Ref. 68.)

following relay in one of several nuclei. Slightly more medial are the lateral and ventral spinothalamic tracts, the latter more properly within the boundaries of the ventrolateral white matter. Spinotectal and spino-olivary tracts are also found ventrolaterally (see Fig. 1). The majority of the area of the lateral white matter is occupied by the fibers of the lateral corticospinal tract. This system, originally bordered by propriospinal fibers medially and the dorsal spinocere-bellar tract laterally, reaches the lateral pial-glial border of the cord at lower lumbar and sacral levels, caudal to the mass of the spinocerebellar system. Its ventral edge is overlapped by the rubrospinal tract, which in man probably does not extend beyond thoracic levels (8). A small but variable number of uncrossed corticospinal fibers are said to descend in the ventral portion of the lateral funiculus as the anterolateral corticospinal tract of Barnes (9).

1. Lateral Corticospinal Tract

It now seems clear that the lateral corticospinal tract originates widely over frontal, parietal, and temporal cortices, with the greatest concentrations of source cells adjacent to, and on both sides of, the fissure of Rolando. Each bundle contains approximately 1 million fibers, of which about 700,000 are myelinated (10). Approximately 90% of the unmyelinated fibers are in the 1-4 μm range. At the other end of the spectrum are 30,000 to 40,000 large fibers 10-22 μm in caliber which undoubtedly arise from the giant pyramidal cells of Betz in the precentral gyrus. This small but specialized contingent of rapidly conducting, high-priority elements achieves its greatest development in man and appears to be concerned with the production of brief periods of reduction in the antigravity tone of extensor muscle masses immediately prior to the inception of a purposeful act (11,12).

Derivation of a significant fraction of corticospinal fibers from the post-Rolandic cortex is underlined by the fact that close to half of its component fiber collaterals and terminals synapse on cells of sensory signature at the base of the dorsal horn in laminae IV, V, and VI (Fig. 4). Corticospinal axons destined for the ventral horn show distribution patterns which are highly species-specific. In the cat terminations are found primarily in and among interneurons (13), whereas in primates and man there is an increasing trend toward direct synaptic linkage with the final common pathway motoneurons (14,15). This trend from indirect to direct synaptic connections between motor cortex and spinal effector cells probably represents another instance of increasing telencephalization of function. In this regard it is interesting that Golgi studies of kitten spinal cord (16) indicate that small numbers of corticospinal terminals can in fact be found on peripheral portions of motoneuronal dendrites where the latter extend into adjacent interneuronal pools (Fig. 4). Located so far from the motoneuronal cell body and the axon hillock, the capacity of these terminals to develop effective levels of facilitatory drive might be considered minimal; thereby proving more

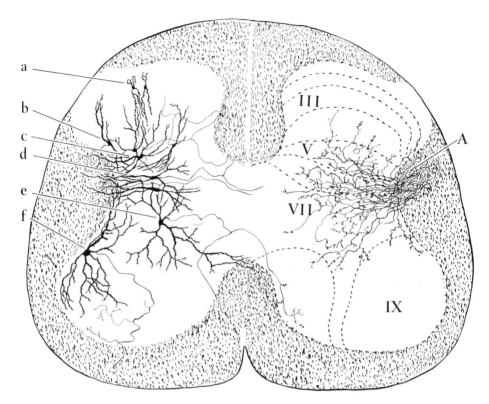

Figure 4 Some of the presynaptic and postsynaptic components of the lateral corticospinal projection upon the lumbar spinal cord of a kitten. Right: Collateral and terminal fibers leaving lateral corticospinal tract (A), terminate in a fan-shaped zone within laminae IV–VII, and impinge slightly on IX. Left: The receptive postsynaptic cell–dendrite groups include elements a–f from the base of the dorsal horn to the ventral horn. Cell f is a motoneuron whose most dorsal running dendrites probably receive contacts from corticospinal terminals. × 65. (From Ref. 16.)

symbolic than functional in that their presence represents the earliest stage of invasion of the motoneuron pool by corticifugal effects (16). On the other hand, notions introduced more recently by Iansek and Redman (17) on the apparently enhanced effectiveness of distally located axodendritic synapses suggest that even this small number of distant synapses might exert significant degrees of synaptic "pressure" on the cell body and the axon hillock–initial segment.

Pyramidal tract control is clearly greater over the more peripherally located muscle systems, compared to those in axial positions; similarly, such control is more effectively expressed upon the upper extremity than upon the lower. Approximately 55% of all pyramidal fibers terminate at cervical cord levels; 20% in the thoracic and 25% at lumbosacral levels (18).

2. Rubrospinal Tract

The rubrospinal tract arises somatotopically from the red nucleus of the midbrain and projects upon all levels of the spinal cord in most mammals, although in man it has not been demonstrated below the thoracic level (8). The system is generally believed to be of greater functional importance in the cat than in the monkey or man; in the latter, in particular, the majority of the fibers are thin and poorly myelinated. Collaterals and terminals enter the internuncial cell pools (laminae V–VII) where they terminate on both cell bodies and dendrites (19). The rubrospinal tract excites flexor motor neurons and inhibits extensor elements via polysynaptic pathways. Red nucleus stimulation enhances flexor muscle activity during the swing phase (20) of a motor act.

3. Dorsal Spinocerebellar Tract

Together with the more ventrally placed ventral spinocerebellar bundle, the dorsal spinocerebellar tract forms the superficial boundary of the lateral white matter, at least from midlumbar levels rostrally. The two tract systems taken together convey information concerning posture and/or movement in individual muscle fibers and muscles and in entire limbs. Synaptic circuitry within the cord differs appreciably for the two tracts, and accordingly accounts for marked differences in their patterns of functional representation.

The dorsal spinocerebellar tract arises from the large cells of the dorsal nucleus of Clarke, which extends from approximately L3 to C8 segments. Located in the internuncial cell pools under the medial portion of the base of the dorsal horn (lamina VII), these large multipolar cells receive collaterals from large dorsal root fibers, primarily of muscle spindle derivation, and send their axons to the ipsilateral border of the white matter where they ascend through the entire length of the cord. The tract first appears at the L3 level and increases in size through C8, at which point the dorsal nucleus of Clarke disappears. The nucleus receives both ascending and descending branches of dorsal root fibers—constituting an afferent influx characterized by large degrees of both convergence and divergence (5,21). Clarke's nucleus actually receives afferent fibers from all parts of the body except the head and neck (dorsal roots C1–C4), but remains functionally related primarily to the caudal portion of the body and the hindlimbs. In view of the massive convergence within the nucleus, it is remarkable that individual dorsal spinocerebellar fibers appear to sort for spindle data from individual muscles and even individual fibers. Conduction velocities of the large fibers are among the most rapid in the central nervous system, varying from 30 to 110 m/sec (22,23).

4. Ventral Spinocerebellar Tract

Anterior to the dorsal spinocerebellar tract and posterior to the site of emergence of ventral root fibers is the ventral or anterior spinocerebellar tract. Originally considered to take origin primarily from cells located on the periphery of the anterior horn at lumbar levels [the spinal border cells of Cooper and Sherrington (24)], it is now felt to originate in large part from rather diffusely organized cell groups in the dorsolateral portion of the anterior gray matter (25) and undoubtedly from laminae V through VII (26). Fibers of this system are almost entirely crossed, of uniformly large diameter (11-20 mμ), and conduct at velocities of 70-120 m/sec. In contrast to the rather fine-grained informational content of dorsal spinocerebellar fibers, axons of the anterior bundle frequently are activated by afferent impulses from Golgi tendon organs with receptive fields involving synergic muscle groups at each joint of the limb. Thus, individual fibers or small groups of fibers may convey information concerning posture or movement of an entire limb.

5. Cuneocerebellar Fibers

The cuneocerebellar fibers convey impulses from group 1a muscle afferents and some cutaneous components from body areas (trunk, arm, and shoulder) above the rostral termination zone of Clarke's nucleus. In the cat at least a rostral spinocerebellar tract has been described (23,27) as the ipsilateral forelimb analog of the anterior spinocerebellar tract. The cell bodies of origin of these fibers are presently unkown.

6. Dorsolateral Fasciculus of Lissauer

Situated just laterally to the entering dorsal roots and crowning the dorsal horn, the dorsolateral fasciculus of Lissauer is probably the only well-defined spinal bundle containing both an admixture of endogenous and exogenously derived (primary sensory, lateral division) fibers. Originally described as containing only fine primary afferents of dorsal root origin by Lissauer (28) and Ranson (29), more recent work has shown that a large proportion of its fibers are of the short propriospinal type from marginal (lamina I) (30) or gelatinosal (laminae II and ?III) cell pools (31). Nonetheless, it seems clear that, in the monkey at least, approximately 50% of the fibers in Lissauer's bundle are primary afferents (32).

7. Lateral Spinothalamic Tract

Lying along the medial surface of the ventral spinocerebellar tract in the more anterior portion of lateral white matter, the lateral spinothalamic tract forms the most important component of the spinothalamic complex. Its well-known role of carrying pain and thermal sensation to the brain stem and thalamus is mediated by small and medium-sized fibers. These gain access to the spinal cord over the lateral division of the dorsal root, enter the dorsolateral tract of Lissauer, in which they course for 1-2 segments, and then synapse on neurons spread rather widely through laminae V through VIII (33-35). From these cells axons arise which cross the midline in the anterior white commissure, often ascending approximately one segment in the process, and then gain the lateral funiculus as the lateral spinothalamic tract. As new fibers reach the bundle from successively more rostral stations, they are added to the medial and anterior face of the fillet, thereby producing a segmental somatotopic representation which is of considerable clinical significance in cases of selective anterolateral cordotomy for intractable pain.

8. Anterior Spinothalamic Tract

The organization of the anterior (or ventral) spinothalamic tract is generally similar to that of the lateral fillet, although it runs in a more anterior position, that is, in the ventral white matter, anteromedial to the ventral root exit zone, is somewhat smaller in size than the lateral spinothalamic tract, has a limited uncrossed component, and mediates sensations of light touch, primarily of an affective nature (36).

A very large and somewhat less easily characterizable group of rather fine-caliber fibers makes up another order of ascending elements. Some of these fibers are named (spinotectal and spino-olivary), but their cells or origin are not yet clear, and their positions in the spinal white matter are less definitive.

C. The Ventral and Medial Columns

The ventral and medial columns contain a group of tracts which, with the exception of ubiquitous propriospinal elements and the very medially placed anterior corticospinal bundle, are all of brain stem derivation. They include the powerful vestibulospinal system, the medial longitudinal fasciculus, and the complex of reticulospinal tracts from the medulla, the pons, and probably the mesencephalon. There are in addition a group of smaller fiber systems, including the tectospinal, interstitiospinal, solitariospinal, and fastigiospinal fibers, plus recently characterized projections from the raphe nuclei and the locus coeruleus. Patterns of termination of these systems are complex and frequently vary among species. The reader is referred to Brodal (37) for a concise but well-documented discussion of these descending elements.

IV. GRAY MATTER

The neuronal ensembles of the spinal gray matter show a diversity of organizational patterns which equals or exceeds that of any part of the neuraxis. The intricacy of the dendritic design can be appreciated only through the use of the

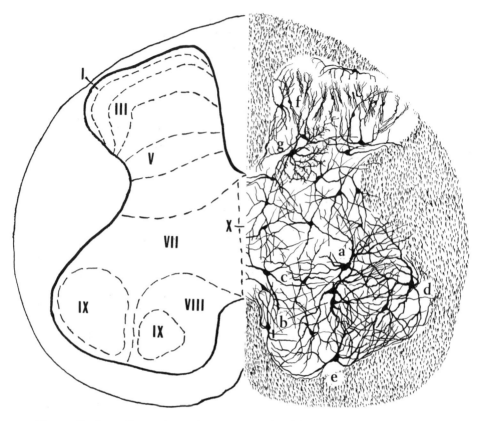

Figure 5 Somewhat schematic cross section of kitten spinal cord showing Rexed's laminae (left) and a limited number of spinal neurons and thin dendritic arbors (right). Cells a–e are interneurons of the anterior horn, g, an interneuron at the base of the dorsal horn, and f, gelatinosal cells of laminae II and III.

Golgi methods, reconstructing and synthesizing the innumerable vignettes offered by this unique method (Fig. 5). More recently, the development of techniques for the introduction of certain dyes (e.g., lucifer yellow) and horse-radish peroxidase directly into individual neurons, which have been recorded intracellularly, provides even richer possibilities for correlating somatodendritic architecture with functional activity. It seems appropriate that the basis for our understanding of spinal cord neuronal organization still rests in the monumental structural studies of Cajal (38). In fact, the reader who is familiar with chapters X through XIV of the classic *Histologie du Système Nerveux de l'Homme et des Vertèbres*, published in 1909, already knows most of the secrets of this complex system. It is therefore all the more remarkable that a Nissl study, first published in 1952 by Rexed (39), employing simple cytoarchitectonic techniques based on comparative cell size and staining intensity has become a classic companion study. The 10 laminar divisions described by visual inspection of transverse and sagittal sections have shown a high degree of correlation with neuronal typology, cell function, and behavior, thus representing a permanent contribution to the literature (Fig. 5). Earlier descriptive morphologic studies provided a terminology which is familiar and, indeed, often used [e.g., substantia gelatinosa (Rolandi), substantia spongiosa, nucleus proprius cornu dorsalis, and so forth], and yet increasingly imprecise for contemporary needs. Rexed's scheme of lamination shall be reviewed briefly for organization and content, with some comments on connectional patterns of particular interest. This provides, in turn, the opportunity to sketch in a few of those structural vignettes that add so richly to our knowledge of the fine structure of the cord while providing substrate for the functions subserved.

The gray matter is made up of two general categories of neurons: (1) tract or column neurons (proprioneurons) whose axons enter the white matter to run varying distances rostrally or caudally, without emerging from the neuraxis; and (2) root neurons whose axons emerge from the spinal axis in ventral roots. Motoneurons of the anterior horn (general somatic efferents) and the smaller sympathomotor cells of the intermediolateral horn at thoracic levels (general visceral efferents) make up this second category. Both are clearly long-axoned (Golgi type I) elements. The problem of short-axoned (Golgi type II) cells in the spinal cord has a long history, and a great deal of both light and heat have been spent in its elucidation. For some years the most popular candidate for short-axoned status appeared to be the Renshaw cells of the medial portion of the anterior horn (40,41).

Despite the compelling nature of some of the physiologic evidence, and the utility of the Renshaw cell concept as a paradigm for recurrent (postsynaptic) inhibition throughout the central nervous system, Golgi studies underlined problems inherent in the circuit model as then conceived (42). Elegant intracellular recording and injection studies by Jankowska (43) supported the results of the earlier Golgi work and helped establish the fact that Renshaw cells are indeed classic long-axoned tract cells not significantly different from other species of propriospinal neurons in the area. The only remaining elements which can presently claim short-axoned status appear to be certain of the smaller (gelatinosal) elements of laminae II and III.

A. Lamina I

Lamina I forms the most dorsal portion of the spinal gray matter, "a thin veil of gray substance" (39) bending around the margins of the dorsal horn. The neurons are somewhat scattered, of varying size, and almost entirely horizontally

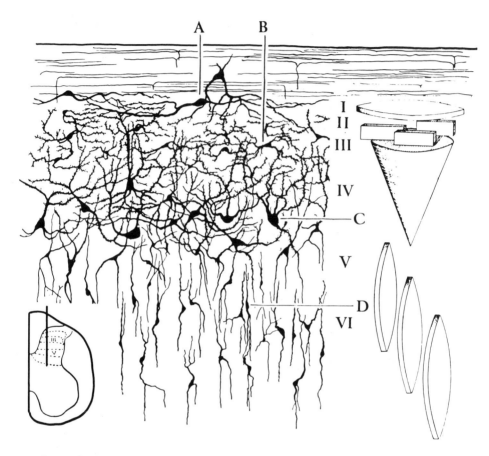

Figure 6 Slightly schematized sagittal section through the dorsal horn of kitten spinal cord showing characteristic patterns of dendrite organization. A, marginal cell of Waldeyer; B, small gelatinosal neuron; C, lamina IV cell; D, interneuron with vertical chiplike dendrite ensemble. Geometric figures on the right give an approximation of the shape of the dendritic domain of the neurons in that layer. Rapid Golgi modification. × 163. (From Ref. 31.)

oriented, with flattened, disclike dendrite domains (Fig. 6). The largest of these elements, the marginal cells of Waldeyer (44), are now known to be responsive to nociceptive information involving tissue destruction, whether of mechanical or thermal nature (45). Their input appears to arise primarily from fine myelinated (and perhaps some unmyelinated) fibers of primary afferent source, and their axons project to the sagittal plane. Spines cover the dendritic branches of these propriospinal pathways.

B. Lamina II

Lamina II corresponds in part, or entirely, to the substantia gelatinosa of the earlier literature. The neurons, which are very small, with only a rim of perinuclear cytoplasm, are aligned in vertical or radial orientation in clumps or miniature palisades. They are most frequently bipolar in structure, with dendritic arrays which are virtually two-dimensional (31,38). The thin, knifelike edge of each dendrite system seen in cross section gives way to elongated hedges of dendrite branches when viewed in the sagittal plane. Spines cover the dendritic branches of these cells, thereby making them, with one exception, the only spine-bearing neurons in the adult mammalian spinal cord (Fig. 7).

C. Lamina III

Lamina III, directly subjacent to lamina II, shows very similar neuronal structure, although the cells tend to become larger with depth. It remains unclear whether these two laminae are really part of the same neuropil field or are discrete entities. Golgi studies emphasize similarities in the structure of the axonal neuropil and the receptive dendritic plexuses (31,38,46,47). Degeneration studies on the other hand can be interpreted as indicating a differential input to the two laminae, the primary afferents of larger diameter being limited to lamina III (32,48). However the problem is finally resolved, one fact remains clear: The architectural pattern of the presynaptic terminals in this zone is unusually exciting and neurologically unique. As might be expected of a complex neuropil field, there are almost as many descriptive variants as there are workers who have attempted the description. Selecting the version with which we are personally familiar (31,49), a characteristic feature is the arc of primary afferent collaterals which sweeps around the ventromedial margin of the gelantinous area from medial division dorsal root fibers and from the posterior columns. These elements lose their myelin sheaths and generate dense flame-shaped arbors whose radial distribution matches that of the dendritic plexuses of gelatinosal cells. It is worthy of note that the sculptured quality of these discrete neuropil patterns, recalling a line of Italian cypress trees, is present only in the areas of the cervical and lumbosacral enlargements. In upper cervical, thoracic, and lower sacral regions the long, individual silhouettes are lost, and the profiles become low and scrublike, resembling an orchard gone to seed. Just as the dendrites of gelatinosal cells assume a different aspect in sagittal section, so also do these tall thin arbors become long, platelike neuropil hedges extending in the rostrocaudal dimension for many hundreds of micrometers. Within these compressed axonal fields lie most of the equally compressed dendritic ensembles of gelatinosal cells, and in these striplike domains, the first central synapses for hair follicle receptors are developed. When one considers the high degree of sensitivity and place specificity of the individual hair receptor on the upper or

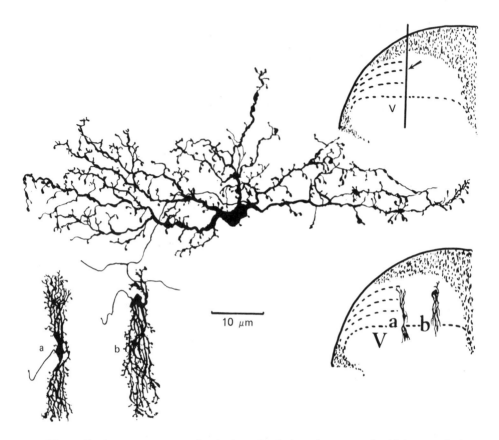

Figure 7 The appearance of spinal cord gelatinosal neurons (a, b) in a typical cross section (lower), and in sagittal section (note plane of section in upper). The familiar compressed, almost two-dimensional dendrite cluster becomes a long, profusely arborizing dendrite system when seen in the sagittal plane. The dendrite spines are long and complex. Drawn from sections of Golgi Cox–stained cat spinal cord × 280. (From Ref. 31.)

lower extremity, it seems all the more remarkable that such individuation of stimuli can be maintained in a long "smeared" field of the sort we are describing. In the kitten and young rodent at least long stalks of ependymal neuroglia extend from ependymal cell bodies lining the vestigial central canal to the pial-glial border (31). As these stalks radiate through laminae II and III they stream between the terminal neuropil fields, effectively isolating adjacent input-output systems (Fig. 8). Assuming that some version of the pattern persists into adult life, one can speculate on its functional significance, providing either isolation of

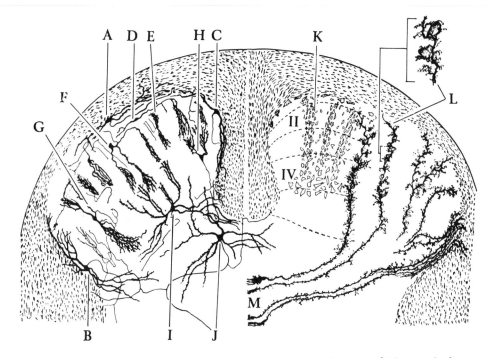

Figure 8 Drawing of a cross section through the dorsal horns of kitten spinal cord showing arrangement of certain neurons and neuroglia. Left: cells A, B, and C are marginal cells of Waldeyer, while D through H are various types of gelatinosal cells of laminae II and III. I and J are larger neurons at the base of the dorsal horn. Right: leafy processes of ependymal neuroglial cells (M) appear to pass between columns of gelatinosal cells, many of which are enfolded by the glial leaves, L. K, columns of neurons in laminae II through IV. Rapid Golgi modification and Nissl stain. × 145. (From Ref. 31.)

individual input-output ensembles or else, like the Golgi epithelial glia of the cerebellar cortex, offering more intensive metabolic support for the energy demands made by this complex neuropil.

Most workers agree that several fine-fiber afferent systems also enter laminae II and III. One group enters the medial side of the substantia gelatinosa from the base of the posterior column (the cornu-commissural zone of Marie (6,32), while a second gains access along the dorsal aspect from the general region of Lissauer's tract. We have suggested that both may be involved in modulation of synaptic processes going on within the main afferent arbors (31).

About 5% of synaptic articulations in this area consist of complex synaptic arrays (50), glomeruli (51), or large synaptic complexes (52). The central terminl is thought by many to arise from a primary afferent collateral, while the surrounding array of axonal, dendritic, and/or dendritic spinous profiles may develop from cells of laminae II through IV. There is little consensus on the physiologic role of this complex, though some workers suspect a gating function for spinothalmic inputs.

D. Laminae IV through VI

Laminae IV through VI make up the bulk of the dorsal horn deep to the gelatinosa. Lamina IV contains a wide range of all types and sizes and it constitutes the greater part of the proper sensory nucleus (nucleus proprius cornu dorsalis of the older terminology). Some of the larger multipolar cells show a particularly intriguing distribution of their dendrites: medial shafts reach toward inputs arriving from the base of the dorsal columns and lateral elements reach toward collaterals of the adjacent lateral corticospinal tract, while dorsal branches ascend into the overlying substantia gelatinosa where they become spine covered and enter into synaptic relations with coarse (and perhaps fine) terminals in laminae III and II (31). Laminae V and VI, constituting the base of the dorsal horn, again show a mixed population of neurons involved in both propriospinal and suprasegmental functions. Many are undoubtedly involved with dorsal root, lateral division fibers, and they may give rise to axons of the spinothalamic tract (34,35). Dendrite systems of many of these cells are bushy and tend to become larger and more profusely branched with greater depth (53).

E. Lamina VII

Lamina VII occupies a broad area at the widest portion of the spinal gray matter and, except for the sometimes interposed pericanalicular lamina X, reaches across the midline, forming the spinal gray commissure. It is the site of a number of important internuncial cell pools as well as source of general visceral efferent innervation for most of the body. This latter role is subserved by the neurons of the intermediolateral nucleus, found between levels T1-L3 and supplying white rami communicantes via the ventral root to sympathetic neurons. Sacral autonomic nuclei occupy a corresponding position in segments S2-S4, and they give rise to preganglionic parasympathetic fibers exiting via ventral roots to form the pelvic nerves. Just medial to these cell pools is the intermediomedial nucleus, a cell system extending the entire length of the spinal cord and believed by some to be recipient to visceral afferent fibers entering in the dorsal root (54). The most conspicuous component of this lamina is undoubtedly the dorsal nucleus of Clarke, found in the medial portion of the zone spanning segments C8 through L2 or L3. Collaterials of dorsal root afferents establish synapses with a high degree of security upon dendrites of this nucleus. The cells are large with prominent coarse Nissl granules and axons which stream laterally to form the dorsal spinocerebellar tract. The dendrite systems appear involuted and coiled within the relatively small field of the nucleus as seen in cross section. Study of sagittal sections, however, reveals very extensive dendrites, frequently running well over a millimeter in the rostrocaudal plane. As might be expected, there is a great deal of dendritic overlap among cells at successive levels along the cord. Additionally, it is now clear that afferent fibers from several levels may converge on the dendrite system of a single neuron (5). Similarly, a single dorsal root may supply afferent fibers to Clarke's column cells in as many as six or seven spinal segments (54). In view of the high degree of demonstrated afferent convergence and divergence, it is surprising that the individual Clarke's cell or its tract axon remains differentially responsive to individual spindle or tendon organ stimulation. Single anterior spinocerebellar fibers on the other hand respond to Golgi tendon organ stimulation with receptive fields which may include one synergic muscle group at each joint of the ipsilateral limb (23,29).

F. Laminae VIII and IX

Together laminae VIII and IX constitute the anterior horn. By definition, the former excludes motoneuron pools and consists entirely of interneurons. Although the axons of virtually all of these cells project via propriospinal tracts to a number of different spinal levels, often as many as 3–5 segments distant, some of their most important functions consist of serving as receptive sites for fibers of suprasegmental origin, whose excitation patterns are then synaptically transferred to nearby motoneurons. In the human spinal cord the vestibulo-spinal, pontine, reticulospinal, and tectospinal tracts and the medial longitudinal fasciculus all synapse on lamina VIII interneurons in order to affect, ultimately, the final common pathway (9,55). In the cat the lateral corticospinal tract still synapses on such cells (13), even though in primates and man the internuncial cell has been largely eliminated from the descending loop.

Lamina IX consists of a number of discrete groups of somatic motoneurons, segregated by function. The neurons are large and usually multipolar in form, ranging from 25 μm to 70 μm or more. The larger cells innervate striated muscle fibers (extrafusals) and are known as alpha (α) motoneurons. Smaller elements innervate the intrafusal fibers of muscle spindles and are known as gamma (γ) motoneurons. General patterns of cellular organization in lamina IX have been described by several authors (56–58). Motoneurons supplying extensor muscles tend to lie more ventral and lateral to those supplying flexors. Similarly, axial muscle nuclei are found most medial and ventral; muscles located most distal on the extremities are supplied by nuclei lying farthest lateral and quite dorsal in the ventral gray matter. Axons leave their nuclei individually and in clusters, emerge from the surface of the cord in the anterolateral sulcus as groups of small rootlets, and then join to form the ventral root. Most of the axons generate one

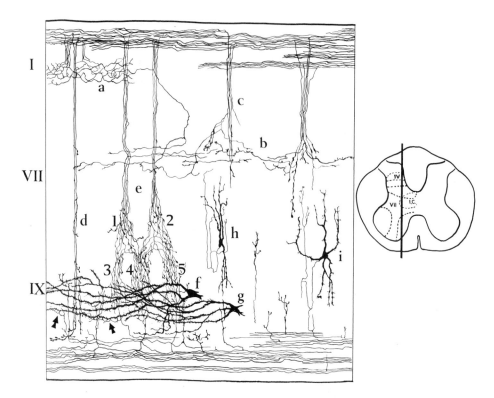

Figure 9 Drawing of sagittal section through the lumbosacral cord of a 40-day-old cat showing selected structural details. Longitudinal axonal neuropil in dorsal horn just below lamina I and in laminae VI–VII is generated by short primary afferent collaterals such as those descending in microbundles c, d, and e. The latter also reach deeply into the internuncial cell pool and the anterior horn where they may terminate on interneurons such as cells h and i or motoneurons such as f and g. Note "primary mix" elements of the microbundles at 1 and 2 and "secondary mix" components at 3, 4, and 5 (see text). Arrows point to sagittally organized axodendritic synapses from terminating ventral column fibers. This pattern markedly differs from the perpendicular course and *en passage* type synapses generated by the primary afferents. Compare the long rostro-caudal dendrite systems of the motoneurons with the predominantly vertically oriented shafts of the interneurons. Only portions of the dendrite systems of these cells have been drawn. Rapid Golgi modification. × 200. (From Ref. 49.)

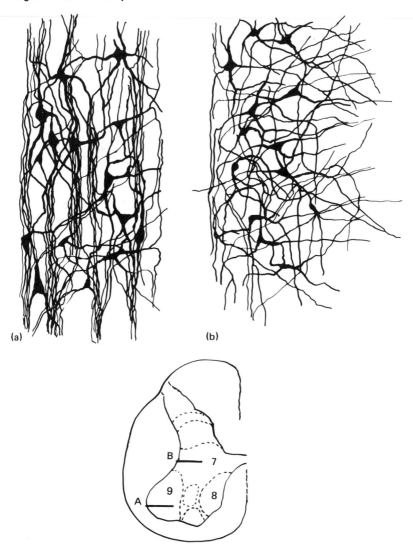

Figure 10 Comparison of the longitudinal dendrite bundle systems of anterior horn motoneurons (a) with the more discrete horizontally arranged dendrite shafts of interneurons (b) in lamina VII. Drawn from Golgi-stained sections of adult cat cord at × 440.

or more recurrent collaterals as they traverse the ventral horn, with the exception of those whose cell bodies are immediately adjacent to the ventral root exit zone.

The motoneuron cell groups resemble elongated footballs when viewed in the sagittal plane. Although the cells themselves are generally multipolar and bear dendritic ensembles of varying pattern, the major dendritic orientation is ordinarily in the rostrocaudal plane, and dendrite systems from a single large human motoneuron may extend for several millimeters. Thus, a longitudinal dendritic neuropil seems characteristic of most spinal motoneurons, an organizational pattern which is very different from that presented by the majority of interneurons with their flattened, coin-shaped dendritic fields, showing the greatest portion of their dendritic array in the transverse section (31,49,59) (Figs. 9 and 10). In fact, the dendritic field organization of neuron groups in various laminae is sufficiently idiosyncratic as to enable a set of geometric patterns to be inscribed about each, thereby characterizing the cell-dendrite system (Fig. 6).

Although we have stressed the segregation by function which marks the organization of each motoneuron pool, it is interesting that the sagittally organized dendrite masses do not seem to recognize such restrictions. We have described complex dendrite bundle systems, often comprising many (3–10) dendrite shafts running in apparent contiguity with each other for hundreds of micrometers, separating, and recombining along the way (60–62). Such bundles are composed of shafts from motor cells supplying different muscles or muscle groups. No detailed functional studies of this structural complex seem yet to have been undertaken, but it would appear that such combinations may include dendrites of cells from agonist groups operating across several joints of an extremity, or alternatively, of agonists and antagonists working across a single joint. The functional implications of such dendrite ensembles have recently been reviewed (63).

V. AXON SYSTEMS

A. Terminal Trajectories

The massive influx of afferent collateral and terminal fibers upon the neuronal core of the spinal cord can only be hinted at in this section. From the propriospinal bundles, shaped against each surface of the gray matter, there is a constant influx of fibers, some seeking their synaptic targets in closely adjacent interneurons, and others crossing much of the dorsal or ventral horn, generating many boutons en passage along the way. The richness of this input is matched by the intricacy of axonal output of most spinal interneurons. Their axons, through multiple bifurcations and branching, may collateralize widely within their own segments, and they may also project axonal branches both upstream and downstream, ipsilateral and contralateral to the cell body of origin. Branches from descending paths of suprasegmental origin also flood in upon the spinal cord, projecting upon interneurons, and often, as in the case of the primate and human corticospinal system, directly upon motoneurons too (13). The breadth of neuronal targets selected by the lateral corticospinal system is particularly interesting. Almost half of the collaterals and terminals of this nominally "motor" tract form their synapses on cells of laminae IV and V in the depths of the dorsal horn (16). This powerful innervation of internuncial cells that are primarily recipient to sensory input exemplifies the modulatory action of cortical centers upon segmental mechanisms. The equally massive terminal neuropil generated in the ventral horn appears to affect both interneurons and motoneurons; techniques are now available, both neurophysiologic and neuro-anatomic, to trace individual fibers from cortical cell of origin to spinal termination.

B. Primary Afferent Collaterals

One of the most interesting organizational patterns is that generated by primary afferent collateral fibers. Entering the dorsolateral surface of the cord as medial division elements of the dorsal root, they run for varying distances in the lateral portion of the posterior column before turning ventrally, either as collaterals or terminals, to drop with almost plumb line directness upon the receptive neuronal matrix below.

Study of Golgi-stained sections cut in either the transverse or sagittal plane reveals that the fibers descend, not individually, but in small tightly formed groups called microbundles (49). These axon ensembles appear to involve combinations of fibers of varying caliber and function, and each microbundle seems to represent a unique "mix" of such elements (49). In addition, it has been noted that in the internuncial cell pools of laminae VI and VII where many of the components of these microbundles may emerge to establish synaptic contacts the remaining axonal elements frequently regroup themselves, thereby establishing a "secondary mix" of primary afferent collaterals which then continue their descent into the ventral horn (Fig. 9). The functional significance of those closely packed fiber complexes is not clear, and they have not yet been subject to extensive ultramicroscopic analysis. Light microscopic study shows the presence of numerous specializations along the component fibers, that is, single and multiple enlargements, often in tiers resembling joints in a bamboo cane, thick pointed excrescences, and so forth. All of these suggest possible structural specializations which may facilitate interaction among the components during their tightly packed course. Conceivably, they might represent a structural substrate for the well-known modulatory effects exerted by flexor reflex afferents on many components of the sensory influx to the spinal cord (64).

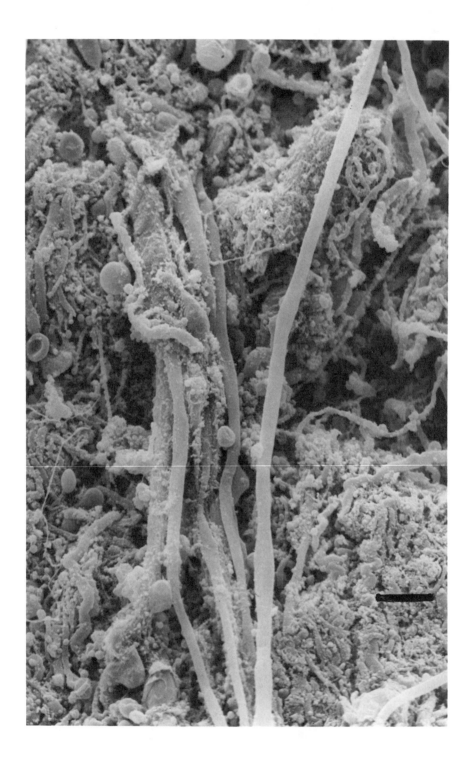

The nature of the terminal patterns established by this fiber contingent upon the receptive motoneuronal dendritic array are of more than passing interest. Although some reports have indicated a parallel, en passage type of iterative axodendritic contact between preterminal afferent fibers and the dendrite shafts along which they ride (57,65), our own Golgi studies have indicated that the primary afferents cross the dendrite shafts virtually at right angles, effecting at most a small, highly localized cluster of terminal contacts on any one shaft. Because of the staggered sequences of motoneurons and their dendrite systems along the rostrocaudal axis, it follows that each dendrite shaft may receive clusters of synaptic contacts from many microbundles of primary afferent collaterals, some close to the somata and some on the most distal dendritic segments. Similarly, as a single primary afferent fiber group "falls through" the dendritic field, it will presumably effect contact with some dendrite shafts very near the soma (or on the cell body itself at times), with some in intermediate positions, and with some far out at the dendritic tips (49). Rall (66,67) has been concerned with the consequences of distribution and degree of effectiveness of synaptic inputs along the soma-dendrite membrane continuum. The presumed attenuation in size and increased time-to-peak as synaptic sites of origin became more remote from the axon hillock–initial segment led us to sketch out a "place" interpretation of spinal dendritic function whereby, for each approaching volley in a presynaptic ensemble, a set of functions is computed by the local group of receptive motoneurons, depending on the anatomic relations of the component elements to the presynaptic domain. However, recent studies by Redman and his colleagues (17) raise serious questions about such a model. They report no apparent relationship between the peak voltage of potentials recorded at the soma and the distance to the site of generation of the excitatory postsynaptic potential, and suggest that differences in "gain" or "sensitivity" of increasingly distal dendritic synapses may make up for their more remote location. They suggest alterations of receptor density with synaptic location as a possible explanation.

From the morphological point of view there is a marked heterogeneity of axonal terminals on the cell body and dendrite surfaces of interneurons and motoneurons. This structural variety undoubtedly reflects, among other factors, the many sources which the impinging terminals represent. Some idea of this pattern and variety can be gained from Figure 12, which shows parts of two

---

Figure 11 Scanning electron microscope photograph of motoneuron dendrite bundle in the anterior horn of the spinal cord of the rat. Note elements both joining and leaving the bundle. Background contains meshwork of axonal neuropil, dendrite segments, and several free erythrocytes. Calibration bar = 10 μm. × 1600 (original magnification).

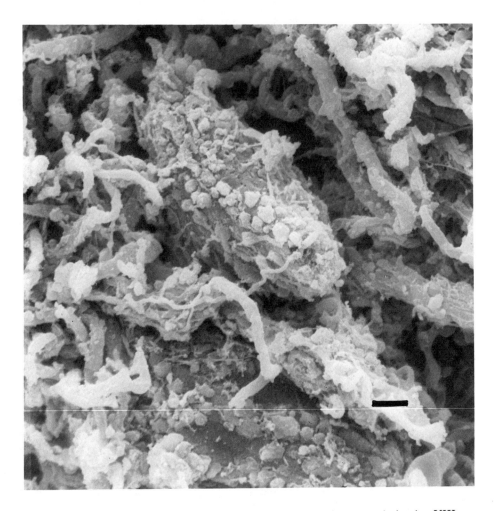

Figure 12 Scanning electron microscope photograph of neurons in lamina VIII of gerbil spinal cord. Dendrite branches apparently have been pulled off the cell body in upper center field during preparation of the tissue. Portion of the surface of a larger cell body is seen at the bottom. Note the varying sizes of axon terminals and the clear, rather dark bare membrane areas. Calibration bar = 5 μm. × 4000 (original magnification).

medium-sized neurons in lamina VIII. Dendrite shafts have apparently been avulsed from the upper cell during preparation, and only part of the surface of the larger element below can be seen. Nonetheless, the range in size and shape of synaptic terminals is considerable, especially of those on the lower element.

Note the crowding of synaptic terminals in some areas and the "clear" areas adjacent. This spotty distribution of terminals characterizes many areas we have studied with the scanning electron microscope. How exciting it will be when we can characterize such structures chemically as we wander among them in a fully tridimensional milieu.

VI. CONCLUSION

Over 100 years of active structural and functional research on the spinal cord have produced an impressive body of information about this most explicitly organized of all noncortical structures. Nonetheless, the gaps in our knowledge remain varied and formidable. For instance, we remain basically uncertain of the patterns of many connectivity systems in the dorsal and ventral horns, of the proportion of interneurons to motoneurons in laminae VIII and IX, of the physiologic nature and chemical characterization of most spinal synapses, and even of the location and nature of many spinal fiber systems ascending to suprasegmental levels. Information of the type sketched out in this chapter can serve, at best, as a preface to the material that follows, and to work by investigators in the decades to come.

REFERENCES

1. Ariëns-Kappers, C. U., Huber, G. C., and Crosby, E. C. (1960). *The Comparative Anatomy of the Nervous System of Vertebrates Including Man*, Hafner, New York, pp. 135–334.
2. Bullock, T. H., and Horridge, G. A. (1965). *Structure and Function of the Nervous System in Invertebrates*, W. H. Freeman, San Francisco, pp. 156–1592.
3. Geschwind, N., and Levitsky, W. (1968). Human brain: Left-right asymmetries in temporal speech region. *Science 161*:186–187.
4. Mountcastle, V. B., and Powell, T. P. S. (1959). Central nervous mechanisms subserving position sense and kinesthesis. *Bull. Johns Hopkins Hosp. 105*: 173–200.
5. Shriver, J. E., Stein, B. M., and Carpenter, M. B. (1968). Central projections of spinal dorsal roots in the monkey. I. Cervical and upper thoracic dorsal roots. *Am. J. Anat. 123*:27–74.
6. Marie, P. (1894). Sur l'origine exogène ou endogène des lésions du cordon postérieur, étudiées comparativement dans le tabes et la pellagre. *Semaine médicale* t.XIV. Quoted from Ramon y Cajal, S. (1909). *Histologie du Système Nerveux de l'Homme et des Vertébrés*, vol. 1, Paris, Maloine, p. 403.
7. Hwang, Y. C., Hinsman, E. J., and Roesel, O. F. (1975). Caliber spectra of fibers in the fasciculus gracilis of the cat cervical cord: a quantitative electron microscopic study. *J. Comp. Neurol. 162*:195–204.

8. Stern, K. (1938). Note on the nucleus ruber magnocellularis and its efferent pathway in man. *Brain 61*:284–289.

9. Carpenter, M. (1976). *Human Neuroanatomy*, 7th ed. Williams and Wilkins, Baltimore, 741 pp.

10. Lassek, A. M. (1954). *The Pyramidal Tract: Its Status in Medicine.* Chas. C Thomas, Springfield, Illinois, 166 pp.

11. Evarts, E. J. (1967). Representation of movements and muscles by pyramidal tract neurons of the precentral motor cortex. In *Neurophysiological Basis of Normal and Abnormal Motor Activities*. Raven, New York, pp. 215–253.

12. Scheibel, M. E., Tomiyasu, U., and Scheibel, A. B. (1977). The aging human Betz cell. *Exp. Neurol. 56*:598–609.

13. Lloyd, D. P. C. (1941). The spinal mechanisms of the pyramidal system in cats. *J. Neurophysiol. 4*:525–546.

14. Bernhard, C. G., Bohm, E., and Petersen, I. (1953). Investigations on the organization of the corticospinal system in monkeys. *Acta Physiol. Scand. 29*:79–103.

15. Kuypers, H. G. J. M. (1960). Central cortical projections to motor and somatosensory cell groups. *Brain 83*:161–184.

16. Scheibel, M. E., and Scheibel, A. B. (1966). Terminal axonal patterns in cat spinal cord. I. The lateral corticospinal tract. *Brain Res. 2*:330–350.

17. Iansek, R., and Redman, S. J. (1973). The amplitude, time course and charge of unitary excitatory post-synaptic potentials evoked in spinal motoneurone dendrites. *J. Physiol. (Lond.) 234*:665–688.

18. Weil, A., and Lassek, A. (1929). A quantitative distribution of the pyramidal tract in man. *Arch. Neurol. Psychiat. 22*:495–510.

19. Nyberg-Hansen, R. (1966). Functional organization of descending supraspinal fiber systems to the spinal cord. Anatomical observations and physiological correlations. *Ergeb. Anat. Entwicklungsgesch. 39*:(No. 2)1–48.

20. Orlovsky, G. N. (1972). Activity of rubrospinal neurons during locomotion. *Brain Res. 46*:99–112.

21. Liu, C. N. (1956). Afferent nerves to Clarke's and the lateral cuneate nuclei in the cat. *Arch. Neurol. Psychiat. 75*:67–77.

22. Lloyd, D. P. C., and McIntyre, A. K. (1950). Dorsal column conduction of group I muscle afferent impulses and their relay through Clarke's column. *J. Neurophysiol. 13*:39–54.

23. Oscarsson, O. (1965). Functional organization of the spino and cuneo cerebellar tracts. *Physiol. Rev. 45*:495–522.

24. Cooper, S., and Sherrington, C. S. (1940). Gower's tract and spinal border cells. *Brain 63*:123–134.

25. Ha, H., and Liu, C. N. (1968). Cell origin of the ventral spinocerebellar tract. *J. Comp. Neurol. 133*:185–205.

26. Hubbard, J. L., and Oscarsson, O. (1962). Localization of the cell bodies of the ventral spinocerebellar tract in lumbar segments of the cat. *J. Comp. Neurol. 118*:199–204.

27. Oscarsson, O., and Uddenberg, N. (1964). Identification of a spinocerebellar tract activated from forelimb afferents in the cat. *Acta Physiol. Scand. 62*: 125–136.

28. Lissauer, H. (1885). Beitrag zur pathogischen Anatomie der tabes dorsalis und sum Faserverlauf im menschlichen Rückenmark. *Neurol. Centralblatt. 4*:245–246.

29. Ranson, S. W. (1914). An experimental study of Lissauer's tract and the dorsal roots. *J. Comp. Neurol. 24*:531–545.

30. Kerr, F. W. L. (1966). The ultrastructure of the spinal tract of the trigeminal nerve and the substantia gelatinosa. *Exp. Neurol. 16*:359–376.

31. Scheibel, M. E., and Scheibel, A. B. (1968). Terminal axonal patterns in cat spinal cord. II. The dorsal horn. *Brain Res. 9*:32–58.

32. LaMotte, C. (1977). Distribution of the tract of Lissauer and the dorsal root fibers in the primate spinal cord. *J. Comp. Neurol. 172*:529–562.

33. Giesler, G. J., Basbaum, A. I., and Menétrey, P. (1977). Projections and origins of the spinothalamic tract in the rat. *Soc. Neurosci. Abstr. 3*:500.

34. Trevino, D. L., Maunz, R. A., Bryan, R. N., and Willis, W. D. (1972). Location of cells or origin of the spinothalamic tract in the lumbar enlargement of cat. *Exp. Neurol. 34*:64–77.

35. Trevino, D. L., Coulter, J. D., and Willis, W. D. (1973). Location of cells of origin of spinothalamic tract in lumbar enlargement of the monkey. *J. Neurophysiol. 36*:750–761.

36. Foerster, O., and Gagel, O. (1932). Die Vorderseitenstrangdurschschneidung beim Menschen. Eine Klinischpathophysiologisch-anatomische Studie. *Ztschr. ges. Neurol. u Psychiat. 138*:1–92.

37. Brodal, A. (1981). *Neurological Anatomy in Relation to Clinical Medicine*, 3rd ed. Oxford University Press, New York, pp. 194–210.

38. Ramon y Cajal, S. (1909). *Histologie du Système Nerveux de l'Homme et des Vertèbrès*, vol. 1, Inst. Cajal, Madrid (reprinted in 1952), pp. 287–419.

39. Rexed, B. (1952). The cytoarchitectonic organization of the spinal cord in the cat. *J. Comp. Neurol. 96*:415–495.

40. Renshaw, B. (1946). Central effects of centripetal impulses in axons of spinal ventral roots. *J. Neurophysiol. 9*:191–204.

41. Eccles, J. C., Fatt, P., and Koketsu, K. (1954). Cholinergic and inhibitory synapses in a pathway from motor-axon collaterals to motoneurones. *J. Physiol. 126*:524–562.

42. Scheibel, M. E., and Scheibel, A. B. (1966). Spinal motoneurones, interneurones and Renshaw cells. A Golgi study. *Arch. Ital. Biol. 104*:328–353.

43. Jankowska, E. (1975). Identification of interneurons interposed in different spinal reflex pathways. In *Golgi Centennial Symposium*, M. Santini (Ed.), Raven, New York, pp. 235–246.

44. Waldeyer, H. (1888). Das Gorilla-Rückenmark. In *Abhanlungen der Preussischen Akademie der Wissenschaften*, Berlin, pp. 1–147.

45. Christensen, B. N., and Perl, E. R. (1970). Spinal neurons specifically excited by noxious or thermal stimuli: Marginal zone of the dorsal horn. *J. Neurophysiol. 33*:293–307.

46. Szentagothai, J. (1964). Neuronal and synaptic arrangements in the substantia gelatinosa Rolandi. *J. Comp. Neurol. 122*:219–240.
47. Beal, J. A., and Fox, C. A. (1976). Afferent fibers in the substantia gelatinosa of the adult monkey (*Macaca mulatta*). A Golgi study. *J. Comp. Neurol. 168*:113–144.
48. Réthelyi, M. (1977). Preterminal and terminal axon arborizations in the substantia gelatinosa of cat's spinal cord. *J. Comp. Neurol. 177*:511–528.
49. Scheibel, M. E., and Scheibel, A. B. (1969). Terminal patterns in cat spinal cord. III. Primary afferent collaterals. *Brain Res. 13*:417–443.
50. Ralston, H. J. (1965). The organization of the substantia gelatinosa Rolandi in the cat lumbrosacral cord. *Z. Zellforsch. 67*:1–23.
51. Kerr, F. W. L. (1975). Neuroanatomical substrates of nociception in the spinal cord. *Pain 1*:325–356.
52. Réthelyi, M., and Szentagothai, J. (1969). The large synaptic complexes of the substantia gelatinosa. *Exp. Brain Res. 7*:258–274.
53. Proshansky, E., and Egger, M. D. (1977). Dendritic spread of dorsal horn neurons in cat. *Exp. Brain Res. 28*:153–166.
54. Carpenter, M. B., Stein, B. M., and Shriver, J. E. (1968). Central projections of spinal dorsal roots in the monkey. V. Lower thoracic lumbrosacral and coccygeal dorsal roots. *Am. J. Anat. 123*:75–118.
55. Brodal, A., Walberg, F., and Blackstad, T. (1950). Termination of spinal afferents to inferior olive in cat. *J. Neurophysiol. 13*:431–454.
56. Romanes, G. J. (1951). The motor cell columns of the lumbosacral spinal cord of the cat. *J. Comp. Neurol. 94*:313–363.
57. Sterling, P., and Kuypers, H. G. J. M. (1967). Anatomical organization of the brachial spinal cord of the cat. I. The distribution of dorsal root fibers. *Brain Res. 4*:1–15.
58. Cruce, W. C. (1974). The anatomical organization of hindlimb motoneurons in the lumbar spinal cord of the frog, *Rana catesbiana*. *J. Comp. Neurol. 74*:59–76.
59. Schoenen, J. (1980). "Organisation Neuronale de la Moelle Épinière de l'Homme," Ph.D. dissertation, Université de Liège, Belgium, 353 pp.
60. Matthews, M. A., Willis, W. D., and Williams, V. (1973). Dendrite bundles in lamina IX of cat spinal cord: a possible source for electrical interaction between motoneurons. *Anat. Rec. 171*:313–328.
61. Scheibel, M. E., and Scheibel, A. B. (1970). Organization of spinal motoneuron dendrites in bundles. *Exp. Neurol. 28*:106–112.
62. Scheibel, M. E., and Scheibel, A. B. (1970). Developmental relationship between spinal motoneuron dendrite bundles and patterned activity in the hind limb of cats. *Exp. Neurol. 29*:328–335.
63. Roney, K. J., Scheibel, A. B., and Shaw, G. L. (1979). Dendritic bundles: survey of anatomical experiments and physiological theories. *Brain Res. Rev. 1*:225–271.
64. Schmidt, R. F. (1971). Presynaptic inhibition in the vertebrate central nervous system. *Ergeb. Physiol. 63*:20–101.

65. Sterling, P., and Kuypers, H. G. J. M. (1967). Anatomical organization of the brachial spinal cord of the cat. II. The motoneuron plexus. *Brain Res.* *4*:16–32.

66. Rall, W. (1962). Theory of physiological properties of dendrites. *Ann. N.Y. Acad. Sci. 96*:1071–1092.

67. Rall, W. (1977). Nervous system. In *The Handbook of Physiology*, E. R. Kendell (Ed.), sect. 1, vol. 1, part 1, Bethesda, Maryland, American Physiological Society, pp. 39–97.

68. Scheibel, M. E., and Scheibel, A. B. (1969). A structural analysis of spinal interneurons and Renshaw cells. In *The Interneuron*, M. A. B. Brazier (Ed.), University of California Press, Los Angeles, pp. 159–208.

3
AFFERENT FIBERS

Robert E. W. Fyffe* *School of Medicine, University of North Carolina at Chapel Hill, Chapel Hill, North Carolina*

I. INTRODUCTION

This chapter will describe the anatomy of the intraspinal axons and terminal arborizations of primary afferent fibers. These central branches are part of a complex entity (the afferent unit) composed of a specialized receptor (transducer) in the periphery, a centrally projecting axon, a cell body in the dorsal root ganglion, and synaptic endings in the spinal cord or brainstem where the afferent signals are transmitted to the appropriate central neurons. Some properties of the afferent unit are very well documented. For a comprehensive review of aspects such as receptor structure, fiber diameter, response properties of units innervating skin and muscle, historical perspective, and classification schemes the reader should consult the detailed accounts published elsewhere (1-7).

It is clear from these studies (e.g., 4,5) that there is currently strong affirmation of the "doctrine of specific nerve energies" attributed to Müller's writings (8) in the mid-nineteenth century. The approach in this review is to consider the central projections of primary afferent fibers from the "specificity" point of

**Present affiliation*: John Curtin School of Medical Research, Australian National University, Canberra, Australia

79

view, an approach which is particularly relevant following the rapidly expanding body of correlative morphologic and functional information which has become available in the last few years.

Classic and modern techniques afford the neuroanatomist a variety of approaches toward defining the patterns of termination of afferent fibers in the spinal cord. The relevant literature published prior to 1973 referring to classic or modern silver impregnation and degeneration methods (9-16) has been reviewed systematically by Réthelyi and Szentágothai (17). Since then, these methods (18-21) and a new generation of neuronal tracing methods employing anterograde and transganglionic transport of markers, such as horseradish peroxidase (HRP) (22-33), cobalt (34), or radioactively labeled amino acids (35-37), which can be visualized autoradiographically, and transganglionic degeneration (38,39) have been used extensively. Several of the more recent studies have also been concerned with defining the ultrastructural features of primary afferent fibers.

Probably the most powerful and significant development has been the introduction of intracellular staining techniques to the neuroanatomist's armamentatrium. In particular, in the mid-1970s, Brown's group (40) and Jankowska and her colleagues (41) described the iontophoretic intracellular injection of HRP into single, functionally identified neurons. Furthermore, the work of Jankowska et al. (41) showed that the labeled neuron could subsequently be analyzed by the electron as well as by light microscope. These techniques have revolutionized neuroanatomic studies, combining as they do the power of the microelectrode with a high resolution, Golgi-like staining of the identified neuron. Full details of the methods and discussion of their advantages and limitations are presented in detail elsewhere (2,40-43). Of relevance to the present review, crucial advances were made when Brown et al. (44) and Light and Perl (43) refined the methodology sufficiently to allow intra-axonal injections of single, identified axons to be performed. Much of the new correlative data to be described in this chapter derives from studies using intra-axonal staining techniques to visualize the intraspinal branches and synaptic boutons of myelinated primary afferent fibers. The myelinated afferent fibers will be discussed systematically according to unit type, but the unmyelinated primary afferents (C-fibers), which have as yet eluded intra-axonal microelectrode recording and staining, will be discussed on the basis of rather more indirect evidence. Analysis of afferent input via trigeminal or visceral nerves (45-53) is considered beyond the scope of this review. The lumbosacral spinal cord has long been the model subject of study in relation to the structural and functional properties of neurons, and this review will concentrate on that area. In discussing the anatomy of the intraspinal branches of afferent fibers in the lumbosacral spinal cord, I will use the cytoarchitectonic subdivisions of the spinal gray matter proposed by Rexed (54,55) as the frame of reference.

II. THE ENTRY OF AFFERENT FIBERS INTO THE SPINAL CORD

Since the work of Bell and Magendie (see 56) the concept (termed the law of separation of function by many neurophysiologists) that the dorsal roots contain only sensory axons and that each ventral root contains only motor (or preganglionic) axons has been accepted as a fundamental principle. In keeping with this idea, the majority of afferent fibers enter the spinal cord through the dorsal roots. What may turn out to be a significant minority (see Sec. II.C) of afferent fibers have been recently rediscovered in the ventral roots; these findings may lead to a reappraisal of Bell and Magendie's law.

A. Bifurcation of Dorsal Root Axons

The fibers which enter the spinal cord via the dorsal roots traditionally were thought to bifurcate into ascending and descending branches close to the entrance zone (17,57). Recent intra-axonal staining studies (see Sec. II and Sec. VII.B) largely confirm this idea, but they illustrate a significant departure in the case of one major group of fibers—the large-diameter hair follicle afferents. These axons (44), and occasionally other large diameter afferents, do not bifurcate on entering the cord, but only have an ascending branch in the dorsal columns. Possible implications of this are discussed by Brown (2).

The course of the dorsal root afferents follow the classically described trajectory (17): the fibers run medially above and parallel to the dorsal border of the dorsal horn and assume, within a few hundred micrometers, their position of ascent or descent in the dorsal columns close to the dorsomedial edge of the dorsal horn. Axons in the dorsal columns frequently follow wavy trajectories but generally become organized in a topographic fashion, as described elsewhere (7,17,58).

Small myelinated and unmyelinated fibers (see Sec. IV) are generally thought to enter Lissauer's tract (17,59,60), where they bifurcate and ascend or descend for short distances in the tract.

B. Segregation of Large and Small Dorsal Root Axons

A longstanding, and controversial, concept that dorsal root fibers become segregated on the basis of their fiber diameter just before entering the spinal cord has recently come under further scrutiny. Lissauer (60) and Ranson (61-65) suggested that the medial division of the dorsal root near the dorsal root entrance zone contains mainly large myelinated fibers, while small fibers congregate in the lateral parts of the root and enter Lissauer's tract. Szentágothai (11) and Snyder (66) felt this idea acceptable, but indicated that the small fibers were in fact radially concentrated at the periphery of the root.

Selective lesions might, therefore, be used to abolish input from one or other of these divisions (61-65), but Wall (67) and others (see 7) contend that technical and other difficulties would so complicate the issue as to make it practically impossible to selectively destroy one subgroup of the coarse or fine fibers or draw valid conclusions from such experimentation.

Snyder (66) has made detailed electron microscopic analyses which support these latter suggestions. With the improved resolution of the electron microscope Snyder (66) demonstrated a lack of segregation of fibers in cat dorsal roots— refuting the concept in that species, whereas in some species of primates, segregation, as described previously, does occur. The latter finding has been utilized in subsequent important anatomic studies (24,25).

C. Ventral Root Afferents

Sherrington (69) described myelinated fibers in ventral roots which survived on the distal side and degenerated on the proximal side of ventral rhizotomy; these were referred to as recurrent fibers. These observations set the scene for investigations many years later in which physiologic recordings and anatomic study established that there are a few myelinated sensory fibers in the ventral roots (70-77). Coggeshall's group studied cat ventral roots with the electron microscope and established that many unmyelinated fibers reacted in the same way as Sherrington's (69) recurrent fibers to ventral rhizotomy (78-80,84). They noted (see also Ref. 86) that up to 30% of the axons in ventral roots from several segments in thoracic, lumbar, and sacral spinal cord were unmyelinated: in thoracic and caudal segments 50% of these are sensory; in lumbosacral segments (i.e., between the sympathetic and parasympathetic outflows) most of the unmyelinated axons are sensory.

Physiologic recording from unmyelinated ventral root axons (74,81-83) confirmed their sensory nature and indicated that they largely innervated visceral receptors, with only a small proportion innervating somatic receptors.

Given the presence of a relatively large number of sensory axons in some ventral roots, the remaining issues concern whether or not they actually enter the cord through the ventral root, and where they terminate. Attempts at resolving these questions are inconclusive. When HRP is injected into the spinal cord, and the dorsal roots are cut, some, predominantly small, cells in the dorsal root ganglion are retrogradely labeled (85,89). However, the number of cells labeled is small and not consistent with the number of presumed sensory (unmyelinated) axons seen anatomically in the ventral root (78-80). Light and Metz (88) applied HRP to the proximal stump of cut ventral roots. They suggested that axons of ventral root origin which terminated in the dorsal horn, including the superficial layers, were the ventral root afferents noted by Coggeshall's group (87). In accord with the earlier anatomic evidence, most of the fibers observed were of small, probably unmyelinated, diameter; some appeared to course eventually into Lissauer's tract. The relatively few fibers observed is inconsistent with the number of afferent fibers in the ventral roots of these segments, giving strength to the suggestions (see 87) that many of the sensory axons recurve and enter via the dorsal roots. Clearly, much anatomic and physiologic study of these axons is required to derive functional implications and to clarify the status of Bell and Magendie's principle.

III. COMMISSURAL AFFERENTS

Cajal's (57) description of presumed primary afferent fiber collaterals which cross the midline of the spinal cord, by way of the dorsal commissure, has been verified by more recent studies. A variety of degeneration studies make brief mention of this aspect of the distribution of afferent fibers at spinal (90-94) and medullary (48,95,96) levels, and Culberson et al. (97) carried out a specific study in several species. Subsequent use of transganglionic transport of HRP (28,31,32), autoradiography (37), anterograde transport of HRP (25), and intra-axonal staining of single identified afferents (43,98,99) have provided further information. The occurrence of contralateral projections is dependent upon segmental and species variation (49,97). They are consistently observed at caudal and high cervical (as well as dorsal column nuclei) levels, but they are rarely seen at lumbar or brachial (except in the oppossum) segments. While there is agreement that collateral branches of primary afferents do cross the midline in the dorsal commissure, there are conflicting views on the location of the terminal fields of these fibers. Some (10,100) postulate direct projections to the contralateral ventral horn, but this has not been confirmed by recent investigations (37,94), including Golgi studies (14). Projections to the marginal zone are frequently observed (10,37). Projections to contralateral laminae III and IV have been reported (94), but these have been denied by others (31,32). Indeed, the latter finding allowed these workers (31,32) to examine the somatotopic organization (bilaterally) of cutaneous nerve projections to these laminae. Lamina V, particularly its lateral part, seems to be a focus for the termination of bilaterally projecting afferents (32,37,43), and the identity of fibers contributing to these terminations can be deduced from intra-axonal injection studies. Light and Perl (43) and Mense et al. (98) demonstrated that small myelinated (AS) fibers innervating mechanical nociceptors in the skin and subcutaneous tissue project across the midline to the marginal zone and lateral lamina V. A few larger diameter fibers, innervating subcutaneous or type I receptors, may also project to contralateral areas of the medial dorsal horn (43,99).

The physiologic correlates of crossed afferent projections in the spinal cord is poorly understood. Their predominance in caudal (tail representation) segments indicated a possible relationship to midline receptive field representation, but this is not supported by the few electrophysiologic studies of neuronal responses in these segments (101,102) in which somatotopy was examined. It has also been tentatively suggested (43) that the contralaterally projecting nociceptive afferents contribute to a pathway (103-105) for nociception and pain that passes rostrally ipsilateral to the afferent input (but contralateral to the cell bodies of origin of the pathway).

IV. AXONS IN THE DORSAL COLUMNS

While most of the axons in the dorsal columns arise from myelinated afferent fibers, the fiber population also includes axons of propriospinal neurons (106), of post synaptic dorsal column neurons (107-115), and, depending upon the species, various types of descending fibers (57,116-121).

A. Ascending Branches of Primary Afferents

There is general agreement from electrophysiologic studies (7,122-126) that the rostral extent of an afferent projection varies according to the type of unit. From the cat hindlimb, only about 25% of the afferents entering the cord at lumbosacral levels actually reach the dorsal column nuclei (127). Components of this group (see 7,126) include all slowly adapting type II units. Most G and T hair units, Pacinian corpuscle and other rapidly adapting foot pad units, and slowly adapting units from around the base of the claws also project directly to the dorsal column nuclei. Only a very small proportion of slowly adapting type I units reach high cervical levels, as is the case for small myelinated (Aδ) fibers (including D-hair and nociceptive units). Muscle and joint afferents do not reach the dorsal column nuclei either (128-130). Species differences in the extent of projection of some afferents, especially the slowly adapting units, may exist (131,132).

The extent of forelimb afferent projections follows a similar pattern (107, 108), but there are important differences. Group I muscle afferents reach the cuneate nucleus directly (133-137), as do slowly adapting type I units (138,139).

The conduction velocity of afferent fibers is reduced as the axon ascends the dorsal columns. This is consistent with the anatomically observed fiber spectrum at high cervical levels which shows most axons in the Aδ range, whereas their peripheral and dorsal root diameters fall in the A$\alpha\beta$ size range (140). Pacinian corpuscle axons generally show less diameter reduction than other afferent types (123,124,141). Some (7,142) interpret conduction velocity (diameter) reduction as a consequence of the issue of collaterals from the fiber, and further, that lack of conduction velocity reduction is indicative of a lack of collateralization. These assumptions are shown to be erroneous by the recent staining of fibers (Pacinian corpuscle afferents [99]) which show little conduction velocity reduction but issue frequent collateral branches at segmental levels. Similar assumptions have been made regarding Pacinian corpuscle axons from visceral nerves (143-146); perhaps intra-axonal staining could resolve this matter, too. All afferent axons in the spinal cord issue collateral branches to the gray matter.

B. Descending Branches of Primary Afferents

Electrophysiologic (147) and anatomic (16) studies have shown that afferents entering the lumbosacral spinal cord may project caudally for up to six or more segments. There is no evidence as to what extent different types of afferent units contribute to these projections. Intra-axonal staining with HRP seldom labels the full extent of the descending branches of any afferent fiber (see 2) and no intra-axonally stained afferents have been seen to end as a projection into the gray matter. The descending branches of afferent axons are usually thinner than the ascending branches (99,148).

V. AXONS IN LISSAUER'S TRACT

The tract of Lissauer (59,60) has been the subject of intensive, often controversial, consideration (see 106,149-151) on the nature of its fiber composition and its functional role. Matters pertinent to this review concern the extent to which afferent fibers are components of the tract, their distribution within the tract, and their likely zones of termination.

A. The Fiber Spectrum of Lissauer's Tract

Coggeshall's group (152,153) has carried out detailed electron microscopic examinations to resolve the morphologic features of the fine fibers present in the tract. Their evidence suggests that most (80–85%) of the axons are unmyelinated. The remaining 15-20% are small myelinated (Aδ) fibers. These findings confirm conclusions made even before the advent of electron microscopy. The unmyelinated and fine myelinated axons are evenly distributed throughout the tract.

B. The Origin of Fibers in Lissauer's Tract

Lissauer (59,60) considered that the axons in the tract were of dorsal root origin. Cajal (57) was less than certain that this was so, and Ranson (61-65), who noted the probable thick/thin fiber segregation in the dorsal roots (see Sec. II.B) and the fine fiber composition of Lissauer's tract, thought that the fine dorsal root axons projected in the medial portion of the tract while the lateral part of the tract mainly contained the fine axons of endogenous neurons. Further confirmation that Lissauer's tract axons were of mixed origin came from the work of Earle (68) and Szentágothai (11), who in fact proposed that the majority of the axons were propriospinal. This shift in opinion was taken further by Wall (154), who denied the presence of any dorsal root fibers in the tract, but later (155) included a few such fibers as components of the tract. Fuller discussion of the development of studies on Lissauer's tract and its composition are given elsewhere (150). The difficulty of interpreting the data (largely from degeneration studies) from which these concepts arose was pointed out by Ranson (62) and more recently by Coggeshall's group (152,153,156). The latter group used electron microscopy to examine the normal tract (see Sec. V.A), and also the effect of single or multiple dorsal rhizotomies. These methods adequately resolve the fine fibers of the tract and generate several conclusions: (1) in the cat approximately one half of the axons are afferent fibers; in the rat and monkey this proportion is around 75–80%. (2) the proportion of the small myelinated and unmyelinated axons which are afferent fibers is approximately the same; furthermore, they are distributed evenly throughout the medial and lateral divisions of the tract. Thus, there is no segregation of endogenous axons in the lateral part of the tract (cf. 155); (3) the afferent fibers ascend and descend from one to three segments from the segment of entry; and (4) the propriospinal axons are somewhat longer and may project from a few millimeters to five to six segments (11).

One final note on this matter arises from the elegant intra-axonal staining of fine myelinated (Aδ) fibers performed by Light and Perl (43). They noted that some of these afferent fibers, both low- and high-threshold types, sent branches into Lissauer's tract *and* into the dorsal columns; sometimes fibers initially ran in Lissauer's tract before coursing medially into the dorsal columns.

The tract is clearly heterogeneous with respect to fiber content and function. The many afferent fibers in the tract subserve a wide spectrum of afferent input; similarly, the endogenous axons are unlikely to be restricted to roles in any one function, such as mediating the phenomenon of presynaptic inhibition of afferent fibers (149,154).

VI. PRIMARY AFFERENT TERMINATIONS—GENERAL PATTERNS

Conflicting hypotheses on the general organization of primary afferent terminations, particularly in the dorsal horn, have been extant for as long as functional concepts on the role of different fiber populations or spinal tracts. Two of the major issues will be discussed here, namely: Are the terminations of large- and small-diameter afferent fibers segregated in the spinal cord? Where do the unmyelinated C-fibers end, and are they segregated from the small myelinated fibers?

Several problems have complicated these issues in the past and much of the morphologic evidence (light and electron microscopy) is somewhat indirect. The various interpretations rely on presumed different degeneration rates of different fibers, relative bouton sizes, and axonal orientation and attempts to trace profiles which often cannot be unequivocally traced back to a parent axon. There is a further conceptual and practical difficulty in defining the superficial layers of the dorsal horn. The marginal zone is now equated with Rexed's lamina I (54,55) and the substantia gelatinosa is now equated with Rexed's lamina II (54,55), and may be further divided into inner (ventral) and outer (dorsal) layers. The ventral boundary of lamina II is rather irregular and often indistinct, which may in part account for some of the differing interpretations of anatomic data.

The small myelinated (Aδ) and unmyelinated (C) afferent fibers in Lissauer's tract have long been associated with the superficial dorsal horn. However, large diameter collaterals were also thought to enter the substantia gelatinosa from the ventral side, and the evidence for this came from Golgi (14,17,57), degeneration (10,11), and HRP transport studies (22). At another extreme, some (12,157) felt that the superficial dorsal horn was largely devoid of primary afferent terminals because few degenerating fibers were observed there following dorsal rhizotomy. This idea has been emphatically refuted since then (15,21).

The "collaterales grosses et profondes de la substance de Rolando" described by Cajal (57) and more recent authors (17) as terminating in the substantia gelatinosa can now be readily identified as the flame-shaped arborizations of hair follicle afferent fibers (see Sec. VII.B). In the adult these fibers do not terminate in the substantia gelatinosa to any great extent but they arborize profusely in lamina III. Other identified large-diameter cutaneous and muscle afferents do not terminate in the substantia gelatinosa either (see Sec. VII, and Ref. 2). Recent Golgi studies of young animals (20) have also failed to demonstrate large-diameter collaterals entering the substantia gelatinosa from the ventral side, although a few single branchlets of lamina III arborizations occasionally do.

On a more general basis, Light and Perl (24,25) have recently made valuable use of the limited degree of segregation of fibers in monkey (*Macaca mulatta*) dorsal roots (66) to demonstrate by anterograde transport of HRP that the fine fibers comprising the lateral division of the root terminate principally in the superficial dorsal horn (laminae I and II), while the thick fibers project predominantly to deeper regions of the spinal gray matter. This finding concurs with other degeneration, autoradiographic, and HRP transport data (36,36) and with the results discussed in Sec. VII.

The evidence, therefore, points to a segregation of input from large- and small-diameter fibers, with the fine fibers predominantly projecting to laminae I and II and the course fibers going to deeper laminae.

This rather simplified concept would be of use in making functional correlations in some situations, but as Light and Perl's (43) elegant intra-axonal staining of fine myelinated (Aδ) afferent fibers has well indicated the matter is slightly more complex. They (43) succeeded in labeling functionally identified Aδ

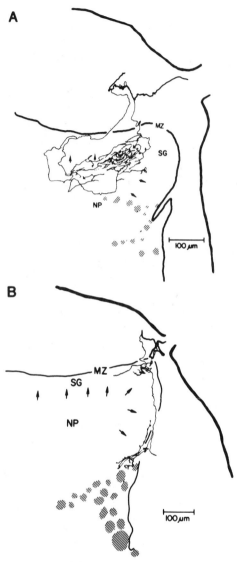

Figure 1 Examples of collateral branches and terminal arborizations arising from thin myelinated afferent fibers. A: This D–hair afferent unit terminated in the ventral part of the substantia gelatinosa and in the immediately subjacent nucleus proprius. B: This high-threshold mechanoreceptive unit ended in the marginal zone, and more ventrally in the lateral part of lamina V. Both reconstructions from cat sacral spinal cord. MZ, marginal zone; SG, substantia gelatinosa; NP, nucleus proprius. Arrows indicate the ventral boundary of the SG. (From Ref. 43.)

afferents innervating D–hair receptors (see 3,176) or high-threshold mechano-receptors (3,158). Each of these groups, like the larger myelinated fibers described in Sec. VII, had quite characteristic and specific central terminal patterns. Most of the D–hair afferent fiber boutons were located in lamina III (like those of the larger diameter half afferents) with some in the most ventral part of lamina II. The high-threshold mechanoreceptors on the other hand projected to lamina I and outer lamina II and also sent branches to lamina V and sometimes across the midline to terminate in the contralateral lamina V (see Fig. 1).

The most reasonable conclusion that can be made to the first point raised in Sec. VI is that any segregation of afferent fiber input that exists is determined not solely by fiber diameter but also by afferent unit type. There is overlap between the terminals of large and small myelinated fibers in the most ventral part of lamina II and in the laminae ventral to that level; only the high-threshold small myelinated fibers segregate part of their terminal field (in lamina I and outer lamina II) from the mass of myelinated afferent fiber terminations.

The question of where the C-fiber terminations fit into this distribution scheme has recently been deduced from electron microscopic studies of degenerating (21) or HRP-labeled (26,156) dorsal root axons in the superficial dorsal horn. Réthelyi (18) had used Golgi techniques and concluded that C-fibers ended in lamina II and Aδ axons ended in lamina I. This concurred with the overall large-small fiber distributions described previously, with the direct evidence of Aδ terminations in lamina I (43) and with evidence from physiologic studies (159,160). The conclusion is supported by Ralston and Ralston (21) and by LaMotte (36), but is opposite to the proposal made by Gobel's group (161, 162) following their analyses of the marginal zone and substantia gelatinosa of the caudal trigeminal nucleus. Furthermore, Gobel et al. (26) have described ultrafine axons and terminals (presumed C-fiber origin) in lamina I of the spinal cord following anterograde transport of HRP from cut dorsal roots. These findings infer that both Aδ and C fibers terminate in lamina I. In relation to the methods used in these analyses it is recognized from electron microscopic examination of identified primary afferents (163–165) that myelinated fibers shed their myelin sheath near their terminal arborizations, become thinner than the parent fiber, and may form quite long unmyelinated branches carrying *en passant* and terminal boutons. Clearly, there would be great advantages in obtaining more direct data on the projections of C-fibers, although to date they have eluded attempts at intra-axonal staining by HRP-filled micropipettes. One might expect that, as for the Aδ fibers, the wide-ranging physiologic properties of different C-fibers (see 3) will determine the precise mode of termination of these fibers.

VII. THE MORPHOLOGY OF FUNCTIONALLY DEFINED PRIMARY AFFERENT FIBER COLLATERALS

In their excellent 1973 review, Réthelyi and Szentágothai (17), following Cajal (57), considered six groups of primary afferent collaterals (plus the commissural afferents considered here in Sec. III). Collaterals to Clarke's column (166-169) include muscle and cutaneous afferents and will not be discussed further because analysis of identified fibers at this level is at a very preliminary stage (170). The other groups of collaterals project to the marginal zone, substantia gelatinosa, center and head of the dorsal horn, and ventral horn. However, it was only possible for Réthelyi and Szentágothai to tentatively assign a functional identity to two types of collaterals; these collaterals were presumed to arise from Ib axons and from the well-known Ia fibers. The situation has changed drastically owing to innovative technical developments (see Sec. VII.A), and there are now at least 10 classes of identified cutaneous or muscle afferent units whose collateral branches in the lumbosacral spinal cord of the cat have been fully described. Some of these give rise to arborizations which can be related to the arborizations described in Golgi material (e.g., 14,17,20), while other axons give rise to patterns that have not been specifically described previously.

A. Methodology

The following accounts draw on data from several laboratories in which intra-axonal staining techniques are used. Employing this common approach, and concentrating on ensuring efficient identification of units, adequate stability, and avoiding spillage so that only one fiber is stained per injection, these groups have produced remarkably consistent results. The individual methods, with appropriate adaptations, are detailed elsewhere (2,40-43) and are summarized here in brief.

Glass microelectrodes filled with a solution (4-10% in Tris buffer with added potassium chloride) of HRP were used to record from single primary afferent axons near the dorsal root entry zone or in the dorsal columns. The unit's responses to appropriate natural or electrical stimulation were identified and the the microelectrode was advanced to attain an intra-axonal penetration. If successful in this attempt (as signaled by a stable membrane potential, of at least 40 mV, and overshooting action potential), HRP was injected into the axon most commonly by iontophoresis (see 2) or pressure (171,357). Rectangular or sinusoidal pulses or direct current (electrode tip positive in all cases) of 5-30 nA amplitude must be passed for one to 20 minutes to provide adequate staining of most fiber types. Histochemical processing by any of several methods (172-174; see also 40) produces reliable visualization of the injected axon and some of its terminal branches and synaptic boutons. Tissue cut in any convenient plane (usually transverse or parasagittal sections) may be examined; greater perspective is gained if a particular type of afferent can be viewed in different planes of section or if it is reconstructed in three dimensions.

B. Collaterals from Afferent Fibers Innervating Hair Follicles

The afferent fibers innervating hair follicles in the skin of the cat and monkey have been classified in terms of their response characteristics and sensitivity, their conduction velocity, and the structure of the hair follicle (175-178). Confusion regarding the nomenclature of the classification schemes has been reviewed elsewhere (2,3,5,7). In this section, the same system as Brown (2) adopted will be used; that is: (1) type D (respond sensitively to movement of down hairs, and conduct in the Aδ range, 10-30 m/sec in the cat and monkey); (2) type G (respond with variable sensitivity to movement of guard hairs and conduct in the A$\alpha\beta$ range, 40-70 m/sec); and (3) type T (respond to movement of tylotrich hairs, highly sensitive and conducting over the same range as type G units, but with a slightly higher mean velocity).

Regardless of the terminology imposed, the hair afferents deliver to the spinal cord a major primary representation of the body surface, and make excitatory connections with many spinal reflex and ascending tract neurons (179-185). Most T and G units have axons that ascend the dorsal columns to the dorsal column nuclei, whereas the axons of D-hair units do not (124-126). The large myelinated T and G units were among the first afferent types to be systematically analyzed by intra-axonal injection of HRP (44), and the smaller (Aδ) D-hair fibers were subsequently successfully labeled also (43). These landmark studies by Brown, Rose, and Snow (44) in Edinburgh, and Light and Perl (43) in Chapel Hill, North Carolina, established the value of the technique for studying both large- and small-diameter afferent fibers. They also established, as will be seen in the following discussion, the specificity of the hair follicle afferent fiber collateral arborizations. All types (T, G, D) generate the same morphologic patterns, independent of the diameter (conduction velocity) of the parent fiber. These patterns are different from any other type of primary afferent arborization in the spinal cord.

1. Collateral Morphology

Analysis of Golgi-impregnated afferent fibers (17,20) indicated that all axons bifurcated into ascending and descending branches as they entered the spinal cord. Surprisingly, it was noted (44) that 75% of large myelinated (types G and T) hair units did not divide, but simply entered and ascended the cord in the dorsal columns. D-hair units (43) usually did bifurcate; their main branches occasionally run in Lissauer's tract before coursing medially into the dorsal columns. All hair afferents give rise to repeated collaterals which arborize in the spinal gray matter. Collaterals arise more frequently in proximity to the entrance zone of the axon, with the frequency dropping off further than about 2 mm from the entry into the cord. The intervals between collaterals range from 100-1400 μm, with an overall mean spacing of about 1 mm. As stated, they are generally closer together near the entrance zone, and when their terminal arborizations are destined to be in the medial part of the dorsal horn as opposed to lateral parts of the dorsal horn.

Collateral branches may penetrate the dorsal horn at any point on its dorsal or medial borders. Usually, the collateral descends directly through the marginal zone and substantia gelatinosa and ventrally to lamina IV or V, where they turn sharply and send recurrent branches dorsally again to form terminal arborizations in laminae III and IV. The characteristic pattern seen in transverse sections can be equated with the "flame-shaped arbors" clearly described by Scheibel and Scheibel (14) and seen in other preparations (12,17,20,57). That these arbors are in fact "end-on" views of a longitudinal plexus of afferent arborizations (12,14,17) has been confirmed (2,44). The longest individual arborizations (from a single collateral) occur in the lateral quarter of the dorsal horn, where they may be up to 1800 μm long; in the medial dorsal horn arborizations are generally 500-800 μm long. The terminal arborizations of adjacent collaterals from a hair afferent axon form a continuous sheet in the parasagittal plane; this sheet of terminals extends over at least the segment of entry of the fiber (see Fig. 2).

There is much more restriction of the transverse spread of an individual arborization, which in the adult cat is usually about 150-400 μm across (44). As expected, this is much wider than the arborizations seen in Golgi material (14,17) from kittens. The position of individual arborizations across the transverse width of the dorsal horn reflects a somatotopic organization (101), where afferents with distal receptive fields project to the medial part of the dorsal horn and axons from proximal receptive fields have arborizations in the lateral parts of the dorsal horn. The location of an axon's terminal arborization across the width of the dorsal horn also determines the frequency of collateral issue: When collaterals are destined for lateral parts of the dorsal horn, there are larger intervals between them than occurs on axons which project to medial parts (2).

The vast majority of the synaptic boutons (discussed later) are located in lamina III, with a few in lamina IV. Only rarely do T- or G-hair afferent collaterals project into lamina II (see Sec. VI); the D-hair afferents, however, sometimes have some boutons in the ventral parts of lamina II.

Ultrastructural studies (163,164) of HRP-labeled hair follicle afferent fiber terminations have confirmed that the structures interpreted as synaptic boutons at the light microscope level (44) are indeed invariably correctly identified as the sole places of synaptic contact in these arborizations. These studies also established that the highly specific morphologic organization of hair afferent and other primary afferent fibers is reflected in specific synaptic arrangements.

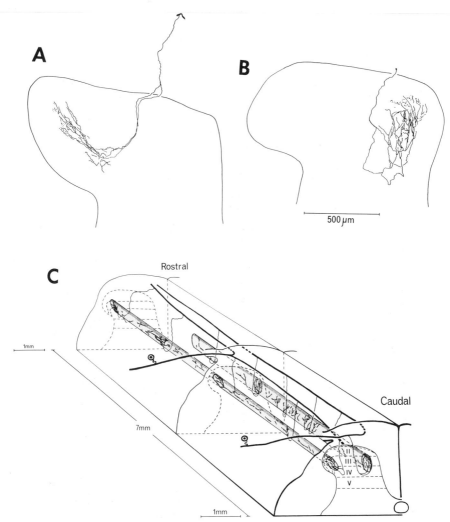

Figure 2 Reconstructions of hair follicle afferent fiber collateral branches in the lumbar spinal cord of the cat. Typical "flame-shaped arborizations" from different axons are seen in the lateral (A) and medial (B) dorsal horn, respectively. A schematic representation (C) of the projections of two hair follicle afferents shows the longitudinally organized terminal arborizations of these fibers. [Scale for A and B = 500 μm.] (From Ref. 42.)

2. Relationships Between Hair Follicle Afferent Fibers and Spinocervical Tract Cells

Brown and Noble (186,187) have recently studied the organization of synaptic contacts made by hair follicle afferents upon spinocervical tract cells. In a direct approach they injected single hair follicle afferent fibers with HRP and then also injected single spinocervical tract cells.

The results were clear. If the primary afferent's receptive field was outside that of the spinocervical tract cell, there was no indication of any synaptic connections between them. If the spinocervical tract cell's receptive field contained that of the primary afferent fiber, then contacts between them were always observed. The number and location of synapses in these cases was correlated with the relative positions of the receptive fields. Where the afferent's field was close to the center of the cell's field, there were many (40-60) contacts and they were on the proximal parts of the dendritic tree. Where the afferent's field was near the periphery of the cell's field there were far fewer contacts and they were located on distal dendrites. The contacts, especially in the former cases, were often of the "climbing" type, formed by several *en passant* boutons apposing a segment of dendrite. While a set of contacts could be spread over several dendritic branches, these branches generally arose from a small number (one to four) of primary dendrites.

Brown and Noble's (186,187) results correlate well with expectations from electrophysiologic studies (181). Together, these pieces of evidence indicate a differential efficacy of distal versus proximal inputs on spinocervical cell dendrites because these cells do not exhibit subliminal fringes to their receptive fields. However, the system is probably complicated by the presence of disynaptic excitation from the same afferents that excite the cell monosynaptically (181); further combined structural-functional studies must be performed to elucidate these matters and perhaps raise the hair follicle–spinocervical tract system to a useful model for the organization of neuronal systems which would complement the well-known Ia-mononeuron model. The "negative" results of Brown and Noble (186,187) indicate that normally ineffective (or "silent") synapses (see 188) do not occur in the hair follicle–spinocervical tract system.

C. Pacinian Corpuscle Afferents

The Pacinian corpuscle is one of the best known cutaneous mechanoreceptors, and it has been intensively studied since its original description (189). The receptor is found in deep dermal or subcutaneous tissue. It is innervated by relatively large (conduction velocity ~50-80 m/sec) myelinated axons, and the unit exhibits characteristic response properties to mechanical transients (177, 190-200). In contrast, the central projections and effects of Pacinian corpuscle stimulation are not so well understood. It is well-known that Pacinian corpuscle afferents project through the dorsal column-medial lemniscal system to the thalamus and, hence, to the cerebral cortex (201-208). The axons reach the dorsal column nuclei with little or no reduction in their conduction velocity (123,124,126,141). Some (142,210) have inferred that this observation, and the lack of segmental effects seen when Pacinian corpuscle afferents from viscera were electrically stimulated (143-146), indicates that these axons do not give off any major collateral branches after entering the spinal cord, but rather ascend directly to the dorsal column nuclei. Other lines of evidence, however, indicate that Pacinian corpuscle afferents are responsible for exciting various types of dorsal horn neurons (209,211,212) including interneurons (209) on the pathway for producing presynaptic inhibition of primary afferent axons (including Pacinian corpuscle afferents themselves) and neurons whose axons also ascend to the dorsal column nuclei (109,110,115). The successful staining of axons innervating Pacinian corpuscles in the glabrous skin of the cat hindlimb (99,165,213) confirms that these afferents do indeed project into the spinal gray matter at segmental levels. These results are discussed in Sec. VII.C.I.

1. Collateral Morphology

The axons innervating Pacinian corpuscles bifurcate into ascending and descending branches shortly after entering the cord, and then assume wavy courses, close to the medial or dorsomedial border of the dorsal horn. The descending branches are usually thinner than the ascending branches of the main axon. Collaterals arise from the ascending and descending axons every 700 μm or so on average; thus, the frequency of collateral branching was about the same as for all the other cutaneous afferent fibers examined (see 2). The ascending branches did not show any noticeable reduction in diameter as they issued successive collaterals, in keeping with the electrophysiologic measurements of the central conduction velocity of these axons.

The collaterals have a characteristic and specific morphology that does not appear to have been previously noted in the literature. The terminal arborizations occupy the medial one third of the dorsal horn; this is in agreement with the somatotopic organization of dorsal horn neurons (101). In this region two distinct terminal zones are observed: the collateral passes ventrally through laminae I and II, or enters lamina III directly from its medial border, and branches profusely in laminae III and IV; the synaptic boutons (see also 165) are distributed mainly in laminae III and IV, with the secondary, smaller, terminal arborization distributed ventrally in laminae V and VI. In general, there is some separation between these two terminal areas. Very few if any boutons are observed in lamina II.

The terminal branches of Pacinian corpuscle afferent fiber collaterals may carry up to 12 boutons of varying size [ranging from small ones ($\sim$1.0 × 1.0 μm)]. The organization of these terminal, bouton-carrying branches was different in the dorsal versus the ventral arborizations. In laminae III and IV the axons usually had a longitudinal orientation and carried many *en passant* boutons; individual collaterals could extend over 400–750 μm in the rostro-caudal direction in these laminae, with occasional continuity or overlap between adjacent collaterals from an axon. In laminae V and VI terminal axons ran in the transverse plane (usually dorsoventrally oriented) and tended to generate regions where small clusters of boutons from one or more terminal branches were formed. These ventral arborizations were much less extensive in both medio-lateral and rostrocaudal spread than the dorsal arborizations (Fig. 3B).

These arrangements are interesting in view of the fact that the arborizations spread over four laminae of the dorsal horn and show a differential organization in different areas. The predominantly rostrocaudal orientation of terminal arborizations in laminae III and IV matches the longitudinal axonal plexus described previously (17) and fits with the longitudinally oriented dendrites of cells in these laminae (17,214). Presumably, the *en passant* boutons of Pacinian corpuscle afferent collateral branches make contact with these dendrites; axosomatic contacts are rarely seen in counterstained sections of the dorsal arborizations. In the ventral parts, however, axosomatic contacts from small clusters of boutons upon small to medium neurons were common. The trans-versely organized terminal axons moreover concur with the perpendicularly oriented degenerating plexuses of laminae V (214) and fit well with the pre-dominant dendritic tree configurations of this area (215,216).

D. Axons Innervating Rapidly Adapting Glabrous Skin Receptors

In addition to the Pacinian corpuscles, another type of rapidly adapting mechanoreceptor occurs in glabrous skin (141,200). This is the Krause (217) ending [or Meissner corpuscle (218) in primate skin]; full details of its structure and response properties are given elsewhere (5,195-200,219). Krause endings are innervated by relatively large-diameter [conduction velocity 45-75 m/sec [123-125,202,207]] myelinated fibers which project centrally in the dorsal columns to high cervical levels, probably to the dorsal column nuclei (225). At the seg-mental level there is little concrete evidence as to the specific types of neuron which may be activated by these afferents (209). They do not excite spino-cervical tract cells (179), but the situation with regard to the spinothalamic tract (105) and the postsynaptic dorsal column system (109,110,115,220) remains equivocal.

1. Collateral Morphology

A very small sample of stained axons are thought (99) to be representative of this population of fibers, and does indicate a distinctive morphology for the collaterals of rapidly adapting foot pad afferents. All of the axons bifurcate shortly after entering the cord and give rise to numerous collaterals from both the ascending and descending branches of the main axon; some of the collaterals begin to subdivide while still within the dorsal columns. They enter the dorsal or dorsomedial part of the dorsal horn and continue to branch to give rise to terminal arborizations in the most medial part of the dorsal horn, almost exclusively in lamina III. Each arborization is narrow in the transverse plane (50-300 μm); relatively restricted rostrocaudally (400-600 μm); and occupies essentially a discrete volume of cord in the medial part of lamina III (Fig. 3A), since there is seldom any overlap between adjacent collaterals from a single fiber. Although in transverse view the collaterals resemble the hair afferent (see Sec. V.B) collaterals in terms of branching and terminal location, an obvious difference is manifest when the sagittal organization is examined: The hair follicle afferents form a continuous column of arborizations, whereas the rapidly adapting glabrous skin afferents do not. These mechanoreceptors (hair afferents and rapidly adapting pad units) clearly also have different functions apart from innervating hairy or glabrous skin. The hair afferents excite many spinocervical tract cells, whereas axons of the rapidly adapting pad units do not.

E. Slowly Adapting Type I Mechanoreceptors

Although there had been several descriptions (221-224) of sensitive, slowly adapting cutaneous mechanoreceptors, Iggo (225,226) was the first to clearly differentiate two distinct classes of receptor in the hairy skin of mammals; these are usually designated type I and type II units. The type II units are discussed in the following section. The type I receptors are found in hairy (176,178,227-234) and glabrous (197,198,209,235-238) skin of several species, and are innervated by myelinated axons whose conduction velocities encompass the A$\alpha\beta$ range (cat: 35-90 m/sec). The receptor in hairy skin is clearly visible under microscopic examination as a dome-shaped structure (225,227,230) analogous to the "Haarscheibe" described at the beginning of this century (239). Each type I receptor is innervated by one large-diameter myelinated fiber; each fiber usually innervates two or three receptors (176,177,227,232). The terminals of the afferent axon are associated with a single layer (up to 50 cells) of specialized epithelial cells that were originally described by Merkel (240; see also 227). No "Haarscheibe" is visible in glabrous skin, but the afferent fiber is again associated with a cluster of 30 or so Merkel cells at the epidermodermal junction (197,198, 218).

Iggo (225) and Tapper (230) independently correlated a particular type of afferent discharge with displacement or deformation of the easily recognizable type I receptor. These important observations were the impetus for much of the experimental examination of receptor specificity and structural-functional relationships which have taken place over the last 20 years.

The physiologic characteristics of the type I afferents have been fully discussed by Burgess and Perl (3). The type I units may signal both velocity and displacement (3). While the central axons of these receptors generally do not reach the dorsal column nuclei directly from hindlimb (123-125), although those of forelimb type I afferents do, some of the information may be relayed to medullary levels via the postsynaptic dorsal column pathway (115).

1. Collateral Morphology

Like most cutaneous and muscle afferent fibers, the majority of type I axons bifurcate shortly after entering the spinal cord. The full extent of their ascending and descending branches in the dorsal columns is not revealed by the intraaxonal HRP staining, and therefore no minimum limit on their rostrocaudal distribution can be inferred. Rostrally, they must extend to high lumbar levels where they excite neurons of the dorsal spinocerebellar tract (183,241).

The main branches issue frequent collaterals [on average, every 600 (glabrous skin units)−700 μm (hairy skin units)] at the segmental level. These give rise to distinctive morphologic arrangements in the dorsal horn. The hairy and glabrous skin type I afferents have essentially the same branching patterns and morphology, and they project to somatotopically appropriate regions of the dorsal horn. Units from galbrous skin thus always terminate in the medial one third of the dorsal horn, whereas units from hairy skin may, if their receptive area is located on proximal skin, project to lateral parts of the dorsal horn.

Collaterals pass directly throught the superficial layers of the dorsal gray matter, or enter the dorsal horn through the medial border of laminae III and IV from axons running deep in the dorsal columns. The branching patterns described by Brown's group (242) do not appear to have been observed in earlier silver-impregnated material, although Hamano et al. (20) in their more recent Golgi study illustrate one collateral (their Fig. 8) which is strikingly similar to some type I afferent fiber collaterals. The important features are that collaterals, especially those entering from the dorsal side, pursue a C- or L-shaped trajectory (convex laterally) through the dorsal four or five laminae. They curve back from their deepest extent (laminae V or VI) and by profuse branching arborize finally in laminae III, IV, and V, mainly in lamina IV. Collaterals entering the dorsal horn through its medial border have somewhat different trajectories (242), but they also arborize in laminae III, IV, and V (Fig. 3C).

The terminal arborizations, when viewed in the transverse plane occupy well-defined, sometimes quite extensive (250-300 μm mediolateral extent and 250-650 μm dorsoventral extent) zones and extend for 100-700 μm (mean ~400 μm) along the longitudinal axis of the cord. There are gaps of 100-500 μm between the arborization of adjacent collaterals from the same axon−thus, the information from type I afferent fibers is delivered to the spinal cord in a discontinuous series of longitudinally aligned, almost spherical lobules.

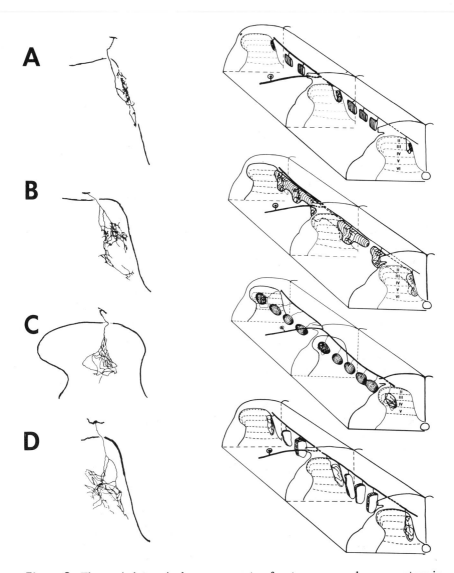

Figure 3 The varied terminal arrangements of cutaneous mechanoreceptors in lumbar spinal cord of cat are shown together with schematic representations of the organization of the collaterals and terminals from these types of afferents (see also Fig. 2). A: Rapidly adapting pad unit (Sec. VII.D); B: Pacinian corpuscle unit (Sec. VII.C); C: Type I unit (Sec. VII.E); and D: Type II unit (Sec. VII.F). Each type of collateral has a characteristic branching pattern and the afferent fibers also present different types of terminal distributions along the long axis of the cord. (Modified from Ref. 356.)

Collaterals from hairy skin type I afferent fibers carry many *en passant* boutons along their terminal branches in the dorsal horn. There is not such a bias toward a longitudinal orientation as occurs in the lamina III arborizations of hair afferents. The predominance of *en passant* boutons in these cases probably accounts for the hairy skin units having a greater bouton density in laminae III and IV than the glabrous skin units, which frequently end as simple terminal boutons.

The distribution of type I afferent fiber boutons is difficult to correlate with functional aspects because so little is known about the central effects of these fibers. At segmental levels neurons in the appropriate part of the dorsal horn have been shown to receive monosynaptic input from type I receptors (185). The role of these neurons is unknown; they could play a part in evoking primary afferent depolarization in primary afferents (209) or in relaying information toward the dorsal column nuclei (109,110,115).

F. Slowly Adapting Type II Mechanoreceptors

The type II (225,226) sense organ is the Ruffini ending (243), which in hairy skin is located in the dermis. These receptors occur in several species, including the cat, the rabbit, and primates (176,177,229,244; see also 3). They are not found in cat glabrous skin, but they probably do exist in primate glabrous skin (178,25,236,245-247). Some are probably situated near the base of the claw in the cat (139,207).

The discharge of type II units during maintained deformation of the skin containing the receptor is regular; this type of discharge, albeit at fairly low levels, is also in evidence when the unit is first isolated for recording (3,244), and it is probably due to stretch of the skin at "rest." The response to skin stretch is directionally sensitive (3), and some (236,247) have proposed a proprioceptive role for these units. Unfortunately, as is the case for the type I units, and despite the easily identifiable response of the afferent unit, there is little information on their central projections. There is no evidence that they excite spinocervical tract cells (179), but they may (183) excite cells of the dorsal spinocerebellar tract at higher lumbar levels. The central axons ascend to the dorsal column nuclei (123-125) and excite neurons which project via the medial lemniscus to the contralateral ventrobasal complex of the thalamus (139,207).

1. Collateral Morphology

Brown et al. (248) recorded type II axons at the dorsal root entrance zone; all of the fibers which were successfully labeled innervated receptors at the claw bases and had peripheral conduction velocities of 41-67 m/sec and central conduction velocities in the dorsal columns (to C2) of lower values (28-51 m/sec), which was in agreement with previous electrophysiologic information (3). It is therefore not known yet whether type II receptors in hairy skin give rise to axons which have different central morphologic features than the units from claw bases.

Most of the fibers bifurcated soon after reaching the entrance zone; indeed, in some cases collaterals destined to enter the dorsal horn directly were issued before the parent fiber bifurcated. The axons ascended or descended, usually in superficial parts of the dorsal columns and, like the other cutaneous afferents, gave off collateral branches every 600 μm or so on average. Collaterals tended to be more closely spaced on the thinner diameter descending axon, and they entered the dorsal horn through the dorsal or dorsomedial border of the gray matter. The collaterals descend toward lamina III and begin to divide profusely to terminate in the medial one third of the dorsal horn. The arborizations ranged from fairly compact ramifications in laminae III and IV to more extensive arborizations which encompassed laminae II, III, IV, and V and even projected into the dorsal part of lamina VI. Most of the terminal axons ran in a dorsolateral to ventromedial orientation in the transverse plane and carried several *en passant* and terminal boutons, the latter often being offset from the terminal branch on a short thin stalk. Each arborization extended for only 100–300 μm in the rostrocaudal direction, and there was seldom any overlap between adjacent collaterals from a single axon. Again, like the type I fibers, the type II fibers project to discrete, separated regions of the cord, which are, however, in line with each other in the longitudinal axis of the cord (see Fig. 3D).

G. Afferent Fibers Innervating Muscle Spindle Primary Endings

Matthews (6) has thoroughly reviewed the properties and functions of muscle spindle and tendon organ afferent fibers (see also 249) and has discussed their probable role in kinesthesia (250,251; see also 332). The structure and innervation of the muscle receptors also received widespread attention, as discussed in detail by Barker (252). This section will deal with the axons innervating the muscle spindle primary endings; the afferents from tendon organs and spindle secondary endings will be considered later (Secs. VII.H and VII.I). The afferents from spindle primary endings will be referred to, in the accepted manner, as group Ia fibers. These fibers form the afferent limb of the intensively studied monosynaptic (or myotatic) reflex pathway to homonymous and synergistic motoneurons (253–255). Recent reviews (256–258) cover in great detail the enormous amount of electrophysiologic data on Ia connections with alpha motoneurons and other spinal interneurons. These intensive investigations, from the classic work of Lloyd (259,260) and of Eccles, Lundberg, and their colleagues (e.g., 261–263; see also 264) to the more recent analyses of single Ia impulse effects on motoneurons (265–270) and the elucidation of interneuronal pathways by Jankowska and her coworkers (271–277; cf. 278), have made the Ia fiber and its synaptic linkages one of the best known neuronal systems in these respects.

The anatomic literature on the central connections of Ia fibers is also abundant, but based mainly on indirect evidence at light and electron microscopic levels it relies on the traditional assumption that only Ia fibers from dorsal roots make monosynaptic connections with motoneurons (10-12,14,279-282). Iles (34) used cobalt labeling of dorsal root fibers in adult cats rather than Golgi or degeneration methods and made allowance in his interpretation of the data for the evidence (see Sec. VII.I) that spindle secondary afferents also make monosynaptic connections with neurons in the ventral horn. Nevertheless, it is still fair to say that the morphologic basis of the organization of Ia connections is poorly understood, even in the light of new ultrastructural data (357,359).

Two general questions require detailed attention at the segmental level. These concern: (1) firm identification of Ia fibers and a detailed description of their anatomic arrangement, and (2) the determination of the number and distribution of synapses from a single Ia afferent on a motoneuron. Intra-axonal staining of Ia fibers and intracellular staining of alpha motoneurons afford direct answers to these problems.

The afferent fiber morphology and structural-functional correlations of the Ia–motoneuron system have been intensively studied in the cat by Brown and Fyffe (283-285), Burke and his colleagues (286), Hongo's group (148,171), and Redman and coworkers (287,288). The criteria for identifying Ia fibers and motoneurons (see 6,148,283) were essentially the same in each study, relying upon peripheral conduction velocity measurement, threshold to electrical stimulation of the muscle nerve, and responses following muscle stretch or twitch contradiction. In the frog spinal cord similar investigations have been carried out by Shapovalov's group (289).

1. Axonal Trajectory and Issue of Collaterals

Thirty-four of 36 stained Ia axons [combined sample of Ishizuka et al. (148) and Fyffe (290)] bifurcated into an ascending and a descending branch on entering the cord; the other two axons only gave rise to ascending branches. The descending branches were always of thinner diameter than the ascending ones (148). The main branches ran medially from their entrance and bifurcation and assumed wavy courses in the dorsal columns, usually in a region close to the dorsomedial border of the dorsal horn and gradually, in both rostral and caudal directions, migrating to deeper regions.

On average, a collateral arises about every millimeter along the axon. The figures of Brown and Fyffe (283) and Ishizuka et al. (148) are very stimilar in this respect and have been independently verified by electrophysiologic methods (291). Munson and Sypert's work (291) provides further evidence that intra-axonal injection of HRP can reveal all the collaterals between the most rostral and most caudal ones stained (see e.g., 2,283). The intervals noted in Golgi studies (14), and utilized by subsequent investigators (34), are much smaller

(100-200 μm), presumably owing to differences in the length of the cord in the newborn and adult cat and possibly also because of the difficulties in reliably tracing single fibers over long distances in silver-impregnated material.

2. Collateral Morphology

Ia afferents from triceps surae, hamstring, plantaris, flexor digitorum longus, and flexor hallucis longus muscles of the cat hindlimb have been described in detail (148,283). The entry of collaterals to the gray matter may be at any point on the medial or dorsal edges of the dorsal horn; the collaterals often have a craniad tilt from their origin in the dorsal columns to their entry into the gray matter. The major collateral branches usually penetrate to laminae V or VI before subdividing. Each collateral distributes terminals to three main zones (see Fig. 4) at or near the segment of entry of the parent fiber: (1) to the medial half of lamina VI, (2) to the dorsolateral parts of lamina VII, and (3) to the motor cell columns (292) in lamina IX. Two groups of Ia afferents have different or additional central projections at the segmental level—hamstring Ia fibers project mainly to the medial and ventral parts of lamina VII and flexor digitorum longus and flexor hallucis longus fibers often have prominent terminal arborizations in laminae III and IV of the dorsal horn as well as in the aforementioned zones (148).

The level and extent of the motoneuron pool (see 292) may influence the morphology of the collaterals. Ishizuka et al. (148) note that soleus Ia afferent collaterals given off caudal to the soleus motor pool terminated only in lamina VI. This feature was not noted by Brown and Fyffe (283) and merits further anatomic and physiologic study.

Different collateral trajectories and terminal zones have been commented on in recent Golgi (14,17) and degeneration (10,12,293) studies and individual collaterals classified (14) on the basis of whether they project to one or more than one motor nucleus. It seems likely that these observations can be largely explained on the basis that collaterals from Ia fibers arising from different muscles project to different interneuronal groups and to different motor cell columns (148,283). There is no evidence (cf. 14) that single collaterals project directly to antagonistic motoneuron pools (see also 17), although there is ample opportunity, given the massive spread of motoneuron dendrites (see e.g., 285, 294,295) for dendritic contacts to be made. The electrophysiologic evidence would argue against even that possibility, and one can conclude that the Ia projections to the motor nuclei are exclusively to homonymous or synergistic motoneuron pools.

3. Projections to Lamina VI

Every Ia afferent fiber collateral gives side branches to the medial part of lamina VI, as would be expected from previous anatomic (17) and electrophysiologic (296) data. The terminal branches in this region carry a variable number (up to

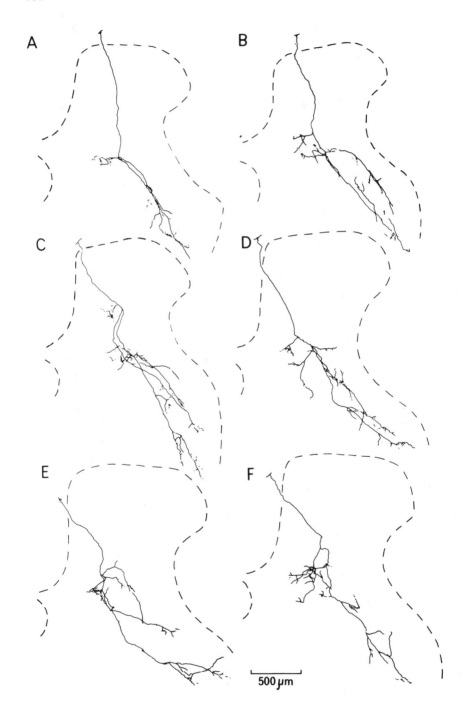

9 or 10) of *en passant* boutons and a terminal bouton (148,283). Some of the boutons are located in the ventral part of lamina V or in the dorsomedial part of lamina VII, but they are mainly concentrated in lamina VI. In this region axosomatic and axodendritic (on proximal dendrites) contacts made by the Ia terminals were frequently observed (148,283).

The lamina VI terminations of Ia collaterals correlates well with the location of the dorsal focal synaptic potential (following stimulation of muscle nerves) recorded by Eccles et al. (296). The functions of the neurons in this area excited by Ia afferents are probably diverse. Some project to supraspinal levels (297) and may complement the dorsal spinocerebellar projection (17,166,298–300) which arises from at least two segments rostral to the segment of entry of the hindlimb muscle Ia fibers studied so far. Another possible ascending pathway receiving activation from the lamina VI Ia arborizations is the ventral spinocerebellar tract; some cells of origin of this tract lie dorsomedially to the ventral horn (301, 302) and could be activated by the Ia terminals in the intermediate region, but it is more likely that Ia input to the ventral spinocerebellar tract is to the spinal border cells (303) in lamina IX (304). In the cat, a subgroup of the postsynaptic dorsal column pathway (115) may also receive direct Ia activation (220). The segmental effects and pathways are complex. Some Ia-activated lamina VI neurons (271) send their axons to the ventral horn and presumably subserve polysynaptic actions upon motoneurons. Other neurons may be concerned with presynaptic inhibitory pathways (see 257).

4. Projections to Lamina VII

After the major collateral branch issues its side branches to lamina VI, it changes direction and runs ventrolaterally, perhaps spitting into two or three thinner branches, toward the motor nuclei. Before reaching the motor pools, the collateral issues up to 10 or so fine branches in the dorsolateral parts of lamina VII. These generate sparse terminations which make juxtasomatic contacts on medium-sized neurons in this region (148,283). Cells located here are probably the interneurons interpolated on the pathway mediating reciprocal [or "direct," see Lloyd (253,259,260)] Ia inhibitory action on antagonistic motoneurons.

Figure 4 Six adjacent collaterals from an Ia afferent fiber are reconstructed sequentially from transverse sections of spinal cord (segment L7). All the collaterals arise from the ascending branch of the Ia fiber in the dorsal columns. A is the most caudal and F is the most rostral collateral shown. The distance between collaterals A and F was 3.2 mm (average intercollateral spacing 640 μm), and the axon is seen to move medially and ventrally on its ascending course. All the collaterals issue synaptic terminals to laminae VI, VII, and IX. (From Ref. 290.)

The characteristics of these neurons were defined by Jankowska and her colleagues (272-276) in an elegant series of experiments that culminated in the intracellular marking of identified Ia inhibitory interneurons (277).

5. Ia Contacts upon Motoneurons

Ia terminals in the motor nuclei (lamina IX) probably make some contacts on cells of origin of the ventral spinocerebellar tract (304) in L6 segments or higher. Their primary targets at the segmental level, however, are the alpha motoneurons innervating the same muscle as the afferent fiber or synergistic motoneurons. The connectivity of Ia fibers upon populations of identified motoneurons has been determined (255,305,306), and it can be concluded that single Ia fibers project to almost all (~90%) of the motoneurons in the homonymous pool and to a smaller proportion (50-60%) of motoneurons in heteronymous or synergistic pools.

However, only 10-20% of the 100-200 boutons which each Ia afferent fiber collateral delivers to the lamina IX region are observed in close proximity (i.e., making presumed axosomatic or axodendritic contacts; see 34) to the cell bodies of motoneurons visualized in counterstained sections (148,283,285). The motoneurons involved in these presumed contacts receive, on average, two to three and a half boutons from a single Ia afferent fiber collateral (148,290). A single collateral could contact from one to 13 motoneuron somata or proximal dendrites (148,290), but would be expected from the known connectivity of the afferents and the frequency of occurrence of collaterals at the level of the target motoneuron pools to contact many more [~50-60 (see 283)]. Clearly, most of the contacts on motoneurons must be on dendritic profiles not seen in the counterstained material.

To visualize these more distally located Ia synapses on motoneurons, Brown and Fyffe (284,285), Burke and his colleagues (286,307,308), and Redman and Walmsley (287,288) have combined intra-axonal labeling of single, identified Ia afferent fibers and intracellular staining (with HRP) of motoneurons thought to be monosynaptically linked to the fiber. In some studies (286,307,308) the target alpha motoneuron was identified as a particular physiologic type (309).

These studies demonstrate the intricate, often complex, microcircuitry of the group Ia-motoneuron system–the "model" for central excitatory synaptic mechanisms. They confirm that Ia afferent fibers make multiple synaptic contacts on the motoneuron surface, sometimes at great distances (>800 μm) from the motoneuron soma. These geometric distances translate into electrotonic distances (see 310,311) of up to 2 (or 4) length constants (λ), depending upon whether high (or low) values for specific membrane resistivities are used (312). Still, these synapses are largely in the proximal geometric half of the dendritic tree (285), and the effectiveness of such distant synapses remains in debate.

In multiple contact systems between a single Ia fiber and a motoneuron the number of boutons ranges from two to six, with a mean around three and a half (285,286), although in more recent studies (312) single Ia fibers were seen to make from three to 17 contacts (average around seven) on individual motoneurons. In the earlier studies (285,286) all the boutons in a multiple contact system arose from terminal axons from one collateral, but in the latter study (312), more than one major collateral contributed the boutons involved. Clearly, the sample sizes are still relatively small and solid numerical analyses must await further experimentation.

The complexity of the bouton distributions in multiple contact systems varied, as would have been expected from the wide range of EPSP (excitatory postsynaptic potential) shapes recorded in motoneurons following activation of single Ia afferents (257,258). Some excitatory postsynaptic potential shapes (255,270,305) are indicative of a restricted synaptic locus, and in the anatomic studies (285,286; see Fig. 5) boutons in some cases ended in a restricted electrotonic region. Furthermore, even when boutons are distributed to different dendritic branches (arising from the same or different primary dendrites) they are often located at similar distances from the cell body. However, in several cases (see 312) the boutons were arranged, not in restricted loci, but in complex patterns with some synapses on proximal and some on distal dendrites. Such distributions are consistent with the widespread distribution of Ia synapses indicated by electrophysiologic studies (255,265,266,270,305,312-314), but they may indeed occur more frequently than these electrophysiologic analyses implied. The correlation between synaptic location and excitatory postsynaptic potential size and shape and the effects of complex preterminal branching patterns needs further analysis of the kind outlined in this section.

H. Tendon Organ Afferent Fibers

Impulses in afferent fibers from Golgi tendon organs produce di- to trisynaptic excitatory or inhibitory effects in alpha motoneurons (6,296,306,315-318), and may excite, monosynaptically, some cells of origin of the dorsal and ventral spinocerebellar tracts (298,319). The structure and physiologic responses of the tendon organ have been detailed elsewhere (6,249,252), and it is now known (320-322) that the tendon organs may be activated by contraction of only a single motor unit in the muscle. The afferent fibers, referred to as group Ib fibers, conduct in the group I range of conduction velocities; in the cat hindlimb muscle nerves these ranges from 72 to 120 m/sec (6,323,324). Rather less is known about the central actions of Ib fibers than for Ia fibers, and the only anatomic information on their central projections was given by Réthelyi and Szentágothai (17), who proposed that the extensive field of arborization of collaterals in the intermediary region (laminae VI and dorsal lamina VII) originated from Ib primary afferents.

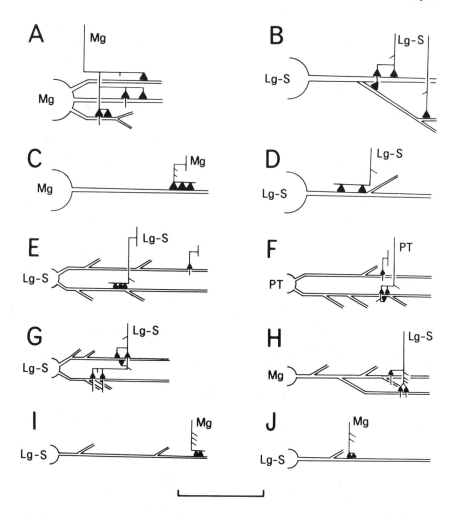

Figure 5 A "wiring diagram" constructed to show the numbers and relative distribution of synapses made by single Ia fibers upon single motoneurons. The muscles innervated by the afferents and motoneurons are indicated: Mg, medial gastrocnemius; Lg/S, lateral gastrocnemius–soleus; PT, the afferent or motor axon ran in the posterior tibial nerve. The scale bar represents 50 μm for A–D and 500 μm for E–J and indicates the distances from the motoneuron soma to the synaptic locations (filled triangles) or to dendritic branch points. The full extent of the dendrites and the preterminal branching of the afferents is not shown. (From Ref. 285.)

1. Ib Collateral Morphology

Intra-axonal staining with HRP (171,325-327) by different groups has detailed information consistent with the available electrophysiologic evidence. These studies confirm Réthelyi and Szentágothai's (17) tentative identification of Ib collateral morphology.

The Ib axons follow courses similar to the Ia fibers after entering the cord and bifurcating into ascending and descending branches in the dorsal columns. The fibers have not yet been traced to their caudal terminations nor to their terminations in Clarke's column (see 298); the current information is from fibers in segments L5-L7, that is, close to their segment of entry. At these levels there is a distinctive and specific anatomic pattern for every collateral. Collaterals arise every 900 μm or so (a spacing close to that of the Ia fibers) and pass directly ventrally through the dorsal horn to lamina V. At this point they break up to form an extensive fan-shaped arborization with terminals in the medial two thirds of lamina VI; occasionally, some terminals lie in laminae V and VII (171,326). Each arborization occupies a discrete zone (up to a maximum of 400 μm in rostrocaudal extent) and there is no overlap between adjacent collaterals from a single axon (Figs. 6 and 7C,D).

Hongo et al. (171) suggested that two types of Ib collaterals exist, perhaps arising from separate populations of Ib fibers. Other evidence (326) suggests that this is unlikely and that the differences are due to the rostrocaudal location of the fiber. In fact, collaterals from a single axon can show differential projections (326), with one projecting only to the intermediate region in the manner described earlier and the next most rostral one projecting additionally to the dorsolateral parts of lamina VII and perhaps even to lamina IX. The lateral projections of more rostral collaterals (e.g. in L6 segment) may be to spinal border cells (303), which can be found as far caudally as L6 (304,328), and some of which receive monosynaptic Ib input for relay in the ventral spinocerebellar tract.

The consistently observed arborization in the medial two-thirds of the intermediate region is presumably associated with the secure activation of interneurons and tract cells in this area (329-331). Such a diversity of actions emphasizes that the Ib afferents should not be solely considered in terms of segmental or reflex effects (316,322).

An interesting phenomenon was reported by Hongo et al. (327), who described interneuronal (or transneuronal) transport of HRP from injected Ib afferent fibers to secondary neurons in laminae V and VI of the spinal cord. This feature has not been observed in other extensive HRP injection studies of primary afferents (2); not only the functional significance, but the mechanisms of this transneuronal staining await further analysis.

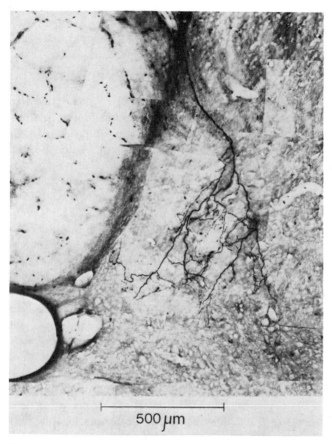

Figure 6 A photomontage from serial transverse sections of the spinal cord, showing the course and branching pattern of a collateral from an Ib afferent fiber. The central canal and the medial edge of the dorsal horn (dorsal columns to the left) can be seen. The terminal branches and boutons of the collateral are in the medial half of lamina VI.

Figure 7 Reconstructions of muscle afferent fiber collaterals (A, C, E) and schematic three-dimensional representations (B, D, F) of the overall projection patterns of these afferents (see Secs. VII.G–VII.I). Ia afferents: A, B; Ib afferents: C, D; Group II afferents: E, F. (Modified from Refs. 2 and 290.)

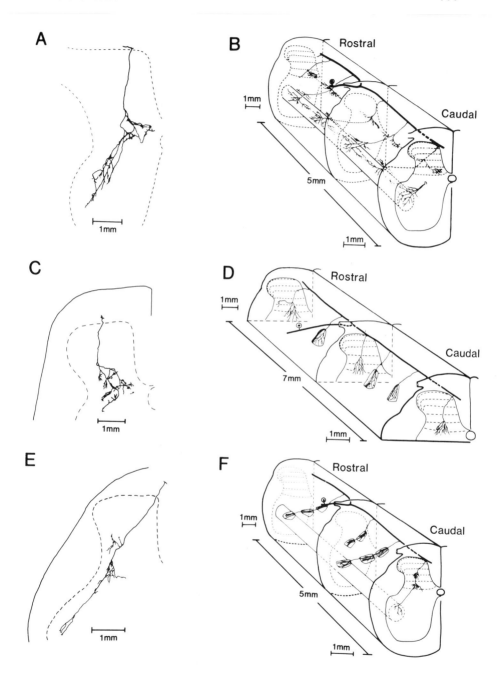

I. Afferent Fibers Innervating Muscle Spindle Secondary Endings

The third type of muscle receptor whose structure and function has been intensively investigated is the secondary ending of the muscle spindle (6). The
receptor is innervated by a group II axon (253) with a peripheral conduction
velocity of 36-72 m/sec (6,324). Characteristic response properties (6,333) as
well as the lower conduction velocity of the afferent fiber make these units
relatively easy to distinguish physiologically from the other muscle receptors.

The postulated role of the group II afferents from muscle has been the
subject of controversial argument. Matthews argued (334-336) that these
afferents contributed to the tonic stretch reflex, and gained support from a
variety of sources (337-341), which indicated that polysynaptic excitatory, or
disinhibition, mechanisms were responsible for the observed effects. Contra-
dictory arguments (342) were thoroughly considered during these investigations.
Then, Kirkwood and Sears (343,344) unexpectedly demonstrated a direct monosynaptic connection of group II axons with motoneurons. This important
finding was confirmed by others (345-451) and it substantiates Matthews' functional ideas. The new information also emphasized that Ia fibers were not the
only afferent fibers projecting to the motoneurons and that significant errors
would arise if anatomic data were interpreted on that assumption.

1. Collateral Morphology

The direct anatomic evidence published so far is very limited (2,352), but it
shows conclusively that muscle group II afferents, like Ia fibers, project directly
to lamina IX, where they have the opportunity to make monosynaptic connections with motoneurons. Like Ia fibers, the group II axons from spindle secondary endings make side projections to more dorsal regions of the spinal gray
matter, although there is little overlap between the areas of termination of these
groups of side branches. Group II afferent fiber collaterals arborize in laminae
III and IV of the dorsal horn and in the lateral parts of laminae V, VI, and VII
as well as in lamina IX (Figs. 7E,F).

The input to lamina IX from these fibers is less extensive that for Ia
afferents, and generally only a few terminal, bouton-carrying branches are seen
(352). This sparse projection is reflected in the lower monosynaptic connectivity
(~50%) with homonymous motoneuron populations (346,348) than is the case
for Ia afferents (255).

The more dorsal levels of termination correlate well with areas in which
focal synaptic potentials and cells reponsive to group II afferent activation are
recorded (353,354). The function of these cells is unknown as yet. Clearly,
however, in view of the now established excitatory link with extensor motoneurons it is unwise (see also 334,346,348) to think of these fibers as having
involvement primarily in flexor reflex afferent systems as was traditionally
thought (317,355).

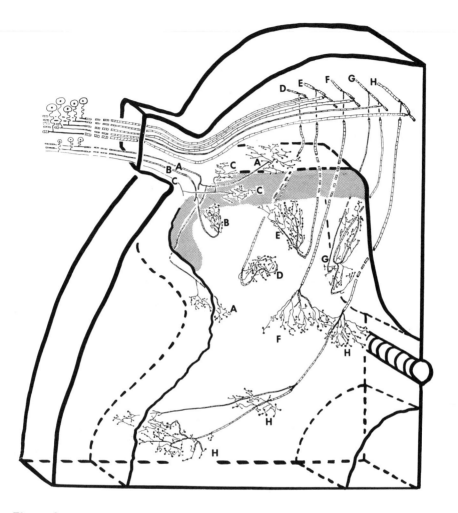

Figure 8 A schematic summary diagram of the spinal terminations of some afferent fibers. The drawing represents a fairly thin (say 500-μm thick) transverse slab of part of one half of the spinal cord. Shading is used to emphasize the superficial dorsal horn. Eight afferent fibers (two Aδ fibers, A and B; one C-fiber, C; five large myelinated fibers, D–H) enter the cord through the dorsal root, birfucate into rostrally and caudally directed branches, and from Lissauer's tract (A–C) or the dorsal columns (D–H) issue collateral branches which arborize in specific fashion in defined regions of the spinal gray matter. Two fibers (A and C) terminate in lamina I and/or lamina II; one of these (A) also sends a major branch to the lateral part of lamina V. Four fibers, including one fine-diameter afferent (B) and three large-diameter fibers (D, E, G) terminate in laminae III–V; functionally, these represent low-threshold mechanoreceptive cutaneous afferents. Large-diameter muscle fibers (F, H) have overlapping terminations in the intermediate region, while Ia afferents (e.g., H) also terminate in the interneuronal and motoneuronal pools of laminae VII and IX.

VIII. CONCLUSIONS

The recent data on identified afferent fiber terminations that form the focus of this review allows us to establish some principles on the organization of afferent input to the spinal cord. The diagram of Figure 8 attempts to illustrate some of the features from which these principles are derived. Eight afferent fibers from different afferent units—three fine-diameter fibers (axons A and B are Aδ fibers, axon C is a C-fiber) enter through the lateral division of the dorsal root (an oversimplification, see Sec. II.B) to Lissauer's tract and five larger myelinated fibers (D–H) enter the dorsal columns, divide, and issue collateral branches to the gray matter. The collaterals of all of these afferent fibers show distinctive terminal arrangements.

The first conclusion (see also 2,151,163,356) is that each afferent fiber terminates in a specific and characteristic manner. The specificity is dependent upon the afferent unit type and extends from the gross branching pattern of the collaterals to the location and distribution of terminals and even to the synaptic arrangements which are formed.

Secondly, it appears on first glance that there is a degree of parcelation of the afferent input, again based on functional properties, to particular layers or levels of the spinal gray matter (see also Ref. 214). Thus, thermal and nociceptive information, carried by fine fibers (Fig. 8A,C) is delivered to lamina I and the outer part of lamina II. Some nociceptive input (A) is however directed to more ventral parts and a more widespread distribution (e.g., to the ventral part of lamina II or even deeper) may emerge when C-fiber projections are definitively visualized. Mechanoreceptive fibers of a wide range of axonal diameters project, somatotopically, to laminae III and IV (Fig. 8B,D,E,F). Deeper still, muscle and tendon organ afferents have overlapping terminations in the intermediate region (Fig. 8G,H), and then in lamina IX the afferents from receptors in muscle spindles (group Ia and Group II fibers) synapse monosynaptically on alpha motoneurons. Ia fibers (e.g., Fig. 7H) also end on inhibitory interneurons in lamina VII.

In dorsal laminae (I, II, and III) the predominant orientation of the neuropil, including the terminal branches of afferent fibers, is along the longitudinal axis of the cord. In deeper laminae, excluding the motor nuclei, dendritic and axonal orientation switch to a somewhat more radial or transverse arrangement. In the motor nuclei both radial and longitudinal dendrites are dominant; the afferent terminations in this region match both these orientations. Most afferent fiber connections are made on the dendrites of the target neurons; hence, soma location is less important than dendritic location and orientation in determining functional connectivities. Finally, given the firm and specific anatomic foundation ensuing from the study of identified neurons (see also 2), dynamic aspects of afferent fiber projections—possible reorganization or modification under certain conditions, the distribution and efficacy of synapses and synaptic mechanisms—can be addressed more directly than in the past.

REFERENCES

1. Andres, K. H., and Von Düring, M. (1973). Morphology of cutaneous receptors. In *Handbook of Sensory Physiology*, vol. II, A. Iggo (Ed.), Springer, New York, pp. 3–28.
2. Brown, A. G. (1981). *Organization of the Spinal Cord*, Springer-Verlag, New York.
3. Burgess, P. R., and Perl, E. R. (1973). Cutaneous mechanoreceptors and nociceptors. In *Handbook of Sensory Physiology*, vol. II, A. Iggo (Ed.), Springer, New York, pp. 29–78.
4. Iggo, A., and Andres, K. H. (1982). Morphology of cutaneous receptors. *Ann. Rev. Neurosci. 5*:1–32.
5. Light, A. R., and Perl, E. R. (1983). Peripheral sensory systems. In *Peripheral Neuropathy*, P. J. Dyck (Ed.), Saunders, Philadelphia.
6. Matthews, P. B. C. (1972). *Mammalian Muscle Receptors and Their Central Actions*, Arnolds, London.
7. Willis, W. D., Coggeshall, R. E. (1978). *Sensory Mechanisms of the Spinal Cord*. Plenum, New York.
8. Müller, J. (1940). *Handbook der Physiologie des Mensachen*, vol. II, J. Hölcher, Coblenz, pp. 249–503.
9. Schimert, J. (1939). Das verhalten der hinter-wurzelkollateralen im Ruckenmark. *Z. Anat. Entwicklungsgesch. 109*:665–687.
10. Sprague, J. M., and Ha, H. (1964). The terminal fields of dorsal root fibers in the lumbosacral spinal cord of the cat, and the dendritic organization of the motor nuclei. In *Progress in Brain Research*, vol. II, *Organization of the Spinal Cord*, Elsevier, Amsterdam, J. C. Eccles (Ed.), pp. 120–152.
11. Szentágothai, J. (1964). Neuronal synaptic arrangement in the substantia gelatinosa Rolandi. *J. Comp. Neurol. 122*:219–240.
12. Sterling, P., and Kuypers, H. G. J. M. (1967). Anatomical organization of the brachial spinal cord of the cat. I. The distribution of dorsal root fibers. *Brain Res. 4*:1–15.
13. Ralston, H. J. (1968). Dorsal root projections to dorsal horn neurons in the cat spinal cord. *J. Comp. Neurol. 132*:303–330.
14. Scheibel, M. E., and Scheibel, A. B. (1969). Terminal patterns in cat spinal cord. III. Primary afferent collaterals. *Brain Res. 13*:417–443.
15. Heimer, L., and Wall, P. D. (1968). The dorsal root distribution to the substantia gelatinosa of the rat with a note on the distribution in the cat. *Exp. Brain Res. 6*:89–99.
16. Imai, Y., and Kusama, T. (1969). Distribution of the dorsal root fibers in the cat. An experimental study with the Nauta method. *Brain Res. 13*: 338–359.
17. Réthelyi, M., and Szentágothai, J. (1973). Distribution and connections of afferent fibers in the spinal cord. In *Handbook of Sensory Physiology*, vol. II, *Somatosensory System*, A. Iggo (Ed.), Springer, New York, pp. 207–252.
18. Réthelyi, M. (1977). Preterminal and terminal axon arborizations in the substantia gelatinosa of cat's spinal cord. *J. Comp. Neurol. 172*:511–528.

19. Beal, J. A., and Fox, C. A. (1976). Afferent fibers in the substantia gelatinosa of the adult monkey (Macaca mulatta): A Golgi study. *J. Comp. Neurol. 168*:113-144.

20. Hamano, K., Mannen, H., and Ishizuka, N. (1978). Reconstruction of trajectory of primary afferent collaterals in the dorsal horn of the cat spinal cord, using Golgi-stained serial sections. *J. Comp. Neurol. 181*: 1-16.

21. Ralston, H. J., and Ralston, D. D. (1979). The distribution of dorsal root axons in laminae I, II and III of the macaque spinal cord: A quantitative electron microscope study. *J. Comp. Neurol. 184*:643-644.

22. Proshansky, E., and Egger, M. D. (1977). Staining of the dorsal root projection to the cat's dorsal horn by anterograde movement of horseradish peroxidase. *Neurosci. Lett. 5*:103-110.

23. Beattie, M. S., Bresnahan, J. C., and King, J. S. (1978). Ultrastructural identification of dorsal root primary afferent terminals after anterograde filling with horseradish peroxidase. *Brain Res. 153*:127-134.

24. Light, A. R., and Perl, E. R. (1977). Differential termination of large-diameter and small-diameter primary afferent fibers in the spinal dorsal gray matter as indicated by labeling with horseradish peroxidase. *Neurosci. Lett. 6*:59-63.

25. Light, A. R., and Perl, E. R. (1979). Reexamination of the dorsal root projection to the spinal dorsal horn including observations on the differential termination of coarse and fine fibers. *J. Comp. Neurol. 186*:117-132.

26. Gobel, S., Falls, W. M., and Humphrey, E. (1981). Morphology and synaptic connections of ultrafine primary axons in lamina I of the spinal dorsal horn: Candidates for the terminal axonal arbors of primary neurons with unmyelinated (C) axons. *J. Neurosci. 1*:1163-1179.

27. Mesulam, M.-M., and Brushart, T. M. (1979). Transganglionic and anterograde transport of horseradish peroxidase across dorsal root ganglia: A tetramethylbenzidine method for tracing central sensory connections of muscles and peripheral nerves. *Neurosci. 4*:1107-1117.

28. Grant, G., Arvidsson, J., Robertson, B., and Ygge, J. (1979). Transganglionic transport of horseradish peroxidase in primary sensory neurons. *Neurosci. Lett. 21*:23-28.

29. Grant, G., Ygge, J., and Molander, C. (1981). Projection patterns of peripheral sensory nerves in the dorsal horn. In *Spinal Cord Sensation*, A. G. Brown and M. Réthelyi (Eds.), Scottish Academic Press, Edinburgh, pp. 33-43.

30. Brown, P. B., and Culberson, J. L. (1981). Dorsal horn projections of cutaneous component of hindlimb dorsal roots. *J. Neurophysiol. 45*: 137-143.

31. Koerber, H. R., and Brown, P. B. (1980). Projections of two hindlimb cutaneous nerves to cat dorsal horn. *J. Neurophysiol. 44*:259-269.

32. Koerber, H. R., and Brown, P. B. (1982). Somatotopic organization of hindlimb cutaneous nerve projections to cat dorsal horn. *J. Neurophysiol. 48*:481-489.

33. Berger, A. J. (1979). Distribution of carotid sinus nerve afferent fibers to solitary tract nuclei of the cat using transganglionic transport of horseradish peroxidase. *Neurosci. Lett. 14*:153–158.

34. Iles, J. F. (1976). Central terminations of muscle afferents on motoneurons in the cat spinal cord. *J. Physiol. (Lond.) 262*:91–117.

35. Cowan, M. M., Gottlieb, P. I., Hendrickson, A. E., Price, J. G., and Woolsey, T. A. (1972). The autoradiographic demonstration of axonal connections in the central nervous system. *Brain Res. 37*:21–51.

36. LaMotte, C. (1977). Distribution of the tract of Lissauer and the dorsal root fibers in the primate spinal cord. *J. Comp. Neurol. 172*:529–562.

37. Réthelyi, M., Trevino, D. L., and Perl, E. R. (1979). Distribution of primary afferent fibers within the sacrococcygeal dorsal horn on audioradiographic study. *J. Comp. Neurol. 185*:603–622.

38. Grant, G., and Arvidsson, J. (1975). Transganglionic degeneration in trigeminal primary sensory neurons. *Brain Res. 95*:265–279.

39. Arvidsson, J., and Grant, G. (1979). Further observations on transganglionic degeneration in trigeminal primary sensory neurons. *Brain Res. 162*:1–12.

40. Snow, P. J., Rose, P. K., and Brown, A. G. (1976). Tracing axons and axon collaterals of spinal neurons using intercellular injection of horseradish peroxidase. *Science 191*:312–313.

41. Jankowska, E., Rastad, J., and Westman, J. (1976). Intracellular application of horseradish peroxidase and its light and electron microscopical appearance in spinocervical tract cells. *Brain Res. 105*:557–562.

42. Brown, A. G., Rose, P. K., and Snow, P. J. (1977). The morphology of spinocervical tract neurones revealed by intracellular injection of horseradish peroxidase. *J. Physiol. (Lond.) 270*:747–764.

43. Light, A. R., and Perl, E. R. (1979). Spinal termination of functionally identified primary afferent neurons with slowly conducting myelinated fibers. *J. Comp. Neurol. 186*:133–150.

44. Brown, A. G., Rose, P. K., and Snow, P. J. (1977). The morphology of hair follicle afferent fiber collaterals in the spinal cord of the cat. *J. Physiol. (Lond.) 272*:779–797.

45. Darian-Smith, I. (1973). The trigeminal system. In *Handbook of Sensory Physiology*, vol. II, A. Iggo (Ed.), Springer, New York, pp. 271–314.

46. Kerr, F. W. L. (1970). The organization of primary afferents in the subnucleus candalis of the trigeminal: A light and electron microscopic study of degeneration. *Brain Res. 23*:147–165.

47. Westrum, L. E., Canfield, R. C., and Black, R. G. (1976). Transganglionic degeneration in the spinal trigeminal nucleus following removal of tooth pulps in adult cats. *Brain Res. 101*:137–140.

48. Beckstead, R. M., and Norgren, R. (1979). An autoradiographic examination of the central distribution of the trigeminal, facial, glossopharyngeal, and vagal nerves in the monkey. *J. Comp. Neurol. 184*:455–472.

49. Marfurt, C. F. (1981). The central projections of trigeminal primary afferent neurons in the cat as determined by transganglionic transport of horseradish peroxidase. *J. Comp. Neurol. 203*:785–798.

50. Hayashi, H. (1980). Distribution of vibrissae afferent fiber collaterals in the trigeminal nuclei as revealed by intra-axonal injection of horseradish peroxidase. *Brain Res. 183*:442–446.

51. Hayashi, H. (1982). Differential terminal distribution of single large cutaneous afferent fibers in the spinal trigeminal nucleus and in the cervical spinal dorsal horn. *Brain Res. 244*:173–177.

52. DeGroat, W. C., Nadelhaft, I., Morgan, C., and Schauble, T. (1978). Horseradish peroxidase tracing of viceral efferent and primary afferent pathways in the cat's sacral spinal cord using benzidine processing. *Neurosci. Lett. 10*:103–108.

53. Morgan, C., Nadelhaft, I., and DeGroat, W. C. (1981). The distribution of visceral primary afferents from the pelvic nerve to Lissauer's tract and the spinal gray matter and its relationship to the sacral parasympathetic nucleus. *J. Comp. Neurol. 201*:415–440.

54. Rexed, B. (1952). The cytoarchitectonic organization of the spinal cord in the cat. *J. Comp. Neurol. 86*:415–495.

55. Rexed, B. (1954). A cytoarchitectonic atlas of the spinal cord in the cat. *J. Comp. Neurol. 100*:297–379.

56. Cranfield, P. F. (1974). *The Way In and the Way Out.* Futura, Mount Kisco, New York.

57. Ramon y Cajal, S. (1909). *Histologie du Système Nerveux de l'Homme et des Vertébrés*, vol. I, Maloine, Paris.

58. Pubols, B. H., Welker, W. I., and Johnson, J. I. (1965). Somatic sensory representation of forelimb in dorsal root fibers of raccoon, coatimundi and cat. *J. Neurophysiol. 28*:312–341.

59. Lissauer, H. (1885). Beitrag zur pathologischen Anatomie der Tabes dorsalis und zum Faserverlauf in menschlichen Ruckenmark. *Neurol. Centralbl. Bd. 4*:245–246.

60. Lissauer, H. (1886). Beitrag zum Faserverlauf im Hinterhorn des menschlichen Ruckenmarks und zum Verhalten desselben bei Tabes dorsalis. *Arch. Psychiat. Nervenkrankh. 17*:377–438.

61. Ranson, S. W. (1913). The course within the spinal cord of the non-medullated fibers of the dorsal roots. A study of Lissauer's tract in the cat. *J. Comp. Neurol. 23*:259–281.

62. Ranson, S. W. (1914). The tract of Lissauer and the substantia gelatinosa Rolandi. *Am. J. Anat. 16*:97–126.

63. Ranson, S. W. (1914). An experimental study of Lissauer's tract and the dorsal roots. *J. Comp. Neurol. 24*:531–545.

64. Ranson, S. W., and Billingsley, P. R. (1916). The conduction of painful impulses in the spinal nerves. *Am. J. Physiol. 40*:571–589.

65. Ranson, S. W., and von Hess, C. L. (1915). The conduction within the spinal cord of afferent impulses producing pain and the vasomotor reflexes. *Am. J. Physiol. 38*:128–152.

66. Snyder, R. (1977). The organization of the dorsal root entry zone in cats and monkeys. *J. Comp. Neurol. 174*:47–70.

67. Wall, P. D. (1962). The origin of a spinal-cord slow potential. *J. Physiol. (Lond.) 164*:508–526.
68. Earle, K. M. (1952). Tract of Lissauer and its possible relation to the pain pathway. *J. Comp. Neurol. 96*:93–111.
69. Sherrington, C. S. (1894). On the anatomical constitution of nerves of skeletal muscles; with remarks on recurrent fibers in the ventral spinal nerve-root. *J. Physiol. (Lond.) 17*:211–258.
70. Dimsdale, J. A., and Kemp, J. M. (1966). Afferent fibers in ventral roots in the rat. *J. Physiol. (Lond.) 187*:25–26P.
71. Kato, M., and Mirata, Y. (1968). Sensory neurons in the spinal ventral roots of the cat. *Brain Res. 7*:479–482.
72. Kato, M., and Tanji, J. (1971). Physiological properties of sensory fibers in the spinal ventral roots in the cat. *Jpn. J. Physiol. 21*:71–77.
73. Ryall, R. W., and Percey, M. F. (1970). Visceral afferent and efferent fibers in sacral ventral roots in cats. *Brain Res. 23*:57–65.
74. Floyd, K., and Morrison, J. F. B. (1974). Splanchnic mechanoreceptors in the dog. *Q. J. Exp. Physiol. 9*:359–364.
75. Loeb, G. E. (1976). Ventral root projections of myelinated dorsal root ganglion cells in the cat. *Brain Res. 106*:159–165.
76. Longhurst, J. C., Mitchell, J. H., and Moore, M. B. (1980). The spinal cord ventral root: An afferent pathway of the hind-limb pressor reflex in cats. *J. Physiol. (Lond.) 301*:467–476.
77. Windle, W. F. (1931). Neurons of the sensory type in the ventral roots of man and of other mammals. *Arch. Neurol. Psychiat. 26*:791–800.
78. Applebaum, M. L., Clifton, G. L., Coggeshall, R. E., Counter, J. D., Vance, W. H., and Willis, W. D. (1976). Unmyelinated fibers in the sacral 3 and caudal 1 ventral roots of the cat. *J. Physiol. (Lond.) 256*:557–572.
79. Coggeshall, R. E., Coulter, J. D., and Willis, W. D. (1974). Unmyelinated axons in the ventral roots of the cat lumbosacral enlargement. *J. Comp. Neurol. 153*:39–58.
80. Emery, D. G., Ito, H, and Coggeshall, R. E. (1972). Unmyelinated axons in thoracic ventral roots of the cat. *J. Comp. Neurol. 172*:37–48.
81. Clifton, G. L., Vance, W. H., Applebaum, D. L., Coggeshall, R. E., and Willis, W. D. (1974). Responses of unmyelinated afferents in the mammalian ventral root. *Brain Res. 82*:163–167.
82. Clifton, G. L., Coggeshall, R. E., Vance, W. H., and Willis, W. D. (1976). Receptive fields of unmyelinated ventral root afferent fibers in the cat. *J. Physiol. (Lond.) 256*:573–600.
83. Coggeshall, R. E., and Ito, H. (1977). Sensory fibers in ventral roots L7 and S1 in the rat. *J. Physiol. (Lond.) 267*:215–235.
84. Coggeshall, R. E., Maynard, C. W., and Lanford, L. A. (1980). Unmyelinated sensory and preganglionic fibers in rat L6 and S1 ventral spinal roots. *J. Comp. Neurol. 193*:41–47.
85. Maynard, C. W., Leonard, R. B., Coulter, J. D., and Coggeshall, R. E. (1977). Central connections of ventral root afferents as demonstrated by

the HRP method. *J. Comp. Neurol. 172*:601–608.

86. Risling, M., Hildesbrand, C., and Aldskogius, H. (1981). Postnatal increase of unmyelinated axon profiles in the feline ventral root L7. *J. Comp. Neurol. 201*:343–351.

87. Coggeshall, R. E. (1980). Law of separation of function of the spinal roots. *Physiol. Rev. 60*:716–755.

88. Light, A. R., and Metz, C. B. (1978). The morphology of the spinal cord efferent and afferent neurons contributing to the ventral roots of the cat. *J. Comp. Neurol. 179*:501–516.

89. Yamamoto, T., Takahashi, K., Satomi, H., and Ise, H. (1977). Origins of primary afferent fibers in the spinal ventral roots in the cat as demonstrated by the horseradish peroxidase method. *Brain Res. 126*:350–354.

90. Corbin, K. B., and Hinsey, J. C. (1935). Intramedullary course of the dorsal root fibers of each of the first four cervical nerves. *J. Comp. Neurol. 63*:119–126.

91. Anderson, F. D. (1960). Distribution of dorsal root fibers in cat spinal cord. *Anat. Rec. 136*:154–155.

92. Sprague, J. M. (1958). The distribution of dorsal root fibers on motor cells in the lumbosacral spinal cord of the cat, and the site of excitatory and inhibitory terminals in monosynaptic pathways. *Proc. R. Soc. Lond. (Biol.) 140*:534–556.

93. Escolar, J. (1948). The afferent connections of the 1st, 2nd and 3rd cervical nerves in the cat. *J. Comp. Neurol. 89*:79–92.

94. Culberson, J. L., and Kimmel, D. L. (1975). Primary afferent fiber distribution at brachial and lumbosacral spinal cord levels in the opossum (Didelphis marsupialis virginiana). *Brain Behav. Evol. 12*:229–246.

95. Hand, P. J. (1966). Lumbosacral dorsal root terminations in the nucleus gracilis of the cat. Some observations on terminal degeneration in other medullary sensory nuclei. *J. Comp. Neurol. 126*:137–156.

96. Rustioni, A., and Macchi, G. (1968). Distribution of dorsal root fibers in the medulla oblongata of the cat. *J. Comp. Neurol. 134*:113–126.

97. Culberson, J. L., Haines, D. E., Kimmel, D. L., and Brown, P. B. (1979). Contralateral projection of primary afferent fibers to mammalian spinal cord. *Exp. Neurol. 64*:83–97.

98. Mense, S., Light, A. R., and Perl, E. R. (1981). Spinal terminations of subcutaneous high-threshold mechanoreceptors. In *Spinal Cord Sensation*, A. G. Brown and M. Réthelyi (Eds.). Scottish Academic Press, Edinburgh, pp. 79–86.

99. Brown, A. G., Fyffe, R. E. W., and Noble, R. (1980). Projections from Pacinian corpuscles and rapidly adapting mechanoreceptors of glabrous skin to the cat's spinal cord. *J. Physiol. (Lond.) 307*:385–400.

100. Szentágothai, J. (1961). Anatomical aspects of inhibitory pathways and synapses. In *Nervous Inhibition*, F. Florey (Ed.), Pergamon, New York, pp. 32–46.

101. Brown, P. B., and Fuchs, J. L. (1975). Somatotopic representation of hindlimb skin in cat dorsal horn. *J. Neurophysiol. 38*:1–19.

102. Wall, P. D. (1960). Cord cells responding to touch, damage and temperature of skin. *J. Neurophysiol. 23*:197–210.
103. Kennard, M. A. (1954). The course of ascending fibers in the spinal cord of the cat essential to the recognition of painful stimuli. *J. Comp. Neurol. 100*:511–524.
104. Trevino, D. L., Coulter, J. D., and Willis, W. D. (1973). Location of cells of origin of spinothalamic tract in lumbar enlargement of the monkey. *J. Neurophysiol. 36*:750–761.
105. Willis, W. D., Trevino, D. L., Coulter, J. D., and Maunz, R. A. (1974). Responses of primate spinothalamic tract neurons to natural stimulation of hindlimb. *J. Neurophysiol. 37*:358–372.
106. Natham, P. W., and Smith, M. C. (1959). Fasciculi proprii of the spinal cord in man. Review of present knowledge. *Brain 82*:610–668.
107. Uddenberg, N. (1968). Differential organization in dorsal funiculi of fibers originating from different receptors. *Exp. Brain Res. 4*:367–376.
108. Uddenberg, N. (1968). Functional organization of long, second-order afferents in the dorsal funiculi. *Exp. Brain Res. 4*:377–382.
109. Angaut-Petit, D. (1975). The dorsal column system. I. Existence of long ascending postsynaptic fibers in the cat's fasciculus gracilis. *Exp. Brain Res. 22*:457–470.
110. Angaut-Petit, D. (1975). The dorsal column system. II. Functional properties and bulbar relay of the postsynaptic fibers of the cat's fasciculus gracilis. *Exp. Brain Res. 22*:471–493.
111. Rustioni, A. (1973). Non-primary afferents to the nucleus gracilis from the lumbar cord of the cat. *Brain Res. 51*:81–95.
112. Rustioni, A. (1974). Non-primary afferents to the cuneate nucleus in the brachial dorsal funiculus of the cat. *Brain Res. 75*:247–259.
113. Rustioni, A. (1977). Spinal cord neurons projecting to the dorsal column nuclei of rhesus monkey. *Science 196*:656–658.
114. Rustioni, A., and Kaufman, A. B. (1977). Identification of cells of origin of non-primary afferents to the dorsal column nuclei of the cat. *Exp. Brain Res. 27*:1–14.
115. Brown, A. G., and Fyffe, R. E. W. (1981). Form and function of spinal neurons with axons ascending the dorsal columns in the cat. *J. Physiol. (Lond.) 321*:31–47.
116. Valverde, F. (1966). The pyramidal tract in rodents, a study of its relations with the posterior column nuclei, dorsolateral reticular formation of the medulla oblongata, and cervical spinal cord (Golgi and electron microscopic observations). *Z. Zellforsch. 71*:297–363.
117. Erulkar, S. D., Sprague, J. M., Whitsel, B. L., Dogan, S., and Jannetta, P. J. (1966). Organization of vestibular projection to the spinal cord of the cat. *J. Neurophysiol. 29*:626–664.
118. Kerr, F. W. L. (1968). The descending pathway to the lateral cuneate nucleus, the nucleus of Clarke and the ventral horn. *Anat. Rec. 160*:375.
119. Dart, A. M. (1971). Cells of the dorsal column nuclei projecting down into the spinal cord. *J. Physiol. (Lond.) 219*:29–30.

120. Kuypers, H. G. J. M., and Marsky, V. A. (1975). Retrograde axonal transport of horseradish peroxidase from spinal cord to brain stem cell groups in the cat. *Neurosci. Lett. 1*:9–14.

121. Burton, H., and Leowy, A. D. (1977). Projections to the spinal cord from medullary somatosensory relay nuclei. *J. Comp. Neurol. 173*:773–792.

122. Wall, P. D. (1960). Two transmission systems for skin senses. In *Sensory Communication*, W. A. Rosenblith (Ed.), Wiley, New York.

123. Brown, A. G. (1968). Cutaneous afferent fibre collaterals in the dorsal columns of the cat. *Exp. Brain Res. 5*:293–305.

124. Petit, D., and Burgess, P. R. (1968). Dorsal column projection of receptors in cat hairy skin supplied by myelinated fibers. *J. Neurophysiol. 31*:849–855.

125. Horch, K. W., Burgess, P. R., and Whitehorn, D. (1976). Ascending collaterals of cutaneous neurons in the fasciculus gracilis of the cat. *Brain Res. 117*:1–17.

126. Brown, A. G. (1973). Ascending and long spinal pathways: Dorsal columns, spinocervical tract and spinothalamic tract. In *Handbook of Sensory Physiology*. vol. II, A. Iggo (Ed.), Springer, New York, pp. 315–338.

127. Glees, P., and Soler, J. (1951). Fiber content of the posterior column and synaptic connections of nucleus gracilis. *Z. Zellforsch. 36*:381–400.

128. Lloyd, D. P. C., and McIntyre, A. K. (1950). Dorsal column conduction of group I muscle afferent impulses and their relay through Clarke's column. *J. Neurophysiol. 13*:39–54.

129. Burgess, P. R., and Clark, F. J. (1969). Dorsal column projection of fibres from the cat knee joint. *J. Physiol. (Lond.) 203*:301–315.

130. Clark, F. J. (1972). Central projection of sensory fibers from the cat knee joint. *J. Neurobiol. 3*:101–110.

131. Whitsel, B. L., Petrucelli, L. M., and Sapiro, G. (1969). Modality representation in the lumbar and cervical fasciculus gracilis of squirrel monkey. *Brain Res. 15*:67–78.

132. Oscarsson, O., Rosen, I., and Uddenberg, N. (1964). A comparative study of ascending spinal tracts activated from hindlimb afferents in monkey and dog. *Arch. Ital. Biol. 102*:137–155.

133. Oscarsson, O., and Rosen, I. (1963). Projection to cerebral cortex of large muscle-spindle afferents in the forelimb nerves of the cat. *J. Physiol. (Lond.) 169*:924–945.

134. Rosen, I. (1969). Localization in caudal brain stem and cervical spinal cord of neurons activated from forelimb group I afferents in the cat. *Brain Res. 16*:55–71.

135. Rosen, I. (1969). Afferent connexions to group I activated cells in the main cuneate nucleus of the cat. *J. Physiol. (Lond.) 205*:209–236.

136. Landgren, S., Sulfvenius, H., and Wolsk, D. (1967). Somato-sensory paths to the second cortical projection area of the group I muscle afferents. *J. Physiol. (Lond.) 191*:543–559.

137. Fyffe, R. E. W., Light, A. R., and Rustioni, A. (1982). Terminal arborizations of primary afferent fibers in the cuneate nucleus of the cat. *J. Physiol. (Lond.) 330*:97P.

138. Brown, A. G., Gordon, G., and Kay, R. H. (1970). Cutaneous receptive properties of single fibers in the cat's medial lemniscus. *J. Physiol. (Lond.)* *211*:37–39P.

139. Brown, A. G., Gordon, G., and Kay, R. H. (1974). A study of single axons in the cat's medial lemniscus. *J. Physiol. (Lond.)* *236*:225–246.

140. Hwang, Y.-C., Hinsman, E. J., and Roesel, O. F. (1975). Caliber spectre of fibers in the fasciculus gracilis of the cat cervical spinal cord: A quantitative electron microscopic study. *J. Comp. Neurol.* *162*:195–204.

141. Jänig, W., Schmidt, R. F., and Zimmerman, M. (1968). Single unit responses and the total afferent outflow from the cat's foot pad upon mechanical stimulation. *Brain Res.* *6*:100–115.

142. Boivie, J. J. G., and Perl, E. R. (1975). Neural substrates of somatic sensation. In *MTP International Review of Science: Physiology*, ser. I, vol. 3, C. C. Hunt (Ed.), University Park Press, Baltimore, pp. 303–411.

143. Widen, L. (1955). Cerebellar representation of high threshold afferents in the splanchnic nerve. *Acta Physiol. Scand.* (Suppl. 117) *33*:1–69.

144. Downman, C. B. B. (1955). Skeletal muscle reflexes of splanchnic and intercostal nerve origin in acute spinal and decerebrate cats. *J. Neurophysiol.* *18*:217–235.

145. Franz, D. N., Evans, M. H., and Perl, E. R. (1966). Characteristics of viscerosympathetic reflexes in the spinal cat. *Am. J. Physiol.* *211*:1292–1298.

146. Pomeranz, B., Wall, P. D., Weber, W. V. (1968). Cord cells responding to fine myelinated afferents from viscera, muscle and skin. *J. Physiol. (Lond.)* *199*:511–532.

147. Wall, P. D., and Werman, R. (1976). The physiology and anatomy of long ranging afferent fibers within the spinal cord. *J. Physiol. (Lond.)* *255*:321–334.

148. Ishizuka, N., Mannen, H., Hongo, T., and Sasaki, S. (1979). Trajectory of group Ia afferent fibers stained with horseradish peroxidase in the lumbosacral spinal cord of the cat: three-dimensional reconstructions from serial sections. *J. Comp. Neurol.* *186*:189–212.

149. Cervero, F., Iggo, A., and Molony, V. (1978). The tract of Lissauer and the dorsal root potential. *J. Physiol. (Lond.)* *282*:295–305.

150. Cervero, F., and Iggo, A. (1980). The substantia gelatinosa of the spinal cord. A critical review. *Brain* *103*:717–772.

151. Perl, E. R. (1981). The superficial dorsal horn: Some ideas from the distant and not so distant past. In *Spinal Cord Sensation*, A. G. Brown and M. Réthelyi (Eds.), Scottish Academic Press, Edinburgh, pp. 59–78.

152. Chung, K. C., and Coggeshall, R. E. (1979). Primary afferent axons in the tract of Lissauer in the cat. *J. Comp. Neurol.* *186*:451–453.

153. Chung, K. C., and Coggeshall, R. E. (1979). Primary afferent fibers in the tract of Lissauer in the rat. *J. Comp. Neurol.* *184*:587–598.

154. Wall, P. D. (1962). The origin of a spinal-cord slow potential. *J. Physiol. (Lond.)* *164*:508–526.

155. Wall, P. D., and Yaksh, T. L. (1979). Effect of Lissauer tract stimulation on activity in dorsal roots and in ventral roots. *Exp. Neurol.* *60*:570–583.

156. Coggeshall, R. E. (1981). Fine structural studies on the tract of Lissauer in rat, cat and monkey. In *Spinal Cord Sensation*, A. G. Brown and M. Réthelyi (Eds.), Scottish Academic Press, Edinburgh, pp. 119–124.

157. Ralston, H. J. (1965). The organization of the substantia gelatinosa Rolandi in the cat lumbosacral spinal cord. *Z. Zellforsch. 67*:1–23.

158. Kruger, L., Perl, E. R., and Sedivec, M. J. (1981). Fine structure of myelinated mechanical nociceptor endings in cat hairy skin. *J. Comp. Neurol. 198*:137–154.

159. Kumazawa, T., and Perl, E. R. (1976). Differential excitation of dorsal horn marginal and substantia gelatinosa neurons by primary afferent units with fine (A & C) fibers. In *Functions of the Skin in Primates with Special Reference to Man,* Y. Zotterman (Ed.), Pergamon, New York, pp. 67–88.

160. Kumazawa, T., and Perl, E. R. (1977). Primate cutaneous sensory units with unmyelinated (C) afferent fibers. *J. Neurophysiol. 40*:1325–1338.

161. Gobel, S., and Binck, J. M. (1977). Degenerative changes in primary trigeminal axons and in neurons in nucleus caudalis following tooth pulp extirpations in the cat. *Brain Res. 132*:347–354.

162. Gobel, S., and Hockfield, S. (1977). An anatomical analysis of the synaptic circuitry of layers I, II and III of trigeminal nucleus caudalis in the cat. In *Pain in the Trigeminal Region*, D. J. Anderson and B. Matthews (Eds.), Elsevier, Amsterdam, pp. 203–211.

163. Réthelyi, M., Light, A. R., and Perl, E. R. (1982). Synaptic complexes formed by functionally defined primary afferent units with fine myelinated fibers. *J. Comp. Neurol. 207*:381–393.

164. Maxwell, D. J., Bannatyne, B. A., Fyffe, R. E. W., and Brown, A. G. (1982). Ultrastructure of hair follicle afferent fiber terminations in the spinal cord of the cat. *J. Neurocytol. 11*:571–582.

165. Egger, M. D., Freeman, N. C. G., Malamed, S., Masarachia, P., and Proshansky, E. (1981). Electron microscopic observations of terminals of functionally identified afferent fibers in cat spinal cord. *Brain Res. 207*: 157–162.

166. Réthelyi, M. (1968). The Golgi architecture of Clarke's column. *Acta Morphol. Acad. Sci. Hung. 16*:311–330.

167. Réthelyi, M. (1970). Ultrastructural synaptology of Clarke's column. *Exp. Brain Res. 11*:159–174.

168. Szentágothai, J., and Albert, A. (1955). The synaptology of Clarke's column. *Acta Morph. Acad. Sci. Hung. 5*:43–51.

169. Grant, G., and Rexed, B. (1958). Dorsal root afferents to Clarke's column. *Brain 81*:567–576.

170. Tracey, D. J., and Walmsley, B. (1982). Anatomy of the connection between identified primary afferents and neurons of the dorsal spinocerebellar tract. *Aust. Phys. Pharm. Soc. Abstr. 13*:134P.

171. Hongo, T., Ishizuka, N., Mannen, H., and Sasaki, S. (1978). Axonal trajectory of single group Ia and Ib fibers in the cat spinal cord. *Neurosci. Lett. 8*:321–328.

172. Metz, C. B., Kavookjian, A., and Light, A. R. (1983). Techniques for HRP intracellular staining of neural elements for light and electron-microscopic analysis. *J. Electrophysiol. Tech. 9*:151-163.

173. Graybiel, A. M., and Devor, M. (1974). A micro-electrophoretic delivery technique for use with horseradish peroxidase. *Brain Res. 68*:167-173.

174. Hanker, J. S., Yates, P. E., Metz, C. B., and Rustioni, A. (1977). A new, specific, sensitive and non-carcinogenic reagent for the demonstration of horseradish peroxidase. *Histochem. J. 9*:789-792.

175. Adrian, E. D. (1931). The messages in sensory nerve fibers and their interpretation. *Proc. R. Soc. Lond. (Biol.) 109*:1-18.

176. Brown, A. G., and Iggo, A. (1967). A quantitative study of cutaneous receptors and afferent fibres in the cat and rabbit. *J. Physiol. (Lond.) 193*:707-733.

177. Burgess, P. R., Petit, D., and Warren, R. M. (1968). Receptor types in cat hairy skin supplied by myelinated fibers. *J. Neurophysiol. 31*:833-848.

178. Perl, E. R. (1968). Myelinated afferent fibers innervating primate skin and their responses to noxious stimuli. *J. Physiol. (Lond.) 197*:593-615.

179. Brown, A. G., and Franz, D. N. (1969). Responses of spinocervical tract neurons to natural stimulation of identified cutaneous receptors. *Exp. Brain Res. 7*:231-237.

180. Brown, A. G. (1971). Effects of descending impulses on transmission through the spinocervical tract. *J. Physiol. (Lond.) 219*:103-125.

181. Hongo, T., and Koike, H. (1975). Some aspects of synaptic organization in the spinocervical tract cell in the cat. In *The Somatosensory System*, H. H. Kornhuber (Ed.), Thieme, Stuttgart, pp. 218-226.

182. Lundberg, A., and Oscarsson, O. (1960). Functional organization of dorsal spino-cerebellar tract in the cat. VII. Identification of units by antidromic activation from the cerebellar cortex with recognition of five functional subdivisions. *Acta Physiol. Scand. 50*:356-374.

183. Mann, M. D. (1971). Axons of dorsal spinocerebellar tract which respond to activity in cutaneous receptors. *J. Neurophysiol. 34*:1035-1050.

184. Brown, P. B., Fuchs, J. L., and Tapper, D. N. (1975). Parametric studies of dorsal horn neurons responding to tactile stimulation. *J. Neurophysiol. 38*:19-25.

185. Tapper, D. N., Brown, P. B., and Moraff, H. (1973). Functional organization of the cat's dorsal horn: Connectivity of myelinated fiber systems of hairy skin. *J. Neurophysiol. 36*:817-826.

186. Brown, A. G., and Noble, R. (1979). Connexions between hair follicle afferent fibres and spinocervical tract neurones in the cat: The synthesis of receptive fields. *J. Physiol. (Lond.) 296*:38-39P.

187. Brown, A. G., and Noble, R. (1982). Connexions between hair follicle afferent fibres and spinocervical tract neurones in the cat. *J. Physiol. (Lond.) 323*77-91.

188. Wall, P. D. (1977). The presence of ineffective synapses and the circumstances which unmask them. *Phil. Trans. Roy. Soc. Lond. (Biol.) 278*:361-372.

189. Pacini, F. (1840). *Nuovi organi scoperti nel corpo umano*. Ciro, Pistoia, Italy.

190. Adrian, E. D., and Umrath, K. (1929). The impulse discharge from the Pacinian corpuscle. *J. Physiol. (Lond.)* 68:139–154.

191. Gray, J. A. B., and Matthews, P. B. C. (1951). A comparison of the adaptation of the Pacinian corpuscle with accommodation of its own axon. *J. Physiol. (Lond.)* 114:454–464.

192. Hunt, C. C. (1961). On the nature of vibration receptors in the hind limb of the cat. *J. Physiol. (Lond.)* 155:175–186.

193. Hunt, C. C. (1974). The Pacinian corpuscle. In *The Peripheral Nervous System*, J. I. Hubbard (Ed.), Plenum, London, pp. 405–420.

194. Loewenstein, W. R., and Mendelson, M. (1963). Components of receptor adaptation in a Pacinian corpuscle. *J. Physiol. (Lond.)* 177:377–397.

195. Malinovsky, L. (1966). Variability of sensory nerve endings in foot pads of a domestic cat (*Felis ocreata L., Felis domestica*). *Acta Anat. (Basel) 64*: 82–106.

196. Lynn, B. (1969). The nature and location of certain phasic mechanoreceptors in the cat's foot. *J. Physiol. (Lond.)* 201:765–773.

197. Jänig, W. (1971). The afferent innervation of the central pad of the cat's hind foot. *Brain Res. 28*:203–216.

198. Jänig, W. (1971). Morphology of rapidly and slowly adapting mechanoreceptors in the hairless skin of the cat's hind foot. *Brain Res. 28*:217–231.

199. Lynn, B. (1971). The form and distribution of the receptive fields of Pacinian corpuscles found in and around the cat's large foot pad. *J. Physiol. (Lond.)* 217:755–771.

200. Iggo, A., and Ogawa, H. (1977). Correlative physiological and morphological studies of rapidly and adapting mechanoreceptors in cat's glabrous skin. *J. Physiol. (Lond.)* 266:275–296.

201. Mountcastle, V. B., Talbot, W. H., Sakata, H., and Hyvärinen, J. (1969). Cortical neuronal mechanisms in flutter vibration studies in unanesthetized monkeys. Neuronal periodicity and frequency discrimination. *J. Neurophysiol. 32*:452–484.

202. Perl, E. R., Whitlock, D. G., and Gentry, J. R. (1962). Cutaneous projection to second order neurons of the dorsal column system. *J. Neurophysiol. 25*:337–358.

203. Hyvärinen, J., and Poranen, A. (1978). Receptive field integration and submodality convergence in the hand area of the post-central gyrus of the alert monkey. *J. Physiol. (Lond.)* 283:539–556.

204. Bennett, R. E., Ferrington, D. G., and Rowe, M. (1980). Tactile neuron classes within second somatosensory area (SII) of cat cerebral cortex. *J. Neurophysiol. 43*:292–309.

205. Douglas, P. R., Ferrington, D. G., and Rowe, M. (1978). Coding of information about tactile stimuli by neurones of the cuneate nucleus. *J. Physiol. (Lond.)* 285:493–513.

206. Bystrzycka, E., Naill, B. S., and Rowe, M. (1977). Inhibition of cuneate neurones: Its afferent source and influence on dynamically sensitive

'tactile' neurones. *J. Physiol. (Lond.) 268*:251-270.

207. Gordon, G., and Jukes, M. G. M. (1964). Dual organization of the extero-receptive components of the cat's gracile nucleus. *J. Physiol. (Lond.) 173*: 263-290.

208. Ferrington, D. G., and Rowe, M. (1982). Specificity of connections and tactile coding capacities in cuneate nucleus of the neonatal kitten. *J. Neurophysiol. 47*:622-640.

209. Jänig, W., Schmidt, R. F., and Zimmerman, M. (1968). Two specific feed-back pathways to the central afferent terminals of phasic and tonic mechanoreceptors. *Exp. Brain Res. 6*:116-129.

210. Wall, P. D. (1973). Dorsal horn electrophysiology. In *Handbook of Sensory Physiology*, A. Iggo (Ed.), vol. II, Springer, New York, pp. 253-270.

211. Armett, C. J., Gray, J. A. B., and Palmer, J. F. (1961). A group of neurones in the dorsal horn associated with cutaneous mechanoreceptors. *J. Physiol. (Lond.) 156*:611-622.

212. Armett, C. J., Gray, J. A. B., Hunsperger, R. W., and Lal, S. (1962). The transmission of information in primary receptor neurones and second order neurones of a phasic system. *J. Physiol. (Lond.) 164*:395-421.

213. Brown, A. G., Fyffe, R. E. W., Heavner, J. E., and Noble, R. (1979). The morphology of collaterals from axons innervating Pacinian corpuscles. *J. Physiol. (Lond.) 292*:24-25P.

214. Réthelyi, M. (1981). Geometry of the dorsal horn. In *Spinal Cord Sensation*, A. G. Brown and M. Réthelyi (Eds.), Scottish Academic Press, Edinburgh, pp. 1-11.

215. Fyffe, R. E. W. (1981). Dendritic trees of dorsal horn cells. In *Spinal Cord Sensation*, A. G. Brown and M. Réthelyi (Eds.), Scottish Academic Press, Edinburgh, pp. 127-136.

216. Proshansky, E., and Egger, M. D. (1977). Dendritic spread of dorsal horn neurons in cats. *Exp. Brain Res. 28*:153-166.

217. Krause, W. (1860). *Die terminalen Korpechen der ernfachen sensiblen Nerven.* Hehn'sche Hofkuchhandlung, Hannover.

218. Cauna, N. (1956). Nerve supply and nerve endings in Meissner's corpuscles. *Amer. J. Anat. 99*:315-350.

219. Munger, B., and Pubols, L. M. (1972). The sensory neuronal organization of the digital skin of the raccoon. *Brain Behav. Evol. 5*:367-393.

220. Jankowska, E., Rastad, J., and Zarjecki, P. (1979). Segmental and supra-spinal input to cells of origin of non-primary fibres in the feline dorsal column. *J. Physiol. (Lond.) 290*:185-200.

221. Frankenhaeuser, B. (1949). Impulses from a cutaneous receptor with slow adaption and low mechanical threshold. *Acta Physiol. Scand. 18*:68-74.

222. Hunt, C. C., and McIntyre, A. K. (1960). Properties of cutaneous touch receptors in cat. *J. Physiol. (Lond.) 53*:88-98.

223. Werner, G., and Mountcastle, V. B. (1965). Neural activity in mechano-receptive cutaneous afferents: Stimulus-response relation. Weber functions, and information transmission. *J. Neurophysiol. 28*:359-397.

224. Witt, I., and Hensel, H. (1959). Afferent Impulse aus der Extremitatenhaut der Katze bei thermischer und mechanischer Reizung. *Pfluegers Arch. 268*: 582–596.

225. Iggo, A. (1963). New specific sensory structures in hairy skin. *Acta Neuroveg. 24*:175–180.

226. Iggo, A. (1966). Cutaneous receptors with a high sensitivity to mechanical displacement. In *Ciba Foundation Symposium on Touch, Heat and Pain*, E. V. S. de Reuck and J. Knight (Eds.), Churchill, London, pp. 237–256.

227. Iggo, A., and Muir, A. R. (1969). The structure and function of a slowly adapting touch corpuscle in hairy skin. *J. Physiol. (Lond.) 200*:763–796.

228. Chambers, M. R., and Iggo, A. (1967). Slowly-adapting cutaneous mechanoreceptors. *J. Physiol. (Lond.) 192*:26–27.

229. Brown, A. G., and Hayden, R. E. (1971). The distribution of cutaneous receptors in the rabbit's hind limb and differential electrical stimulation of their axons. *J. Physiol. (Lond.) 213*:495–506.

230. Tapper, D. N. (1963). The cutaneous slowly-adapting mechanoreceptor of the cat. *Physiologist 6*:288.

231. Tapper, D. N. (1964). Input-output relationships in a skin tactile sensory unit of the cat. *Trans. N.Y. Acad. Sci. 26*:697–701.

232. Tapper, D. N. (1965). Stimulus-response relationships in the cutaneous slowly-adapting mechanoreceptor in hairy skin of the cat. *Exp. Neurol. 13*:364–385.

233. Lindblom, U., and Tapper, D. N. (1967). Terminal properties of vibrotactile sensor. *Exp. Neurol. 17*:1–15.

234. Harrington, T., and Merzenich, M. M. (1970). Neural coding in the sense of touch: Human sensations of skin indentation compared with the responses of slowly adapting mechanoreceptive afferents innervating the hairy skin of monkeys. *Exp. Brain Res. 10*:251–264.

235. Kenton, B., Kurger, L., and Woo, M. (1971). Two classes of slowly adapting mechanoreceptor fibers in reptile cutaneous nerve. *J. Physiol. (Lond.) 212*:21–44.

236. Knibestöl, M., and Vallbo, A. B. (1970). Single unit analysis of mechanoreceptor activity from the human glabrous skin. *Acta Physiol. Scand. 80*: 178–195.

237. Smith, K. R. (1967). The structure and function of *Haarscheibe*. *J. Comp. Neurol. 13*:459–474.

238. Smith, K. R. (1970). The ultrastructure of the human *Haarscheibe* and Merkel cell. *J. Invest Dermatol. 54*:150–159.

239. Pinkus, F. (1904). Uber Hautsinnesorgane neben den menschlichen Harr (Harrscheiben) udd ihre vergeichend anatomische Bedeutung. *Arch. Mikrosk. Anat. Entw. Mech. 65*:121–179.

240. Merkel, F. (1875). Tastzellen und Tastkörperchen bei den Haustieren und beim Menschen. *Arch. Mikrosk. Anat. Entw. Mech. 11*:636–652.

241. Mann, M. D., Kasprzak, H., and Tapper, D. N. (1971). Ascending dorsolateral pathways relaying type I afferent activity. *Brain Res. 27*:176–178.

242. Brown, A. G., Rose, P. K., and Snow, P. J. (1978). Morphology and organization of axon collaterals from afferent fibers of slowly adapting type I units in cat spinal cord. *J. Physiol. (Lond.) 277*:15–27.

243. Ruffini, A. (1894). Sur un nouvel organe nerveux terminal et sur la presence des corpuscles Golgi-Mazzoni dans le conjonctif sous-cutane de la pulpe des doigts de l'homme. *Arch. Ital. Biol. 21*:249–265.

244. Chambers, M. R., Andres, K. H., Van Duering, M., and Iggo, A. (1972). The structure and function of the slowly adapting type II mechanoreceptor in hairy skin. *Q. J. Exp. Physiol. 57*:417–445.

245. Talbot, W. H., Darian-Smith, I., Kornhuber, H. H., and Mountcastle, V. B. (1968). The sense of flutter-vibration: Comparison of the human capacity with response patterns of mechanoreceptive afferents from the monkey hand. *J. Neurophysiol. 31*:301–334.

246. Knibestöl, M. (1975). Stimulus-response functions of slowly adapting mechanoreceptors in the human glabrous skin area. *J. Physiol. (Lond.) 245*: 63–80.

247. Johansson, R. S. (1978). Tactile sensibility in the human hand: Receptive field characteristics of mechanoreceptive units in the glabrous skin area. *J. Physiol. (Lond.) 281*:101–123.

248. Brown, A. G., Fyffe, R. E. W., Rose, P. K., and Snow, P. J. (1981). Spinal cord collaterals from axons of type II slowly adapting units in the cat. *J. Physiol. (Lond.) 316*:469–480.

249. Hunt, C. C. (1974). The physiology of muscle receptors. In *Handbook of Sensory Physiology*, C. C. Hunt (Ed.), Springer, Berlin, pp. 191–234.

250. Matthews, P. B. C. (1977). Muscle afferents and kinaesthesia. *Br. Med. Bull. 33*:137–142.

251. Matthews, P. B. C. (1982). Where does Sherrington's 'muscular sense' originate? Muscles, joints, corrolary discharges? *Ann. Rev. Neurosci. 5*: 189–218.

252. Barker, D. (1974). The morphology of muscle receptors. In *Handbook of Sensory Physiology*, C. C. Hunt (Ed.), vol. III/2, Springer, Berlin, pp. 1–190.

253. Lloyd, D. P. C. (1946). Integrative pattern of excitation and inhibition in two-neuron reflex arcs. *J. Neurophysiol. 9*:439–444.

254. Renshaw, B. (1940). Activity in the simplest spinal reflex pathways. *J. Neurophysiol. 3*:373–387.

255. Mendell, L. M., and Henneman, E. (1971). Terminals of Ia fibers: Location, density and distribution within a pool of 300 homonymous motoneurons. *J. Neurophysiol. 34*:171–187.

256. McIntyre, A. K. (1974). Central actions of impulse in muscle afferent fibers. In *Handbook of Sensory Physiology*, C. C. Hunt (Ed.), vol. III/2, Springer, Berlin, pp. 235–288.

257. Burke, R. E., and Rudomín, P. (1977). Spinal neurons and synapses. In *Handbook of Physiology*, vol. I, E. R. Kandel (Ed.), American Physiological Society. Bethesda, Maryland, pp. 877–944.

258. Redman, S. J. (1979). Junctional mechanisms at group Ia synapses. *Prog. Neurobiol.* *12*:33–83.

259. Lloyd, D. P. C. (1943). Reflex action in relation to pattern and peripheral source of afferent stimulation. *J. Neurophysiol.* *6*:111–120.

260. Lloyd, D. P. C. (1943). Neuron patterns controlling transmission of ipsilateral hind limb reflexes in cat. *J. Neurophysiol.* *6*:293–315.

261. Eccles, J. C., and Pritchard, J. J. (1937). The action potential of motoneurones. *J. Physiol. (Lond.)* *89*:43–45P.

262. Eccles, J. C., and Rall, W. (1951). Repetitive monosynaptic activation of motoneurones. *Proc. R. Soc. Lond. (Biol.)* *138*:475–498.

263. Eccles, J. C., Eccles, R. M., and Lundberg, A. (1957). Synaptic actions on motoneurones in relation to the two components of the group I muscle afferent volley. *J. Physiol. (Lond.)* *136*:527–546.

264. Eccles, J. C. (1964). *The Physiology of Synapses*. Springer, New York.

265. Kuno, M. (1964). Quantal components of excitatory synaptic potentials in spinal motoneurones. *J. Physiol. (Lond.)* *175*:81–99.

266. Kuno, M. (1964). Mechanism of facilitation and depression of the excitatory synaptic potential in spinal motoneurones. *J. Physiol. (Lond.)* *175*:100–112.

267. Kuno, M., and Miyahara, J. T. (1969). Non-linear summation of unit synaptic potentials in spinal motoneurones of the cat. *J. Physiol. (Lond.)* *201*:465–477.

268. Kuno, M., and Miyahara, J. T. (1969). Analysis of synaptic efficacy in spinal motoneurones from 'quantum' aspects. *J. Physiol. (Lond.)* *201*:479–493.

269. Burke, R. E. (1967). Composite nature of the monosynaptic excitatory postsynaptic potential. *J. Neurophysiol.* *30*:1114–1136.

270. Jack, J. J. B., Miller, S., Porter, R., and Redman, S. J. (1971). The time course of minimal excitatory post-synaptic potentials evoked in spinal motoneurones by group Ia afferent fibers. *J. Physiol. (Lond.)* *215*:353–380.

271. Czarkowska, J., Jankowska, E., and Sybirska, E. (1976). Axonal projections of spinal interneurones excited by group I afferents in the cat, revealed by intracellular staining with horseradish peroxidase. *Brain Res.* *118*:115–118.

272. Hultborn, H., Jankowska, E., and Lindström, S. (1971). Recurrent inhibition from motor axon collaterals of transmission in the Ia inhibitory pathway to motoneurones. *J. Physiol. (Lond.)* *215*:591–612.

273. Hultborn, H., Jankowska, E., and Lindström, S. (1971). Recurrent inhibition of interneurones monosynaptically activated from group Ia afferents. *J. Physiol. (Lond.)* *215*:613–636.

274. Hultborn, H., Jankowska, E., and Lindström, S. (1971). Relative contribution from different nerves to recurrent depression of Ia IPSP's in motoneurones. *J. Physiol. (Lond.)* *215*:637–664.

275. Jankowska, E., and Roberts, W. J. (1972). An electrophysiological demonstration of the axonal projections of single spinal interneurones in the cat. *J. Physiol. (Lond.) 222*:597–622.
276. Jankowska, E., and Roberts, W. J. (1972). Synaptic actions of single interneurones mediating reciprocal Ia inhibition of motoneurones. *J. Physiol. (Lond.) 222*:623–642.
277. Jankowska, E., and Lindström, S. (1972). Morphology of interneurones mediating Ia reciprocal inhibition of motoneurones in the spinal cord of the cat. *J. Physiol. (Lond.) 226*:805–823.
278. Eccles, J. C., Fatt, P., and Landgren, S. (1956). Central pathway for direct inhibitory action of impulses in largest afferent nerve fibers to muscle. *J. Neurophysiol. 19*:75–98.
279. Szentágothai, J. (1948). Anatomical considerations of monosynaptic reflex arcs. *J. Neurophysiol. 11*:445–454.
280. Illis, L. (1967). The relative densities of monosynaptic pathways to the cell bodies and dendrites of the cat ventral horn. *J. Neurol. Sci. 4*:259–270.
281. Conradi, S. (1969). On motoneuron synaptology in adult cats. *Acta Physiol. Scand.* (Suppl. 332) *78*:1–115.
282. McLaughlin, B. J. (1972). Dorsal root projections to the motor nuclei in the cat spinal cord. *J. Comp. Neurol. 144*:461–474.
283. Brown, A. G., and Fyffe, R. E. W. (1978). Morphology of group Ia afferent fibre collaterals in the spinal cord of the cat. *J. Physiol. (Lond.) 274*:111–127.
284. Brown, A. G., and Fyffe, R. E. W. (1978). Synaptic contacts made by identified Ia afferent fibres upon motoneurones. *J. Physiol. (Lond.) 284*:43–44P.
285. Brown, A. G., and Fyffe, R. E. W. (1981). Direct observations on the contacts made between Ia afferent fibres and alpha motoneurones in the cat's lumbosacral spinal cord. *J. Physiol. (Lond.) 313*:121–140.
286. Burke, R. E., Walmsley, B., and Hodgson, J. A. (1979). HRP anatomy of group Ia afferent contacts on alpha motoneurones. *Brain Res. 160*:347–352.
287. Redman, S. J., and Walmsley, B. (1980). A combined electrophysiological and anatomical location of single group Ia fibre connexions with cat spinal motoneurones. *J. Physiol. (Lond.) 308*:99P.
288. Redman, S. J., and Walmsley, B. (1981). The synaptic basis of the monosynaptic stretch reflex. *Trends in Neuroscience 4*:248–251.
289. Grantyn, R., Shapovalov, A. I., and Shiriaev, B. I. (1982). Combined morphological and electrophysiological description of connections between single primary afferent fibers and individual mononeurons in the frog spinal cord. *Exp. Brain Res. 48*:459–462.
290. Fyffe, R. E. W. (1981). "Spinal Cord Terminations of Afferent Fibres from Cat Hind Limb Muscles." Ph.D. dissertation, University of Edinburgh.

291. Munson, J. B., and Sypert, G. W. (1979). Properties of single central Ia afferent fibres projecting to motoneurones. *J. Physiol. (Lond.) 196*:315–327.

292. Romanes, G. J. (1951). The motor cell columns of the lumbosacral cord of the cat. *J. Comp. Neurol. 94*:313–364.

293. Carpenter, M. B., Stein, B. M., and Shriver, J. E. (1968). Central projections of spinal dorsal roots in the monkey. II. Lower thoracic, lumbosacral and coccygeal dorsal roots. *Amer. J. Anat. 123*:75–118.

294. Rose, P. K. (1982). Branching structure of motoneuron stem dentrites: A study of neck muscle motoneurons intracellularly stained with horseradish peroxidase in the cat. *J. Neurosci. 2*:1596–1607.

295. Ulfhake, B., and Kellerth, J.-P. (1981). A quantitative light microscopic study of the dendrites of cat spinal alpha-motoneurons after intracellular staining with horseradish peroxidase. *J. Comp. Neurol. 202*:571–583.

296. Eccles, J. C., Fatt, P., Landren, S., and Wusburg, G. J. (1954). Spinal cord potentials generated by volleys in the large muscle afferents. *J. Physiol. (Lond.) 125*:590–606.

297. Aoyama, M., Hongo, T., and Kudo, N. (1973). An uncrossed ascending tract originating from below Clarke's column and conveying group I impulses from the hindlimb muscles in the cat. *Brain Res. 62*:237–241.

298. Oscarsson, O. (1973). Functional organization of spinocerebellar paths. In *Handbook of Sensory Physiology*, A. Iggo (Ed.), vol. II, Springer, New York, pp. 340–380.

299. Szentágothai, J. (1961). Somatotopic arrangement of synapses of primary sensory neurons in Clarke's column. *Acta Morph. Acad. Sci. Hung. 10*:307–311.

300. Lundberg, A., and Winsbury, G. J. (1960). Functional organization of the dorsal spino-cerebellar tract in the cat. VI. Further experiments on excitation from tendon organ and muscle spindle afferents. *Acta Physiol. Scand. 49*:165–170.

301. Ha, H., and Liu, C.-N. (1968). Cell origin of the ventral spinocerebellar tract. *J. Comp. Neurol. 133*:185–206.

302. Hubbard, J. I., and Oscarsson, O. (1962). Localization of the cell bodies of the ventral spinocerebellar tract in lumbar segments of the cat. *J. Comp. Neurol. 118*:199–204.

303. Cooper, S., and Sherrington, C. S. (1940). Gower's tract and spinal border cells. *Brain 63*:123–134.

304. Burke, R. E., Lundberg, A., and Weight, F. (1971). Spinal border cell origin of the ventral spinocerebellar tract. *Exp. Brain Res. 12*:283–294.

305. Munson, J. B., and Sypert, G. W. (1979). Properties of single fibre excitatory post-synaptic potentials in triceps surae motoneurones. *J. Physiol. (Lond.) 296*:329–342.

306. Watt, D. G. D., Stauffer, E. K., Taylor, A., Reinking, R. M., and Stuart, D. G. (1976). Analysis of muscle receptor connections by spike triggered averaging. I. Spindle primary and tendon organ afferents. *J. Neurophysiol. 39*:1375–1392.

307. Burke, R. E. (1980). Structural-functional relations in monosynaptic group Ia action on spinal alpha-motoneurones. *Proc. I.U.P.S. Budapest XIV*:72-73.

308. Burke, R. E., Pinter, M. J., Lev Tov, A., and O'Donovan, M. J. (1980). Anatomy of monosynaptic contacts from group Ia afferents to defined types of extensor alpha-motoneurons in the cat. *Soc. Neurosci. Abstr. 6*:713.

309. Burke, R. E., Levine, D. N., Tsairis, P., and Zajac, F. E. (1973). Physiological types and histochemical profiles in motor units of the cat gastrocnemius. *J. Physiol. (Lond.) 234*:723-748.

310. Rall, W. (1977). Core conductor theory and cable properties of neurons. In *Handbook of Physiology*, E. R. Kandel (Ed.), sect. I, vol. I, American Physiological Society, Bethesda, Maryland, pp. 39-97.

311. Jack, J. J. B., Noble, D., and Tsien, R. W. (1975). Electric current flow in excitable cells. *Oxford University Press*, Oxford.

312. Glenn, L. L., Burke, R. E., Fleshman, J. W., and Lev-Tov, A. (1982). Estimate of electrotonic distance of group Ia contacts on cat alpha-motoneurons: An HRP morphological study. *Soc. Neurosci. Abstr. 8*:995.

313. Rall, W., Burke, R. E., Smith, T. G., Nelson, P. G., and Frank, K. (1967). Dendritic location of synapses and possible mechanisms for the monosynaptic EPSP in motoneurons. *J. Neurophysiol. 30*:1169-1193.

314. Nelson, S. G., and Mendell, L. M. (1978). Projection of single knee flexor Ia fibers to homonymous and heteronymous motoneurons. *J. Neurophysiol. 41*:778-787.

315. Eccles, J. C., Eccles, R. M., and Lundberg, A. (1957). Synaptic actions on motoneurones caused by impulses in Golgi tendon organ afferents. *J. Physiol. (Lond.) 138*:227-252.

316. Granit, R. (1950). Reflex self-regulation of muscle contraction and autogenetic inhibition. *J. Neurophysiol. 13*:351-372.

317. Eccles, R. M., and Lundberg, A. (1959). Synaptic actions in motoneurones by afferents which may evoke the flexion reflex. *Arch. Ital. Biol. 97*:199-221.

318. Laporte, Y., and Lloyd, D. P. C. (1952). Nature and significance of the reflex connections established by large afferent fibers of muscular origin. *Am. J. Physiol. 169*:609-621.

319. Lundberg, A. (1971). Function of the ventral spinocerebellar tract: A new hypothesis. *Exp. Brain Res. 12*:317-330.

320. Jansen, J. K. S., and Rudjord, T. (1965). Fusimotor activity in a flexor muscle of decerebrate cat. *Acta Physiol. Scand. 63*:236-246.

321. Alnaes, E. (1967). Static and dynamic properties of Golgi tendon organs in the anterior tibial and soleus muscle of the cat. *Acta Physiol. Scand. 70*:176-187.

322. Houk, J., and Henneman, E. (1967). Responses of Golgi tendon organs to active contractions of the soleus muscle of the cat. *J. Neurophysiol. 30*:1482-1493.

323. Bradley, K., and Eccles, J. C. (1953). Analysis of the fast afferent impulses from thigh muscles. *J. Physiol. (Lond.) 122*:462–473.

324. Hunt, C. C. (1954). Relation of function to diameter in afferent fibers of muscle nerves. *J. Gen. Physiol. 38*:111–131.

325. Brown, A. G., and Fyffe, R. E. W. (1978). The morphology of group Ib muscle afferent fiber collaterals. *J. Physiol. (Lond.) 277*:44–45P.

326. Brown, A. G., and Fyffe, R. E. W. (1979). The morphology of group Ib afferent fiber collaterals in the spinal cord of the cat. *J. Physiol. (Lond.) 296*:215–228.

327. Hongo, T., Kudo, N., Yamashita, M., Ishizuka, N., and Mannen, H. (1981). Transneuronal passage of intra-axonally injected horseradish peroxidase (HRP) from group Ib and II fibers into the secondary neurons in the dorsal horn of the cat spinal cord. *Biomed. Res. 2*:722–727.

328. Lundberg, A. A., and Weight, F. (1971). Functional organization of connexions to the ventral spinocerebellar tract. *Exp. Brain Res. 12*:295–316.

329. Lucas, M. E., and Willis, W. D. (1974). Identification of muscle afferents which activate interneurons in the intermediate nucleus. *J. Neurophysiol. 37*:282–293.

330. Eccles, R. M. (1965). Interneurons activated by higher threshold group I muscle afferents. In *Studies in Physiology*, D. R. Curtis, and A. K. McIntyre (Eds.), Springer, New York, pp. 59–64.

331. Lindström, S., and Schomburg, E. D. (1974). Group I inhibition in Ib excited ventral spinocerebellar tract neurones. *Acta Physiol. Scand. 90*: 166–185.

332. Sherrington, C. S. (1906). *The Integrative Action of the Nervous System*. Yale University Press, New Haven, Connecticut.

333. Matthews, P. B. C. (1963). The response of de-efferented muscle spindle receptors to stretching at different velocities. *J. Physiol. (Lond.) 168*: 660–678.

334. Matthews, P. B. C. (1969). Evidence that the secondary as well as the primary endings of the muscle spindles may be responsible for the tonic stretch reflex of the decerebrate cat. *J. Physiol. (Lond.) 204*:365–393.

335. Matthews, P. B. C. (1970). A reply to criticism of the hypothesis that the group II afferents contribute excitation to the stretch reflex. *Acta Physiol. Scand. 79*:431–433.

336. McGrath, G. J., and Matthews, P. B. C. (1973). Evidence from the use of vibration during procaine nerve block that the spindle group II fibres contribute excitation to the tonic stretch reflex of the decerebrate cat. *J. Physiol. (Lond.) 235*:371–408.

337. Westbury, D. R. (1972). A study of stretch and vibration reflexes of the cat by intracellular recording from motoneurones. *J. Physiol. (Lond.) 226*:37–56.

338. Kanda, K., and Rymer, W. Z. (1977). An estimate of the secondary spindle receptor afferent contribution to the stretch reflex in extensor muscles of the decerebrate cat. *J. Physiol. (Lond.) 264*:63–87.

339. Fromm, C., Haase, J., and Wolf, E. (1977). Depression of the recurrent inhibition of extensor motoneurons by the action of group II afferents. *Brain Res. 120*:459–468.

340. Lundberg, A., Malmgren, K., and Schomburg, E. D. (1973). Characteristics of the excitatory pathway from group II muscle afferents to alpha motoneurones. *Brain Res. 88*:538–542.

341. Cook, W. A., and Duncan, C. C. (1971). Contribution of group I afferents to the tonic stretch reflex of the decerebrate cat. *Brain Res. 33*:509–513.

342. Grillner, S. (1970). Is the tonic stretch reflex dependent upon group II excitation? *Acta Physiol. Scand. 78*:431–432.

343. Kirkwood, P. A., and Sears, T. A. (1974). Monosynaptic excitation of motoneurones from secondary endings of muscle spindles. *Nature 252*: 242–244.

344. Kirkwood, P. A., and Sears, T. A. (1975). Monosynaptic excitation of motoneurones from muscle spindle secondary endings of intercostal and triceps surae muscles in the cat. *245*:64–66P.

345. Lundberg, A., Malmgren, K., and Schomberg, E. D. (1977). Comments on reflex actions evoked by electrical stimulation of group II muscle afferents. *Brain Res. 122*:551–555.

346. Stauffer, E. K., Watt, D. G. D., Taylor, A., Reinking, R., and Stuart, D. G. (1976). Analysis of muscle receptor connections by spike-triggered averaging. II. Spindle group II afferents. *J. Neurophysiol. 39*:1393–1402.

347. Zengel, J. E., Munson, J. B., Fleshman, J. W., and Sypert, G. W. (1981). Projections of individual medial gastrocnemius spindle group II afferents to type-identified motoneurons. *Soc. Neurosci. Abstr. 7*:409.

348. Munson, J. B., Fleshman, J. W., and Sypert, G. W. (1980). Properties of single-fiber spindle group II EPSP's in triceps surae monotneurons. *J. Neurophysiol. 44*:713–725.

349. Lüscher, H.-R., Ruenzel, P., Fetz, E., and Henneman, E. (1980). Postsynaptic population potentials recorded from ventral roots perfused with isotonic sucrose: Connections of groups Ia and II spindle afferent fibers with large populations of motoneurons. *J. Neurophysiol. 42*: 1146–1164.

350. Sypert, G. W., Fleshman, J. W., and Munson, J. B. (1980). Comparison of monosynaptic actions of medial gastrocnemius group Ia and group II muscle spindle afferents on triceps surae motoneurons. *J. Neurophysiol. 44*:726–738.

351. Fu, T. C., and Schomburg, E. D. (1974). Electrophysiological investigation of the projection of secondary muscular spindle afferents in the cat spinal cord. *Acta Physiol. Scand. 91*:314–329.

352. Fyffe, R. E. W. (1979). The morphology of group II muscle afferent fibre collaterals. *J. Physiol. (Lond. 296*:39–40P.

353. Fu, T. C., Santini, M., and Schomburg, E. D. (1974). Characteristics of spinal focal synaptic potentials generated by group II muscle afferents. *Acta Physiol. Scand. 91*:298–313.

354. Fukushima, K., and Kato, M. (1975). Spinal interneurons responding to group II muscle afferent fibers in the cat. *Brain Res. 90*:307–312.

355. Holmquist, B., and Lundberg, A. (1961). Differential supraspinal control of synaptic actions evoked by volleys in the flexion reflex afferents in alpha motoneurones. *Acta Physiol. Scand.* (Suppl. 186) *54*:1–51.

356. Brown, A. G. (1981). The terminations of cutaneous nerve fibres in the spinal cord. *Trends Neurosci. 4*:64–67.

357. Conradi, S., Cullheim, S., Gollvik, L., and Kellerth, J.-O. (1983). Electron microscopic observations on the synaptic contacts of group Ia muscle spindle afferents in the cat lumbosacral spinal cord. *Brain Res. 265*:31–39.

358. Fyffe, R. E. W., and Light, A. R. (1984). The ultrastructure of group Ia afferent fiber synapses in the lumbosacral spinal cord of the cat. *Brain Res.* in press.

4
SYNAPTIC CONNECTIVITY
IN THE SPINAL DORSAL HORN

Miklós Réthelyi *Semmelweis University Medical School, Budapest, Hungary*

I. DEFINITION OF THE DORSAL HORN

In the classic descriptions (1,2) the spinal gray matter has been divided into three main regions: dorsal horn (Hinterhorn, corne postérieure), ventral horn (Vorderhorn, corne antérieure), and intermediate zone (pars intermedia, substance grise intermédiaire). No special effort was exerted to set clear borders between these regions. With the introduction of the laminar arrangement of perikarya (3,4) the dorsal horn in the cat became spontaneously defined as laminae I through VI, that is, the entire outbulging of the gray matter in the dorsal direction. The renaissance of the Golgi technique, which started in the 1960s, and the introduction of geometric shapes and analogies into the analysis of the neuropil initiated a basically new concept in the structure of the spinal gray matter. Golgi-Kopsch–impregnated spinal cord sections of adult cats revealed that the spinal gray matter consists of two rodlike structures on the two sides of the central canal [central core (5,6,7)], surrounded by the "appendages," that is, dorsal, lateral, and ventral horns (Fig. 1). The whole arrangement is reminiscent of the composite pillars of Gothic churches from the twelfth and thirteenth centuries.

The unequivocal separation of the central core from the appendages is manifest in the difference of the main orientation pattern of the neuropil. This

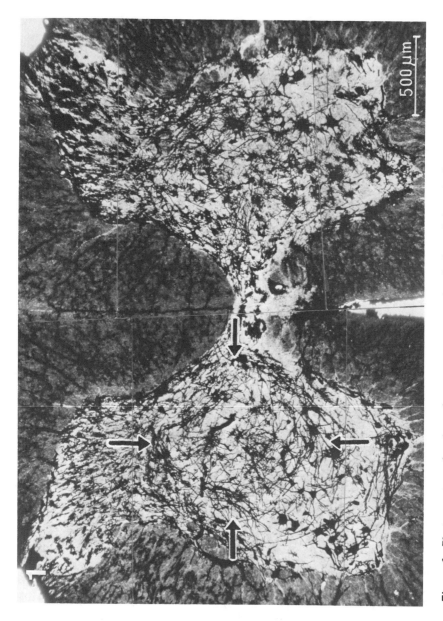

Figure 1 Photomontage showing a low-power cross-sectional view of the spinal gray matter at segment L5. The central core (indicated by arrows at left) is easily visualized on both sides. Golgi–Kopsch stain, adult cat. (From Ref. 5.)

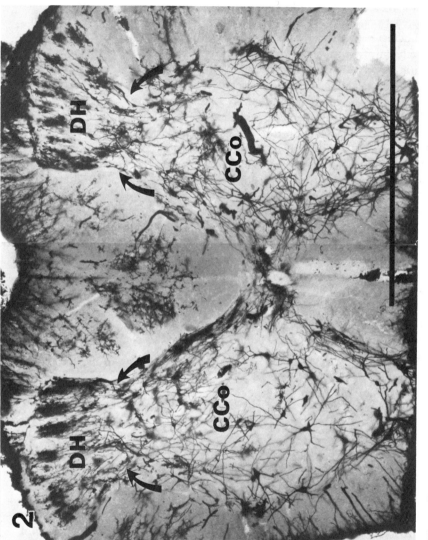

Figure 2 Low-power photomontage showing a cross section of the spinal cord of the rat: upper thoracic region. Arrows point to the transitional zone between the dorsal horn (DH) and the central core (CCo). Golgi–Kopsch impregnation. Scale: 1 mm.

was clearly shown first by Scheibel and Scheibel (8) on sagittal Golgi sections prepared from the spinal cord of kittens. It turned out that the overwhelming longitudinal orientation of dendrites and terminal axon arborizations changes abruptly into a transverse and dorsoventral direction at the border between laminae IV and V. This separation line could be documented later in the dendritic tree distribution in the spinal cord of adult cats (5). The dorsally bent outline of the central core can be clearly seen also on transverse Golgi specimens prepared from the spinal cord of adult rats (Fig. 2). The distribution of dorsal root fibers following dorsal rhizotomy matches well with the orientation pattern of dendritic trees (9,10). This structural peculiarity of dendrites and axons, which has been confirmed repeatedly in the course of recent studies of horseradish peroxidase (HRP)-stained dorsal horn neurons and single dorsal root fibers (discussed later), suggested a definition of the dorsal horn to consist of laminae I through IV of Rexed (3). In this way, the dorsal horn is seen to form a coherent structural unit with neuronal circuitries subserving mechano-, thermo-, noci-, and visceroreceptive sensory mechanisms.

The dorsal horn consists of the marginal zone, substantia gelatinosa, and nucleus proprius (i.e., head and neck of the dorsal horn) of the classic literature. The extraction of laminae V and VI from the dorsal horn and their inclusion in the intermediate zone (central core) is harmonious with the participation of the neurons of these laminae in proprioceptive mechanisms (11). One has to admit, however, that functional properties of neurons show an admixture at the transition zone between the dorsal horn and the central core.

II. SURVEY OF CELLULAR AND FIBER STRUCTURE OF THE DORSAL HORN

Although the cellular and fiber arrangement of the dorsal horn will be covered fully in Chapter 2, a brief survey of the light microscopic structure of neuronal components would be necessary to correctly appreciate the synapses made and/or received by them. The drawings in Figure 3 represent the summary diagrams of several classic and recent contributions (12-25). With certain minor discrepancies, they may be applied to both cat and monkey spinal dorsal horn. The neuronal structure of human dorsal horn (26) appears to be more complicated, while the neuronal structure of the dorsal horn of rodents is less well described.

In the following description the neurons will be reviewed first because they form the framework of the dorsal horn. The empty spaces of the lattice of dendrites and perikarya are filled with axons and axon terminals: They will be discussed subsequently. The glial cells and their processes will be disregarded for practical reasons.

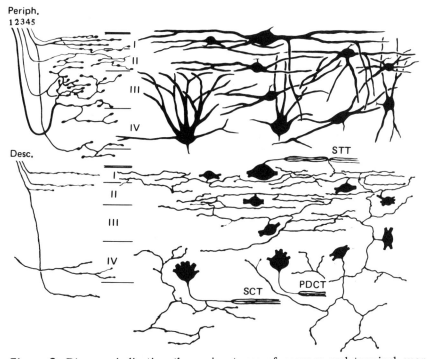

Figure 3 Diagram indicating the major types of neurons and terminal axon arborizations in the dorsal horn (laminae I–IV) in the sagittal plane. Upper left: Central branches of primary sensory neurons (Periph.). From left to right: 1. Coarse cutaneous myelinated fiber (Aβ) terminating in laminae III and IV. 2. Fine cutaneous myelinated fiber (Aδ) terminating in lamina III. 3. Unmyelinated C-fiber terminating in lamina II. 4. Fine cutaneous myelinated fiber (Aδ) terminating in lamina I and at the border of laminae IV and V. 5. Unmyelinated C-fiber terminating in lamina I. Upper right: Large-, medium-sized, and small neurons with their dendritic arborizations. Many dendrites are studded with irregular protrusions (omitted from the diagram). Lower left: Descending connections (Desc.). Corticospinal tract fibers terminate in lamina IV; medullospinal fibers terminate in laminae I and II as well as at the border between laminae IV and V. Lower right: Axon trajectories of the same neurons as shown above (dendrites are omitted). Ascending tract neurons are labeled STT: spinothalamic tract neuron; SCT: spinocervical tract neuron; PDCT: postsynaptic dorsal column tract neuron.

A. Neurons of the Dorsal Horn

The size of the perikarya in the dorsal horn represents a complete range from small to large neurons (8–45 μm in diameter). While small- and medium-sized perikarya occur ubiquitously, larger neurons prevail only in laminae I and IV.

1. Large Neurons in Lamina I

Large neurons (Waldeyer's cells, posteromarginal cells, Marginalzellen) occur scattered in lamina I or sometimes in the adjacent white matter. The far-reaching dendrites of these neurons are largely confined to lamina I, but some of the dendrites dip down to more ventral portions of the dorsal horn (1,8,13,20,27,28). Since large neurons in lamina I could be labeled by HRP from the contralateral thalamus in the cat and monkey (29), from the cerebellum in the rat, cat, and squirrel monkey (30), and from various spinal cord segments in the cat (31–34), they seem to establish long-distance connections.

2. Large Neurons in Lamina IV

Neurons with thick dendrites projecting predominantly dorsally are regular components of Golgi specimens prepared from the spinal cord of different experimental animals (1,8,13,18). Some of these neurons give off axons to the spinocervical tract (SCT) (35,36); others belong to the postsynaptic dorsal column tract (PDCT) (37). The distribution of the dendritic trees differs in these two groups of tract cells: the dendrites of the spinocervical tract neurons do not penetrate lamina II, those of the polysynaptic DCT neurons do (17,38).

3. Small- and Medium-sized Neurons

Small- and medium-sized neurons by far constitute the largest proportion of nerve cells in all parts of the dorsal horn. In laminae II and III they are the only cellular components. Neurons with longitudinally oriented quasi-symmetric dendritic arborizations represent the most familiar variety of small- and medium-sized cells. They occur mostly in lamina II (islet cells of Ramon y Cajal [1]), but similar neurons can be seen all over the dorsal horn (18,28). Another variety of medium-sized neurons has a fan-shaped dendritic tree, namely, the limitroph cells of Ramon y Cajal (1) at the border of laminae I and II and the antenna neurons in lamina III (10); the dorsoventrally oriented dendrites of these latter cells merge in lamina II. A third type of small neuron is the star-shaped cell (23). Some other dorsal horn neurons with small or medium-sized perkarya in laminae III and IV have perpendicularly oriented dendritic arborizations (39).

B. Fiber Architecture of the Dorsal Horn

Terminal axon arborizations of the dorsal horn originate from three main sources: dorsal root ganglia (central branches of primary sensory neurons), supraspinal centers (fibers of descending tracts), and spinal cord neurons (axons of short- and long-range propriospinal neurons). All these fibers generate elaborate terminal arborizations.

1. Termination Pattern of the Central Branches of Primary Sensory Neurons

Only a short summary will be presented here to emphasize the laminar arrangement of functionally different fibers (Fig. 3). A large variety of Aβ cutaneous mechanoreceptor fibers and mechanosensitive fine myelinated Aδ fibers terminate in laminae III and IV and to some extent also in the dorsal part of the central core region (38,40,41). Aδ nocireceptor fibers (high-threshold mechanoreceptor or mechanical nocireceptor fibers [42]) terminate partly in lamina I, in the adjacent portion of lamina II, and partly at the junction of the dorsal horn and central core. Additional termination areas of some of these latter fibers include a midline nucleus dorsal to the central canal and the contralateral lamina V (41). Several pieces of indirect evidence suggest that C-mechanoreceptor fibers terminate in the cat in the wider ventral portion of lamina II (43,44), while polymodal C-nocireceptor fibers seem to be arranged similarly as Aδ nocireceptor fibers (44). Morphologic analysis of the dorsal horn distribution of thermosensitive primary sensory neurons is still lacking. A considerable number of primary sensory neurons from the pelvic viscera contribute strictly to lamina I (45).

2. Sources of Propriospinal Connections

With the exception of some lamina I cells (31) the dorsal horn neurons do not participate in long-range propriospinal links (33,34). This means that large portions of the axon arborizations of small- and medium-sized neurons remain within the confines of the segment in which the perikarya are located (13-16, 46,47). In a manner similar to the dendritic organizational patterns, axon arborizations may be stretched either rostrocaudally or dorsoventrally. The rostrocaudal orientation characterizes the axon trees of neurons in laminae I through III, while the dorsoventral pattern occurs with neurons in laminae III and IV. Neurons with dorsoventrally oriented axon arborizations are good candidates to connect the dorsal horn to the central core because their axon trees often cross the border between laminae IV and V (16).

Another source of propriospinal connections is the local collaterals of ascending tract neurons. The best known are the initial arborizations of the axons of the spinocervical tract neurons (17,48), which form another kind of link between the dorsal horn and the central core.

3. Termination of Descending Tract Fibers in the Dorsal Horn

Beside a small fraction of corticospinal fibers that terminate in lamina IV (49, 50), the superficial laminae of the dorsal horn are the main targets of some descending medullospinal pathways (19,51). The single fiber studies of Light (25) revealed that some raphe-spinal descending axons give off collaterals in the superficial dorsal horn as they course toward the posterior commissure.

Corticospinal fibers originating from the forelimb representation area in the postcentral cortex of macaque were traced to the medial part of laminae I and II of the brachial spinal cord (51a).

III. SYNAPTOLOGY OF FUNCTIONALLY IDENTIFIED NEURONS

In contrast to Sec. II, the discussion of synaptic connections of dorsal horn neurons will start with the axons and proceed to the dendrites and perikarya.

This reversed order is more suitable to follow the sequence of impulse transmission through the synapses.

The dorsal horn, or parts of it (most frequently lamina II, or substantia gelatinosa), has been the subject of several ultrastructural analyses in the past 20 years (cat: 46,52,53; rat: 54,55; monkey: 56). Certain synaptologic features emerged from these studies (e.g., the lack of axosomatic synapses on small perikarya, the ubiquitous occurrence of glomerular synapses, the differential distribution of axon terminals with different synaptic and dense-core vesicles), but these investigations were plagued by the interwoven lattice of dendrites of several types of neurons.

The introduction of HRP labeling of functionally identified neurons (57–61) became a unique technique to assess the synaptic connections of individual neurons and to relate these connections to functional properties. In the spinal dorsal horn the technique has been especially successful because of the easy access to the main axonal input (i.e., dorsal root fibers), and especially difficult because of the small size of many perikarya.

In this review, the synaptic connections of the dorsal horn will be described on the basis of single neuron studies. This necessarily restricts the survey to the components so far analyzed, but the unequivocal nature of this kind of information yields a solid basis for further physiologic interpretations. Any new types of neurons or terminal axon arborizations to be studied in the future could be easily added to the existing charts. It is needless to stress that the ultrastructural analysis of HRP-stained, functionally identified neurons have not yielded any new kinds of profiles in the electron micrographs. Instead, these studies have made it possible to go back to the well-known ultrastructural descriptions of the dorsal horn, both at the spinal (52,53,56,62,63) and medullary levels (64), and to identify certain profiles and synaptic connections and to assign functional significance to them.

A. The Presynaptic Components of Synaptic Connections (Axon Terminals and Vesicle-Containing Dendrites)

Practically all kinds of cutaneous myelinated primary sensory fibers have been injected with HRP in the cat, and some types of fibers have also been injected with HRP in the monkey, but so far only a few of these fibers have been studied with the electron microscope.

1. Aβ Fibers

At present, little preliminary data have been published about the synaptic ultrastructure of thick cutaneous mechanoreceptor fibers. Ralston (65) described the terminations of HRP-labeled G-2 hair follicle afferent fibers synapsing on small- to medium-sized dendrites in the monkey dorsal horn. The large-sized HRP-labeled boutons occasionally received axoaxonic synapses from ovoid vesicle-containing (F-type) axon endings. Essentially similar synapses were found in connection with type I slowly adapting mechanoreceptor and Pacinian corpuscle afferent fibers in the cat lamina IV (66). Hair follicle afferent fibers with thick myelinated axons terminate in the cat dorsal horn with boutons containing circular synaptic vesicles 35-60 nm in diameter. The boutons form asymmetric axodendritic synapses (Fig. 4). Axon terminals containing ovoid synaptic vesicles form axoaxonic synapses with the primary endings (67).

Intra-axonally labeled Pacinian corpuscle afferent fibers and rapidly adapting afferent fibers from Krause corpuscles were found to synapse with one to three dendritic shafts and spines, and received axoaxonic synapses in the cat lumbosacral spinal cord. Additionally, the HRP-labeled boutons contacted profiles reminiscent of vesicle-containing dendrites. Synaptic arrangements by sensory fibers from Pacinian and Krause corpuscles are less complicated than glomerular complexes, but usually more complicated than terminations of hair follicle afferents (67a).

2. Aδ Fibers

The synaptic connections of two functionally different kinds of Aδ fibers were studied by Réthelyi et al. (68,69). One kind belonged to the sensitive D-hair follicle receptors (70), the other to the high-threshold mechanoreceptors [mechanical nocireceptors (42)]. As it was briefly described previously, the terminal axon arborizations of the two kinds of Aδ fibers terminate with multiple *en passant* and terminal boutons in separate regions of the dorsal horn and the adjacent parts of the central core. As a consequence of this arrangement, various types of Aδ fibers synapse with two different kinds of dorsal horn neurons. Only neurons with dorsoventrally oriented dendritic arborizations (e.g., polysynaptic dorsal column tract neurons) may be the joint targets of both low- and high-threshold fine myelinated primary afferent fibers.

The synaptic connections of D-hair follicle receptor fibers in lamina III consist of axon-spine, axodendritic, axoaxonic, and dendrodendritic synapses. These connections are arranged in synaptic glomeruli.

There is a large-sized (up to 5-6 μm in diameter) axon terminal that is densely filled with spherical synaptic vesicles and mitochondria in the center of the glomerulus: This is the *en passant* or terminal enlargement of the primary fiber. The large axon terminal is completely surrounded by smaller profiles, identified as dendritic spines, dendrites, and axons (Fig. 5). The dendrites and dendritic spines are postsynaptic, while the ovoid synaptic vesicle-containing small axon profiles are presynaptic to the primary axon terminals. Dendritic spines often contain pleomorphic synaptic vesicles and synapse with adjacent spines.

Fine myelinated high-threshold mechanoreceptor fibers have two different kinds of synaptic arrangements at their two termination fields in the cat and monkey: glomerular in the superficial region and nonglomerular at the transitional territory between the dorsal horn and the central core.

The glomeruli in lamina I [the terminal arborizations often reach the underlying narrow portion of lamina II, called outer region (71) or IIa (72)] include axon-spine, axodendritic, axoaxonic, dendroaxonic, and dendrodendritic synapses in the cat, and only axon-spine, axodendritic, and axoaxonic synapses

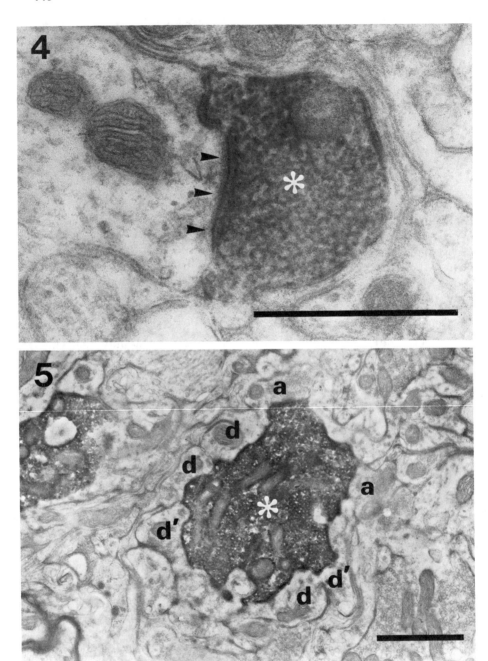

in the monkey. The central component of the glomerulus is the *en passant* or terminal bouton of a Aδ nocireceptor fiber. The surface of the bouton is contacted by groups of smaller neuronal processes (Fig. 6).

The primary axon terminals are presynaptic to dendrites and dendritic spines, and postsynaptic to small axon terminals containing ovoid synaptic vesicles and small- to medium-sized profiles that contain small clusters of pleomorphic synaptic vesicles. In some glomeruli these latter profiles, tentatively identified as vesicle-containing dendrites (53,64,73), synapse only with the primary axon terminal. In some other glomeruli these dendrites synapse with both the axon and one of the dendrites that is postsynaptic to the primary axon (Figs. 7A,B).

Occasionally, small *en passant* enlargements can also be seen along the arborizations of Aδ mechanical nocireceptor fibers. They appear to be small boutons filled with spherical synaptic vesicles. They synapse with dendritic shafts.

At the junction of the dorsal horn and central core the boutons of the myelinated mechanical nocireceptor fibers synapse with dendritic shafts or irregular dendritic appendages. They receive multiple axoaxonic synapses from small axon terminals.

Parallel to the lack of vesicle-containing dendrites in the monkey dorsal horn (56), synaptic glomeruli formed by fine myelinated nocireceptor fibers do not contain these kind of profiles (69). Axoaxonic synapses occurred more frequently in these glomeruli in the monkey than in the cat (Figs. 8A,B).

3. C-Fibers

Special fine-tip and high-resistance glass microelectrodes (74) and high-impedance electrometers (75) were necessary to impale fine myelinated fibers (41). Unmyelinated C-fibers, however, have been too fine in diameter to be impaled regularly using even the highest level of present-day sophistication in experimental technique.

Occasionally, the activity of single C-fibers can be recorded in the spinal cord of the monkey, and one such fiber has been stained with HRP (76). The parent fiber generated an elaborate arborization, mainly in lamina II (Fig. 9A),

---

Figure 4 Electron micrograph showing an HRP-labeled bouton (*) of a G–hair follicle receptor fiber synapsing with a dendritic shaft (arrowheads). Scale: 0.5 μm. (Courtesy of D. J. Maxwell.)

Figure 5 Low-power electron micrograph showing an HRP-labeled bouton (*) of a D–hair follicle receptor fiber. It is surrounded by the enlarged heads of dendritic protrusions (d), some of which contain pleomorphic synaptic vesicles (d'), and by axon terminals (a). Cat. Scale: 1 μm.

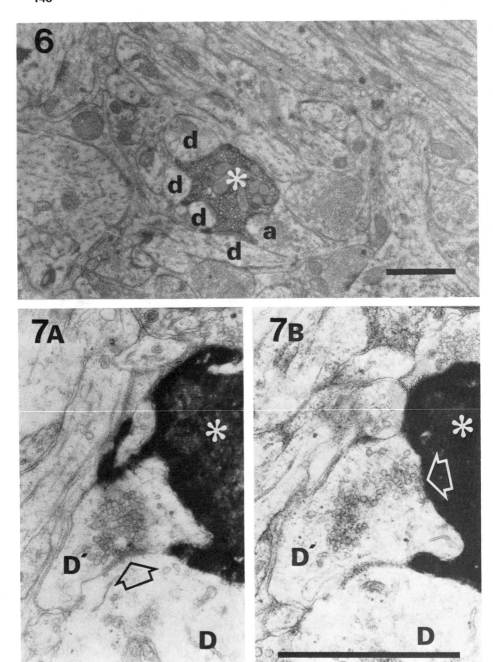

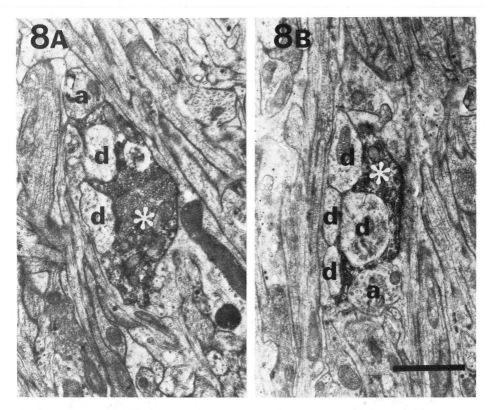

Figure 8 Low-power serial electron micrographs showing a bouton (*) of a myelinated high-threshold mechanoreceptor fiber. It is surrounded by dendritic protrusions (d) and axon terminals (a). Monkey. Scale: 1 μm.

Figure 6 Low-power electron micrograph showing an HRP-labeled bouton (*) of a myelinated high-threshold mechanoreceptor fiber. It is surrounded by dendritic protrusions (d) and by an axon terminal (a). Cat. Scale: 1 μm.

Figure 7 High-power serial electron micrographs showing the synaptic connections between an HRP-labeled bouton (*) of a myelinated high-threshold mechanoreceptor fiber, a dendritic shaft (D), and a vesicle-containing dendrite (D'). The latter is presynaptic to the dendritic shaft (arrow in A) and to the primary bouton (arrow in B). The synapse between the primary bouton and the dendritic shaft (D) takes place on subsequent sections of the series. Cat. Scale: 1 μm.

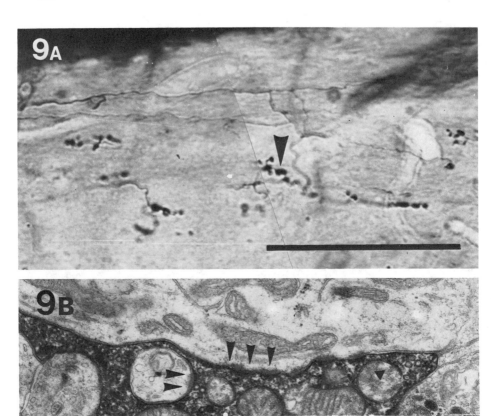

Figure 9 Light and electron microscopic demonstrations of the spinal cord termination of an HRP-labeled C-fiber. A: The fiber generates a longitudinal arborization in lamina I and in the outer part of lamina II. Large terminal and *en
passant* boutons can be seen at the end of the preterminal fibers. One of them
(arrowhead) is shown on B. Monkey, sagittal section. Scale: 100 μm. B: Electron

reminiscent of the presumed C-fiber axon trees seen in Golgi specimens prepared from cat spinal cord (43). Also, the size and distribution of *en passant* and terminal enlargements of the HRP-stained arborization were almost identical to the enlargements of the C-fibers in Golgi sections. Serial electron micrographs prepared from the boutons revealed that they contained spherical synaptic vesicles as well as dense-core vesicles. The boutons formed glomerular synaptic complexes with several dendrites and dendritic protrusions (Fig. 9B). Large-sized axon terminals filled with spherical and dense-core vesicles were found in direct apposition with the HRP-stained boutons. Symmetric desmosomelike specializations could be detected between the two boutons.

The individual boutons of the stained fiber showed similar synaptic organization all along the arborization. Unfortunately, the short duration of intracellular recording impeded the functional characterization of the fiber. The mere fact, however, that an unmyelinated primary afferent fiber could be impaled and successfully stained intracellularly with HRP forecasts the time when identification and histologic analysis of all kinds of primary afferent fibers will be a routine technique.

The axoaxonic attachments between the primary afferent boutons and other, apparently similar, axon terminals seem to suggest that the connections of unmyelinated primary afferent fibers differ in certain significant aspects from those of myelinated fibers.

4. Review of the Termination of Primary Afferent Fibers (Synaptic Glomeruli)

From the time of the first ultrastructural analyses of the spinal gray matter (52, 77) up to the most recent comprehensive reviews (e.g., 78) the synaptic glomeruli in the dorsal horn seemed to be the key structures to understand the impulse transmission of primary sensory neurons.

There is a general consensus that the large axon terminals in the center of the glomeruli correspond to enlargements of primary sensory fibers, and that the smaller profiles belong to dorsal horn neurons. Individual descriptions vary, however, in the interpretation of the origin of smaller profiles. Willis and Coggeshall (78) summarized the structural differences found by different authors in the construction of the glomeruli. To date, the ultrastructural analysis of functionally identified primary afferent fibers have revealed that synaptic glomeruli are formed predominantly around the boutons of both fine myelinated and

---

micrograph of one of the boutons (*) of the arborization (marked by arrowhead on A). It synapses with dendritic shafts and dendritic protrusions (arrowheads). A desmosomelike attachment (triangle) can be seen between the HRP-labeled and an unlabeled axon terminal (Ax). Both axons contain spherical synaptic and dense-core vesicles. Scale: 1 μm.

unmyelinated fibers. Coarse myelinated fibers tend to terminate with simple synapses. Furthermore, the components of the glomeruli and their synaptic interconnections vary according to the functional capacity of the primary sensory fiber.

In the glomeruli the activity of the primary afferent fibers is transmitted to several neurons, mainly through their dendritic protrusions, the shape of which permits sudden changes of ionic equilibrium of the dendritic membrane and the amplification of the postsynaptic potential (79). At nonglomerular synapses the primary afferent fibers synapse with the smooth surface of the dendritic shaft. Axoaxonic synapses seem to control the activity of the peripheral fibers in both cases, similar to other nonglomerular primary afferent axon terminals in the spinal cord (80,81). In the case of the fine myelinated Aδ nocireceptor fibers, the dendroaxonic synaptic connections are probably another component exerting presynaptic inhibitory control on some of the boutons of the arborization (but see Ref. 82). The dendrodendritic synapses between apparently identical dendritic protrusions in the glomeruli around D-hair follicle receptor fibers may enhance the synaptic efficacy of transmission from the the peripheral fiber to the second-order neuron.

Viewing the situation from the angle of the connectivity, the main difference between glomerular and nonglomerular terminations of fibers would mean quasi-linear versus divergent transmission between individual boutons and postsynaptic components. Functionally, this difference could be translated as synaptic connections assuring straightforward one neuron to few neurons, or the somewhat indistinct one neuron to several neurons projections. Tactile peripheral impulses arriving at the dorsal horn along the fast fibers are likely to be transmitted to a relatively small group of second-order neurons within the termination area of the fiber through axodendritic synapses. Similar kinds of impulses traveling along the slow (fine myelinated and unmyelinated) mechanoreceptor fibers arrive much later in the dorsal horn, and they seem to be transmitted to a larger number of neurons within the confines of the arborizations. Since only fine fibers carry the peripheral messages of both thermo- and nocireception (83–85), the extension of the previous reasoning would suggest that the first spinal analysis of these impulses is carried out by a relatively great number of neurons in a less straightforward way.

5. Termination of Intrinsic Axons

Figure 3 illustrates that the intrinsic axon terminals of the dorsal horn comprises *en passant* and terminal boutons of segmental interneurons that are located in laminae I through IV, and the local axon arborizations of ascending tract neurons. There is one published report in which Gobel et al. (86) demonstrated the synaptic connections of three substantia gelatinosa neurons in the cat. They have found that axon endings of islet cells contain oval and flattened synaptic vesicles. Of the two reported endings, one synapsed with a dendritic shaft, another with a spine. The axon endings of the observed stalked (limitroph) neuron contained dense-core as well as spherical and ovoid synaptic vesicles.

In collaboration with Perl and Light, we have been studying the synaptology of functionally identified dorsal horn neurons (87,88). The axon arborizations of dorsal horn interneurons, irrespective of the dominant peripheral input to the neuron, have several small enlargements (0.1–0.5 μm in diameter) that are densely packed with spherical or somewhat flattened synaptic vesicles and few dense-core vesicles. The enlargements formed simple axodendritic synapses with small- or large-caliber dendritic profiles. Often, the bouton considerably surrounded the postsynaptic profile (Figs. 10A,B). No evidence has

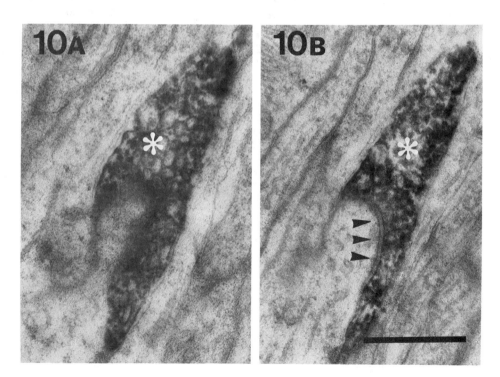

Figure 10 High-power serial electron micrographs showing an *en passant* bouton (*) from the axon arborization of a lamina I islet cell. The postsynaptic component is a fine dendrite, although it could be misinterpreted as a dendritic spine if only a single section of the series (A) were seen. Arrowheads mark the synaptic connection. Cat. Scale: 0.5 μm.

been found to indicate the participation of the axon terminals found in our studies in axoaxonic synapses.

Another source of intrinsic axon terminals in the dorsal horn comes from the local collateral arborizations of ascending tract neurons. We have described an axon of a Waldeyer cell issuing a local collateral to lamina I (88). More complete information, including ultrastructural analysis, is available about the local boutons of two HRP-labeled spinocervical tract neurons (48,89). The local collaterals are distributed over laminae IV and V. Four fifths of the boutons with diameters of 1.0–1.5 μm synapse on dendritic shafts (rarely on protrusions); the remaining one fifth synapse on perikarya (rarely on somatic spines). In the axodendritic synapses the axon often halfway surrounds the dendrite. The boutons do not participate in axoaxonic or dendroaxonic synapses. The boutons in axodendritic synapses contact mainly one dendrite, rarely two, and occasionally three. In the axosomatic synapses the soma is the only postsynaptic structure. Eighty to 90% of the boutons proved to be *en passant* enlargements; the higher figure refers to the axosomatic synapses.

The synaptic vesicles are spherical or slightly ovoid. Sophisticated quantitative analysis revealed statistically significant differences in the appearance of synaptic vesicles in the enlargements belonging to the two spinocervical tract neurons (90).

6. Synapses Made by Descending Fibers

Light (25) described the dorsal horn termination of descending fibers originating from the rostral medulla of the cat. Out of a larger series six descending fibers were reported to issue collaterals to lamina I and the outer portion of lamina II along their course to laminae V and X. These fibers could be orthodromically activated from the most rostral extent of the nucleus raphe magnus. The larger part of medullary descending fibers in Light's study terminated in the central core region without issuing any collateral branches to the dorsal horn.

The ultrastructural analysis of the HRP-stained descending raphe-spinal fibers showed enlarged (0.8–1.0 μm) portions of the fibers that were filled with round or oval synaptic vesicles and occasional dense-core vesicles. They synapsed on both large and small dendritic shafts (25).

7. Vesicle-Containing Dendrites as Presynaptic Components in the Dorsal Horn

Several ultrastructural studies indicated the occurrence of vesicle-containing dendrites in the dorsal horn neuropil of the cat (53,73), in contrast to the monkey (56). They also seem to represent regularly occurring components in the synaptic glomeruli of the medullary substantia gelatinosa (64). Vesicle-containing dendrites were mentioned previously (Sec. III.A) in connection with glomerular synapses of primary sensory neurons. Further observations on functionally identified and HRP-labeled dorsal horn neurons (87,88) suggested that

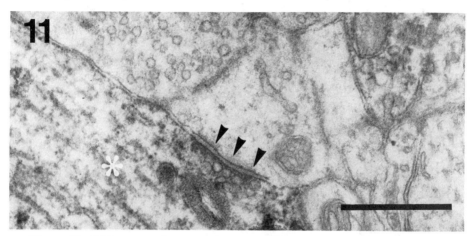

Figure 11 High-power electron micrograph showing a portion of a dendritic shaft (*) of an HRP-labeled lamina II islet cell. It contains a small cluster of spherical synaptic vesicles and a dense-core vesicle, and synapses with an adjacent dendritic profile (arrowheads). Cat. Scale: 0.5 μm.

the vesicle-containing dendritic processes in the glomeruli of D–hair follicle afferent fibers belong to mechanosensitive interneurons of laminae II and III. Synaptic vesicles appear in the dendritic shafts of neurons with similar functional properties (Fig. 11; Ref. 91), a finding consistent with the observations of Gobel et al. (86). Synaptic membrane specializations were seen between adjacent dendrites at these sites.

No direct evidence is available about the origin of vesicle-containing dendritic processes establishing dendroaxonic synapses in the glomeruli around the axon enlargements of myelinated mechanical nocireceptor fibers.

B. The Postsynaptic Components of Synaptic Connections (Perikarya and Dendrites)

Of the neuronal population of the dorsal horn two kinds of large-sized neurons, Waldeyer cells in lamina I and the spinocervical tract neurons in lamina IV, can be described separately, while the rest of the neurons (small and medium-sized cells distributed over the entire dorsal horn) will be treated jointly.

1. Waldeyer Cells

Two neurons with large perikarya have been seen in lamina I in our studies on HRP labeling of functionally identified neurons in the dorsal horn (88). Their

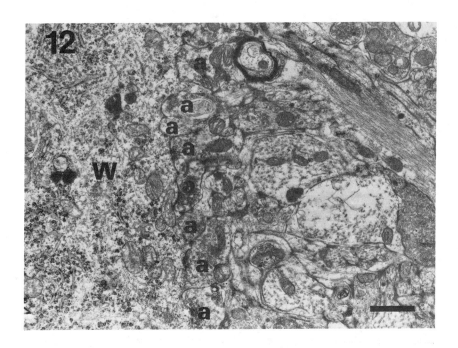

Figure 12 Low-power electron micrograph showing detail from an HRP-labeled Waldeyer cell (W). A large number of small axon terminals (a) synapse with the neuron. Cat. Scale: 1 μm.

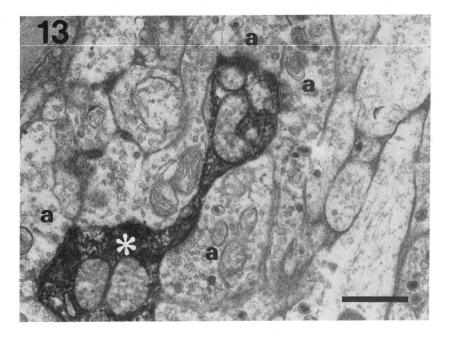

widespread dendrites were mostly also confined to lamina I. Some dendritic branches could be traced toward the intermediate zone of the spinal gray matter (central core), following the lateral curvature of lamina I.

With the exception of the aforementioned features, the two neurons varied remarkably in dendritic structure and synaptic connections. The smooth dendrites and the perikaryon of one of them were uninterruptedly covered with small axon terminals that contained either spherical or ovoid synaptic vesicles (Fig. 12). Both the dendritic shafts and the long, irregular dendritic protrusions of the other neuron were contacted by axon terminals. A type of large-sized boutons that were loosely filled with spherical synaptic and dense-core vesicles prevailed among the axon terminals (Fig. 13). The perikaryon of this latter neuron possessed an elaborate system of somatic protrusions that represented postsynaptic sites.

2. Spinocervical Tract Cells

Functionally identified and HRP-labeled spinocervical tract neurons in cat spinal cord were recently studied with the electron microscope by Maxwell et al. (92). They described two types of synaptic boutons that contacted the soma and dendrites of the neurons: One type contained round, clear synaptic vesicles, and another type flattened synaptic vesicles. Boutons with round vesicles occurred more frequently (63%) than those with flattened vesicles (37%). The boutons varied with the morphology of the synaptic contacts (asymmetric for boutons with round vesicles and symmetric for those with flattened vesicles) and in their distribution (boutons with flattened vesicles were preferentially located on proximal dendrites). It has been presumed that some of the boutons with round synaptic vesicles may belong to hair follicle afferent fibers. Both physiologic data (93) and the ultrastructure of the axon enlargements (67) make this assumption tenable. The origin of the boutons with flattened synaptic vesicles is unknown. They may be the substrate for the postsynaptic inhibition that is regularly exerted on spinocervical tract neurons (94).

3. Small- and Medium-Sized Neurons in the Dorsal Horn

Neurons in the dorsal horn with small perikarya vary morphologically in the orientation of the dendritic arborizations (Fig. 3). Physiologically, they differ in the origin of the dominant peripheral input. Thus, a dorsal horn neuron may function as a mechanoreceptive, thermoreceptive, or nocireceptive second-order

---

Figure 13 Electron micrograph showing a protrusion (*) of an HRP-labeled Waldeyer cell (different from that shown in Figure 12). The protrusion receives several synaptic connections from axon terminals (a) of similar vesicle content. Cat. Scale: 1 μm.

neuron, or various sensory modalities may converge on it. (The functional classification of dorsal horn neurons has been reviewed thoroughly recently [78].)

Gobel et al. (86) studied the afferent synaptic connections of two islet cells and one limitroph cell in the substantia gelatinosa of the cat (lumbar region). In their descriptions islet cells have no or few axosomatic synapses. Large scalloped axon endings as well as three kinds of simple axon endings that terminate on dendritic spines and shafts provide the afferent impulses to the neurons. As was mentioned earlier, dendrites and dendritic spines of islet cells contain clusters of synaptic vesicles and enter dendrodendritic and dendroaxonic connections. The stalked (limitroph) cell showed somewhat more axosomatic synapses than the perkarya of islet cells did. The major synaptic input on the dendritic spines are the scalloped endings. Simple axodendritic synapses occurred infrequently. Stalked cells received dendrodendritic synapses, probably from the dendrites of islet cells.

The synaptologic analysis of 14 small- to medium-sized functionally identified dorsal horn neurons in the caudal spinal cord of the cat permitted us (87,88, 91) to study the afferent synaptic connections of the neurons on a larger sample, and to come to a preliminary level of generalization.

Functionally, the neurons were classified as nocireceptive or mechanoreceptive, depending on their dominant peripheral input (the functional characterizations of the neurons have been described in previous publications [95-97]). At the light microscopic level the neurons fell into several categories based upon the orientation pattern of the dendritic arborization.

The perikarya of the neurons are generally devoid of synaptic onnections (Fig. 14), yet one nocireceptive and one mechanoreceptive neuron displayed numerous axosomatic synapses. The small-sized axon terminals contained flattened synaptic vesicles (Fig. 15).

All but one neuron had dendrites richly studded with irregular protrusions. They were found to invariably represent postsynaptic sites. In contrast to the findings of others (82), large-sized axon terminals, that formed synaptic glomeruli (scalloped enlargements) and simple boutons synapsed equally with the dendritic protrusions. Parallel with the structural diversity of the glomeruli found in various laminae, the dendritic protrusions participated in various types of glomeruli. In lamina I the glomerulus with one or more dendritic protrusions of HRP-stained nocireceptive neurons resembled those found at the end of fine myelinated mechanical nocireceptor fibers (Fig. 16). In the middle of lamina II the dendritic protrusions of some mechanoreceptive neurons joined the classic substantia gelatinosa glomeruli (46,52,54,55,64; Fig. 17). At the border of laminae II and III the dendritic protrusions and, occasionally, dendritic shafts participated in a third type of glomeruli that comprised numerous axoaxonic synapses (Fig. 18). On the other hand, dendritic protrusions all over the dorsal horn might be contacted by simple axon terminals that contained spherical

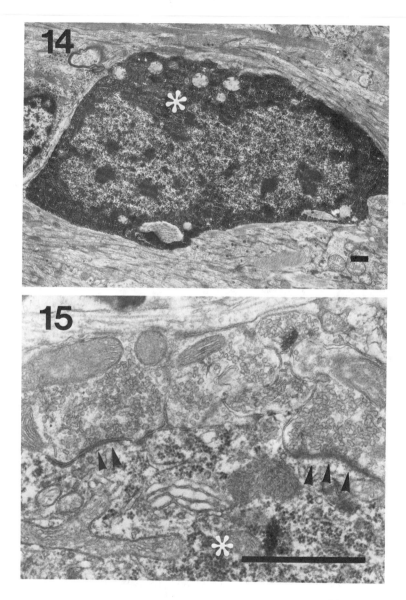

Figure 14 Low-power electron micrograph showing the perikaryon (*) of an HRP-stained lamina I islet cell. Cat. Scale: 1 μm.

Figure 15 Electron micrograph showing a detail from the perikaryon (*) of an HRP-labeled lamina III islet cell. Axon terminals containing flattened vesicles synapse with the perikaryon (arrowheads). Cat. Scale: 1 μm.

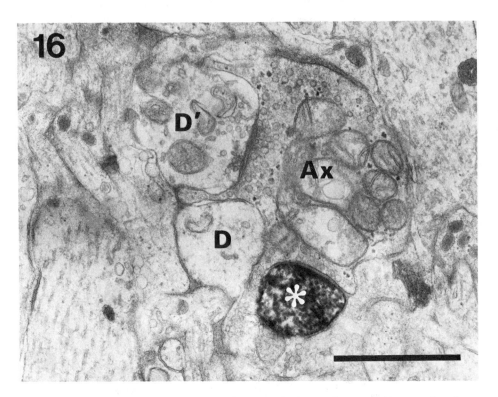

Figure 16 Electron micrograph showing a glomerular synaptic complex in lamina I. An unlabeled axon terminal (Ax) synapses on a vesicle-containing dendrite (D′), and two other dendritic protrusions. One of which (*) is HRP-labeled and belongs to a lamina I islet cell. The other (D) is unlabeled. The synaptic connection between the axon and this latter protrusion is seen on another section of the series. Cat. Scale: 1 µm.

synaptic vesicles (Figs. 19A,B). Occasionally, the long neck of the protrusion was the target of synapsing axon endings.

Dendritic shafts were covered to a variable extent with boutons that contained various kinds of synaptic vesicles. An almost complete cuff of axon terminals surrounded the vertically oriented dendrites of some of the lamina III neurons (Fig. 20).

As was mentioned previously, some mechanoreceptive neurons contained synaptic vesicles in their dendritic tree, some did not. Also, some of the nocireceptive neurons received dendrodendritic synapses (Figs. 21A,B), some did not.

The limited sample of small- and medium-sized dorsal horn neurons studied with the aid of intracellular injection of HRP furnished one important conclusion:

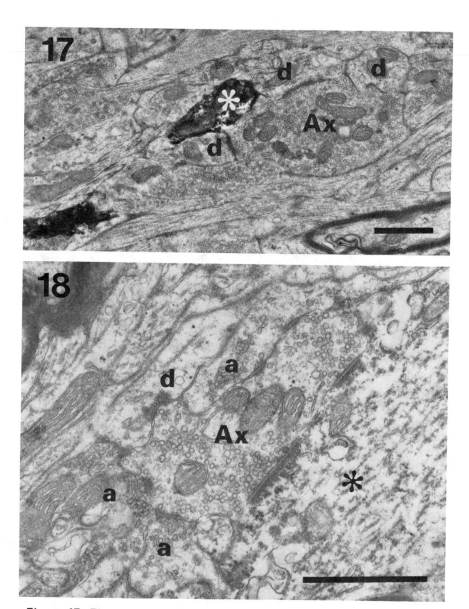

Figure 17 Electron micrograph showing a glomerular synaptic complex in lamina II. An unlabeled axon terminal (Ax) synapses with several dendritic protrusions (d), one of which (*) belongs to an HRP-labeled lamina II islet cell. A portion of the dendritic shaft from which the protrusion emanated is seen in the lower left corner. Cat. Scale: 1 μm.

Figure 18 Electron micrograph showing a glomerular synaptic complex in lamina III. The unlabeled axon terminal (Ax) synapses with a thick dendrite (*) of a lamina III islet cell and with an unlabeled small dendritic profile (d). Several small axon terminals (a) are presynaptic to the large bouton. Cat. Scale: 1 μm.

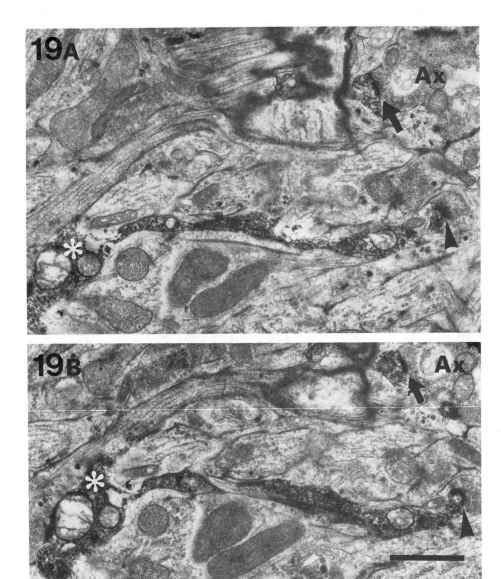

Figure 19 Serial electron micrographs showing details of the dendritic arborization of a limitroph cell. The asterisk marks a portion of a dorsoventrally oriented dendrite in lamina II. The fine terminal dilatation of a long protrusion receives a synapse from an axon enlargement (arrowheads in A and B), while the head of another protrusion is a postsynaptic component of a classic lamina II glomerulus (arrows in A and B). Cat. Scale: 1 μm.

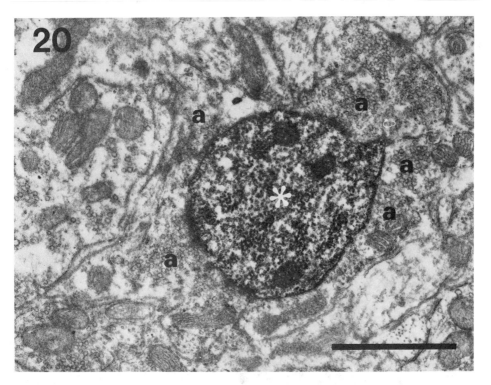

Figure 20 Electron micrograph showing a dendritic cross section (*) of an HRP-labeled lamina III neuron with vertically oriented dendritic arborization. The dendrite is covered by several synapsing axon terminals (a). Cat. Scale: 1 μm.

These neurons are different from each other in their afferent synaptic connections. As will be described in detail (91), neurons of identical functional features and similar morphologic appearance differ enormously in the distribution of various kinds of synapsing axon terminals along the somatodendritic regions. As a corollary of this statement, certain synaptic connections occur repeatedly along the dendritic branches of one neuron, while others were not seen even after observing a large number of ultrasections. The best example to illustrate this observation has been provided by HRP-stained neurons, the dendrites of which were distributed in lamina II. Of the 10 neurons of this subgroup, the dendrites of only three were seen to be arranged in the classic synaptic glomeruli of this lamina.

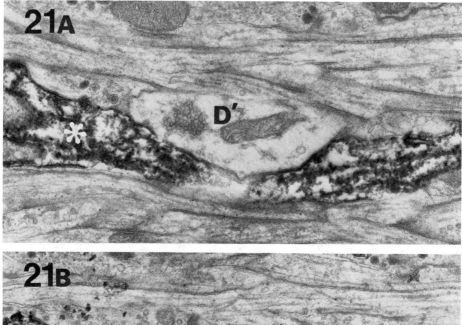

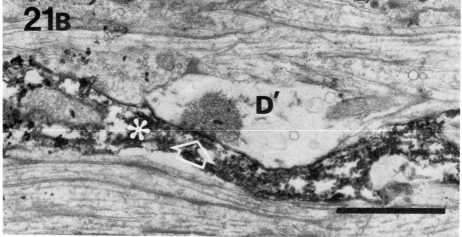

Figure 21 Serial electron micrographs showing a dendrodendritic synapse (arrow) between an unidentified dendritic profile (D′, presynaptic component) and the dendrite (*) of a nocireceptor specific limitroph cell. Cat. Scale: 1 μm.

IV. INTERNEURONAL CONNECTIONS IN THE DORSAL HORN

Neuronal circuits in the dorsal horn start with the primary sensory neurons. Their impulses are eventually transmitted to long ascending tract neurons, either directly or indirectly through one or several interneurons. The activity of spinal inhibitory neurons and that of descending tracts may influence the flow of impulses along this chain of neurons at various locations. In addition, connections to spinal reflex centers may branch off from various components of the circuits.

The neuronal networks of the dorsal horn are responsible for the initial analysis and processing of sensory impulses from cutaneous mechano-, thermo-, and nocireceptors (83-85). Furthermore, a large portion of visceral afferent fibers (45) and high-threshold mechanoreceptor fibers from deep structures (muscles, tendons, fasciae, joint capsules) terminate mainly in the superficial regions of the dorsal horn (98).

The differential distribution of primary sensory fibers of various receptor characteristics and that of dorsal horn neurons responding to various kinds of peripheral stimulation (21,22,95-97,99) indicate that in the cat and to some extent in the monkey the narrower superficial portion of the dorsal horn (lamina I and outer region of lamina II) incorporates thermo-, noci-, and visceroreceptive neuronal circuits. Consequently, neurons that form mechanoreceptive circuits are confined to the larger ventral portion of the dorsal horn (inner region of lamina II, laminae III and IV). Neurons receiving a convergence of mechano-, thermo-, and nocireceptive impulses can also be found in the dorsal horn, but their preferential location is lamina V, that is, the transition zone between the dorsal horn and the central core or the central core itself (see Ref. 78).

To date, not enough ultrastructural data are available to devise elaborate circuits for the various functional attributes of the dorsal horn. Certain aspects of the neuronal interconnections emerge, however, from the single neuron HRP studies and from the electron microscopic immunohistochemical detection of various transmitters or modulator substances in axon terminals.

The forwarding of peripheral messages to the second-order neurons, be they interneurons or tract neurons, seems to be determined primarily by the location and arborization pattern of primary afferent fibers, and by other orientational principles of the dorsal horn neuropil. Since predominantly the ultrastructural aspects of the dorsal horn synaptology has been covered in this chapter, these aspects of the circuits will not be detailed further. A hypothesis emphasizing the functional significance of glomerular versus nonglomerular termination of various classes of primary sensory fibers has been given earlier.

An important problem in the dorsal horn circuits is the position of the inhibitory interneurons included in the networks. Unexpectedly, each fine axon ending of HRP-stained functionally identified neurons in our sample (91) contained spherical or slightly ovoid synaptic vesicles. In contrast, the islet cells in the substantia gelatinosa (86) possessed axon terminals with oval or flattened synaptic vesicles that conformed to the suggested inhibitory character of similar neurons in the medullary substantia gelatinosa (100). However, unconditional application of Uchizono's observation (101) in the functional interpretation of axon terminals in the spinal gray matter appears to be hazardous. Rastad (102)

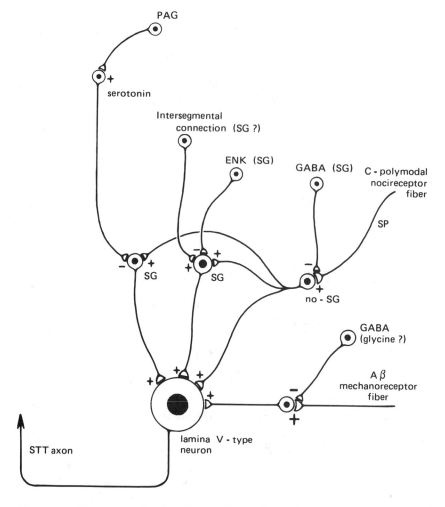

Figure 22 Diagram indicating the position of dorsal horn neurons in a hypothetic circuit between a C–polymodal nocireceptor fiber and lamina V–type
neuron. The neuronal connections are based on physiologic and pharmacologic observations (see text). The activity of the C-fiber is inhibited presynaptically by GABA-ergic neurons (GABA). The C-fiber terminates on interneurons,
which excite the lamina V–type neuron, either directly or indirectly through
other interneurons. The segmental enkephalinergic neurons (see Ref. 134)
inhibit one group of these interneurons, while the descending serotoninergic
fibers inhibit another group. The perikarya of the descending serotonergic
neurons in the raphe nuclei receive excitatory connection from neurons of the
mesencephalic periaqueductal gray (PAG) matter (135). Also facilitatory short
intersegmental neurons of the dorsal horn may connect to the groups of

showed recently that the physiologically identified Ia inhibitory interneurons in lamina VII had local axon enlargements with spherical or slightly ovoid synaptic vesicles. This is all the more interesting because there are a great number of flattened vesicle-containing axon terminals in the ventral horn (80,103). In this analogy, some of the HRP-stained dorsal horn neurons may be inhibitory.

The weight of presynaptic versus postsynaptic inhibition in the spinal cord, and in a more restricted sense in the sensory pathways, was measured in several review articles (104-106). The almost ubiquitous occurrence of small-sized axon terminals that synapsed on the boutons of primary afferent fibers (not necessarily on all boutons of the arborization of a given fiber) offers a reliable structural basis for presynaptic inhibition as it was proposed by Eccles (107) and Gray (108). Immunohistochemical studies indicated that in the rat small axon terminals (or one group of them) in axoaxonic contact with the primary afferent boutons contain glutamic acid decarboxylase (GAD), the enzyme mediating the synthesis of γ-aminobutyric acid (GABA) from glutamic acid (109,110). Similarly, small-sized axon terminals could be labeled by tritiated GABA in the rat (111). The perikarya of these GABA-ergic neurons are located in laminae II and III (110). It is tempting to consider these axoaxonic synapses as the morphologic substrate for segmental (or afferent) inhibition of peripheral impulses (104,112,113).

A number of studies disclosed that noxious heat- or C-fiber–evoked activity of lamina V–type convergent neurons (11) could be suppressed by opioids that act at the spinal level (114-117), or by stimulation of descending brain stem pathways (118-121). The activity of dorsal horn units was increased also by the administration of the opioid antagonist naloxone (122,123). Consequently, parenteral administration of naloxone lowered the threshold of the hot-plate and tail-flick tests in rats (124). The diagram in Figure 22 shows hypothetic connections between a C-polymodal nocireceptor fiber (a fiber with noxious heat-sensitive receptors) and a lamina V–type neuron. Although this latter neuron is outside the dorsal horn, physiologic and pharmacologic studies hinted that the activity of the primary fiber is relayed through groups of dorsal horn interneurons (114,115,125,126).

---

interneurons on which the inhibitory influences are manifested. Many of the neurons shown on the diagram are located in the substantia gelatinosa (SG) or less strictly speaking, are identical to the small- and medium-sized neurons of the dorsal horn. The lamina V–type neuron receives another peripheral input from an Aβ mechanoreceptor fiber through interneurons. GABA- or glycine-containing inhibitory neurons are effective at the central end of the primary afferent fiber. The axon of the lamina V–type neuron contribute to the spino-thalamic tract (STT). +, excitatory synaptic connections; –, inhibitory synaptic connections.

It is very probable that C-polymodal nocireceptor fibers contain substance P (127). The segmental presynaptic inhibition mediated by GABA-ergic neurons seems to operate at the spinal cord termination of the primary sensory neuron (125,128). The C-fiber synapses on substance P-sensitive interneurons that are apparently outside the confines of the substantia gelatinosa (114). These interneurons connect directly or indirectly through further interneurons to the lamina V-type neuron. It is not unlikely that both segmental enkephalinergic and descending serotoninergic inhibition is effective through these interneurons, as shown schematically in Figure 22.

Direct connections between enkephalinergic as well as serotoninergic fibers and lamina V-type neurons is improbable because the sensitive mechano-receptors' induced activity of the neurons is unaffected during opioid adminis-tration or during the stimulation of descending pathways (but see 129). A pre-synaptic type of inhibition (i.e., inhibitory axon terminals synapsing with the primary afferent terminals) could be ruled out because of the prevailing axo-dendritic synapses made by both enkephalinergic and serotoninergic terminals (130,131).

It has also been suggested that the segmental opioid and descending sero-toninergic inhibition operates on two distinct neuronal subsystems of the dorsal horn (125,132). None of these subsystems appears to be active during segmental inhibition (115,128).

All these physiologic and pharmacologic implications require an extensive population of interneurons in the dorsal horn. Since each neuron seems to have an individual position in various subsystems (in addition to inhibitory circuits; also, facilitatory connections have been reported through axons of Lissauer's tract; 133), the large diversity of synaptic connections found on the dorsal horn neurons may furnish an adequate structural basis for the diverse functional roles.

V. ACKNOWLEDGMENTS

This work was supported by a cooperative research program sponsored by the Hungarian Academy of Sciences and the United States National Science Founda-tion, and by grant NS10321 and facilities provided by grant NS14899 from the National Institute of Neurological and Communicative Disorders and Stroke of the United States Public Health Service.

REFERENCES

1.   Ramon y Cajal, S. (1909). *Histologie du Système Nerveux de l'Homme et des Vertébrés*, vol. I, Maloine, Paris.
2.   Bok, S. T. (1928). Das Rückenmark. In *Handbuch der mikroskopischen Ana-tomie des Menschen*, Bd. IV, Teil I, W. Möllendorf (Ed.), Springer, Berlin.

3. Rexed, B. (1954). A cytoarchitectonic atlas of the spinal cord in the cat. *J. Comp. Neurol. 100*:297-379.

4. Rexed, B. (1952). The cytoarchitectonic organization of the spinal cord in the cat. *J. Comp. Neurol. 96*:415-495.

5. Réthelyi, M. (1976). Central core in the spinal gray matter. *Acta Morph. Acad. Sci. Hung. 24*:63-70.

6. Réthelyi, M. (1981). Geometry of the dorsal horn. In *Spinal Cord Sensation*, A. G. Brown and M. Réthelyi (Eds.), Scottish Academic Press, Edinburgh, pp. 1-11.

7. Szentágothai, J. and Réthelyi, M. Cyto- and neuropil architecture of the spinal cord. In *New Developments in Electromyography and Clinical Neurophysiology*, vol. III, J. E. Desmedt (Ed.), Karger, Basel, pp. 20-37.

8. Scheibel, M. E., and Scheibel, A. B. (1968). Terminal axonal patterns in cat spinal cord. II. The dorsal horn. *Brain Res. 9*:32-58.

9. Sterling, P., and Kuypers, H. G. J. M. (1967). Anatomical organization of the brachial spinal cord of the cat. I. The distribution of dorsal root fibers. *Brain Res. 4*:1-15.

10. Réthelyi and Szentágothai, J. (1973). Distribution and connections of afferent fibers in the spinal cord. In *Handbook of Sensory Physiology*, vol. II, A. Iggo (Ed.), Springer, New York, pp. 237-252.

11. Wall, P. D. (1967). The laminar organization of dorsal horn and effects of descending impulses. *J. Physiol. (Lond.) 188*:403-423.

12. Pearson, A. A. (1952). Role of gelatinous substance of spinal cord in conduction of pain. *Arch. Neurol. Psychiatr. 68*:515-529.

13. Szentágothai, J. (1964). Neuronal and synaptic arrangement in the substantia gelatinosa Rolandi. *J. Comp. Neurol. 122*:219-240.

14. Mannen, H., and Sugiura, Y. (1976). Reconstruction of neurons of dorsal horn proper using Golgi stained serial sections. *J. Comp. Neurol. 168*: 303-312.

15. Sugiura, Y. (1975). Three dimensional analysis of neurons in the substantia gelatinosa Rolandi. *Proc. Jap. Acad. 51*:336-341.

16. Matsushita, M. (1969). Some aspects of the interneuronal connections in cat's spinal gray matter. *J. Comp. Neurol. 136*:57-80.

17. Brown, A. G., Rose, P. K., and Snow, P. J. (1977). The morphology of spinocervical tract neurones revealed by intracellular injection of horseradish peroxidase. *J. Physiol. (Lond.) 270*:747-764.

18. Beal, J. A., and Cooper, M. H. (1978). The neurons in the gelatinosal complex (laminae II and III) of the monkey (Macaca mulatta): A Golgi study. *J. Comp. Neurol. 179*:89-121.

19. Basbaum, A. I., Clanton, C. H., and Fields, H. L. (1978). Three bulbospinal pathways from the rostral medulla of the cat: An autoradiographic study of pain modulating systems. *J. Comp. Neurol. 178*:209-224.

20. Beal, J. A. (1979). The ventral dendritic arbor of marginal (lamina I) neurons in the adult primate spinal cord. *Neurosci. Lett. 14*:201-206.

21. Price, D. D., Hayashi, H., Dubner, R., and Ruda, M. A. (1979). Functional relationships between neurons of marginal and substantia gelatinosa layers of primate dorsal horn. *J. Neurophysiol. 42*:1590-1608.

22.   Bennett, G. J., Abdelmoumen, M., Hayashi, H., and Dubner, R. (1980). Physiology and morphology of substantia gelatinosa neurons intracellularly stained with horseradish peroxidase. *J. Comp. Neurol. 194*: 809-827.

23.   Bicknell, H. R., and Beal, J. A. (1981). Star shaped neurons in the substantia gelatinosa of the adult cat spinal cord. *Neurosci. Lett. 22*: 37-41.

24.   Molony, V., Steedman, W. M., Cervero, F., and Iggo, A. (1981). Intracellular marking of identified neurones in the superficial dorsal horn of the cat spinal cord. *Q. J. Exp. Physiol. 66*:211-223.

25.   Light, A. R. (1982). Spinal projections of physiologically identified axons from the rostral medulla of cats. In *Proceedings of the IIIrd World Congress of Pain*, J. J. Bonica, U. Lindblom, and A. Iggo (Eds.), Raven, New York, pp. 373-379.

26.   Schoenen, J. (1980). *Organisation Neuronale de la Moelle Épinière de l'Homme*. Ph.D. dissertation, Université de Liège, Belgium, 353 pp.

27.   Waldeyer, H. (1888). Das Gorilla-Rückenmark. *Abhandlungen der Preussischen Akademie der Wissenschaften*, Berlin, pp. 1-147.

28.   Beal, J. A., Penny, J. E., and Bicknell, H. R. (1981). Structural diversity of marginal (lamina I) neurons in the adult monkey (Macaca mulatta) lumbospinal cord: A Golgi study. *J. Comp. Neurol. 202*:237-254.

29.   Trevino, D. L., and Carstens, E. (1975). Confirmation of the location of spinothalamic neurons in the cat and monkey by the retrograde transport of horseradish peroxidase. *Brain Res. 98*:177-182.

30.   Snyder, R. L., Faull, R. L. M., and Mehler, W. R. (1978). A comparative study of the neurons of origin of the spinocerebellar afferents in the rat, cat and squirrel monkey based on the retrograde transport of horseradish peroxidase. *J. Comp. Neurol. 181*:833-852.

31.   Burton, H., and Loewy, A. D. (1976). Descending projections from the marginal cell layer and other regions of the monkey spinal cord. *Brain Res. 116*:485-491.

32.   Matsushita, M., Hosoya, Y., and Ikeda, M. (1978). Anatomical organization of the spinocerebellar system in the cat, as studied by retrograde transport of horseradish peroxidase. *J. Comp. Neurol. 184*:81-105.

33.   Skinner, R. D., Coulter, J. D., Adams, R. J., and Remmel, R. S. (1979). Cells of origin of long descending propriospinal fibers connecting the spinal enlargements in cat and monkey determined by horseradish peroxidase and electrophysiological techniques. *J. Comp. Neurol. 188*:443-454.

34.   Molenaar, I., and Kuypers, H. G. J. M. (1978). Cells of origin of propriospinal fibers and of fibers ascending to supraspinal levels. A HRP study in cat and Rhesus monkey. *Brain Res. 152*:429-450.

35.   Craig, A. D. (1976). Spinocervical tract cells in cat and dog, labeled by the retrograde transport of horseradish peroxidase. *Neurosci. Lett. 3*:173-177.

36.   Brown, A. G., House, C. R., Rose, P. K., and Snow, P. J. (1976). The morphology of spinocervical tract neurones in the cat. *J. Physiol. (Lond.) 260*: 719-738.

37.   Rustioni, A., and Kaufman, A. B. (1977). Identification of cells of origin of non-primary afferents to the dorsal column nuclei of the cat. *Exp. Brain Res. 27*:1-14.

38. Brown, A. G. (1981). *Organization in the Spinal Cord*, Springer, New York.
39. Fyffe, R. E. W. (1981). Dendritic trees in dorsal horn cells. In *Spinal Cord Sensation*. A. G. Brown and M. Réthelyi (Eds.), Scottish Academic Press, Edinburgh, pp. 127–136.
40. Brown, A. G., Fyffe, R. E. W., Rose, P. K., and Snow, P. J. (1981). Spinal cord collaterals from axons of type II slowly adapting units in the cat. *J. Physiol. (Lond.) 316*:469–480.
41. Light, A. R., and Perl, E. R. (1979). Spinal termination of functionally identified primary afferent neurons with slowly conducting myelinated fibers. *J. Comp. Neurol. 186*:133–150.
42. Burgess, P. R., and Perl, E. R. (1967). Myelinated afferent fibers responding specifically to noxious stimulation of the skin. *J. Physiol. (Lond.) 190*:541–562.
43. Réthelyi, M. (1977). Preterminal and terminal axon arborizations in the substantia gelatinosa of cat's spinal cord. *J. Comp. Neurol. 172*:511–528.
44. Réthelyi, M. (1981). Anatomy of afferent terminals concerned with nocireception. In *Advances of Physiological Sciences*, vol. 16, E. Grastyán and P. Molnár (Eds.), Akadémiai Kiadó, Budapest, pp. 151–160.
45. Morgan, C., Nadelhaft, I., and DeGroat, W. C. (1981). The distribution of visceral primary afferents from the pelvic nerve to Lissauer's tract and the spinal gray matter and its relationship to the sacral parasympathetic nucleus. *J. Comp. Neurol. 201*:415–440.
46. Réthelyi, M., and Szentágothai, J. (1969). The large synaptic complexes of the substantia gelatinosa. *Exp. Brain Res. 7*:258–274.
47. Gobel, S. (1975). Golgi studies of the substantia gelatinosa neurons in the spinal trigeminal nucleus. *J. Comp. Neurol. 162*:397–416.
48. Rastad, J., Jankowska, E., and Westman, J. (1977). Arborization of initial axon collaterals of spinocervical tract cells stained intracellularly with horseradish peroxidase. *Brain Res. 135*:1–10.
49. Nyberg-Hansen, R., and Brodal, A. (1963). Sites of termination of corticospinal fibers in the cat. *J. Comp. Neurol. 120*:369–391.
50. Scheibel, M. E., and Scheibel, A. B. (1966). Terminal axonal patterns in cat spinal cord. I. The lateral corticospinal tract. *Brain Res. 2*:333–350.
51. Basbaum, A. I., and Fields, H. L. (1979). The origin of descending pathways in the dorsolateral funiculus of the spinal cord of the cat and rat: Further studies on the anatomy of pain modulation. *J. Comp. Neurol. 187*:513–532.
51a. Cheema, S., Whitsel, B. L., and Rustioni, A. (1983). Corticospinal projections from pericentral and supplementary cortices in macaque as revealed by anterograde transport of horseradish peroxidase. *Neurosci. Lett. Suppl. 14*:S62.
52. Ralston, H. J., III. (1965). The organization of the substantia gelatinosa Rolandi in the cat lumbosacral spinal cord. *Z. Zellforsch. 67*:1–23.
53. Ralston, H. J., III. (1968). The fine structure of neurons in the dorsal horn of the cat spinal cord. *J. Comp. Neurol. 132*:275–302.
54. Knyihár, E., László, I., and Tornyos, S. (1974). Fine structure and fluoride resistant acid phosphatase activity of electron dense sinusoid terminals in the substantia gelatinosa Rolandi of the rat after dorsal root transection. *Exp. Brain Res. 19*:529–544.

55. Coimbra, A., Sodré-Borges, B. P., and Magalhaes, M. M. (1974). The substantia gelatinosa Rolandi of the rat. Fine structure, cytochemistry (acid phosphatase) and changes after dorsal root section. *J. Neurocytol.* *3*:199–217.

56. Ralston, H. J., III. (1979). The fine structure of laminae I, II, and III of the Macaque spinal cord. *J. Comp. Neurol.* *184*:619–642.

57. Light, A. R., and Durkovic, R. G. (1976). Horseradish peroxidase: An improvement in intracellular staining of single, electrophysiologically characterized neurons. *Exp. Neurol.* *53*:847–850.

58. Jankowska, E., Rastad, J., and Westman, J. (1976). Intracellular application of horseradish peroxidase and its light and electron microscopical appearance in spinocervical tract. *Brain Res.* *105*:557–562.

59. Kitai, S. T., Kocsis, J. D., Preston, R. J., and Sugimori, M. (1976). Monosynaptic inputs to caudate neurons identified by intracellular injection of horseradish peroxidase. *Brain Res.* *109*:601–606.

60. Snow, P. J., Rose, P. K., and Brown, A. G. (1976). Tracing axons and axon collaterals of spinal neurons using intracellular injection of horseradish peroxidase. *Science* *191*:312–313.

61. Cullheim, S., and Kellerth, J.-O. (1976). Combined light and electron microscopic tracing of neurons, including axons and synaptic terminals, after intracellular injection of horseradish peroxidase. *Neurosci. Lett. 2*: 307–313.

62. Ralston, H. J., III. (1968). Dorsal root projections to dorsal horn neurons in the cat spinal cord. *J. Comp. Neurol.* *132*:303–330.

63. Ralston, H. J., Ralston, D. D. (1979). The distribution of dorsal root axons in laminae I, II and III of the Macaque spinal cord: A quantitative electron microscopic study. *J. Comp. Neurol.* *184*:643–683.

64. Gobel, S. (1974). Synaptic organization of the substantia gelatinosa glomeruli in the spinal trigeminal nucleus of the adult cat. *J. Neurocytol.* *3*:219–243.

65. Ralston, H. J. (1981). The synaptic organization of the Macaque dorsal horn. In *Spinal Cord Sensation*, A. G. Brown and M. Réthelyi (Eds.), Scottish Academic Press, Edinburgh, pp. 13–21.

66. Egger, M. D., Freeman, N. C. G., Malamed, S. M., Masarachia, P., and Prosohansky, E. (1981). Electron microscopic observations of terminals of functionally identified afferent fibers in cat spinal cord. *Brain Res.* *207*:157–162.

67. Maxwell, D. J., Bannytyne, B. A., Fyffe, R. E. W., and Brown, A. G. (1982). Ultrastructure of hair follicle afferent fibre terminations in the cat's spinal cord. *J. Neurocytol.* *11*:571–582.

67a. Maxwell, D. J., Bannatyne, B. A., Fyffe, R. E. W., and Brown, A. G. (1984). Fine structure of primary afferent axon terminals projecting from rapidly adapting mechanoreceptors of the toe and foot pads of the cat. *Quart. J. Exp. Physiol. 169*.

68. Réthelyi, M., Light, A. R., and Perl, E. R. (1979). Ultrastructure of synaptic terminations of functionally identified fine myelinated afferent fibers. *Soc. Neurosci. Abstr. 5*:728.

69. Réthelyi, M., Light, A. R., and Perl, E. R. (1982). Synaptic complexes formed by functionally defined primary afferent units with fine myelinated fibers. *J. Comp. Neurol. 207*:381–393.

70. Brown, A. G., and Iggo, A. (1967). A quantitative study of cutaneous receptors and afferent fibres in the cat and rabbit. *J. Physiol. 193*:707–738.

71. Light, A. R., and Perl, E. R. (1979). Reexamination of the dorsal root projection to the spinal dorsal horn including observations on the differential termination of coarse and fine fibers. *J. Comp. Neurol. 186*:117–131.

72. Gobel, S., and Falls, W. M. (1979). Anatomical observations of horseradish peroxidase–filled terminal primary axonal arborizations in layer II of the substantia gelatinosa of Rolandi. *Brain Res. 175*:335–340.

73. Ralston, H. J., III. (1971). The synaptic organization in the dorsal horn of the spinal cord and in the ventrobasal thalamus in the cat. In *Oral-Facial Sensory and Motor Mechanisms*, R. Dubner and Y. Kawamura (Eds.), Appleton-Century-Crofts, New York, pp. 229–250.

74. Brown, K. T., and Flaming, D. G. (1977). New microelectrode techniques for intracellular work in small cells. *Neuroscience 2*:813–827.

75. Jochem, W. J., Light, A. R., and Smith, D. (1981). A high-voltage electrometer for recording and iontophoresis with fine-tipped, high resistance microelectrodes. *J. Neurosci. Methods 3*:261–269.

76. Light, A. R., Réthelyi, M., and Perl, E. R. unpublished.

77. Réthelyi, M., and Szentágothai, J. (1965). On a peculiar type of synaptic arrangement in the substantia gelatinosa of Rolandi. In *Proceedings of the 8th International Congress of Anatomists*, Stuttgart, Thieme, p. 99.

78. Willis, W. D., and Coggeshall, R. E. (1978). *Sensory Mechanisms of the Spinal Cord*, Plenum, New York.

79. Grubard, K., and Calvin, W. H. (1979). Presynaptic dendrites: Implications of spikeless synaptic transmission and dendritic geometry. In *The Neurosciences, Fourth Study Program*, F. O. Schmitt and F. G. Worden (Eds.), MIT Press, Cambridge, Massachusetts, pp. 317–331.

80. Conradi, S. (1969). Ultrastructure and distribution of neuronal and glial elements on the motoneuron surface in the lumbosacral spinal cord of the adult cat. *Acta Physiol. Scand.* (Suppl.) *332*:5–48.

81. Réthelyi, M. (1970). Ultrastructural synaptology of Clarke's column. *Exp. Brain Res. 11*:159–174.

82. Gobel, S. (1976). Dendroaxonic synapses in the substantia gelatinosa glomeruli of the spinal trigeminal nucleus of the cat. *J. Comp. Neurol. 167*:165–176.

83. Burgess, P. R., and Perl, E. R. (1973). Cutaneous mechanoreceptors and nocireceptors. In *Handbook of Sensory Physiology*, vol. II, A. Iggo (Ed.), Springer, New York, pp. 29–78.

84. Iggo, A. (1974). Cutaneous receptors. In *The Peripheral Nervous System*, J. I. Hubbard (Ed.), Plenum, New York, pp. 347–404.

85. Perl, E. R., and Burgess, P. R. (1973). Classification of afferent dorsal root fibers: Mammals. In *Biology Data Book*, vol. II, P. L. Altman and D. S. Dittmer (Eds.), *Fed. Am. Soc. Exp. Biol.* Bethesda, Maryland, pp. 1141–1149.

86. Gobel, S., Falls, W. M., Bennett, G. J., Abdelmoumene, M., Hayashi, H., and Humphrey, E. (1980). An EM analysis of the synaptic connections of horseradish peroxidase-filled stalked cells and islet cells in the substantia gelatinosa of adult cat spinal cord. *J. Comp. Neurol.* *194*:781-807.

87. Light, A. R., Réthelyi, M., and Perl, E. R. (1981). Ultrastructure of functionally identified neurones in the marginal zone and the substantia gelatinosa. In *Spinal Cord Sensation*, A. G. Brown and M. Réthelyi (Eds.), Scottish Academic Press, Edinburgh, pp. 97-106.

88. Réthelyi, M., Light, A. R., and Perl, E. R. (1981). In *Proceedings of the IIIrd World Congress of Pain*, J. J. Bonica, U. Lindblom, and A. Iggo (Eds.), Raven, New York, pp. 111-118.

89. Rastad, J. (1981). Morphology of synaptic vesicles in axo-dendritic and axo-somatic collateral terminals of 2 feline spinocervical tract cells stained intracellularly with horseradish peroxidase. *Exp. Brain Res.* *41*:390-398.

90. Rastad, J. (1981). Quantitative analysis of axodendritic and axosomatic collateral terminals of 2 feline spinocervical tract cells. *J. Neurocytol.* *10*:475-496.

91. Réthelyi, M., Light, A. R., and Perl, E. R. in preparation.

92. Maxwell, D. J., Fyffe, R. E. W., and Brown, A. G. (1982). Fine structure of spinocervical tract neurones and the synaptic boutons in contact with them. *Brain Res.* *233*:394-399.

93. Brown, A. G., and Noble, R. (1982). Connections between hair follicle afferent fibers and spinocervical tract neurones in the cat: The synthesis of receptive fields. *J. Physiol. (Lond.)* *323*:77-91.

94. Hongo, T., Jankowska, E., and Lundberg, A. (1968). Post-synaptic excitation and inhibition from primary afferents in neurones of the spinocervical tract. *J. Physiol. (Lond.)* *199*:569-592.

95. Christensen, B. N., and Perl, E. R. (1970). Spinal neurons specifically excited by noxious or thermal stimuli: Marginal zone of the dorsal horn. *J. Neurophysiol.* *33*:293-307.

96. Kumazawa, T., and Perl, E. R. (1978). Excitation of marginal and substantia gelatinosa neurons in the primate spinal cord: Indications of their place in dorsal horn functional organization. *J. Comp. Neurol.* *177*:417-434.

97. Light, A. R., Trevino, D. L., and Perl, E. R. (1979). Morphological features of functionally defined neurons in the marginal zone and substantia gelatinosa of the spinal dorsal horn. *J. Comp. Neurol.* *186*:151-171.

98. Mense, S., Light, A. R., and Perl, E. R. (1981). Spinal terminations of subcutaneous high-threshold mechanoreceptors. In *Spinal Cord Sensation*, A. G. Brown and M. Réthelyi (Eds.), Scottish Academic Press, Edinburgh, pp. 76-86.

99. Cervero, F., Molony, V., and Iggo, A. (1979). Ascending projections of nocireceptor driven lamina I neurones in the cat. *Exp. Brain Res.* *35*:135-149.

100. Gobel, S., and Hockfield, S. (1977). An anatomical analysis of the synaptic circuitry of layers I, II and III of trigeminal nucleus caudalis in the cat. In *Pain in the Trigeminal Region*, D. J. Anderson and B. Matthews (Eds.), Elsevier Biomedical Press, New York, pp. 203-211.

101. Uchizono, K. (1955). Characteristics of excitatory and inhibitory synapses in the central nervous system of the cat. *Nature (Lond.) 207*:642–643.
102. Rastad, J. (1981). Ultrastructural morphology of axon terminals of an inhibitory interneurone in the cat. *Brain Res. 223*:397–401.
103. Bodian, D. (1975). Origin of specific synaptic types in the motoneuron neuropil of the monkey. *J. Comp. Neurol. 159*:225–244.
104. Schmidt, R. F. (1973). Control of the access of afferent activity of somatosensory pathways. In *Handbook of Sensory Physiology*, vol. II, A. Iggo (Ed.), Springer, New York, pp. 151–206.
105. Boivie, J. J. G., and Perl, E. R. (1975). Neural substrates of somatic sensation. In *Neurophysiology*, C. C. Hunt (Ed.), University Park Press, Baltimore, pp. 303–411.
106. Levy, R. A. (1977). The role of GABA in primary afferent depolarization. *Prog. Neurobiol. 9*:211–267.
107. Eccles, J. C. (1965). *The Physiology of Synapses*, Springer, Berlin.
108. Gray, E. G. (1962). A morphological basis for presynaptic inhibition? *Nature 193*:82–83.
109. McLaughlin, B. J., Barber, R., Saito, K., Roberts, E., and Wu, J.-Y. (1975). Immunocytochemical localization of glutamate decarboxylase in rat spinal cord. *J. Comp. Neurol. 164*:305–322.
110. Barber, R. P., Vaugh, J. E., Saito, K., McLaughlin, B. J., and Roberts, E. (1978). GABAergic terminals are presynaptic to primary afferent terminals in the substantia gelatinosa of the rat spinal cord. *Brain Res. 141*:35–55.
111. Ribeiro-da-Silva, A., and Coimbra, A. (1980). Neuronal uptake of ^{3}H GABA and ^{3}H glicine in laminae I-II (substantia gelatinosa Rolandi) of the rat spinal cord. An autoradiographic study. *Brain Res. 188*:449–464.
112. Whitehorn, D., and Burgess, P. R. (1973). Changes in polarization of central branches of myelinated mechanoreceptor and nocireceptor fibers during noxious and innocuous stimulation of the skin. *J. Neurophysiol. 36*:226–237.
113. Jänig, W., Schmidt, R. F., and Zimmermann, M. (1968). Single unit responses and the total afferent outflow from the cat's foot pad upon mechanical stimulation. *Exp. Brain Res. 6*:100–115.
114. Duggan, A. W., Griersmith, B. T., Headly, P. M., and Hall, J. G. (1979). Lack of effect by substance P at sites in the sunstantia gelatinosa where Met-enkephalin reduces the transmission of nocireceptive impulses. *Neurosci. Lett. 12*:313–317.
115. Duggan, A. W., Johnson, S. M., and Morton, C. R. (1981). Differing distributions of receptors for morphine and Met^5-enkephalinamine in the dorsal horn of the cat. *Brain Res. 229*:379–387.
116. LeBars, D., Guilbaud, G., Chitour, D., and Besson, J. M. (1980). Does systemic morphine increase descending inhibitory controls of dorsal horn neurones involved in nociception? *Brain Res. 202*:223–228.
117. Johnson, S. M., and Duggan, A. W. (1981). Evidence that opiate receptors of the substantia gelatinosa contribute to the depression by intravenous morphine of the spinal transmission of impulses in unmyelinated primary afferents. *Brain Res. 207*:223–228.

118. Oliveras, J. L., Besson, J. M., Guilbaud, G., and Liebsekind, J. C. (1974). Behavioral and electrophysiological evidence of pain inhibition from midbrain stimulation in the cat. *Exp. Brain Res. 20*:32–44.

119. Fields, H. L., Basbaum, A. I., Clanton, C. H., and Anderson, S. D. (1977). Nucleus raphe magnus inhibition of spinal cord dorsal horn neurons. *Brain Res. 126*:441–453.

120. Guilbaud, G., Oliveras, J. L., Giesler, G., and Besson, J. M. (1977). Effects induced by simulation of the centralis inferior nucleus of the raphe on dorsal horn interneurons in cat's spinal cord. *Brain Res. 126*:355–360.

121. Willis, W. D., Haber, L. H., and Martin, R. F. (1977). Inhibition of spinothalamic tract cells and interneurons by brain stem stimulation in the monkey. *J. Neurophysiol. 40*:968–981.

122. Henry, J. L. (1979). Naloxone excites nociceptive units in the lumbar dorsal horn of the spinal cat. *Neuroscience 4*:1485–1491.

123. Fitzgerald, M., and Woolf, C. J. (1980). The stereospecific effect of naloxone on rat dorsal horn neurones; inhibition in superficial laminae and excitation in deeper laminae. *Pain 9*:293–306.

124. Yaksh, T. L., Huang, S. P., Rudy, T. A., and Frederickson, R. C. A. (1977). The direct and specific opiate-like effect of met[5]-enkephalin and analogs on the spinal cord. *Neuroscience 2*:593–596.

125. Headly, P. M., Duggan, A. W., and Griersmith, B. T. (1978). Selective reduction of noradrenaline and 5-hydroxytryptamine of nociceptive responses of cat dorsal horn neurones. *Brain Res. 145*:185–189.

126. Griersmith, B. T., and Duggan, A. W. (1980). Prolonged depression of spinal transmission of nocireceptive information by 5-HT administered in the substantia gelatinosa: Antagonism by methysergide. *Brain Res. 187*:231–236.

127. Yaksh, T. L., Jessell, T. M., Gamse, R., Mudge, A. W. and Leeman, S. E. (1980). Intrathecal morphine inhibits substance P release from mammalian spinal cord in vivo. *Nature (Lond.) 286*:155–157.

128. Johnston, S. E., and Davies, J. (1981). Descending inhibitions from the nucleus raphe magnus and adjacent reticular formation to the dorsal horn of the rat are not antagonized by biculline or strychnine. *Neurosci. Lett. 26*:43–47.

129. Ruda, M. A. (1982). Opiates and pain pathways: Demonstration of enkephalin synapses on dorsal horn projection neurons. *Science 215*:1523–1525.

130. Hunt, S. P., Kelly, J. S., and Emson, P. C. (1980). The electron microscopic localization of methionine-enkephalin within the superficial layers (I and II) of the spinal cord. *Neuroscience 5*:1871–1890.

131. Ruda, M. A., and Gobel, S. (1980). Ultrastructural characterization of axonal endings in the substantia gelatinosa which take up ^{3}H serotonin. *Brain Res. 184*:57–83.

132. Reddy, S. V. R., and Yaksh, T. L. (1980). Spinal noradrenergic terminal system mediates antinociception. *Brain Res. 189*:391–401.

133. Dubuisson, D., and Wall, P. D. (1980). Descending influences on receptive fields and activity of single units recorded in laminae 1, 2 and 3 of cat spinal cord. *Brain Res. 199*:283–298.

134. Glazer, E. J., and Basbaum, A. I. (1981). Immunohistochemical localization of leucine-enkephalin in the spinal cord of the card: Enkephalin-containing marginal neurons and pain modulation. *J. Comp. Neurol. 196*: 377–389.

135. Behbehani, M. M., and Fields, H. L. (1979). Evidence that an excitatory connection between the periaqueductal gray and nucleus raphe magnus mediates stimulation produced analgesia. *Brain Res. 170*:85–93.

5

TYPES OF SYNAPTIC CONNECTIONS IN THE CORE OF THE SPINAL GRAY MATTER

Miklós Réthelyi *Semmelweis University Medical School, Budapest, Hungary*

I. INTRODUCTION

Golgi architectural studies (1), neuroembryologic observations, and synaptologic considerations (2) gave rise to ideas which resulted in the delineation of a double cylinder-shaped area in the spinal gray matter which incorporates the neurons of the spinal segmental apparatus (3). In the first and mainly speculative description, Szentágothai (2) called this part of the gray matter the *central reticular core*. He also elaborated the main input and output connections of the central core. The input connections are mainly from primary afferent neurons, various descending fiber tracts, and collaterals of axons of dorsal horn neurons, while the output of the central core is directed mainly toward the motoneurons but also toward higher brain regions via ascending tracts. In addition to the connections, the central core region contains large numbers of intrinsic neurons (4).

Subsequent Golgi studies on adult cat spinal cord (5) clearly showed a remarkable orientation of dendrites in the intermediate zone, arranged to form a circle or an elliptic area in cross sections. The dorsal periphery of the circular area reaches the dorsal border of Rexed's lamina V (6). Ventrally, the circle touches the dorsal or dorsomedial border of the motoneuronal cell group. Medially, especially ventromedially, the situation is equivocal. It is not quite certain if all neurons of lamina VIII are to be included in the circle (see Chap. 4,

179

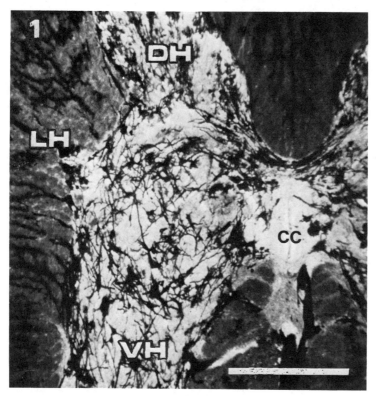

Figure 1 Microphotograph showing the orientation of dendrites in the inter-mediate zone at segment T2. Surrounded by the dorsal horn (DH), ventral horn (VH), and lateral horn (LH), the dendrites of the intermediate zone neurons encircle the central core. CC, central canal. Golgi-Kopsch stain, adult cat. Scale: 500 μm. (Modified from Ref. 5.)

Figure 1). This dendritic arrangement is also present in the thoracic segments. The intermediolateral (sympathetic) nucleus (lateral horn) is located outside the circle, while the area of Clarke's column is somewhat arbitrarily incorporated in it (Fig. 1), in spite of the radical differences in its primarily longitudinally oriented dendritic arborizations (7).

The circular or elliptic area includes large portions of lamina V, all of lamina VI and VII, and parts of lamina VIII of Rexed (6). This central core of the spinal gray matter seems to form two uninterrupted columns on each side of the central canal along the entire cord. The dorsal, lateral, and ventral horns (columns) are attached to the central core as crestlike appendages at its dorsal, lateral, and ventral (ventrolateral) circumferences (2,5). The neuropil of the central core is well separated from that of the horns because of the prevailing transverse orientation pattern of axons and dendrites (5,8-11).

Ultrastructural characterization of synaptic structures in the central core (intermediate zone of earlier literature) is fragmentary, and is restricted largely to synapses made by primary sensory fibers and descending tract fibers that terminate in the dorsal portion of the central core (laminae V-VI).

II. NEURONAL CONNECTIVITY IN THE CENTRAL CORE

Neurons in the central core fall into small, medium, and rarely large categories (6). (Histologic data in this and the following sections refer to the spinal cord of cats if not otherwise specified.) They have three to seven main dendrites which radiate up to 1 mm (average: 600-700 μm; [12]). The size of the dendritic tree is commensurate with the number of primary dendrites in the dog (13), and apparently this relationship is true for other laboratory animals as well. The entire dendritic tree is mainly confined to the transverse plane (9,10,16). But there are a few exceptions, for example, the rostrocaudally oriented dendrites of Ia inhibitory interneurons (14) and the spinothalamic tract neurons in the ventromedial portion of the central core (15). The axon may originate from the perikaryon, but more frequently it arises from a main dendrite and joins the lateral or ventral funiculi. Some of the axons cross the midline and enter the contralateral ventral funiculus (7,12). Before leaving the gray matter a large number of the axons issue local collaterals (16,17), which are more profuse over the motoneuronal cell group and less dense near to their origin in the central core (18). Dendritic arborization and axonal pathways of different groups of neurons in the central core have been studied recently by intracellular labeling of functionally identified neurons [ventral spinocerebellar tract neurons (19), dorsal spinocerebellar tract neurons (20), spinothalamic tract neurons (15), and interneurons of both segmental reflex pathways and descending tracts (21)]. In a systematic analysis, six types of interneurons could be distinguished in laminae V through VI based upon axon trajectory. Axon trajectories of patterns 1 and 2 projected to motoneurons, patterns 3, 4, and 5 to neurons of laminae V through VII (intrinsic neurons of the central core), and pattern 6 represented axons crossing in the anterior commissure. Seventy-five percent of these neurons were funicular cells (22). Interneurons in lamina VII mediating Ia reciprocal inhibition to motoneurons (23) proved to be funicular neurons, too, with axons joining the ipsilateral ventral or lateral funiculus. Initial axon collaterals within the ventral horn were seen only occasionally (14). Neurons of the central core giving rise to long ascending pathways do not have initial collaterals (15,19,20), unlike similar neurons located in the dorsal horn (24,25).

The central core is the termination area of at least three axon systems: (1) primary afferent fibers, (2) long descending fibers, and (3) propriospinal fibers.

2

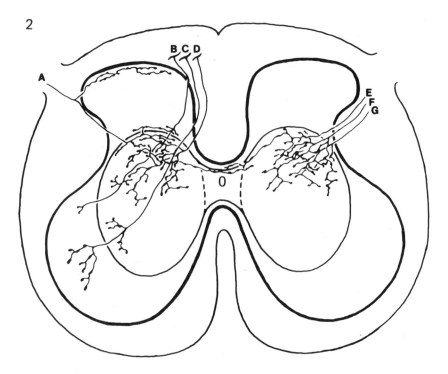

Figure 2 Schematic drawing illustrating the course of primary afferent fibers (left) and descending fibers (right) arborizing entirely or partially in the central core. A, fine myelinated nocireceptor fiber; B, group II muscle afferent fiber; C, group Ia muscle afferent fiber; D, group Ib muscle afferent fiber; E, raphespinal fiber; F, corticospinal fiber; G, rubrospinal fiber. The two eliptic areas represent the central core.

A. Primary Afferent Fibers

Primary afferent fibers terminate in most of the entire central core as shown with degeneration techniques (8,26–28; monkey cord: 29,30) and autoradiography (31; monkey cord: 32). Several types of primary afferent collaterals have been identified in Golgi preparations and subsequently by the use of single-fiber horseradish peroxidase (HRP) injections (Fig. 2). Group Ia muscle afferent fibers issue two sets of collateral branches on their way to the motoneuron cell group, one in medial lamina VI and another in lamina VII at the border of the motoneuron nucleus (18,33,34). Group Ib muscle afferent fibers arborize over large portions of the central core (3,35). Group II muscle afferent fibers show variability in branching and terminal arborization. They have three arborization territories: one centered in lamina V (reaching occasionally more dorsal laminae and lamina VI as well), another in the lateral portion of laminae VI through VII, and a sparse terminal arborization in the motor nucleus (36). Some large-caliber cutaneous fibers terminate in the dorsal part of the central core (see 37), while fine myelinated mechanical nocireceptor fibers from the skin (38) and muscles (39) arborize along the border of the dorsal horn and central core. Primary sensory fibers entering the spinal cord via the ventral roots (40) travel across the central core toward their termination site in the dorsal horn (41).

B. Long Descending Fibers

Long descending fibers arborize and terminate in the central core from several discrete paths in the lateral and ventromedial funiculi. Experimental degeneration, autoradiography, and more recently fluorescent and immunohistochemical techniques have often been used to disclose the extensively overlapping termination territories of descending tracts (for details see 42–49; monkey spinal cord: 50–52). In the following description the course, branching pattern, and termination of individual fibers will be reviewed (Fig. 2). Earlier Golgi information has been complemented in increasing extent by the analysis of functionally identified and HRP-stained descending fibers.

Golgi-stained spinal cord sections revealed that the fibers of the *lateral corticospinal tract* vary in diameter between less than 1 μm and 4–5 μm. They possess several collaterals capped with single or multiple boutons along their course in the gray matter (53,54). The light microscopic analysis of single physiologically identified and HRP-stained corticospinal tract axons completes the previous picture by demonstrating that a collateral branch of the stem fiber bifurcates several times before entering the gray matter across the lateral border of lamina V. Within the gray matter the termination field of a collateral branch is triangular in lamina VI and VII on transverse sections at the high cervical level. The rostrocaudal extent of the arborization of a single collateral branch may span 1.3–3.0 mm (55).

The diameter of stem axons in the *rubrospinal tract* varies between 4 and 9 μm. Functionally identified and HRP-stained rubrospinal fibers issue collaterals that enter the gray matter through laminae V through VII. The collateral branches arborize and terminate in the central core with prominent rostrocaudal arborizations (up to 5.1 mm in length). Small swellings can be seen at the end of the short side branches (56).

HRP-stained descending fibers from the midline medullary-pontine region (*raphe-spinal tract*) appear to divide and terminate in *en passant* and terminal boutons in the central core area. One group of the raphe-spinal fibers issues collaterals which course toward the superficial dorsal horn as well (57).

C. Propriospinal Fibers

Forming long and short intraspinal connections, the propriospinal fibers originate mainly from the neurons of the central core itself (4,58–60). Matching

Golgi information and the results of experimental degeneration techniques, Szentágothai (53) concluded that axon collaterals traversing the intermediate region in a rather straight course belong to the propriospinal system. Short side branches of these axons terminate in small terminal knobs.

III. FRAGMENTS OF THE ULTRASTRUCTURE OF THE CENTRAL CORE

The ultrastructural (synaptologic) description of the central core, as does that of any other part of the central nervous system, relies on studies made on intact animals as well as studies in which certain axon components or groups of neurons had been labeled. For many years the transection of axons or destruction of perikarya and the ensuing anterograde degeneration were the techniques of choice to distinguish a single system of axons. The technique of axoplasmic transport of radio-labeled proteins and the autoradiographic detection of labeled axon terminals on ultrathin sections has been introduced more recently (61), but this procedure has not received such widespread application as the degeneration technique. Recently, it has been realized that the ultrastructural analysis of functionally identified and HRP-stained neurons and terminal axon arborizations is undoubtedly the best way to characterize synaptic structures given or received by individual neurons. In these cases, the neurons retain their normal relationships to the neighboring components of the neuropil and as a rule, the cytoplasmic organelles are well preserved.

Since the notion of a central core is relatively new, no ultrastructural study is available which describes the entire area. Moreover, it is very probable that the synaptic structure of the central core is heterogeneous with regard to the origin and termination of different pathways or groups of neurons. In the following paragraphs, synaptic connections will be reviewed in the dorsal half of the central core (laminae V and VI) because this area is the joint arborization territory of primary afferent fibers and descending fibers that course in the lateral funiculus. The latter fibers terminate predominantly in the lateral basilar region of Ramon y Cajal (7). This area denotes the lateral portion of laminae V and VI. Synapses made by certain types of propriospinal neurons and those found in Clarke's column will also be outlined.

A. Dorsal Half of the Central Core

The neuropil of the dorsal half of the central core of the spinal gray matter (laminae V–VI, including the lateral basilar region) contains numerous myelinated axons. Synapsing axon terminals in part contact perikarya, in part dendrites, and on occasion axon terminals. Comparing the frequency of various synaptic formations, the dorsal half of the central core contains more axosomatic and fewer axoaxonic synapses than laminae I through III. The shape of synaptic vesicles may be round or flattened (62).* The main type of synaptic connections in the lateral basilar region is formed by axon terminals that contain round synaptic vesicles and terminate on dendrites. One fifth to one quarter of the boutons contain flattened vesicles, and few terminals could be seen with dense-core vesicles. Axosomatic (12-14% of all synaptic connections) and axoaxonic synapses (1.0-3.4% of all synaptic connections) occur as well (63-65). The elongated terminals on the proximal dendrites, the perikarya with multiple synaptic contacts (65), and the glomerular synapses (63) all appear to be rarities in the lateral basilar region and may belong to neighboring territories.

Synaptic terminals of primary afferent fibers were selectively labeled by dorsal rhizotomy and by HRP injection. Degenerating boutons occurred both in lamina V and VI; about twice as much in the latter than in the former. They synapsed on perikarya and dendrites of large- and medium-sized neurons (40-50 μm and 20-25 μm in diameter, respectively), but avoided small-sized neurons. Degenerating boutons participated in axoaxonic synapses as postsynaptic components (66). (The author has lumped laminae IV through VI together. Details relevant to laminae V and VI have been extracted from the original papers.) It must be remembered that vesicle-containing dendrites had not been recognized (albeit anticipated) at the time of the ultrastructural descriptions of Ralston (62,66). It remains to be clarified to what extent vesicle-containing profiles belong to dendritic arborizations.

HRP injection into individual neurons has permitted the ultrastructural analysis of functionally identified primary afferent fibers. Although much has to be done (the excellent light microscopic analyses of various types of primary sensory fibers in the central core area [37] suggest that ultrastructural results will soon be available), the synaptic articulations of some thick and fine-diameter cutaneous primary afferent fibers at the junction of the dorsal horn and central core have been described. Boutons of fine myelinated mechanical nocireceptor fibers (67) synapse on dendritic shafts or sometimes on irregular dendritic appendages. Small-sized, flattened vesicle-containing boutons, presumed to be axon terminals, frequently contact the synaptic enlargements of primary fibers (68; Fig. 3). Interestingly, the same mechanical nocireceptor fiber has another terminal arborization in the superficial dorsal horn where the boutons participate in synaptic complexes of several dendritic protrusions, axon terminals, and vesicle-containing dendritic profiles (see Chap. 4, and 68).

Small- and large-sized boutons that contain round synaptic vesicles that originate from thick myelinated sensory fibers of type I slowly adapting cutaneous mechanoreceptors synapse on relatively large dendrites (69). Indications that axoaxonic synapses in which the primary bouton would be the presynaptic component have been presented by the same authors (69).

Boutons of corticospinal fibers, which make up approximately 10% of all terminals in the lateral basilar region, are located mainly on dendrities (65). There are conflicting views as to whether the terminals are evenly distributed

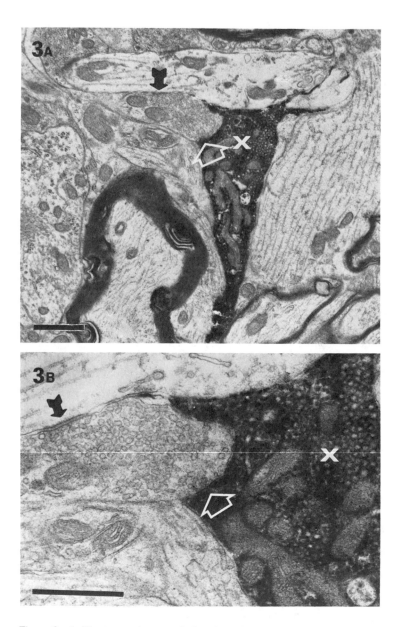

Figure 3 A: Electron micrograph showing a horseradish peroxidase labeled bouton (x) of a fine myelinated nocireceptor fiber from the transition zone between the dorsal horn and the central core. The bouton synapses with a dendrite (the synaptic specialization is better seen on adjacent serial sections), whereas it receives an axoaxonic synapse (white arrow) from an adjacent small axon terminal containing flattened synaptic vesicles. The latter synapses with the same dendrite (black arrow). B: Higher power detail from the synaptic junctions as seen on the adjacent serial section. Lettering as above. Scales: 1 μm.

along the dendrites (65) or whether they form groups of adjacent terminals that contact the same dendrite (63).

Terminals of rubrospinal fibers synapse predominantly on dendrites and occasionally on neuronal perikarya. Almost 10% of all axon terminals in the lateral basilar region appears to belong to rubrospinal fibers (70). Degenerating rubrospinal axon terminals appear to contain mostly round synaptic vesicles (64), but the distortion of the boutons during the process of degeneration has made it difficult to ascertain the shape of the vesicles with certainty.

Synapsing boutons of cortico- and rubrospinal fibers are similar in size (1.4-1.5 μm, mean diameter) and in distribution along the dendrites of the neurons (71).

Preliminary results of ultrastructural investigations of HRP-stained cortico-spinal tract axons (72) have shown that the *en passant* and terminal boutons are 1.0-2.0 μm in diameter, and many of them may synapse with the same dendrite (Fig. 4). A bouton usually forms only one synaptic junction with a dendrite or perikaryon, occasionally two dendrites were contacted by the same bouton (72).

Rubrospinal terminals in the rat measured 0.5-1.0 μm in diameter and synapsed with small-caliber dendrites (73). Identical axon terminals in the opossum are even smaller (0.5-0.7 μm in diameter), and contacted small (apparently distal) dendrites in the lateral basilar region. More medially, they synapse on larger (probably proximal) dendritic shafts (74).

Raphe-spinal descending fibers from the medullary-pontine region terminate with several boutons that contain round or oval synaptic vesicles, and occasional dense-core vesicles 60-70 nm in diameter terminate on dendritic shafts. Synaptic boutons of descending fibers were regularly found in the vicinity of dendritic appendages (57).

Collateral branches of the axons of the spinocervical tract neurons that arborize at the transition zone of the dorsal horn and central core have been labeled with HRP and studied with the electron microscope. The boutons measured 1.0-1.5 μm in diameter, contained round or slightly elliptic synaptic vesicles, and synapsed mostly on dendrites and occasionally on perikarya (75). Terminal boutons of group Ia muscle spindle afferent fibers in lamina VI synapse with somata and large dendritic shafts. They frequently received axoaxonic contacts from small axon terminals containing flattened synaptic vesicles (75a).

B. Synaptic Connections Made by Propriospinal Neurons

Both degeneration and HRP studies have been used to identify the axon ter-minals of propriospinal neurons. Although axon collaterals of these neurons terminate abundantly in the central core (22), ultrastructural studies available preferentially described boutons synapsing in the ventral horn which mainly contact motoneurons.

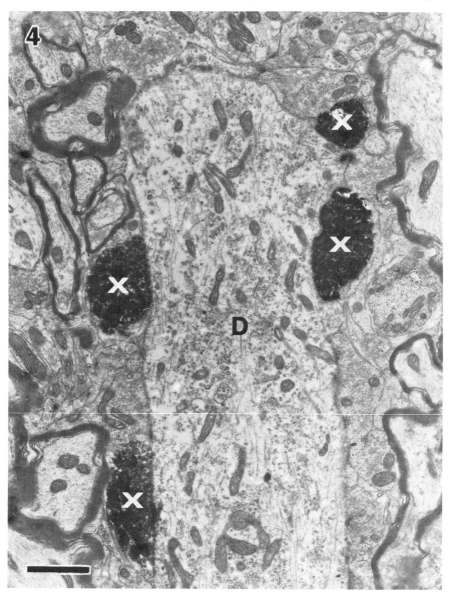

Figure 4 Electron micrograph showing four boutons (x) of a horseradish peroxidase–labeled corticospinal tract fiber contacting the same dendrite (D) in lamina VI. Scale: 1 μm. (Courtesy of D. J. Maxwell.)

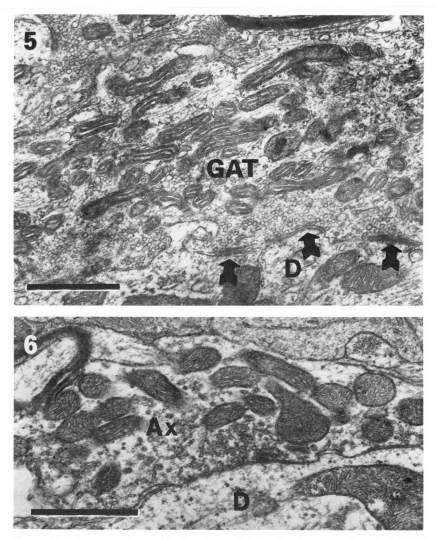

Figure 5 Electron micrograph showing a detail of a giant axon terminal (GAT) contacting a dendrite (D) in Clarke's column. Arrows point to three of the many synaptic contacts between the axon terminal and the dendrite. Scale: 1 μm. (Modified from Ref. 79.)

Figure 6 Enlarged portion of a fine fiber (Ax) with flattened synaptic vesicles synapsing with a dendrite (D) in Clarke's column. Scale: 1 μm. (Modified from Ref. 79.)

Axons of propriospinal neurons coursing in the lateral and ventral funiculi terminate with relatively large-sized terminals (up to 5.3 μm in diameter) on proximal dendrites and perikarya of the neurons in the ventral horn (71). Axon collaterals of lamina VII interneurons mediating Ia reciprocal inhibition to motoneurons arborize among motoneurons (lamina IX) and establish axodendritic and axosomatic synapses. The small-sized boutons contacted several postsynaptic structures and contained polymorphic synaptic vesicles. The length:width ratio of the vesicles was 1:3, which is only marginally greater than a similar figure in the spinal cord terminals of excitatory spinocervical tract neurons (76).

C. Synapses in Clarke's Column

Although Clarke's column is completely isolated from the adjacent gray matter and has a predominantly longitudinal orientation pattern (7,77), it is confined to the central core along the thoracic and upper lumbar segments. Early silver impregnation techniques showed unusually large-sized axon terminals that synapsed with dendrites and perikarya of large Clarke's neurons (78). Indeed, later ultrastructural analyses demonstrated giant axon terminals that contained round synaptic vesicles and formed repeated synaptic connections with the neurons (79,80; Fig. 5). Giant axon terminals were often found to be contacted by small, flattened vesicle-containing boutons in the form of axoaxonic synapses (Fig. 7). At slight variance with these findings Saito (80) described similar synapses with pleomorphic vesicles in the small boutons. Small-sized boutons

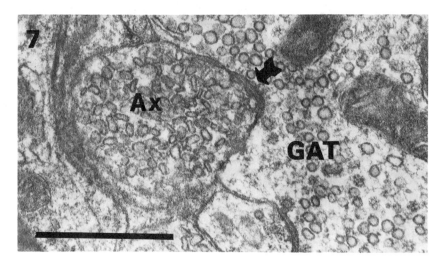

Figure 7 Axoaxonic synapse (arrow) from Clarke's column between a giant axon terminal (GAT) and a smaller axon containing flattened synaptic vesicles (Ax). Scale: 0.5 μm.

with round synaptic vesicles and fusiform *en passant* enlargements of fine axons that contained flattened synaptic vesicles (Fig. 6) were distinguished synapsing with the neurons of Clarke's column. These axons proved to belong to propriospinal neurons (79). Later on, the types of axon terminals were raised to six based on differences in size and vesicle content (80). Recent analysis of synaptic connections on physiologically identified dorsal spinocerebellar tract neurons in Clarke's column confirmed earlier ultrastructural data (80a).

IV. CONCLUSIONS

As was indicated earlier, it is still a premature task to summarize the synaptology of the central core. The relatively simple structure of the neuropil (i.e., axodendritic and axosomatic synapses without any peculiar arrangement, like synaptic glomeruli) has not attracted investigators to perform ultrastructural synaptologic studies. Degeneration analyses that demonstrate the termination of long descending and propriospinal systems have been handicapped by the uncertainties in identifying the degenerating axon terminals. Clumping of synaptic vesicles and the accumulation of neurofibrils in the boutons as early signs of degeneration are ambiguous indicators. The darkening of the cytoplasm as a more obvious sign of degeneration occurred infrequently, and those degenerating boutons were often completely surrounded by glial processes. It is easy to envisage that with the upsurge of intracellular staining of functionally identified neurons the synaptic ultrastructure of the central core region will be really understood in the near future.

The ultrastructural details available suggest that the neurons of the central core receive synaptic input from primary afferent, descending, and propriospinal fibers through simple synapses. Presynaptic control over peripheral impulses (81,82) may be assumed as the axoaxonic synapses are found on the terminations of primary sensory fibers. Lack of axoaxonic synapses on the terminal boutons of descending fibers may indicate that their impulses can be controlled only postsynaptically, although electrophysiologic evidence of presynaptic modulation of the activity of rubropsinal tract fibers has been recently considered (83).

Comparing synapses in the dorsal horn with those in the central core, one is surprised by the large degree of divergence in the dorsal horn (one fiber has numerous boutons compressed into relatively restricted spaces; a large portion of the boutons synapse with numerous postsynaptic processes in the form of synaptic glomeruli, see 84). This two-level divergent termination of fibers keeps a fair balance with the necessary, although not too extensive, convergence (85) manifesting on the neurons. This arrangement makes the impression that the connections among neurons and the ensuing function of the neuronal networks are equally determined by the wiring (what is connected to what) and by the synapses themselves (geometry of the contacts) in the dorsal horn. In contrast, in the central core the wiring seems to be the decisive factor in the interneuronal connections. A wealth of data obtained by neurophysiologic experiments indicate that preterminal fiber systems and neurons in the central core are interconnected to ensure abundant and ample convergence of impulses from various sources and of both excitatory and inhibitory characters [86-92; for a thorough analysis of integrative neuronal activities in the central core region, the reader is referred to Baldissera et al. (93)]. The apparently simple and straightforward synaptic connections *per se* do not seem to add much to the integrative capacity of the circuits. In contrast to the neuronal structure of the dorsal horn, divergent connections, that is, spread of impulses of descending and propriospinal neurons that terminate in the central core are assured by their multisegmental or multilevel (within one segment) termination pattern (4,94,95).

Synaptic structure of primary afferent terminals (large boutons with multiple synaptic sites) and unit responses in Clarke's column (large excitatory postsynaptic potentials evoked in the neurons) correlate fairly well (96). The significance of synaptic terminals from other sources has to be analyzed.

ACKNOWLEDGMENTS

The author thanks Dr. János Szentagothai for his suggestions while reading the manuscript. Technical help was provided by Mrs. A. Fervagñer.

REFERENCES

1. Leontovich, T. A., and Zhukova, G. P. (1963). The specificity of the neuronal structure and topography of the reticular formation in the brain and spinal cord or carnivora. *J. Comp. Neurol. 121*:347–380.

2. Szentágothai, J. (1967). The anatomy of complex integrative units in the nervous system. In *Results in Neuroanatomy, Neurochemistry, Neuropharmacology and Neurophysiology*, K. Lissák (Ed.), Akadémiai Kiadó, Budapest, pp. 9–45.

3. Réthelyi, M., and Szentágothai, J. (1973). Distribution and connections of afferent fibres in the spinal cord. In *Handbook of Sensory Physiology*, vol. II, A. Iggo (Ed.), Springer, New York, pp. 237–252.

4. Szentágothai, J. (1951). Short propriospinal neurons and intrinsic connections of the spinal gray matter. *Acta Morph. Acad. Sci. Hung., 1*:81–94.

5. Réthelyi, M. (1976). Central core in the spinal gray matter. *Acta Morph. Acad. Sci. Hung. 24*:63–70.

6. Rexed, B. (1952). The cytoarchitectonic organization of the spinal cord in in the cat. *J. Comp. Neurol. 96*:415–495.

7. Ramon y Cajal, S. (1909). *Histologie du Système Nerveux de l'Homme et des Vertébrés*, vol. I., Maloine, Paris.

8. Sterling, P., and Kuypers, H. G. J. M. (1967). Anatomical organization of the brachial spinal cord of the cat. I. The distribution of dorsal root fibers. *Brain Res. 4*:1–15.

9. Scheibel, M. E., and Scheibel, A. B. (1968). Terminal axonal patterns in cat spinal cord. II. The dorsal horn. *Brain Res. 9*:32–58.
10. Szentágothai, J., and Réthelyi, M. (1973). Cyto- and neuropil architecture of the spinal cord. In *New Developments in Electromyography and Clinical Neurophysiology*, vol. III, J. E. Desmedt (Ed.), Karger, Basel, pp. 20–37.
11. Mannen, H. (1975). Reconstruction of axonal trajectory of undividual neurons in the spinal cord using Golgi-stained serial sections. *J. Comp. Neurol. 159*:357–374.
12. Matsushita, M. (1970). Dendritic organization of the ventral spinal gray matter in the cat. *Acta Anat. 76*:263–288.
13. Galfan, S., Kao, G., and Ruchkin, D. S. (1970). The dendritic tree of spinal neurons. *J. Comp. Neurol. 139*:385–412.
14. Jankowska, E., and Lindström, S. (1972). Morphology of interneurones mediating Ia reciprocal inhibition of motoneurones in the spinal cord of the cat. *J. Physiol. (Lond.) 226*:805–823.
15. Meyers, D. E. R., and Snow, P. J. (1982). The morphology of physiologically identified deep spinothalamic tract cells in the lumbar spinal cord of the cat. *J. Physiol. (Lond.) 329*:373–388.
16. Scheibel, M. E., and Scheibel, A. B. (1966). Spinal motoneurons, interneurons and Renshaw cells. A Golgi study. *Arch. Ital. Biol. 104*:328–353.
17. Matsushita, M. (1969). Some aspects of the interneuronal connections in cat's spinal gray matter. *J. Comp. Neurol. 136*:57–80.
18. Szentágothai, J. (1967). Synaptic architecture of the spinal motoneuron pool. In *Recent Advances in Clinical Neurophysiology. Electroencephalography and Clinical Neurophysiology* (Suppl. 25), L. Widén (Ed.), Elsevier, Amsterdam, pp. 6–19.
19. Jankowska, E., and Lindström, S. (1970). Morphological identification of physiologically defined neurones in the cat spinal cord. *Brain Res. 20*: 323–326.
20. Randic, M., Miletic, V., and Loewy, A. D. (1981). A morphological study of cat dorsal spinocerebellar tract neurons after intracellular injection of horseradish peroxidase, *J. Comp. Neurol. 198*:453–470.
21. Jankowska, E., and Lindström, S. (1970). Intracellular staining of physiologically identified interneurones in the cat spinal cord. *Acta Physiol. Scand. 78*:4A–5A.
22. Czarkowska, J., Jankowska, E., and Sybirska, E. (1976). Axonal projections of spinal interneurones excited by group I afferents in the cat, revealed by intracellular staining with horseradish peroxidase. *Brain Res. 118*:115–118.
23. Hultborn, H., Jankowska, E., and Lindström, S. (1971). Recurrent inhibition of interneurones monosynaptically activated from group Ia afferents. *J. Physiol. (Lond.) 215*:613–636.
24. Rastad, J., Jankowska, E., and Westman, J. (1977). Arborization of initial axon collaterals of spinocervical tract cells stained intracellularly with horseradish peroxidase. *Brain Res. 135*:1–10.

25. Brown, A. G., and Fyffe, R. E. W. (1981). Form and function of spinal neurones with axons ascending to the dorsal columns in the cat. *J. Physiol. (Lond.) 321*:31–47.

26. Schimert, J. (1939). Das Verhalten der Hinterwurzelkollateralen im Rückenmark. *Z. Anat. Entwicklungsgesch. 109*:665–687.

27. Sprague, J. M. (1958). The distribution of dorsal root fibres on motor cells in the lumbosacral spinal cord of the cat, and the site of excitatory and inhibitory terminals in monosynaptic pathways. *Proc. R. Soc. (Lond.) 140*:534–556.

28. Imai, Y., and Kusama, T. (1969). Distribution of the dorsal root fibers in the cat. An experimental study with the Nauta method. *Brain Res. 13*: 338–359.

29. Shriver, J. E., Stein, B. M., and Carpenter, M. B. (1968). Central projections of spinal dorsal roots in the monkey. I. Cervical and upper thoracic dorsal roots. *Am. J. Anat. 123*:27–74.

30. Carpenter, M. B., Stein, B. M., and Shriver, J. E. (1968). Central projections of spinal dorsal roots in the monkey. II. Lower thoracic, lumbosacral and coccygeal dorsal roots. *Am. J. Anat. 123*:75–118.

31. Réthelyi, M., Trevino, D. L., and Perl, E. R. (1979). Distribution of primary afferent fibers within the sacrococcygeal dorsal horn: An autoradiographic study. *J. Comp. Neurol. 185*:603–622.

32. Ralston, H. J., and Ralston, D. D. (1979). Identification of dorsal root synaptic terminals on monkey ventral horn cells by electron microscopic autoradiography. *J. Neurocytol. 8*:151–166.

33. Brown, A. G., and Fyffe, R. E. W. (1978). The morphology of group Ia afferent fibre collaterals in the spinal cord of the cat. *J. Physiol. (Lond.) 274*:111–127.

34. Ishizuka, N., Mannen, H., Hongo, T., and Sasaki, S. (1979). Trajectory of group Ia afferent fibers stained with horseradish peroxidase in the lumbosacral spinal cord of the cat: Three dimensional reconstructions from serial sections. *J. Comp. Neurol. 186*:189–212.

35. Brown, A. G., and Fyffe, R. E. W. (1979). The morphology of group Ib afferent fibre collaterals in the spinal cord of the cat. *J. Physiol. (Lond.) 296*:215–228.

36. Fyffe, R. E. W. (1979). The morphology of group II muscle afferent fibre collaterals. *J. Physiol. (Lond.) 296*:39–40.

38. Brown, A. G. (1981). *Organization in the Spinal Cord.* Springer, New York.

39. Light, A. R., and Perl, E. R. (1979). Spinal termination of functionally identified primary afferent neurons with slowly conducting myelinated fibers. *J. Comp. Neurol. 186*:133–150.

39. Mense, S., Light, A. R., and Perl, E. R. (1981). Spinal terminations of subcutaneous high-threshold mechanoreceptors. In *Spinal Cord Sensation*, E. G. Brown and M. Réthelyi (Eds.), Scottish Academic Press, Edinburgh, pp. 79–86.

40. Coggeshall, R. E., Coulter, J. D., and Willis, W. D. (1974). Unmyelinated axons in the ventral roots of the cat lumbosacral enlargement. *J. Comp. Neurol. 153*:39–58.

41. Light, A. R., and Metz, C. B. (1978). The morphology of the spinal cord efferent and afferent neurons contributing to the ventral roots of the cat. *J. Comp. Neurol. 179*:501–516.

42. Szentágothai-Schimert, J. (1941). Die Endigundsweise der absteigenden Rückenmarksbahnen. *Z. Anat. Entwicklungsgesch. 111*:322–330.

43. Nyberg-Hansen, R. (1966). Functional organization of descending supra-spinal fibre systems to the spinal cord. Anatomical observations and physiological correlations. *Ergebn. Anat. Entwicklungsgesch. 39*:1–48.

44. Petras, J. M. (1967). Cortical, tectal and tegmental fiber connections in the spinal cord of the cat. *Brain Res. 6*:275–324.

44. Chambers, W. W., and Liu, C. C. (1957). Corticospinal tract of the cat. An attempt to correlate the pattern of degeneration with deficits in reflex activity following neocortical lesions. *J. Comp. Neurol. 108*:23–55.

45. Edwards, S. B. (1972). The ascending and descending projections of the red nucleus in the cat: An experimental study using an autoradiographic tracing method. *Brain Res. 48*:45–63.

47. Basbaum, A. I., Clanton, C. H., and Fields, H. L. (1978). Three bulbo-spinal pathways from the rostral medulla of the cat: An autoradiographic study of pain modulating systems. *J. Comp. Neurol. 178*:209–224.

48. Bobillier, P., Seguin, S., Petitjean, F., Saévert, D., Touret, M., and Jouvet, M. (1976). The raphe nuclei of the cat brain stem: A topographical atlas of their efferent projections as revealed by autoradiography. *Brain Res. 113*:449–486.

49. McLachlan, E. M., and Oldfield, B. J. (1981). Some observations on the catecholaminergic innervation of the intermediate zone of the thoraco-lumbar spinal cord of the cat. *J. Comp. Neurol. 200*:529–544.

50. Liu, C. N., and Chambers, W. W. (1964). An experimental study of the cortico-spinal system in the monkey (Macaca mulatta). The spinal path-ways and preterminal distribution of the degenerating fibres following discrete lesions of the pre- and postcentral gyri and bulbar pyramid. *J. Comp. Neurol. 123*:257–284.

51. Kuypers, H. G. J. M. (1973). The anatomical organization of the descend-ing pathways and their contributions to motor control especially in primates. In *New Developments in Electromyography and Clinical Neuro-physiology*, vol. III, J. E. Desmedt (Ed.), Karger, Basel, pp. 38–68.

52. Swanson, L. W., and McKellar, S. (1979). The distribution of oxytocin- and neurophysin-stained fibers in the spinal cord of the rat and monkey. *J. Comp. Neurol. 188*:87–106.

53. Szentágothai, J. (1964). Propriospinal pathways and their synapses. In *Progress in Brain Research*, vol. 11, J. C. Eccles and J. P. Schadé (Eds.), Elsevier, Amsterdam, pp. 155–177.

54. Scheibel, M. E., and Scheibel, A. B. (1966). Terminal axonal patterns in cat spinal cord. I. The lateral corticospinal tract. *Brain Res. 2*:333–350.

55. Futami, T., Shinoda, Y., and Yokota, J. (1979). Spinal axon collaterals of corticospinal neurons identified by intracellular injection of horseradish peroxidase. *Brain Res. 164*:279–284.

56. Shinoda, Y., Yokota, J.-I., and Futami, T. (1982). Morphology of physiologically identified rubrospinal axons in the spinal cord of the cat. *Brain Res. 242*:321–325.

57. Light, A. R. (1982). Spinal projections of physiologically identified axons from the rostral medulla of cats. In *Proceedings of the IIIrd World Congress of Pain*, J. J. Bonica, U. Lindblom, and A. Iggo (Eds.), Raven, New York, pp. 373–379.

58. Molenaar, I., and Kuypers, H. G. J. M. (1978). Cells of origin of propriospinal fibers and of fibers ascending to supraspinal levels. A HRP study in cat and rhesus monkey. *Brain Res. 152*:429–450.

59. Matsushita, M., Ikeda, M., and Hosoya, Y. (1979). The location of spinal neurons with long descending axons (long descending propriospinal tract neurons) in the cat: A study with the horseradish peroxidase technique. *J. Comp. Neurol. 184*:63–80.

60. Skinner, R. D., Coulter, J. D., Adams, R. J., and Remmel, R. S. (1979). Cells of origin of long descending propriospinal fibers connecting the spinal enlargements in cat and monkey determined by horseradish peroxidase and electrophysiological techniques. *J. Comp. Neurol. 188*:443–454.

61. Hendrickson, A. (1972). Electron microscopic distribution of axoplasmic transport. *J. Comp. Neurol. 144*:381–397.

62. Ralston, H-J., III (1968). The fine structure of neurons in the dorsal horn of the cat spinal cord. *J. Comp. Neurol. 132*:275–302.

63. Dyachkova, L. N., Kostyuk, P. G., and Pogorelaya, N. Ch. (1971). An electron microscopic analysis of pyramidal tract terminations in the spinal cord of the cat. *Exp. Brain Res. 12*:105–119.

64. Kostyuk, P. G., and Skibo, G. G. (1975). An electron microscopic analysis of rubrospinal tract termination in the spinal cord of the cat. *Brain Res. 85*:511–516.

65. Hanaway, J., and Smith, J. M. (1979). Synaptic fine structure and the termination of corticospinal fibers in the lateral basal region of the cat spinal cord. *J. Comp. Neurol. 183*:471–436.

66. Ralston, H. J., III (1963). Dorsal root projections to dorsal horn neurons in the cat spinal cord. *J. Comp. Neurol. 132*:303–330.

67. Burgess, P. R., and Perl, E. R. (1967). Myelinated afferent fibers responding specifically to noxious stimulation of the skin. *J. Physiol. (Lond.) 190*:541–562.

68. Réthelyi, M., Light, A. R., and Perl, E. R. (1982). Synaptic complexes formed by functionally defined primary afferent units with fine myelinated fibers. *J. Comp. Neurol. 207*:381–393.

69. Egger, M. D., Freeman, N. C. G., Malamed, S., Masarachia, P., and Proshansky, E. (1981). Electron microscopic observations of terminals of functionally identified afferent fibers in cat spinal cord. *Brain Res. 207*:157–162.

70. Hanaway, J., and Smith, J. M. (1978). Fine structure of the rubrospinal terminals in the cervical cord of the cat. *J. Neurol. Sci. 39*:31–36.

71. Skibo, G. G., and Pogorelaya, N. Ch. (1979). Structural features of synaptic connections between descending systems and spinal neurons in the cat. *Neuroscience 4*:965–971.

72. Brown, A. G., Fyffe, R. E. W., Maxwell, D. J., and Ralston, H. J., III. (1982). The morphology of physiologically identified corticospinal axons in the cat. *Soc. Neurosci. Abstr. 8*:877.

73. Brown, L. T. (1974). Rubrospinal projections in the rat. *J. Comp. Neurol. 154*:169–188.

74. Goode, G. E., and Sreesai, M. (1978). An electron microscopic study of rubrospinal projections to the lumbar spinal cord of the opossum. *Brain Res. 143*:61–70.

75. Rastad, J. (1981). Morphology of synaptic vesicles in axo-dendritic and axo-somatic collateral terminals of 2 feline spinocervical tract cells stained intracellularly with horseradish peroxidase. *Exp. Brain Res. 41*: 390–398.

75a. Maxwell, D. J., and Bannatyne, B. A. (1983). Ultrastructure of muscle spindle afferent terminations in lamina VI of the cat spinal cord. *Brain Res. 288*:297–301.

76. Rastad, J. (1981). Ultrastructural morphology of axon terminals of an inhibitory interneurone in the cat. *Brain Res. 223*:337–401.

77. Réthelyi, M. (1968). The Golgi architecture of Clarke's column. *Acta Morph. Acad. Sci. Hung. 16*:311–330.

78. Szentágothai, J., and Albert, A. (1955). The synaptology of Clarke's column. *Acta Morph. Acad. Sci. Hung. 5*:43–51.

79. Réthelyi, M. (1970). Ultrastructural synaptology of Clarke's column. *Exp. Brain Res. 11*:159–174.

80. Saito, K. (1974). The synaptology and cytology of the Clarke cell in nucleus dorsalis of the cat: An electron microscopic study. *J. Neurocytol. 3*:179–197.

80a. Houchin, J., Maxwell, D. J., Fyffe, R. E. W., and Brown, A. G. (1983). Light and electron microscopy of dorsal spinocerebellar tract neurones in the cat: and intracellular horseradish peroxidase study. *Quart. J. Exp. Physiol. 68*:719–732.

81. Eccles, J. C. (1964). Presynaptic inhibition in the spinal cord. In *Progress in Brain Research*, vol. 12, J. C. Eccles and J. P. Schadé (Eds.), Elsevier, Amsterdam, pp. 65–91.

82. Schmidt, R. F. (1973). Control of the access of afferent activity to somatosensory pathways. In *Handbook of Sensory Physiology*, vol. II, A. Iggo (Ed.), Springer, New York, pp. 151–208.

83. Rudomin, P., and Jankowska, E. (1981). Presynaptic depolarization of terminals of rubrospinal tract fibers in intermediate nucleus of cat spinal cord. *J. Neurophysiol. 46*:517–531.

84. Réthelyi, M. Synaptic connectivity in the spinal dorsal horn. Chap. 4, this volume.

85. Réthelyi, M. (1983). Specificity versus convergence of nociceptive and mechanoreceptive impulses in the spinal dorsal horn. Fortschritte der Zoologie, Bd. 28. Multimodal Convergences in Sensory Systems, E. Horn (Ed.), Gustav Fisher Verlag, Stutgart, New York, pp. 33–46.

86. Hongo, T., Jankowska, E., and Lundberg, A. (1966). Convergence of excitatory and inhibitory action on interneurones in the lumbosacral cord. *Exp. Brain Res. 1*:338–358.

87. Pomeranz, P., Wall, P. D., and Weber, W. V. (1968). Cord cells responding to fine myelinated afferents from viscera, muscle and skin. *J. Physiol. (Lond.) 199*:511–532.

88. Selzer, M., and Spencer, W. A. (1969). Interactions between visceral and cutaneous afferents in the spinal cord: Reciprocal primary afferent fiber depolarization. *Brain Res. 14*:349–366.

89. Lundberg, A. (1969). Convergence of excitatory and inhibitory action in interneurons in the spinal cord. In *The Interneurone*, M. A. B. Brazier (Ed.), University of California Press, Los Angeles, pp. 231–265.

90. Bayev, K. V., and Kostyuk, P. G. (1973). Convergence of cortico- and rubrospinal influence on interneurones of cat cervical spinal cord. *Brain Res. 52*:159–171.

91. Hancock, M. B., Foreman, R. D., and Willis, W. D. (1975). Convergence of visceral and cutaneous input onto spinothalamic tract cells in the thoracic spinal cord of the cat. *Exp. Neurol. 47*:240–248.

92. Jankowska, E., Johannisson, T., and Lipski, J. (1981). Common interneurones in reflex pathways from group Ia and Ib afferents of ankle extensors in the cat. *J. Physiol. (Lond.) 310*:381–402.

93. Baldissera, F., Hultborn, H., and Illert, M. Integration in spinal neuronal systems. In *Handbook of Physiology–The Nervous System II Motor Control*. V. B. Brooks (Ed.), Williams & Wilkins, Baltimore.

94. Sterling, P., and Kuypers, H. G. J. M. (1968). Anatomical organization of the brachial spinal cord of the cat. III. The propriospinal connections. *Brain Res. 7*:419–443.

95. Hayes, N. L., and Rustioni, A. (1981). Descending projections from brain stem and sensorimotor cortex to spinal enlargements in the cat. Single and double retrograde tracer studies. *Exp. Brain Res. 41*:89–107.

96. Kuno, M., Munoz-Martinez, E. J., and Randic, M. (1973). Synaptic action on Clarke's column neurones in relation to afferent terminal size. *J. Physiol. (Lond.) 228*:343–360.

6
MEMBRANE PROPERTIES
OF CAT SPINAL MOTONEURONS

Peter C. Schwindt   *University of Washington School of Medicine, and Veterans Administration Medical Center, Seattle, Washington*

Wayne E. Crill   *University of Washington School of Medicine, Seattle, Washington*

I. INTRODUCTION

This chapter will focus on the membrane properties which underly the conversion of graded postsynaptic input into frequency coded spike output. We first describe the passive and active responses of motoneurons to intracellular injected current along with some important aspects of their cable properties. Studies of spike components have indicated that the motoneuron is organized into interactive functional compartments, and this organization governs the flow of information through the cell. Studies of repetitive firing properties have determined the input–output characteristics of the cell. Studies of cable properties have shed light on how synaptic input is filtered, shaped, and weighted; that is, in what sense synaptic input is integrated by the motoneuron. The present knowledge of these three factors—compartmental organization, input-output characteristics, and cable properties—allows considerable understanding of the function of motoneurons. Next, we present our current understanding of the voltage-dependent ionic conductances that underly motoneuron excitability. Lastly, we describe the roles of the passive properties and the voltage-dependent conductances in determining motoneuron firing characteristics. We also note here that recent extensive reviews have been published which cover many aspects of motoneuron behavior (1,2).

II. FUNCTIONAL PROPERTIES OF MOTONEURONS

A. Motoneuron Anatomic Structure

Alpha motoneurons are located in the anterior horn of the spinal gray matter, and the neurons innervating single muscles form longitudinal columns extending over 1-3 spinal segments. The diameter of the lumbar motoneuron cell bodies, or perikarya, varies from 30 to 70 μm (3,4). Attached to the soma of each motoneuron are five to 22 major dendritic trunks and a single axon (5,6). The branching dendrites frequently extend at least 1 mm [but see Rose (7) for morphologic characteristics of motoneurons that innervate neck muscles]. Dendritic branching occurs predominantly in the longitudinal direction (8). The axon hillock is a conical protrusion of the soma, relatively free of Nissl substance, where the axon arises. The segment of axon between the axon hillock and the beginning of the myelin sheath is termed the initial segment. The dendrites, soma, axon hillock, and initial segment of spinal motoneurons are covered with synaptic boutons that originate from the spinal interneurons, segmental primary afferent fibers, and some descending fibers from higher centers. Spinal motoneurons have dendrites that lack spines and are relatively smooth.

B. The Ionic Basis of Resting Potential

The resting potential of quiescent or nonspiking motoneurons in the cat and primates range between -55 and -80 mV. Because it is difficult to change quantitatively intercellular and extracellular ionic concentration, we know little about the specific ionic mechanisms responsible for their resting membrane potential. Analysis is also complicated since the motoneuron is never at "rest" in the same sense as an axon. Continuous synaptic bombardment is present in the intact animal even when it is deeply anesthetized. The use of tissue culture or slice methods should solve many of these problems because there is less tonic synaptic bombardment, and extracellular fluid ionic concentrations are under experimental control in the in vitro preparations. In the case of mammalian spinal motoneurons, it is generally assumed that the potassium conductance at resting potential is much higher than the sodium and chloride conductances. However, raising extracellular potassium concentration from 3 mM (the normal value) to as high as 8 mM is reported to have little or no effect on resting membrane potentials, indicating that spinal neurons, in contrast to spinal glial cells, do not behave like an ideal, Nernstian, potassium electrode near resting potential (9). Experiments such as those of Ito and Oshima (10-12), in which various ions are injected into motoneurons, are difficult to interpret because intracellular ionic concentration is not known. Nevertheless, since chloride injection has no effect upon resting potential, the resting chloride conductance is probably low. The occurrence of depolarization at lower temperatures has been interpreted as evidence compatible with the presence of an electrogenic sodium pump current contributing to the resting potential, although its role is probably relatively minor (13). Evidence has also been presented suggesting the presence of a non-electrogenic chloride pump (14).

C. Motoneuron Spike Components

In the earliest intracellular studies an inflection on the rising phase of the moto-neuron action potential was noted (15). The inflection is more prominent on antidromic than on orthodromic spikes. If two antidromic spikes are evoked in succession within an interval of 10-20 msec, the inflection is exaggerated, and further shortening of the stimulus interval causes the second antidromic stimulus to evoke only a smaller response (Fig. 1). This small spike also fails in all-or-nothing manner if the stimulus interval is made very short (15-18). Similar decomposition of the motoneuron spike into two all-or-none components can be accomplished by artificially hyperpolarizing the cell. The small spike has been termed the A or IS (initial segment) spike, and the larger component, which has the longer refractory period, has been termed the B or SD spike. Several kinds of observations have suggested that the A spike originates on the axon side of the soma (16-18). One of the most straightforward of these is the demonstration that the A spike, when evoked orthodromically in isolation, can collide with and occlude an antidromic spike evoked from the motor axon (Fig. 1). It has been postulated that the A spike originates in the axon initial segment (thus the desig-nation IS spike), and the B spike is generated on the soma-dendritic membrane (thus, SD spike). Although the A spike is postulated to be full size in the initial segment region, it appears smaller when recorded in the soma, principally because of the shunt, or relative short circuit, provided by the large, passive, parallel input conductance and capacitance which the soma-dendritic region presents to the limited local circuit current generated in the small initial segment region.

Since the inflection on the rising phase of the action potential is caused by invasion of the B region (and triggering of the B spike) by the A spike, and since the inflection is seen on orthodromic as well as antidromic spikes, the implica-tion is that the A or initial segment region is the lowest threshold region of the cell. This has also been shown directly by intracellular current injection (16,18). That is, the A region serves as the "trigger zone" for spike initiation because orthodromic depolarization brings the initial segment region to its spike threshold before the soma-dendritic spike threshold is reached. The A spike initiated in the initial segment region will travel down the axon orthodromically and will simultaneously antidromically invade the soma-dendritic region, where it provides enough depolarization (20-40 mV) to initiate the high-threshold soma-dendritic spike. Notice that the initial segment region is downstream from

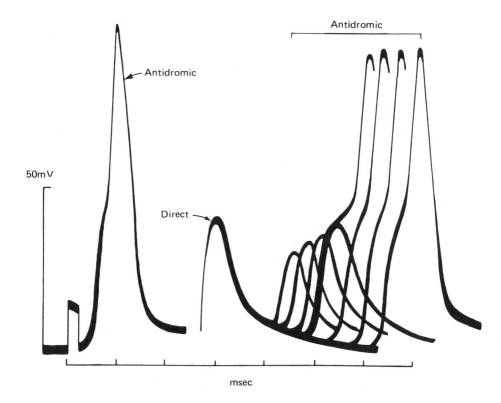

Figure 1 A (or IS) and B (or SD) components of motoneuron's action potential. Superimposed traces of action potentials in a cat lumbar spinal motoneuron evoked successively by antidromic, intracellular, and antidromic stimulation. It is possible to evoke the A spike (the second spike of the sequence) in isolation by intracellular stimulation because the B spike remains refractory for a considerable time following the first, antidromic, AB spike. The latency of the last antidromic stimulus was varied by stimulating at different times in relation to the first two stimuli. An antidromically evoked action potential which follows the intracellularly evoked A spike with a latency of < 1.5 msec will collide with the orthodromically propagated, intracellularly evoked A spike. Thus, the A spike must originate on the axon side of the soma. (After Ref. 18.)

all synaptic input and, thus, it "sees" a weighted average of all synaptic input, where the weighting function depends upon the amplitude of the synaptic input and the cable properties of the dendritic tree (see Sec. III).

Motoneuron spikes have two afterpotentials, both of which are associated with the B or soma-dendritic spike and are not seen following the A or initial segment spike (15-17). The least functionally important afterpotential is the delayed depolarization (DD) which occurs at the trailing foot of the B spike. The delayed depolarization sometimes appears as a small hump at the foot of the spike and sometimes as an abrupt termination of the rapid spike repolarization into a subsequent slow decay of membrane potential (19,20). Postulated mechanisms for the delayed depolarization include active or passive invasion of the dendrites by the soma-dendritic spike (21), or a residual depolarization following from the initial segment spike (22). Computer simulations based on voltage clamp data (see Sec. IV.A) also suggest that the persistance of inward ionic currents together with the decay of a fast outward ionic current could play a role.

A prolonged after-hyperpolarization (AHP) follows the B spike, and a decline in input resistance occurs during the after-hyperpolarization (23-26). The after-hyperpolarization amplitude decreases as the cell is hyperpolarized, and extrapolating the relation between after-hyperpolarization amplitude and membrane potential allows an estimate of after-hyperpolarization reversal potential. The extrapolated reversal potential is consistent with a plausible value of the Nernst equilibrium potential for potassium (27,28). For these reasons, the after-hyperpolarization has been assumed to reflect a prolonged increase in potassium conductance following the B spike (29). The after-hyperpolarization duration varies from about 50 to 180 msec among different motoneurons, but the variation is not entirely random. Motoneurons that innervate motor units with slower twitch times tend to have a longer duration after-hyperpolarization (28,37,38). These same cells have slower axon conduction velocities and higher input resistances and, therefore, a smaller size (6,39). They also are the first cells recruited into rhythmic firing on graded, tonic, natural stimulation (40). These observations indicate that the membrane conductances underlying the after-hyperpolarization are not uniform across the motoneuron population but vary in relation to cell function. The after-hyperpolarization following a spike evoked from rest has little function beyond providing a mild depression of excitability for a period following a spike, but the conductances underlying the after-hyperpolarization play a major role in governing rhythmic firing (see Sec. V.B).

D. Repetitive Firing Properties

Intracellular injection of a constant current pulse is a convenient experimental paradigm used to mimic a tonic synaptic current. The amplitude of the minimal long-lasting constant current pulse that evokes a single spike is called rheobase. If the current pulse is incremented to a value ~1.4 times rheobase, sustained, pacemakerlike, repetitive firing ensues, starting at a minimum steady firing rate that varies from ~5 to 20 Hz among different cells. However, the cell does not

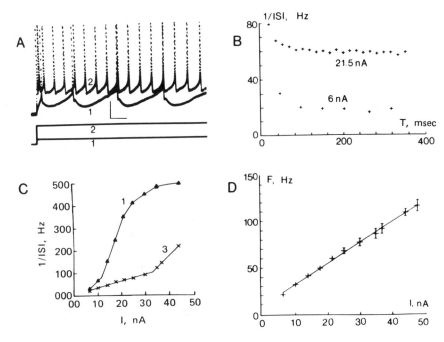

Figure 2 Example of repetitive firing characteristics of lumbar motoneurons. A: Superimposed records of the initial portion of the rhythmic responses of a motoneuron (upper) to like-numbered, long-lasting injected current pulses (lower). Top of spikes are clipped. Motoneuron impaled with two microelectrodes. Calibration is 10 mV, 25 nA, 20 msec. B: Plot of instantaneous firing rate (1/ISI) vs. time (T) for the cell in A during application of constant currents resulting in slow (6.0 nA) and fast (21.5 nA) firing rates. C: Plot of instantaneous firing rate (1/ISI) vs. injected current (I) from cell of A for the first (1) and third (3) interspike intervals (ISIs). D: Plot of mean, steady firing rate (F) vs. injected current (I) in same cell. Line gives least squares fit to data points. Error bars indicate standard deviation from mean rate, which is significant only at faster firing rates. Notice that steady F-I relation (D) in this cell consists of a single linear segment in spite of more complex relations for different ISIs during adaptation (C). Compare with steady F-I relation of Figure 12C.

reach its steady firing rate immediately; interspike intervals (ISIs) at the start of the current pulse are shorter (firing rate is faster) than the final steady value. This slowing of the firing rate over time is called adaptation (31,33). As seen in Figure 2A,B, the initial period of adaptation in motoneurons is usually rather brief, lasting only ~100-200 msec. However, if the current pulse is applied for several seconds, a subsequent, very slow decline of firing rate, termed "slow adaptation" (31), is usually observed. A plot of firing rate versus injected current (the F-I curve) can usually be fit adequately by one or more linear segments. This is true both for the steady firing rate and the "instantaneous" firing rate (computed as the reciprocal of the interspike interval) during adaptation. The F-I curve for the first one or two interspike intervals has an S shape, as seen in Figure 2C, but the initial part of the curve at smaller injected currents is adequately fit by two straight lines (30). As adaptation progresses, the two-line fit describes progressively more of the total F-I curve, but the slope of the two lines decreases from interspike interval to interspike interval (Fig. 2C). The transition firing rate (the rate at which the F-I plot suddenly steepens) remains roughly constant from interspike interval to interspike interval (30-32; see Fig. 2C). The range of firing rates described by the line of smaller slope has been termed the "primary range" of firing, and the steeper line covers the "secondary range" (30). It can be appreciated from Figure 2C,D that the slope of the F-I relationship for the first interval may be considerably steeper than that obtained during steady firing. The slope of the line segments describing the F-I relationship represents the "gain" of the cell's input–output relationship, measured as spikes per second obtained per nA of current. There is a sudden increase in this gain if firing enters the secondary range.

The F-I relationship of many motoneurons during steady (adapted) firing is best described by one linear segment (31,33; see Fig. 2D); other cells retain the secondary range even during steady firing (30,34,35; see Fig. 12C). The latter are generally the smaller cells, judging by input resistance (35). A minority of cells have been observed to retain the S-shaped F-I relationship, which is typical of the first interspike interval in all cells, during steady firing (35). The slope of the primary range F-I curve during steady firing varies from 1 to 3 Hz/nA and the secondary range slope from 3 to 8 Hz/nA among different cells (31,35). There appears to be no clear relationship between primary and secondary range slope or between slope and input resistance in the range 0.5-2.5 MΩ (35,36). However, cells with longer after-hyperpolarization tend to fire at slower minimum and maximum firing rates, and cells of higher input resistance tend to require a smaller current to initiate repetitive firing (32,36).

E. Accommodation Properties

Spinal motoneurons also show accommodation, which is a decrease in excitability or an increase in spike threshold related to the time rate of change of a depolarizing current. That is, in many excitable cells the spike threshold for a rapidly rising current is lower than for a more slowly rising depolarizing current (41-44). In axons accommodation is a result primarily of the inactivation of available sodium conductance by membrane depolarization (45). At resting potential 30-50% of the sodium conductance channels of axons are inactivated (46). Further sodium inactivation by depolarizing current is one reason axons do not show sustained firing to a constant depolarizing current (47). One measure of accommodation is the minimum current gradient for excitation. This is the minimum time rate of change of depolarizing current that will still excite a cell. Healthy motoneurons with normal repetitive firing properties have no minimum current gradient; they will always fire even with the slowest rising current (44). However, accommodation does occur. Threshold for slowly rising currents is higher than for more rapidly rising currents. Because the motoneuron spike is initiated in the initial segment, the accommodative properties of motoneurons likely reflect the accommodative properties of the initial segment.

III. CABLE PROPERTIES

Because motoneuron dendrites are long, narrow, branching structures, synaptic current or voltage recorded at the soma is likely to be significantly attenuated compared to its initial value at synaptic sites remote from the soma. Recall that spike initiation in motoneurons occurs in the initial segment. Thus, adequate depolarization of the initial segment is critical for action potential initiation. Early investigators (29,48) felt that dendrites could be modeled as "infinite" cables. If the dendrites behaved as passive core conductors, synaptic input far out in the dendritic tree would have little effect on the impulse generation in the initial segment in this model. However, the degree of attenuation of remote synaptic input will depend critically on the value of dendritic specific membrane resistance (R_m). Obviously, if R_m were infinite, no attenuation would occur whatever the dendritic length. An appropriate parameter for evaluating electrical (rather than physical) dendritic length is the "space constant" (λ) of a dendritic segment. This is the length over which a steady voltage applied to a point would decay to $1/e$ of the applied value if the dendritic segment were extended to infinity and is given by λ equals $\sqrt{rR_m/2\ R_a}$, where r is the dendritic radius and R_a is the specific cytoplasmic resistance. R_a is low and rather similar among different neurons. For a given r, λ will depend upon R_m. If R_m is large, the dendrite will be short electrically even if it is long and narrow physically. Thus, in order to evaluate the degree of attenuation of distal synaptic input it is necessary to determine R_m or λ and related parameters for motoneuron dendrites.

Because of the aforementioned considerations, it became important to evaluate core conductor properties of dendrites. A major advance occurred when Rall approached the problem by modeling the motoneuron as an isopotential soma attached to cable segments representing dendrites (2,49-52). He found that the mathematic analysis is greatly simplified by representing the entire dendritic tree as a single "equivalent" cylinder of finite length, and he showed that this model could represent a real motoneuron if the following conditions held: (1) the sum of the diameters of the dendritic daughter branches to the 3/2 power equals the diameter of the parent branch to the 3/2 power; (2) all branches end at the same electrotonic distance from the soma; and (3) all branches have the same kind of end termination. Although the assumptions that allow this simplification apparently do not hold in real motoneurons (see below), the model has had great practical and heuristic value. For example, one can assume parameters such as electrotonic length and then determine how remote postsynaptic potentials (PSPs) appear at the soma (51,53). With the use of additional assumptions, it is possible to estimate how far from the soma a postsynaptic potential occurred using shape parameters measured from the postsynaptic potential recorded at the soma (53–56). From the viewpoint of the present chapter, the equivalent cylinder model has the advantage that, if applicable, the passive electrical properties of a motoneuron could be completely described by only four parameters: (1) input resistance at the soma (R_N); (2) membrane time constant (τ_m); (3) dendritic to somatic input conductance ratio (ρ); and (4) equivalent electrotonic length (L). The latter is the length of the equivalent cylinder in terms of space constants rather than dimensional length. Furthermore, these parameters could be estimated by analyzing the time course of membrane potential transients in response to injected current pulses applied to the *soma* (52,57,58). The latter advantage is particularly important because motoneurons can be impaled reliably only at the soma, so any analysis of dendritic electrical properties must be determined by somatic recording and current injection.

A variety of investigators (59,60) have applied the methods suggested by Rall (49–52) or they have developed their own methods (61) based on his model to estimate the aforementioned parameters from somatic recordings of voltage transients in response to injected current. Estimates of membrane time constants have ranged from 2 to 10 msec, with a value of 4-6 msec being typical (6,52,56, 59,61). The parameter ρ was estimated to lie between five and 10 (6,36,49, 50,60,62,63). Because ρ is large, motoneurons are said to possess "dendritic dominance." That is, most current injected into the soma flows into the dendrites, and the input resistance measured is mainly influenced by the dendritic tree rather than the somatic membrane. A large ρ also implies that transient responses are similarly influenced greatly by dendritic properties. All studies have estimated that L lies between one and two space constants (6,52, 59,60,62,63). This is significant because it implies that motoneurons are relatively compact electrically even though their dendritic tree is extensive spatially.

Even though the studies cited previously have obtained similar estimates of the electrical parameters, there remains some uncertainty about the applicability of the equivalent cylinder model because of its stringent requirements for dendritic branching patterns and end terminations. In the last decade motoneuron cable parameters have been examined more directly by making transient and steady-state electrical measurements at the soma and then examining the

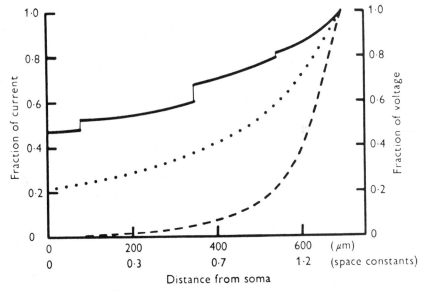

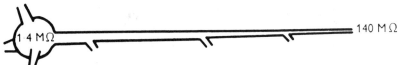

Figure 3 Calculated spatial distribution of current (left ordinate) and voltage change (right ordinate) caused by a steady current injected at the tip of a reconstructed dendrite (neuron 5 of Barrett and Crill [6]) 1.6 space constants long. The solid line is the fraction of injected current remaining intracellularly along the dendrite. Discontinuities are caused by dendritic branches. Dashed line is normalized voltage along the reconstructed dendrite. Dotted line is fraction of current along a semi-infinite equivalent membrane cylinder. Bottom is a schematic representation of the dendrite showing the calculated input impedance at the soma and the dendritic tip. (From Ref. 65.)

anatomic structure of the same neuron. This was first accomplished in moto-neurons by Lux et al. (62) using radioautography and by Barrett and Crill (6,64) using Procion dye injection. In the experiments of Barrett and Crill (6,64) the subthreshold passive response of a lumbar motoneuron was measured and then the cell was injected with the fluorescent dye Procion yellow. After fixation, and using extreme care to minimize and identify tissue shrinkage, a reconstruction of the neuron studied electrophysiologically was prepared from serial sections of the spinal cord. Detailed geometric measurements were made of the soma and dendrites. Because of the variations in length and diameter of the dendrites, the

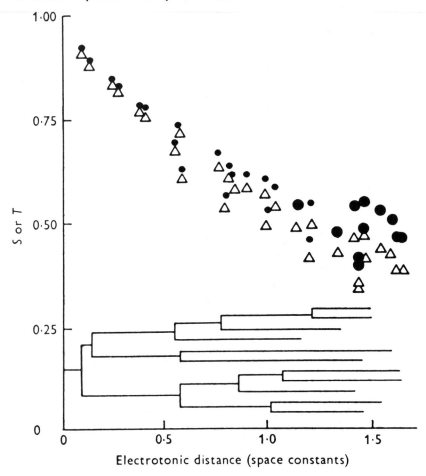

Figure 4 The effectiveness of a unit synaptic conductance change at various points along a reconstructed dendrite (neuron 5 of Barrett and Crill [6]). Circles are normalized fraction of injected charge that reaches the soma (T). Large circles denote values for terminal branches. Triangles are synaptic effectiveness (S), which is the time integral of the voltage change produced at the soma by a unit conductance change divided by the time integral of the somatic voltage change expected if the same conductance occurred on the soma. (From Ref. 65.)

tree was divided into uniform short cylinders. The summed diameter of the dendrites to the 3/2 power showed a rapid decrease near the soma, followed by a less but constant decrease throughout the extent of the dendrites. This decrease was caused both by tapering and by termination of dendritic branches. Cytoplasmic resistivity was measured at 70 ± 15 Ω cm. The specific membrane resistivity was measured by calculating the input conductance of the distal segments assuming the value of R_m varying from 500 to 5000 Ω cm^2. The input conductance of each segment became the terminal conductance of the next segment and the input conductance as a function of R_m at the proximal end was again calculated. These calculations were iteratively repeated until values for the input conductance for the soma and the entire dendritic tree as a function of R_m was determined. Since the input resistance, R_n, had been measured from the reconstructed cell, the value of a uniform R_m giving the corresponding R_n could be obtained directly from the plot of R_n versus R_m. For 10 motoneurons studied in this manner, R_m was 1770 ± 380 Ω cm^2 assuming the dendritic terminals were sealed, and 2520 ± 660 Ω cm^2 assuming they extended to infinity at their terminating diameter. For 116 different primary dendrites in 10 neurons the mean electrotonic length (L) was 1.4 ± 0.27 space constants. Dendritic to soma conductance ratio (ρ) was 9.3 ± 3.3 for closed-end dendrites. Furthermore, the cells with the largest surface area and fastest axon conduction velocity had the smallest soma input conductance, as would be expected.

Barrett and Crill (65) used their measurements of the geometry and specific membrane properties to calculate the effectiveness of synaptic input at various distances from the soma. Based on the assumption that the passive properties of the dendrites and the soma are the same, the fraction of injected synaptic current that reaches the soma from a bouton located at any point on the dendrite can be calculated. As shown in Figure 3, the actual dendrite is more effective in charge transfer than the equivalent cylinder model. This large effective current transfer occurs because of the low input impedance offered by the soma and other dendrites proximal to the synaptic site. Because the input resistance at the dendritic tip may be 100 times the value at the soma, unitary postsynaptic potentials far from the soma are theoretically very large, and there is a large voltage attenuation of the postsynaptic potentials. However, the critical measure of effectiveness is charge transfer. Figure 4 shows charge transfer calculated for a quantal conductance change at various points along a single reconstructed dendrite.

Although the reconstructions of motoneurons reveal significant differences from the conceptional model of Rall (2) [e.g., dendrites not all the same electrotonic length and a progressive decrease in the dendritic trunk parameter (Σ diameters to 3/2 power) with distance from the soma], the measurements of the key parameters of dendritic passive properties of Lux et al. (62) and of Barrett and Crill (6,65) are remarkably similar to the values initially estimated by Rall (50,51). It is conceivable that the transient responses of real motoneurons to injected currents are insensitive to the exact branching and termination characteristics of the dendrites, even though the simplicity obtained in the mathematic analysis which led to Rall's model (2) is very sensitive to these characteristics.

IV. VOLTAGE-DEPENDENT IONIC CONDUCTANCES

A. Application of the Voltage Clamp Technique to Motoneurons

A great deal has been learned about the electrical properties of motoneurons and their functional input/output characteristics using intracellular current injection ("current clamp") techniques. Following the lead of earlier investigators (66,67), a recent series of experiments has applied the voltage clamp technique to lumbar motoneurons. Although the voltage clamp technique has been extremely successful in elucidating the precise mechanism underlying excitability in many neurons, it is unlikely that similar success will ever be attained in mammalian central nervous system neurons because of several severe theoretic and technical problems. In a mammalian neuron the voltage is controlled only at a "point" (presumably the soma and some unknown fraction of proximal dendrites) on a complex, cablelike structure. For this reason, the whole cell is not isopotential with the command voltage applied at the "point." If significant active currents are generated beyond the region of effective voltage control, the apparent time and voltage dependence of the evoked ionic currents would be inaccurate at best and nonsense at worst. However, if most of the active conductances are located at the controlled "point," and if most of the dendritic tree were passive, the latter would merely constitute a linear, "leak" conductance which is approximately equivalent to the neuronal input conductance in cells like motoneurons which have a large dendritic dominance. In this case, the accuracy of the measured active ionic currents would be unaffected. The latter condition appears to hold approximately in normal motoneurons, and probably is the major factor responsible for the success of the experiments. Some indications that the measured ionic currents are reasonably accurate and actually determine somatic membrane potential in the unclamped condition are: (1) the behavior of the currents is reasonable and consistent from cell to cell; (2) electrical activity, such as the action potential, can be reconstructed from quantitative measurements; and (3) cell behavior (such as voltage thresholds, depolarization levels, firing behavior) in the unclamped condition is consistent with the voltage clamp data obtained in the same cell.

Even if the theoretic problems remain hypothetic, a variety of practical problems limit the type of information that can be obtained. Most severe is the difficulty of altering the extracellular environment in a controlled way in vivo so that conductance components and equilibrium potentials may be altered. These manipulations have proven invaluable in the investigation of invertebrate neurons. Even if the lack of a "space clamp" does not distort the ionic currents, it does result in a long decay time of the capacitance-charging transient, even if the voltage rise is instantaneous (52). This long transient, then, may obscure or distort current components with fast onset (such as sodium) as well as the fast tail currents used to determine accurately equilibrium potentials. An additional practical problem is that the cells must be impaled with separate voltage-recording and current-injecting microelectrodes. In our experience, the great majority of the cells examined are damaged after impalement with the two microelectrodes, since their resting and action potentials and rhythmic firing characteristics are usually subnormal compared to cells penetrated with a single microelectrode. As a consequence, only a few cells can be held in good condition long enough to make the many measurements required for quantitative descriptions of conductances. A large variation is seen in the precise behavior of the current components from cell to cell. This is expected from the known variation of membrane properties such as after-hyperpolarization duration or rhythmic firing characteristics, but it may also be due to injury in the voltage clamp experiments. Both of these factors make it virtually impossible to confidently quote, for example, a time constant or conductance value as typical of all motoneurons. Although the qualitative data are quite consistent, the quantitative data so far obtained should be considered as indicative of the true values rather than as definitive results. In spite of these problems, the voltage clamp results provide considerable insight, which cannot be gained by other methods, into the mechanisms underlying motoneuron excitability and the functional role of the active conductances. The properties of the major ionic current components of lumbar motoneurons are summarized below (Secs. IV.B–E), and our current understanding of their role in cell excitability is discussed further in Sec. V.

B. Subthreshold Response

One assumption of cable theory is that the subtreshold response of the motoneuron is determined by passive, linear membrane elements. In fact, it has been long known that the subthreshold response displays both voltage and time dependence, although this behavior is not likely to negate the main conclusions of cable analysis. The time dependence of the response, first described by Ito and Oshima (68), is indicated by the ultimate "sag" in membrane potential seen during the application of a long-lasting hyperpolarizing current pulse (Fig. 5B) and a subsequent small depolarizing oscillation after the current is terminated. A mirror image of these slow oscillations are often seen for long, depolarizing current pulses (Fig. 5B). In our experience, the response is invariably seen upon hyperpolarization, though it may not appear upon depolarization in all cells. A subthreshold voltage dependence (rectification) has been described by several investigators (27,68,69), who found that input resistance increases when the cell is depolarized and decreases when it is hyperpolarized (Fig. 5A). Since this behavior is opposite to that predicted by the Goldman constant field equation (70), it is often called "anomalous" rectification. Similar time- and voltage-dependent responses are seen in pyramidal cells of the neocortex and the hippocampus and, thus, may be a general property of mammalian neurons (71–73).

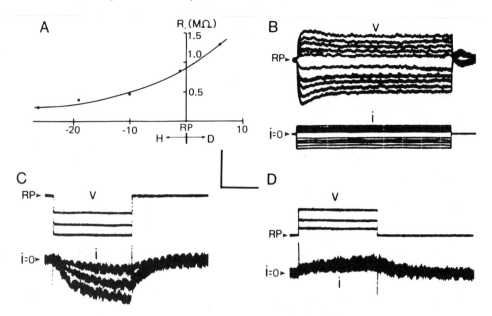

Figure 5 Subthreshold time- and voltage-dependent membrane properties of lumbar motoneurons. A: An example of the variation of input resistance in the subthreshold region around resting potential (RP) in one motoneuron. Intracellularly injected current was used to artificially depolarize (D) and hyperpolarize (H) the cell and to measure input resistance (R). (After Ref. 69.) B: Superimposed records of membrane potential (upper) in response to long-lasting, subthreshold, hyperpolarizing and depolarizing injected current pulses (lower) in a different cell. Note prominent "overshoots" of membrane potential in responses to pulses in either direction and membrane potential oscillation of opposite sign after termination of current pulse. C,D: Voltage clamp records from cell of B. Upper traces are superimposed records of voltage steps imposed from a D.C. clamp at the same natural resting potential as B and traversing the same range of potentials as in B. Lower traces are superimposed records of the ionic membrane currents activated by the corresponding voltage steps. Current "tails" which persist after termination of the voltage steps are caused by relaxation of the activated conductances to their rest values. Here and in subsequent voltage clamp records the ohmic, "leak" current has been electronically subtracted before photography; only active currents are shown. Here and in subsequent records outward ionic current is taken as positive. Hyperpolarizing steps (C) activate a slow, inward current, termed I_{AR}, and depolarizing steps (D) activate a slow outward current, termed I_{Ks} (see text). The persistent inward current (I_i) is likely mixed with I_{Ks} and results in the constant amplitude of the outward current as voltage is stepped up, since I_i becomes dominant at slightly more depolarized voltage steps (not shown). (See text for further explanation.) Calibration: 20 mV for B–D; 8 nA for C, D; 50 nA for B; 100 msec for B–D.

Some insight into the mechanisms underlying these subthreshold responses has been provided by voltage clamp studies.

The mechanism resulting in the increased input conductance upon hyperpolarization is different from the mechanism causing the decreased input conductance upon depolarization. When a motoneuron is depolarized by voltage clamp, its steady current-voltage (I-V) curve exhibits a region of decrementing and, ultimately, negative slope conductance over a voltage range below spike threshold (74,75) (Fig. 8A). The decrease of slope conductance is caused by the activation of a persistent, inward, calcium current (see Sec. IV.E) which is superimposed on the outward "leak" and potassium currents. The decreased slope conductance will be reflected as a increased input resistance when current clamp techniques are used. When a motoneuron is hyperpolarized by voltage clamp an inward current develops slowly during the clamp and decays slowly afterward (Fig. 5C). The development of this current is consistent with an increased membrane conductance upon hyperpolarization. This current component was first described by Barrett et al. (76) and termed "anomalous rectification current" (I_{AR}). Similar currents are seen in neocortical and hippocampal neurons (77; C. E. Stafstrom, unpublished data, 1983). I_{AR} develops with time constants on the order of 40-60 msec which remain approximately constant for hyperpolarization to 50 mV negative to rest, and its reversal potential is near rest. It is unaffected in motoneurons or neocortical cells by intra- or extracellular sodium or potassium conductance blockers, calcium-blocking divalent cations, barium, or increased intracellular chloride. In motoneurons it is difficult to detect a difference in the instantaneous current jumps at the onset or termination of the clamp in spite of the large current developed. This suggests that a fast-acting, voltage-dependent, electrogenic pump could play a role as originally suggested by Ito and Oshima (68), although this has not been directly tested. Whatever is the basis of this current, it is clear that it is responsible both for the rectification in the hyperpolarizing direction and the accompanying, slow membrane potential oscillations seen in current clamp studies.

The slow membrane potential oscillations often seen upon depolarization result from the activation of a small, slow outward current in cells in which this current dominates or is activated at lower potentials than the persistent inward current (Fig. 5D). At present, it is not entirely clear whether this slow outward current is a reversed I_{AR} or a separate, slow potassium current (see Sec. IV.D). Overall, the voltage clamp results indicate that there is really no voltage range where the membrane behaves strictly passively, but the subthreshold active currents are small and rather slowly activated.

C. The Sodium Conductance

The fast, transient, inward sodium current (I_{Na}) of motoneurons was first observed by Araki and Terzuolo (66) and has recently been analyzed quantitatively

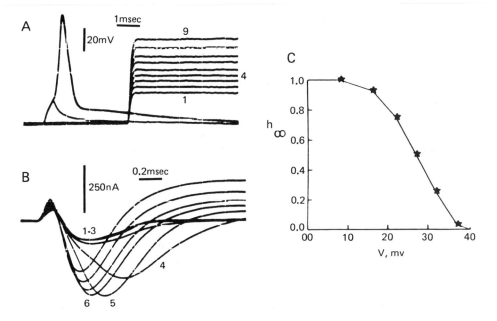

Figure 6 An example of the fast, transient sodium current of lumbar moto-neurons. A: Superimposed traces of an action potential and subthreshold response to a brief current pulse and subsequent voltage steps imposed on the same motoneuron. B: Superimposed records of the fast, transient, inward, active currents activated by the like-numbered voltage steps in A. Steps 1-3 activate only an all-or-none, uncontrolled inward current resulting from firing of the axon initial segment. This current is the same for all voltage steps. Sodium current is not clearly apparent until step 4. C: A plot of the steady sodium inactivation characteristic (h_∞) for a different cell vs. depolarization from resting potential (V). Resting potential was ~-75 mV in this cell.

by Barrett and Crill (78). As seen in Figure 6A, when voltage is stepped positive from resting potential the first current waveform observed is a brief, all-or-none, uncontrolled, transient inward current whose amplitude is unrelated to the size of the voltage step (Fig. 6A,B, steps 1-3). This waveform likely represents firing of the initial segment, since a similar current is seen when an isolated initial segment spike is clamped near resting potential (66). The axon-evoked initial segment current can be occluded by collision with the soma-evoked initial segment current. The initial segment current usually has a peak amplitude of about 100 nA and a duration of about 1 msec or less.

The somatic sodium current does not appear until the voltage is stepped 25-40 mV positive to rest (Fig. 6A,B, step 4). The relatively high activation threshold of this conductance component is consistent with the findings (see

Sec. II.C) that the soma-dendritic spike is triggered by the large somatic depolarization caused by the initial segment spike. The sodium current is graded with depolarization, and in the best cells reaches a maximum value of 400–600 nA ~50 mV positive to rest (66,78). However, we have also observed cells having considerably smaller peak sodium currents which still generate 60–70 mV spikes. Apparently, spike height also depends somewhat upon passive cell properties, as will be discussed in Sec. V.A.

This current appears to be carried by sodium, since it is eliminated by extracellular tetrodotoxin (TTX) (78) and intracellular QX314 (79), agents which are known to block identified sodium currents in other preparations. Its apparent equilibrium potential (E_{Na}) is also consistent with sodium being the main charge carrier. A value of ~120 mV positive to rest is obtained in cells having resting potentials of –60 – –70 mV (66,78). This value (~+60 mV absolute) is similar to that obtained in squid axon. However, the true value of E_{Na} is less certain in motoneurons because of a number of technical problems, one of which is that the capacitative transient becomes enormous at large depolarizations. It can obscure the small I_{Na} at these potentials and necessitates the use of extrapolation of the peak I_{Na}-voltage relation to determine E_{Na}.

The presence of the long capacitative transient and the superimposed initial segment current makes it difficult to quantitatively describe I_{Na} activation kinetics. However, I_{Na} activation is nonlinear (78), and a satisfactory motoneuron I_{Na} onset can be reproduced using third-order kinetics with time constants similar to those for squid axon at about $12°C$ in a Hodgkin-Huxley formulation (76,78). Scaling squid or frog node kinetics to $37°C$ results in much too fast an I_{Na} onset or spike upstroke.

It is far easier technically to measure I_{Na} inactivation characteristics. The inactivation process has first-order kinetics with a time constant of 1–2 msec near rest and ~0.2 msec 60 mV positive to rest (78). Motoneurons which exhibit normal rhythmic firing characteristics (i.e., comparable to those observed after single microelectrode penetration) have a steady-state inactivation characteristic like that in Figure 6C. That is, they show minimal I_{Na} inactivation to ~20 mV positive to rest. It can be appreciated that such inactivation characteristics are required to enable spike generation during rhythmic firing because the membrane potential between rhythmic spikes remains depolarized during the interspike interval and can traverse potentials 20 mV or greater before spike initiation (Figs. 2A, 9A, and 10). In addition, to generate a spike I_{NA} must overcome a large outward leak current as well as potassium currents (see Sec. IV.D), which are activated below spike threshold. Spike threshold increases with firing rate (see Sec. V.B), and it has been found that the maximum firing rate is obtained when firing level reaches the potential when I_{Na} is about half inactivated. Thus, I_{Na} inactivation probably governs the maximum firing rates attainable in motoneurons.

Implicit in the data of Barrett et al. (76), and also observed in subsequent studies, is the fact that the sodium activation and inactivation characteristics [analogous to the m_∞ and h_∞ curves of Hodgkin and Huxley (80)] overlap over a certain voltage range (e.g., from 30 mV to 40 mV positive to resting potential). The degree of overlap varies from cell to cell, but its presence implies that a steady, depolarizing I_{Na} can occur, since I_{Na} will be activated but not fully inactivated in the region of m and h overlap.

D. The Potassium Conductances

Examples of the outward, potassium currents of motoneurons are shown in Figure 7A and B. These currents were first examined in detail and analyzed quantitatively by Barrett et al. (76). One of their major findings was that there are two kinetically separable outward current components, one having fast kinetics (I_{Kf}), and the other (I_{Ks}) having time constants ~10 times slower. The disparity in time constants is great enough that onset or decay of the two components may be recognized by inspection of the current records (Fig. 7A). Not only can the outward current be separated mathematically into two components, but each component can be activated independently in special circumstances (76). One indication of their kinetic independence can be seen in Figure 7A, where, after the earliest downstep, I_{Kf} is decaying while I_{Ks} is still increasing at the downstep potential.

A second major finding was that the outward currents are indeed persistent. The transient potassium current, I_A, which is so prominent in molluscan somata (81), appears to be absent in motoneurons. A very fast transient outward current is seen in some cells, particularly those with high resting potential (75), but at present, it is not clear whether it results from a true conductance increase or whether it is an artifact resulting from lack of a space clamp of the initial segment. If it is real, its kinetics are so fast that it would have the same functional role as I_{Kf}, operating to help repolarize the spike in those neurons in which it is found.

I_{Kf} has nonlinear activation kinetics and seems best described as a fourth-order process. Its activation time constants vary rapidly with voltage from a maximum of 4 or 5 msec somewhat positive to rest to ~1 msec near 60 mV positive to rest (76). I_{Kf} first becomes strongly activated slightly positive to the potential where I_{Na} first appears, but other current components (see below and Sec. IV.E) may mask its more moderate activation at potentials closer to rest. Overall, I_{Kf} closely resembles the delayed rectifier of squid or frog axon.

I_{Ks} is well described by first-order kinetics; its activation time constants decrease slowly with voltage, at least within 20 mV or so of resting potential (78). Within this range time constants as long as 50 msec can be observed, but the time constants vary from cell to cell as does the after-hyperpolarization for

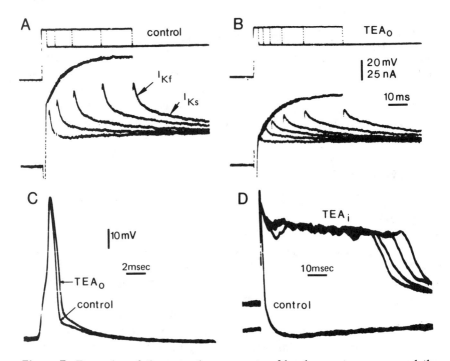

Figure 7 Examples of the potassium currents of lumbar motoneurons and the effect of TEA application on the outward currents and the action potential. A, B: Superimposed records of imposed voltage steps (upper) and corresponding, active, outward, ionic currents (lower) before (A) and after (B) extracellular iontophoresis of TEA. The voltage step paradigm consists of a prepulse of variable duration and of amplitude sufficient to activate the potassium conductances followed by a downstep to the same potential at various times after the prepulse. Because their time constants are so different, the kinetically separable, fast (I_{Kf}) and slow (I_{Ks}) components of the potassium current can easily be seen to develop (in A) with a fast and slow time course during the prepulse and to decay with markedly different time courses after the downstep. Notice also from the tail currents amplitudes that I_{Kf} is nearly fully activated by the shortest prepulse, whereas I_{Ks} continues to grow as the prepulse is lengthened. Extracellular TEA iontophoresis (B) greatly diminishes I_{Kf} but leaves I_{Ks} unaffected. C: Superimposed records of spikes evoked by brief current pulses immediately before the corresponding voltage clamp records of A and B were taken. In this cell the persistent inward current (I_i) (see text) had deteriorated owing to impalement injury, and the great decrement of I_{Kf} by TEA had little effect on spike duration. D: Superimposed records of spikes evoked by brief current pulses before (control—top of spike clipped) and after (TEA_i) intracellular TEA injection in a different cell where the persistent inward current remained present during the time that TEA diminished the outward currents. In this situation, a prolonged plateau action potential eventually develops. (Intracellular TEA also typically causes the cells to depolarize as also seen in the record.) Voltage calibration in C also applies to D.

which the component is responsible (76). Its time constants decrease with depolarization, but for technical reasons are difficult to measure accurately at large depolarizations. However, the quick establishment of a steady outward current at large depolarizations (82) suggests that the time constants become much faster. I_{Ks} is first activated about 10 mV or less positive to rest. As discussed in Sec. IV.B, its activation apparently results in the membrane potential "sag" often seen during injection of long subthreshold current pulses and the subsequent small hyperpolarization that follows the termination of the current pulse.

Both I_{Kf} and I_{Ks} have linear instantaneous I-V relations, at least in the voltage range positive to rest where tail currents are clear and the instantaneous I-V relation can be measured. The linear I-V relations are fortunate, since E_K must again be obtained by extrapolation. This is because the long capacitative transient obscures the small, brief I_{Kf} tails at potentials negative to rest, while I_{Ks} only reaches a local minimum because hyperpolarizing steps activate the "anomalous rectification current," I_{AR}, described in Sec. IV.B, which has time constants similar to I_{Ks}. In addition, the decay of a persistent inward current (see Sec. IV.E), which is activated by any prepulse that activates I_K, distorts and decrements the true outward current tail, particularly for large downsteps. For these reasons, the E_K value obtained is variable from cell to cell, and probably represents an upper bound to the true E_K. The extrapolated reversal potential is usually 15-20 mV negative to rest, but less negative values are also obtained (76).

The negative apparent reversal potential is consistent with I_{Kf} and I_{Ks} being potassium currents. More direct evidence is provided by the positive shift of the apparent reversal potential when extracellular potassium is raised by iontophoresis (82), or if intracellular potassium is decreased by injection of an impermeant cation (83). In addition, the outward currents are depressed by intra- or extracellular iontophoresis of a variety of agents known to block identified, voltage-dependent potassium currents in other cells. However, I_{Kf} is predominantly affected by most of the blocking agents that have been tried. Intracellular iontophoresis of tetraethylammonium (TEA), 4-aminopyridine, or QX314 depresses the outward currents (75,79). I_{Kf} is affected initially, but I_{Ks} is also depressed upon prolonged injection, possibly because these relatively impermeant cations displace internal potassium and shift E_K. Both internal and external Ba^{2+} rapidly depress I_{Kf}, though external Ba^{2+} apparently has to enter the cell to exert its action (79). Although extracellular Ba^{2+} in calcium-free solutions is an effective blocker of slow potassium currents in a variety of invertebrate and vertebrate neurons, it is far less effective on I_{Ks} than on I_{Kf} in vivo motoneurons in which calcium is still present extracellularly. One indication of this is that normal after-hyperpolarizations follow prolonged "Ba^{2+} spikes" in cells showing no sign of I_{Kf} (79). Perhaps the clearest pharmacologic separation of I_{Kf} from I_{Ks} occurs with extracellular iontophoresis of TEA (82). An example is shown in Figure 7.

These experiments have shown that I_{Kf} and I_{Ks} are pharmacologically as well as kinetically separable, at least in the sense that I_{Kf} can be depressed much more effectively than I_{Ks} by these agents. One way this could happen is if I_{Ks} were predominantly dendritic and, thus, out of range of perisomatic iontophoresis. This cannot be discounted, but a number of other factors argue against this. For example, if this were true, it is difficult to understand how I_{Ks} could be activated by much smaller somatic depolarizations than I_{Kf}. In addition, extracellular iontophoresis of calcium-blocking divalent cations (Co^{2+}, Mn^{2+}, Ni^{2+}) effectively depress both I_{Kf} and I_{Ks} to a similar extent (82).

The effect of the divalent cations is of interest because slow potassium currents like I_{Ks} have been found to be activated by calcium entry, rather than voltage, in a variety of vertebrate and invertebrate neurons, and these potassium currents can be blocked by extracellular divalent cations or an intracellular calcium chelator. There is considerable indirect evidence that motoneurons possess such calcium-mediated potassium conductance. Intracellular calcium injection decreases motoneuron input resistance near rest in a manner consistent with an increased potassium permeability (84). Extracellular iontophoresis of calcium-blocking divalent cations or intracellular iontophoresis of the calcium chelator (EGTA) selectively depresses the after-hyperpolarization and its associated increase in input conductance, whereas spike duration is essentially unaltered by these agents (85,86). A similar effect is seen in frog motoneurons when calcium-blocking divalent cations are applied or when extracellular calcium concentration is lowered (87).

Curiously, extracellular iontophoresis of divalent cations depresses both I_{Kf} and I_{Ks} equally well when these currents are examined under voltage clamp, even though only the after-hyperpolarization appears to be affected when the same cells are examined under current clamp (82). It turns out that spike repolarization is relatively insensitive to large changes in I_{Kf} (see Fig. 7A–C), whereas the after-hyperpolarization is quite sensitive to changes in I_{Ks}, which makes the technique of comparing alterations of spike and after-hyperpolarization potentials a rather poor measure of the specificity of a blocking agent. Since the divalent cations act nonselectively on I_{Kf} and I_{Ks}, they may also be acting nonspecifically, that is, in ways unrelated to calcium blockade, especially since it is very unlikely that I_{Kf} is calcium mediated. One nonspecific mechanism involves an I-V curve shift due to an interaction by extracellular cations with voltage-dependent channels. Large shifts can be produced in frog axon by relatively small divalent cation increments (88), and a similar effect appears to occur in motoneurons with large iontophoresis (82). On the other hand, large depolarizations of motoneurons reveal a region of negative slope conductance with the concomitant disappearance of the I_{Ks} tail current (89). Such behavior in invertebrate cells is caused by the decrease in a calcium-mediated potassium current as the membrane potential approaches E_{Ca}, but it is not certain that the same explanation holds for this behavior in motoneurons.

Because of the abovementioned uncertainties and contradictions, and the lack of a direct test, it remains unclear whether I_{Ks} is calcium mediated. Recently, a slowly activating, voltage-dependent potassium current (the "m current"), which clearly is *not* calcium-mediated, has been found in sympathetic ganglion neurons (90) and hippocampal pyramidal cells (91). It is possible that I_{Ks} is also such a current, but appropriate tests have not yet been performed.

E. The Calcium Conductance

In healthy motoneurons a persistent inward current, which has been termed I_i, is activated by relatively small voltage steps positive to resting potential (75). An example of I_i behavior is shown in Figure 8. Since I_i is persistent, it results in a region of negative slope conductance, and often, a region of net inward current on the steady I-V curve of motoneurons (Fig. 8A). This current component has been difficult to study in detail, principally because it is extremely sensitive to the damage caused by impalement with two microelectrodes, and it deteriorates within a short time in most cells. The deterioration is likely caused by release of calcium from internal stores or calcium leakage around the microelectrodes (see later). In spite of this technical problem, some general properties of I_i have been discovered, and these are consistent from cell to cell.

I_i is first clearly activated about 10 mV positive to resting potential, which is well below threshold for the somatic I_{Na}. Near its activation threshold I_i does not decrement during prolonged voltage steps, and in most cells it activates very slowly with a smooth waveform (Fig. 8C, step 1). Its time course may be fit by a single exponential having a time constant on the order of 15-20 msec, though time constants of 50 msec have been observed in some cells. In other cells I_i appears to reach a steady value within ~10 msec, but there are clear signs of potassium current being mixed with I_i in these cells, and this mixture probably determines the apparent I_i time course. In fact, I_i appears to be mixed with potassium currents at every potential where it can be observed, and this is the main factor that has precluded a quantitative description of I_i. Currents must be observed in isolation for a quantitative analysis to be meaningful.

The onset of I_i becomes much more rapid, and its amplitude becomes much greater as voltage is stepped above I_i activation threshold (Fig. 8C, steps 2,4). I_i clearly activates rapidly at larger depolarizations (75). Although the true I_i time course cannot be discovered because of contaminating potassium currents, the time course of I_i onset, together with evidence for lack of I_i inactivation, suggests that the curve describing the variation of I_i time constants with voltage would resemble a rectangular hyperbola. The time constants would be quite long at small depolarizations but they would rapidly decrease with increments of depolarization. Beyond the knee of the hyperbola, ~20-30 mV positive to rest, the time constants would remain quite short. Such behavior is also seen for the calcium conductance of certain molluscan neurons (92,93).

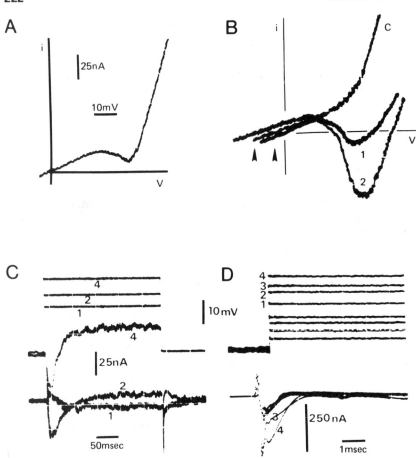

Figure 8 Examples of the persistent, inward calcium current (I_i) of lumbar motoneurons and the effect of extracellular barium. A: Quasi–steady-state membrane current-voltage (I–V) relation of a motoneuron measured by application of a ramp voltage clamp which rises slowly enough that the sodium current reaches its steady inactivation valve at each potential. The linear portion of the curve near resting potential (origin of the plot) is determined principally by ohmic, "leakage" conductance. At larger depolarization, a persistent inward current is activated. It superimposes on the linear, "leak" I–V relation and results in the negative slope conductance and inward-going portion of the I–V relation. At still larger depolarizations, the potassium currents become dominant; they restore the positive-slope characteristic and result in the large, outward "delayed rectification" portion of the I–V relation. B: Effect of extracellular iontophoreses of Ba^{2+} on a motoneuron I–V relation. In this cell I_i had "deteriorated" (the inward charge transfer could no longer be detected) owing to impalement injury. Thus, no negative slope characteristic is seen in the

Peak I_i amplitude usually occurs 20–30 mV positive to rest, which is still below I_{Na} threshold in most cells. Little is known about the variation of the underlying conductance with voltage except that the maximum chord conductance, G_i, must be quite small given that peak I_i is usually 25 nA or less and the driving potential $(E\text{-}E_{Ca})$ is probably on the order of 200 mV.

As voltage is stepped higher I_i appears to become transient and smaller until it is no longer visible for steps beyond 40–50 mV positive to rest (in the range where I_{Kf} becomes strongly activated). In spite of this behavior, there are several pieces of indirect evidence indicating that I_i does not totally inactivate, or does so very slowly, for depolarizations to ~70 mV positive to rest (75). For example, after internal TEA injection prolonged plateau action potentials can develop which keep the cell depolarized for 100 msec or more (Fig. 7D), and voltage clamp analysis has shown that I_i is responsible for maintaining this depolarization subsequent to the depression of potassium currents by TEA (75). Therefore, I_i appears to be transient at larger depolarizations in normal cells simply because the coactivated potassium currents become large enough to obscure the underlying I_i.

Two lines of indirect evidence suggest that I_i is carried predominantly by calcium ions: (1) I_i remains present after I_{Na} is eliminated by intracellular QX314 (79), and (2) I_i is enhanced by external iontophoresis of Ba^{2+}. The latter carries charge through Ca^{2+} channels more effectively than Ca^{2+} itself. An example of the Ba^{2+} effect is shown in Figure 8B. Notice that I_i had "deteriorated" in this cell before Ba^{2+} application. However, the Ba^{2+} effect indicates that the Ca^{2+} channels were still present; it was merely that the inward charge transfer (I_i) could not be detected prior to Ba^{2+} application, possibly owing to an injury-induced rise in intracellular Ca^{2+}. Because the Ba^{2+} current that flows through I_i channels can be made very large by adequate Ba^{2+} iontophoresis, and

---

control record, but two successive, Ba^{2+} applications (curve 1: 150 nA, 50 sec; curve 2: 250 nA, 45 sec) result in a negative slope conductance and large, net-inward currents. Ba^{2+} is effectively carrying charge through the Ca^{2+} channels that normally generate I_i. C: Time course of I_i in response to voltage steps in a different cell. Like-numbered voltage steps (upper) and ionic current traces (lower) correspond. Notice slow onset and persistence of I_i activated by step 1. At larger depolarizations I_i appears to be transient (step 2) and ultimately becomes unrecognizable (step 4). D: Fast, transient inward currents at start of same series of voltage steps. Like-numbered traces in C and D are identical, but are shown at faster sweep speed in D. Sodium current is not clearly activated until steps 3 and 4. Smaller voltage steps only trigger all-or-none initial segment current (see text), which is identical for all voltage steps. Note by comparison of C and D that I_i is first activated, and is most prominent, at voltages below sodium activation threshold. Voltage calibration in A also applies to B.

because Ba^{2+} also depresses potassium conductance (see Sec. IV.D), it was possible to observe I_{Ba} over a much greater voltage range than is possible with I_i because of contaminating potassium currents. Thus, the experiments with Ba^{2+} verify more directly the previous conclusions that I_i is, at most, slowly inactivating over a large voltage range and in normal cells is hidden by the large potassium currents that develop as the cell is depolarized.

Calcium conductances have now been found in the soma/dendritic region of virtually every cell type that has been examined. Like I_i, the calcium currents in these cells are found to be slowly inactivating when contaminating potassium currents are removed. In most cells the calcium conductance is not activated until large depolarizations are imposed. I_i differs in that it is first activated at small depolarizations from rest. In this way, and also in its postulated kinetics, it resembles more closely a calcium current component of certain molluscan bursting pacemakers (92,93). These latter cells also appear to have a separate, fast-activated calcium current which is first activated at large depolarizations, and which is mainly responsible for activating their calcium-mediated potassium conductance (92). It is possible that motoneurons also possess a similar separate calcium conductance that activates I_{Ks}, but at present, we have no evidence less tenuous than the negative slope conductance at large depolarizations which was mentioned earlier. However, the Ba^{2+} current appears to activate very rapidly at all potentials (79), which may indicate the existence of some fast-activating calcium channels in motoneurons. Unless I_i kinetics become much faster at large depolarization than they appear to be in the voltage range where I_i can be observed, it would appear to be physically impossible for I_i to activate sufficient potassium during the brief depolarization provided by the spike to result in a significant after-hyperpolarization. As also mentioned earlier, I_{Ks} may not be calcium-activated after all. One indication of this is that a slow outward current can be seen clearly in many motoneurons at voltages below the apparent threshold for I_i activation (Fig. 5D).

Although I_i appears to resemble the slow calcium current of molluscan bursting pacemakers, motoneurons do not normally engage in self-sustained bursting activity. It should be kept in mind that I_i is an inward current *component*. It is superimposed on the large, outward "leak" current and on the potassium currents so that the total current is net-outward at all voltages in most cells (see Fig. 8A). As has been discussed elsewhere (83), when the total ionic current is net-inward, the existence of bursting behavior and its character will depend strongly upon the voltage dependence of I_i and each of the outward currents and, most importantly, on the kinetics of each current component. I_i can maintain prolonged, self-sustained bursting in motoneurons, but this occurs only after potassium currents have been depressed by drugs or by a raised E_K during spinal seizures (83).

V. ROLE OF ACTIVE AND PASSIVE MEMBRANE PROPERTIES IN FIRING BEHAVIOR

A. Action Potential Generation

Using measured sodium and potassium parameters in a Hodgkin-Huxley formulation (78) for the ionic currents together with measured passive characteristics, Barrett et al. (76) were able to satisfactorily reproduce the action potential, and after-hyperpolarization, and low-frequency rhythmic firing of the cell from which the data were obtained. Not surprisingly, I_{Na} caused the spike upstroke and I_{Kf} was involved in spike repolarization, whereas I_{Ks} was responsible for the after-hyperpolarization and controlled the rhythmic firing rate. The delayed depolarization was basically caused by the passive properties of the dendritic tree. Subsequent experiments and computer simulations based on voltage clamp data have provided additional insight into the factors influencing motoneuron excitability. For example, in cells in which I_i has deteriorated a large reduction in I_{Kf} by TEA or Ba^{2+} has a relatively minor effect on action potential duration (79,82; see Fig. 7C), and the same result is obtained in computer simulations. Fractional I_{Ks} activation together with the large leak conductance of motoneurons is enough to rapidly repolarize the cell. However, I_i is present in normal cells, and when potassium currents are depressed in the presence of I_i (or I_{Ba}) a prolonged depolarization plateau follows the upstroke of the spike (75,79; see Fig. 7D). Thus, while I_{Kf} apparently is not required for rapid spike repolarization *per se*, it is necessary in order to rapidly overcome any I_i activated during the spike and to prevent the development of a prolonged action potential.

A striking finding of Barrett et al. (76) is that the chord conductances governing the potassium currents are quite small, generally having peak values only a few times greater than leak conductance (the *slope* conductances can, of course, be much larger). In fact, the peak potassium conductance of their exemplar cell is 1–4 μS smaller than subsequently seen in other, presumably more "healthy," cells (our own data), but the order of magnitude seems correct. One may wonder how such small active conductances could actually "drive" the large leak conductance and capacitance of a motoneuron and produce normal electrical activity.

The most apt comparison may be with a frog node of Ranvier. There, the currents generated by the miniscule node must "drive" the passive load provided by the axon and depolarize the next node to threshold, just as the motoneuron soma must "drive" the passive load provided by the dendritic tree during an action potential. For the node the important passive load is not its small leak conductance but the passive input resistance of the axon, which is on the order of 10 MΩ. The ratio of peak sodium conductance to this axon "leak" conductance is 7.5:1, whereas the ratio for potassium is only 1.3:1 (94). Clearly, the

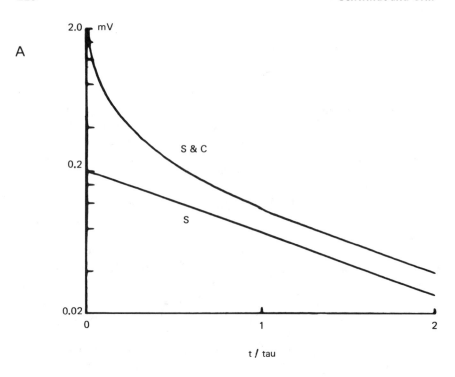

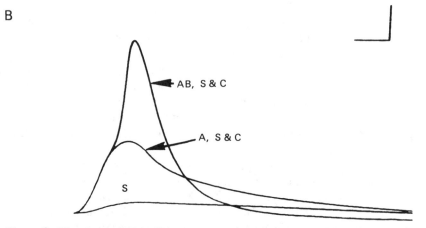

Figure 9 The theoretic impulse responses of two neuron models and their influence on the voltage response produced by membrane current. A: The impulse response of a neuron modeled as an isopotential soma (S) and a soma plus finite, uniform, equivalent cylinder combination (S&C). Each model had a 1 MΩ input resistance and τ_M = 5 msec. The S&C model had ρ = 10 and L = 1.5⋅λ; its impulse

motoneuron is better off, since this ratio for total potassium conductance varies from 3:1 to 7:1 (76) for a 1 MΩ input conductance. However, the effective capacitance of the motoneuron is much greater than that seen by a node in the axon (6). Thus, the transient characteristics of the passive load (as measured by its frequency response or impulse response) will also play a major role in determining how well the active conductances can impose a particular voltage response on the passive system.

In order to account for passive cable properties without having to resort to some arbitrary, assumed cable structure, Barrett et al. (76) measured the impulse response of the motoneuron and convolved this with the active currents computed from the Hodgkin–Huxley formulations at each point in time during the reconstruction. The rationale for this procedure is that the impulse response of a linear, time invariant system (properties usually assumed for the passive cable properties of motoneurons) completely determines its transfer function no matter how complex is the system. No formal network models of the system need to be made. The convolution of the impulse response with any arbitrary "input" current (in this case, the computed ionic currents plus any injected current) will give the voltage response of the system. However, the key assumption in performing this convolution is that the active currents are generated at the "point" (the isopotential compartment) where the impulse response is measured, namely, the soma and some unknown fraction of proximal dendrites approximately isopotential with the soma. This is equivalent to assuming that the currents are generated in the somatic compartment and the dendrites provide merely a shunting, linear cable network. Apparently, the assumption is approximately correct, since reconstruction of electrical activity from voltage clamp data is successful using the convolution technique.

As mentioned previously, because the active conductances and currents are small and the passive conductance and capacitance is large, the precise voltage response of a cell to ionic currents will depend greatly upon its precise impulse response. How the impulse response can vary with the cable structure of a

---

response was computed from equations 4.17–4.22 of Rall (2). Its peak response is off scale at 2.2 mV. B: Computer reconstruction of the "antidromic" voltage response using Hodgkin-Huxley–like formulations based on voltage clamp data for ionic currents, a simulated "A" or "IS" current modeled as a triangular inward current of 70 nA amplitude and 1 msec duration, and the two passive models of A. Only the S&C model allows the membrane potential to reach somatic sodium conductance threshold and trigger a full "AB" spike in response to the brief "IS" current. The same current applied to the S model only results in a small depolarization and passive decay. When sodium conductance is deleted in the reconstruction, the S&C model also produces a much more realistic "A spike" than the S model. Calibration: 0.5 msec, 20 mV.

neuron is shown in Figure 9A, where the impulse responses of an isopotential soma (S) and a soma plus finite cable (S&C) are compared. In each case, the "neuron" has the same input resistance and membrane time constant, but the peak and the total area of the soma-plus-cable impulse response is much larger. The difference this can make in voltage behavior is seen in Figure 9B, where the computed response of the models, each having identical conductances, to a simulated initial segment current is shown. The superior impulse response provided by the cable/soma model allows the initial segment current to trigger a somatic action potential, whereas the "low pass filter" characteristics of the soma-only model does not allow the voltage to reach threshold in response to the brief initial segment current.

B. Factors Influencing Rhythmic Firing

The motoneuron after-hyperpolarization contrasts markedly with the short, sometimes nonexistent after-hyperpolarization of motor axons. It was recognized very early that the after-hyperpolarization implies the existence of a repolarizing conductance with very long time constants, and that the long after-polarization allows motoneurons to fire repetitively at the very low minimum firing rates of which they are capable (29,38). One has merely to observe the after-hyperpolarization and the pacemaker potential at minimum firing rate to become convinced that the former is smoothly transformed into the latter. Indeed, a strong correlation is found between after-hyperpolarization duration and minimum firing rate (32). Thus, attention has naturally focused on the conductance underlying the after-hyperpolarization in trying to understand the mechanisms governing rhythmic firing. The problem has been to determine how the conductance underlying the after-hyperpolarization, and any other relevant factors, govern the *whole range* of firing rates of which a motoneuron is capable, including the steady secondary range firing observed in many motoneurons.

A variety of theoretic models have been presented to account for motoneuron rhythmic firing (94–102). Each of these models is based partly on data obtained from current clamp studies and partly on assumed parameters, and each more or less successfully reproduces one or more aspects of motoneuron rhythmic firing. Interesting, the assumptions used to characterize active and passive properties differ significantly from model to model, and also differ in significant ways from the voltage clamp results. Apparently, there are a variety of mechanisms which *could* produce motoneuronlike rhythmic firing. The voltage clamp results have provided some insight into which mechanisms actually are involved in the control of rhythmic firing, although a complete solution to the problem is far from being in view.

The assumption that the conductance underlying the after-hyperpolarization (G_{Ks}) provides the foundation for rhythmic firing behavior has been fully supported by experimental results. Control of rhythmic firing by a slow potassium conductance in frog motoneurons has been demonstrated directly by experimental manipulation of this conductance component (87), and as mentioned previously, reconstruction of firing behavior from cat voltage clamp data indicates that G_{Ks} governs this activity. Although the voltage clamp data merely supports a long held assumption, the direct demonstration is important because it has shown that the transient potassium conductance, G_A, which governs rhythmic firing in gastropod somata (80) and certain crustacean axons (103) plays no role in and is not required for motoneuron rhythmic firing. Thus, there are significant species differences in rhythmic firing mechanisms.

The voltage clamp data has also made it possible to describe more precisely how G_{Ks} governs rhythmic firing, even in qualitative terms. This may be appreciated by referring to the schematic representation of the steady-state G_{Ks} activation curve ($G_{Ks\infty}$) in Figure 10 and by considering the action potential to be a brief rectangular depolarization. The shape of the $G_{Ks\infty}$ curve is known from the voltage clamp results. When rhythmic firing is initiated G_{Ks} will try to reach the $G_{Ks\infty}$ value at the peak of the "spike" (V_S in Fig. 10). Whether it succeeds will depend upon its time constants at large depolarizations. These are difficult to measure accurately in motoneurons for technical reasons, but if they follow the progression of low voltage time constants they must be considerably slower than assumed in various models, and they would have to be faster than I_{Na} time constants to reach the $G_{Ks\infty}$ curve during the brief depolarization provided by the spike. Consequently, the G_{Ks} value attained will fall far short of the $G_{Ks\infty}$ curve (point 3 in Fig. 10). However, the exact G_{Ks} value reached during the spike will influence the depth and duration of the pacemaker potential following the spike because the G_{Ks} value obtained during the spike will decay exponentially toward the appropriate value of the $G_{Ks\infty}$ curve during the interspike interval. [Of course, I_{Ks} will not be exponential because of the variation of driving potential, $(E-E_K)$, during the interspike interval.] Since the pacemaker potentials do not hyperpolarize (Figs. 2A and 12A), and since G_{Ks} is activated just positive to rest (as indicated by the $G_{Ks\infty}$ curve), neither voltage nor G_{Ks} will return to zero (path 4-5 in Fig. 10). During the next spike, G_{Ks} approaches the $G_{Ks\infty}$ curve from a nonzero value. Therefore, the same ΔG_{Ks} produced by the spike will bring it closer to the $G_{Ks\infty}$ curve, and larger G_{Ks} will be attained (point 7 in Fig. 10). However, the next interspike interval will be longer because of this larger peak G_{Ks}, and G_{Ks} will decay more (as a percentage of peak G_{Ks}) than during the first interval (path 8-9 in Fig. 10). It should be realized, by considering several cycles of this behavior, that a limit will be reached where the values of G_{Ks} attained during the spike and at the end of the interspike interval will remain constant, and so will the interspike interval. The incremental activation of G_{Ks} until a limit cycle is reached plays a major role in firing rate adaptation at low firing rates, and has been proposed as an adaption

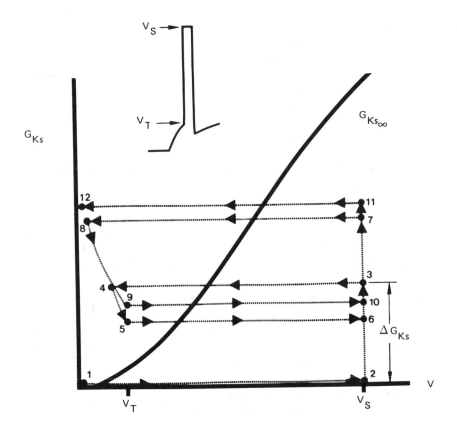

Figure 10 Highly simplified diagram indicating the variation of slow potassium conductance (G_{Ks}) during the onset of rhythmic firing at a slow rate in response to injected current. For purposes of illustration, the spike is assumed to be a brief rectangular depolarization having constant threshold V_T and peak voltage V_S (see inset). The curve labeled G_{Ks_∞} represents the steady-state slow potassium activation curve. The path taken by G_{Ks} and voltage during the initial few cycles of firing in this simplified construct, considering that the cell is initially depolarized from rest (point 1), may be examined by following the labeled points (1–12) in sequence. Paths 2–3, 6–7, and 10–11 are traversed at the peak of the spike. They will be traversed rapidly because the G_{Ks} time constants are short, and the latter will determine the length (ΔG_{Ks}) of these paths. Paths 4–5, 8–9, 12, etc., are traversed during the ISI. They will be traversed slowly because G_{Ks} time constants are slow near rest. (See text for further explanation.)

mechanism in several models (95,96,101) where the phenomenon is called "summation" of the after-hyperpolarization conductance. In practice, the limit cycle is reached rapidly since adaptation in lumbar motoneurons is rather brief (30; see Fig. 2B).

In the simple construct of Figure 10, the peak value of G_{Ks} reached during the spike will determine the peak G_{Ks} available during the interspike interval. The amount of I_K developed by G_K together with the outward, ohmic, "leak" current and the injected current will determine the firing rate. The peak G_{Ks} activated during the spike will depend on the G_{Ks} time constants at large depolarizations. The persistence of G_{Ks} during the interspike interval will depend upon the G_{Ks} time constants at small depolarizations and on the $G_{Ks\infty}$ curve at these potentials. It should be noticed that if G_{Ks} should reach the $G_{Ks\infty}$ curve during a spike, the peak G_{Ks} value following a spike would appear to "saturate" when spikes are evoked at closer intervals, even though the $G_{Ks\infty}$ curve is far from its saturation value. An apparent saturation of after-hyperpolarization voltage and associated input conductance (slope conductance) has been observed in some cells when two spikes are evoked at close intervals (97), but factors such as incremental I_i activation (see below) can also cause an apparent after-hyperpolarization saturation.

From the previous considerations, it can also be realized that the degree of G_{Ks} activation during the interspike interval will be influenced secondarily, but importantly, by spike height and duration, and thus by I_{Na} characteristics together with the cell's passive properties. One lesson from computer reconstruction has been that each conductance component and passive properties can influence rhythmic firing characteristics, directly or indirectly.

There are several additional important factors that influence actual rhythmic firing which the simple construct of Figure 10 does not include. Both spike threshold and mean depolarization during the interspike interval increase drastically with firing rate in motoneurons (see Fig. 11). Since G_{Ks} increases exponentially with voltage in the subthreshold range, and since G_{Ks} time constants decrease with voltage, ever more G_{Ks} will be activated during the interspike interval as firing rate increases, even if G_{Ks} activated during the spike remains constant. In fact, the latter quantity will tend to increase (if G_{Ks} does not reach the $G_{Ks\infty}$ curve during the spike) because G_{Ks} at the start of a spike will be at a larger value for fast firing rates than for slow firing rates. Opposing the tendency of G_{Ks} to increase with firing rate is the fact that rhythmic spikes become smaller and broader as firing rate increases (34,35,104). Because of this, G_{Ks} activated during the spike becomes relatively less important and G_{Ks} activated during the interspike interval becomes relatively more important. Overall, G_{Ks} becomes increasingly and more "tonically" activated the faster the firing

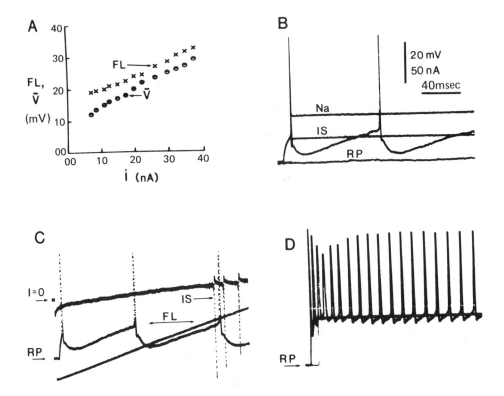

Figure 11 Variation of spike threshold with firing rate during rhythmic firing and the relation of spike threshold to the accommodative properties of the axon initial segment. A: Variation of spike threshold (FL) and average depolarization between spikes ($\overline{V}$) during steady rhythmic firing vs. injected current (i) in a motoneuron. Both FL and $\overline{V}$ are plotted with respect to resting potential. B: Superimposed records of a low-rate rhythmic response to injected current in another cell and two voltage steps imposed after the rhythmic firing record was obtained. Step IS first activated firing of the axon initial segment and step Na was the step where somatic sodium current was first clearly activated (ionic current records are not shown). Notice that step IS corresponds to threshold of the first spike but not the subsequent spikes. C: Superimposed records of a low-rate rhythmic response of the same cell as B, a ramp voltage command which starts at a hyperpolarized potential and which rises at the same rate as the pacemaker potentials, and the ionic current (upper) activated by the ramp command. The three brief downward (inward) deflections on the membrane current trace are repetitive all-or-none, uncontrolled initial segment currents triggered by the rising someatic voltage. Notice that the somatic voltage at which the first initial segment current is triggered corresponds to spike threshold (FL) of rhythmic spikes subsequent to the first spike. The initial segment has accommodated during the slowly rising ramp voltage. D: Superimposition of the fastest rhythmic response recorded in this cell and voltage step "Na" of B. Only at the fastest firing rates does spike threshold approach somatic sodium activation threshold. Calibrations in B also apply to B–D.

rate. Computer simulations have shown that at fast firing rates the variation of I_{Na} and I_{Kf} become as significant as I_{Ks} in determining the precise firing behavior attained (102).

The two independent microelectrodes used for voltage clamp allow accurate measurement of the true D.C. variation of spike threshold and pacemaker potentials with firing rate. As mentioned previously, it has been found that both spike threshold and the mean depolarization in the interspike interval can double as steady firing rate progresses from minimum to maximum (104). This behavior can be appreciated by inspection of Figure 11A. Spike threshold also shows a significant variation over time at a given injected current strength, particularly at fast firing rates (104). The variation in spike threshold has been investigated using the voltage clamp technique, as illustrated in Figure 11B–D, by observing the imposed somatic voltage level at which the all-or-none initial segment current is triggered under different imposed voltages and comparing this voltage to rhythmic spike threshold in the unclamped condition. The somatic voltage at which the initial segment current is triggered appears to be identical to rhythmic spike threshold when the time course and magnitude of the imposed conditioning voltage is similar to the behavior of the pacemaker potentials (Fig. 11B, and C). In general, spike threshold is far below somatic sodium threshold except at the fastest firing rates; only at these rates could the spike be triggered directly by somatic I_{Na} activation (Fig. 11D). Over most of the firing range, the rhythmic spikes are triggered by the initial segment, but the latter apparently has accommodative properties similar to those of motor axons (44,105), and its accommodation causes the drastic rise of spike threshold with steady firing rate and time.

The rise of spike threshold with firing rate has several major consequences. The time it takes for a given pacemaker potential to again cross spike threshold after a preceding spike determines firing rate, and how far the pacemaker potential must rise to cross threshold can greatly influence the actual firing rate attained in response to a given injected current. This can be appreciated by considering the greatly different firing rates that would be attained if the potential "P" in Figure 12A had to reach the threshold corresponding to potential "S." Thus, the firing rates (the F-I curve) produced by a given set of active conductances and injected currents could vary radically, depending upon the precise behavior of spike threshold with firing rate. Conversely, even if the active and passive properties of a neuron were known in detail, it would be impossible to predict its precise firing behavior without the additional knowledge of how its spike threshold varies with injected current strength and time.

The complications provided to the simple construct of Figure 10 by the rise in spike threshold has been discussed earlier in terms of G_{Ks} activation. A more profound complication is provided by I_i activation. First, it can be realized that even if the pacemaker potentials themselves do not provide enough depolarization to activate I_i, it will be at least fractionally activated (like G_{Ks}) by the brief

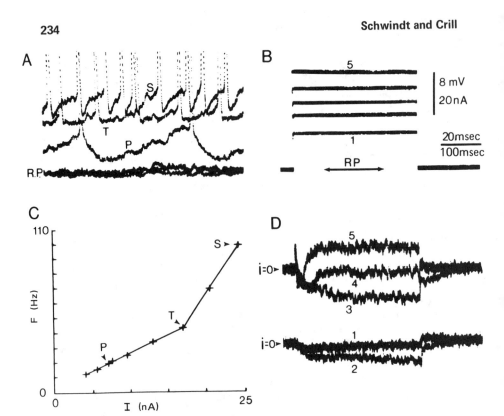

Figure 12 Ionic currents activated at voltages traversed by the pacemaker potentials in a cell which exhibits both a "primary" and "secondary" range during steady rhythmic firing. A: Pacemaker potentials during steady rhythmic firing corresponding to like-labeled points in C. B: Voltage steps imposed from a D.C. clamp at resting potential. The voltages in A and B may be compared directly. C: Plot of steady firing rate (F) vs. injected current (I) for this cell. D: Active ionic currents (leakage current subtracted) activated by like-numbered voltage steps of B. Note that the persistent inward current is strongly activated and is present for the duration of the step at voltages corresponding to the whole excursion of the pacemaker potentials during secondary range firing. 20 msec calibration in B refers to A; 100 msec calibration refers to B and D. (From Ref. 104.)

but large depolarization provided by the spikes. It will subsequently decay during the interspike interval, but during this time it will oppose I_{Ks} and alter the interspike interval from the value that would be determined by G_{Ks} alone. It has, in fact, been found (104) that the pacemaker potentials at the lowest firing rates do not enter the voltage range where I_i is activated, or do so only partially. If there were no increase in spike threshold, this situation would hold at all firing rates. Instead, the rise in spike threshold together with the increase in mean depolarization during the interspike interval (due to the pacemaker potentials becoming shallower) ensures that I_i is activated during the entire excursion of the pacemaker potentials at faster firing rates (Fig. 12).

In cells such as that shown in Figure 12, which have a secondary range during steady firing, the secondary range commences when the pacemaker potentials traverse the voltage range where I_i is strongly and tonically activated. The effect of this tonic I_i activation is to provide, starting at a certain firing rate, a steady, depolarizing, ionic current which aids the injected current in opposing I_{Ks}. The result is a sudden steepening of the F-I curve. Activation of I_i at voltages corresponding to pacemaker potentials at fast firing rates is also found in cells which do not exhibit the secondary range during steady firing, but in these cells there is clear evidence that I_{Ks} is mixed with and largely counters I_i. Owing to the I_i/I_{Ks} mix, the apparent amplitude of the inward component is much smaller than in cells like that shown in Figure 12; the mixed current is inward-going over a smaller voltage range, and I_i appears to decrement rather than remain steady because of the I_{Ks}/I_i mix (104). Based on these observations, it has been hypothesized (104) that the relative strength (the mixture) of I_{Ks} and I_i over the relevant voltage range will determine whether a cell does or does not exhibit a secondary range during steady firing.

It has been further hypothesized (104) that the main role of I_i is more basic than providing a secondary range. In order to increase firing rate and result in a linear F-I curve, increments of injected current must counter not only the large, linear leak conductances but also I_{Ks}, which increases more than linearly with firing rate (i.e., mean depolarization), as discussed earlier. It would appear that the major role of I_i is to counter the everincreasing I_{Ks} so that the F-I curve can increase linearly rather than plateau at larger injected current strengths (larger mean depolarization). Such a plateau of the F-I curve is seen in cells where I_i has deteriorated (104) and in computer simulations where I_i is not included. Some support for the hypothesis that I_i can govern the slope of the F-I curve is provided by comparison with cat neocortical cells in vitro (106). These cells have a slow outward current very similar to I_{Ks} of motoneurons, but the slope of their F-I curve is 10-20 times greater. The difference in firing behavior may result from the fact that the slow outward current of the cortical cells is opposed by a persistent inward current, relatively much stronger than I_i, starting at minimum firing rate. According to this hypothesis, a major factor determining the low primary range slope of motoneurons is the existence of a significant voltage range where the persistent inward current (I_i) is *not* tonically activated.

VI. CONCLUSIONS

After 30 years of experimentation using intracellular recording together with a variety of other techniques and theory, we are able to understand in considerable detail how lumbar motoneurons transform graded, postsynaptic input into frequency-coded output signaled by all-or-none spikes. The discovery that the motoneuron is organized into functional compartments (initial segment, soma, dendrites) defined the pathway of information flow through the cell. Measurement of passive parameters and cable properties together with the development of practical, simplified models has provided insight into how synaptic input is filtered, summated, and viewed by the spike trigger zone. Measurement of rhythmic firing and accommodation properties have provided a quantitative description of motoneuron input/output properties, that is, the output frequency code corresponding to the amount of filtered, summated, synaptic input reaching the trigger zone. More recently, application of the voltage clamp technique has provided the first glimpses of the ionic mechanisms underlying the input/output transformation. The knowledge gained about the integrative function of the lumbar motoneuron is useful both in understanding its role as the "final common pathway" in motor control and in providing a basis for comparison of the integrative function of other mammalian central nervous system neurons.

ACKNOWLEDGMENT

Supported by the Veterans Administration, and NIH Grant NS 16972.

REFERENCES

1. Burke, R. E., and Rudomín, P. (1977). Spinal neurons and synapses. In *Handbook of Physiology*. vol. 1, *Cellular Biology of Neurons*. E. R. Kandel (Ed.), American Physiological Society, Bethesda, Maryland, pp. 877–944.
2. Rall, W. (1977). Core conductor theory and cable properties of neurons. In *Handbook of Physiology*, vol. I, E. R. Kandel (Ed.), American Physiological Society, Bethesda, Maryland, p. 39.
3. Van Buren, J. M., and Frank, K. (1965). Correlation between the morphology and potential field of a spinal motor nucleus in the cat. *Electroencephal. Clin. Neurophysiol. 19*:112–126.
4. Zwaagstra, B., and Kernell, D. (1981). Sizes of soma and stem dendrites in intracellularly labelled α-motoneurones of the cat. *Brain Res. 204*:295–309.
5. Aitken, J. T., and Bridger, J. E. (1962). Neuron size and neuron population density in the lumbosacral region of the cat's spinal cord. *J. Anat. 95*: 38–53.
6. Barrett, J. N., and Crill, W. E. (1974). Specific membrane properties of cat motoneurones. *J. Physiol. (Lond.) 239*:301–324.

7. Rose, P. K. (1981). Distribution of dendrites from Biventer Cervicis and Complexus motoneurons stained intracellularly with horseradish peroxidase in the adult cat. *J. Comp. Neurol. 197*:395–409.
8. Dekker, J. J., Lawrence, D. G., and Kuypers, H. G. J. M. (1973). The location of longitudinally running dendrites in the ventral horn of the cat spinal cord. *Brain Res. 51*:319–325.
9. Lothman, E. W., and Somjen, G. G. (1975). Extracellular potassium activity, intracellular and extracellular potential responses in the spinal cord. *J. Physiol. (Lond.) 252*:115–136.
10. Ito, M., and Oshima, T. (1964). The electrogenic action of cations on cat spinal motoneurons. *Proc. Roy. Soc. Lond. (Biol.) 161*:92–108.
11. Ito, M., and Oshima, T. (1964). The extrusion of sodium from cat spinal motoneurons. *Proc. Roy. Soc. Lond. (Biol.) 161*:109–131.
12. Ito, M., and Oshima, T. (1964). Further study on the active transport of sodium across the motoneuronal membrane. *Proc. Roy Soc. Lond. (Biol.) 161*:132–141.
13. Klee, M. R., Pierau, F. K., and Faber, D. S. (1974). Temperature effects on resting potential and spike parameters of cat motoneurons. *Exp. Brain Res. 19*:478–492.
14. Lux, H. D. (1971). Ammonium and chloride extrusion: Hyperpolarizing synaptic inhibition in spinal motoneurons. *Science 173*:555–557.
15. Brock, L. G., Coombs, J. S., and Eccles, J. C. (1953). Intracellular recording from antidromically activated motoneurones. *J. Physiol. (Lond.) 122*: 429–461.
16. Coombs, J. S., Curtis, D. R., and Eccles, J. C. (1957). The interpretation of spike potentials of motoneurones. *J. Physiol (Lond.) 139*:198–231.
17. Coombs, J. S., Curtis, D. R., and Eccles, J. C. (1957). The generation of impulses in motoneurones. *J. Physiol. (Lond.) 139*:232–249.
18. Fuortes, M. G. F., Frank, K., and Becker, M. C. (1957). Steps in the production of motoneuron spikes. *J. Gen. Physiol. 40*:735–752.
19. Granit, R., Kernell, D., and Smith, R. S. (1963). Delayed depolarization and the repetitive response to intracellular stimulation of mammalian motoneurones. *J. Physiol. (Lond.) 168*:890–910.
20. Kernell, D. (1964). The delayed depolarization in cat and rat motoneurones. *Prog. Brain Res. 12*:42–55.
21. Nelson, P. G., and Burke, R. E. (1967). Delayed depolarization in cat spinal motoneurons. *Exp. Neurol. 17*:16–26.
22. Baldissera, F. (1976). Relationships between the spike components and the delayed depolarization in cat spinal neurones. *J. Physiol. (Lond.) 259*: 325–338.
23. Baldissera, F., and Gustafsson, B. (1970). Time course and potential dependence of the membrane conductance change during the afterhyperpolarization in the cat's motoneurones. *Brain Res. 17*:365–368.
24. Baldissera, F., and Gustafsson, B. (1974). Regulation of repetitive firing in motoneurons by the afterhyperpolarization conductance. *Brain Res. 30*: 431–434.

25. Baldissera, F., and Gustafsson, B. (1974). Afterhyperpolarization conductance time course in lumbar motoneurones of the cat. *Acta Physiol. Scand.* *91*:512–527.

26. Mauritz, K. H., Schlue, W. R., Richter, D. W., and Nacimiento, A. C. (1974). Membrane conductance course during the spike intervals and repetitive firing in cat spinal motoneurones. *Brain Res. 76*:223–233.

27. Coombs, J. S., Eccles, J. C., and Fatt, P. (1955). The electrical properties of the motoneurone membrane. *J. Physiol. (Lond.) 130*:291–325.

28. Kuno, M. (1959). Excitability following antidromic activation in spinal motoneurones supplying red muscles. *J. Physiol. (Lond.) 149*:374–393.

29. Eccles, J. C. (1957). *The Physiology of Nerve Cells.* Johns Hopkins Press, Baltimore.

30. Kernell, D. (1965). High-frequency repetitive firing of cat lumbosacral motoneurones stimulated by long-lasting injected currents. *Acta Physiol. Scand. 65*:74–86.

31. Kernell, D. (1965). The adaptation and the relation between discharge frequency and current strength of cat lumbosacral motoneurones stimulated by long-lasting injected currents. *Acta Physiol. Scand. 65*:65–73.

32. Kernell, D. (1965). The limits of firing frequency in cat lumbosacral motoneurones possessing different time course of afterhyperpolarization. *Acta Physiol. Scand. 65*:87–100.

33. Granit, R., Kernell, D., and Shortess, G. K. (1963). Quantitative aspects of repetitive firing of mammalian motoneurones caused by injected currents. *J. Physiol. (Lond.) 168*:911–931.

34. Schwindt, P. C., and Calvin, W. H. (1972). Membrane potential trajectories between spikes underlying motoneuron rhythmic firing. *J. Neurophysiol. 35*:311–325.

35. Schwindt, P. C. (1973). Membrane potential trajectories underlying motoneuron rhythmic firing at high rates. *J. Neurophysiol. 36*:434–449.

36. Kernell, D. (1966). Input resistance, electrical excitability and size of ventral horn cells in cat spinal cord. *Science 152*:1637–1639.

37. Burke, R. E. (1967). Motor unit types of cat triceps and surae muscle. *J. Physiol. (Lond.) 193*:141–160.

38. Eccles, J. C., Eccles, R. M., and Lundberg, A. (1958). The action potentials of the alpha motoneurones supplying fast and slow muscles. *J. Physiol. (Lond.) 142*:275–291.

39. Kernell, D., and Zwaagstra, B. (1981). Input conductance, axonal conduction velocity and cell size among hindlimb motoneurones of the cat. *Brain Res. 204*:311–326.

40. Henneman, E., Somjen, G. G., and Carpenter, D. O. (1965). Functional significance of cell size in spinal motoneurons. *J. Neurophysiol. 28*:599–620.

41. Bradley, K., and Somjen, G. G. (1961). Accommodation in motoneurones of the rat and the cat. *J. Physiol (Lond.) 156*:75–92.

42. Frank, K., and Fuortes, M. G. F. (1960). Accommodation of spinal motoneurones of cats. *Arch. Ital. Biol. 98*:165–170.

43. Sasaki, K., and Otani, T. (1961). Accommodation in spinal motoneurons of the cat. *Jap. J. Physiol. 11*:443–456.

44. Schlue, W. R., Richter, D. W., Mauritz, K.-H., and Nacimiento, A. C. (1974). Response of cat spinal motoneuron somata and axons to linearly rising currents. *J. Neurophysiol. 37*:303–309.

45. Frankenhauser, B., and Vallbo, A. B. (1965). Accommodation in myelinated nerve fibers of *Ninopus Laevis* as computed on the basis of voltage clamp data. *Acta Physiol. Scand. 63*:1–20.

46. Hille, B. (1977). Ionic basis of resting and action potentials. In *Handbook of Physiology*, vol. I, E. R. Kandel (Ed.), American Physiological Society, Bethesda, Maryland, p. 99.

47. Stein, R. B. (1967). The frequency of nerve action potentials generated by applied currents. *Proc. Roy. Soc. (Lond.) (Biol.) 167*:64–86.

48. Lorenté de No, R., and Condouris, G. A. (1959). Decremental conduction in peripheral nerve: Integration of stimuli in the neuron. *Proc. Natl. Acad. Sci. U.S.A. 45*:592–617.

49. Rall, W. (1959). Branching dendritic trees and motoneuron membrane resistivity. *Exp. Neurol. 1*:491–527.

50. Rall, W. (1960). Membrane potential transients and membrane time constant of motoneurons. *Exp. Neurol. 2*:503–532.

51. Rall, W. (1962). Theory of physiological properties of dendrites. *Ann. N.Y. Acad. Sci. 96*:1071–1092.

52. Rall, W. (1969). Time constants and electronic length of membrane cylinders and neurons. *Biophys. J. 9*:1483–1508.

53. Rall, W., Burke, R. E., Smith, T. G., Nelson, P. G., and Frank, K. (1967). Dendritic location of synapses and possible mechanisms for the monosynaptic EPSP in motoneurons. *J. Neurophysiol. 30*:1169–1193.

54. Rall, W. (1970). Cable properties and effects of synaptic location. In *Excitatory Synaptic Mechanisms*, P. Andersen and J. K. S. Jansen (Eds.), Universitetsforlaget, Oslo, pp. 175–187.

55. Jack, J. J. B., Miller, S., Porter, R., and Redman, S. J. (1970). The distribution of group Ia synapses on lumbrosacral spinal motoneurones in the cat. In *Excitatory Synaptic Mechanisms*, P. Andersen and J. K. S. Jansen (Eds.), Universitetsforlaget, Oslo, pp. 199–205.

56. Jack, J. J. B., Miller, S., Porter, R., and Redman, S. (1971). The time course of minimal excitatory post-synaptic potentials evoked in spinal motoneurone by group Ia afferent fibres. *J. Physiol. (Lond.) 215*:353–380.

57. Jack, J. J. B., and Redman, S. J. (1971). An electrical description of the motoneurone, and its application to the analysis of synaptic potentials. *J. Physiol. (Lond.) 215*:321–352.

58. Jack, J. J. B., and Redman, S. J. (1971). The propagation of transient potentials in some linear cable structures. *J. Physiol. (Lond.) 215*:283–320.

59. Burke, R. E., and ten Bruggencate, G. (1971). Electrotonic characteristics of alpha motoneurones of varying size. *J. Physiol. (Lond.) 212*:1–20.

60. Nelson, P. G., and Lux, H. D. (1970). Some electrical measurements of motoneuron parameters. *Biophys. J. 10*:55–73.

61. Iansek, R., and Redman, S. J. (1973). An analysis of the cable properties of spinal motoneurones using a brief intracellular current pulse. *J. Physiol. (Lond.) 234*:613–636.

62. Lux, H. D., Schubert, P., and Kreutzberg, G. W. (1970). Direct matching of morphological and electrophysiological data in cat spinal motoneurons. In *Excitatory Synaptic Mechanisms*, P. Andersen and J. K. S. Jansen (Eds.), Universitetsforlaget, Oslo, pp. 189–198.

63. Iansek, R., and Redman, S. J. (1973). The amplitude, time course and charge of unitary excitatory post-synaptic potentials evoked in spinal motoneurone dendrites. *J. Physiol. (Lond.) 234*:665–688.

64. Barrett, J. N., and Crill, W. E. (1971). Specific membrane resistivity of dye-injected cat motoneurons. *Brain Res. 28*:556–561.

65. Barrett, J. N., and Crill, W. E. (1974). Influence of dendritic location and membrane properties on the effectiveness of synapses in cat motoneurones. *J. Physiol. (Lond.) 239*:325–345.

66. Araki, T., and Terzuolo, C. A. (1962). Membrane currents in spinal motoneurons associated with the action potential and synaptic activity. *J. Neurophysiol. 25*:772–789.

67. Frank, K., Fuortes, M. G. F., and Nelson, P. G. (1959). Voltage clamp of motoneuron soma. *Science 130*:38–39.

68. Ito, M., and Oshima, T. (1965). Electrical behaviour of the motoneurone membrane during intracellularly applied current steps. *J. Physiol. (Lond.) 180*:607–635.

69. Nelson, P. G., and Frank, K. (1967). Anomalous rectification in cat spinal motoneurons and effect of polarizing currents on excitatory postsynaptic potential. *J. Neurophysiol. 30*:1097–1113.

70. Hodgkin, A. L., and Katz, B. (1949). The effect of sodium ions on the electrical activity of the giant axon of the squid. *J. Physiol. (Lond.) 108*: 37–77.

71. Hotson, J. R., Prince, D. A., and Schwartzkroin, P. A. (1979). Anomalous rectification in hippocampal neurons. *J. Neurophysiol. 42*:889–895.

72. Koike, H., Okada, Y., Oshima, T., and Takahashi, K. (1968). Accommodative behavior of cat pyramidal tract cells investigated with intracellular injection of currents. *Exp. Brain Res. 5*:173–188.

73. Takahashi, K. (1965). Slow and fast groups of pyramidal tract cells and their respective membrane properties. *J. Neurophysiol. 28*:908–924.

74. Schwindt, P. C., and Crill, W. E. (1977). A persistent negative resistance in cat lumbar motoneurons. *Brain Res. 120*:173–178.

75. Schwindt, P. C., and Crill, W. E. (1980). Properties of a persistent inward current in normal and TEA-injected motoneurons. *J. Neurophysiol. 43*: 1700–1724.

76. Barrett, E. F., Barrett, J. N., and Crill, W. E. (1980). Voltage sensitive outward currents in cat motoneurones. *J. Physiol. (Lond.) 304*:251–276.

77. Halliwell, J. V., and Adams, P. R. (1982). Voltage clamp analysis and muscarinic excitation in hippocampal neurons. *Brain Res. 250*:71–92.

78. Barrett, J. N., and Crill, W. E. (1980). Voltage clamp of cat motoneurone somata: Properties of the fast inward current. *J. Physiol. (Lond.) 304*: 231–249.

79. Schwindt, P. C., and Crill, W. E. (1980). Effects of barium on cat spinal motoneurons studied by voltage clamp. *J. Neurophysiol. 44*: 827–846.

80. Hodgkin, A. L., and Huxley, A. F. (1952). The dual effects of membrane potential on sodium conductance in the giant axon of *Loligo. J. Physiol. (Lond.) 116*:497–506.

81. Connor, J. A., and Stevens, C. F. (1971). Voltage clamp studies of transient outward membrane current in gastropod neural somata. *J. Physiol. (Lond.) 213*:21–30.

82. Schwindt, P. C., and Crill, W. E. (1981). Differential effects of TEA and cations on the outward ionic currents of cat motoneurons. *J. Neurophysiol. 46*:1–15.

83. Schwindt, P. C., and Crill, W. E. (1980). Role of a persistent inward current in motoneuron bursting during spinal seizures. *J. Neurophysiol. 43*:1296–1318.

84. Krnjević, K., and Lisiewicz, A. (1972). Injections of calcium ions into spinal motoneurones. *J. Physiol. (Lond.) 225*:363–390.

85. Krnjević, K., Lamour, Y., MacDonald, J. F., and Nistri, A. (1978). Motoneuronal after-potentials and extracellular divalent cations. *Can. J. Physiol. Pharmacol. 56*:516–520.

86. Krnjević, K., Puil, E., and Werman, R. (1978). EGTA and motoneuronal after potentials. *J. Physiol. (Lond.) 275*:199–223.

87. Barrett, E., and Barrett, J. N. (1976). Separation of two voltage sensitive potassium currents and demonstration of a tetrodotoxin-resistant calcium current in frog motoneurons. *J. Physiol. (Lond.) 255*:737–774.

88. Århem, P. (1980). Effects of some heavy metal ions on the ionic currents of myelinateal fibres from *Xenopus Laevis. J. Physiol. (Lond.) 306*:219–231.

89. Schwindt, P. C., and Crill, W. E. (1981). Negative slope conductance at large depolarizations in cat spinal motoneurons. *Brain Res. 207*:471–475.

90. Brown, D. A., and Adams, P. R. Muscarinic suppression of a novel voltage-sensitive K^+ current in a vertebrate neurone. *Nature 283*:673–676.

91. Adams, P. R., Brown, D. A., and Halliwell, J. V. (1981). Cholinergic regulation of M-current in guinea pig hippocampal neurons. *J. Physiol. (Lond.) 317*:29–30P.

92. Adams, D. J., Smith, S. J., and Thompson, S. H. (1980). Ionic currents in molluscan soma. *Annu. Rev. Neurosci. 3*:141–167.

93. Eckert, R., and Lux, H. D. (1976). A voltage sensitive persistent calcium conductance in neural somata of *Helix. J. Physiol. (Lond.) 254*:129–151.

94. Hille, B. (1971). Voltage clamp studies on myelinated nerve fibers. In *Biophysics and Physiology of Excitable Membranes*, W. J. Adelman, Jr. (Ed.), Van Nostrand, New York.

95. Baldissera, F., and Gustafsson, B. (1974). Firing behaviour of a neurone model based on the afterhyperpolarization conductance time course. First interval firing. *Acta Physiol. Scand. 91*:528–544.

96. Baldissera, F., and Gustafsson, B. (1974). Firing behaviour of a neurone model based on the afterhyperpolarization conductance time course and algebraical summation. Adaptation and steady-state firing. *Acta Physiol. Scand. 92*:27–47.

97. Baldissera, F., Gustafsson, B., and Parmiggiani, F. (1978). Saturating summation of the afterhyperpolarization conductance in spinal motoneurones. A mechanism for secondary range repetitive firing. *Brain Res. 146*:69–82.

98. Baldissera, F., and Parmiggiani, F. (1979). After hyperpolarization conductance time-course and repetitive firing in a motoneurone model with early inactivation of the slow potassium conductance system. *Biol. Cybern. 34*: 233–240.

99. Kernell, D. (1968). The repetitive impulse discharge of a simple neurone model compared to that of spinal motoneurones. *Brain Res. 11*:685–687.

100. Kernell, D., and Sjoholm, H. (1972). Motoneurone models based on voltage clamp equations for peripheral nerve. *Acta Physiol. Scand. 86*: 546–562.

101. Kernell, D., and Sjoholm, H. (1973). Repetitive impulse firing comparisons between neurone models based on "voltage clamp equations" and spinal motoneurones. *Acta Physiol. Scand. 87*:40–56.

102. Traub, R. D., and Llínas, R. (1977). The spatial distribution of ionic conductances in normal and axotomized motoneurones. *Neuroscience 2*:829–849.

103. Connor, J. A. (1975). Neural repetitive firing. A comparative study of membrane properties of crustacian walking leg axons. *J. Neurophysiol. 38*:922–932.

104. Schwindt, P. C., and Crill, W. E. (1982). Factors influencing motoneuron rhythmic firing: Results from a voltage clamp study. *J. Neurophysiol. 48*: 875–890.

105. Richter, D. W., Schlue, W. R., Mauritz, K.-H., and Nacimiento, A. C. (1974). Comparison of membrane properties of the cell body and the initial part of the axon of phasic motoneurones in the spinal cord of the cat. *Exp. Brain Res. 21*:193–206.

106. Stafstrom, C. E., Schwindt, P. C., and Crill, W. E. (1982). Negative slope conductance due to a persistent subthreshold sodium current in cat neocortical neurons *in vitro*. *Brain Res. 236*:221.

7

DENDRITES AND
MOTONEURONAL INTEGRATION

Peter L. Carlen, David A. McCrea,* and Dominique Durand[†]
University of Toronto, Toronto, Ontario, Canada

I. MOTONEURON DENDRITES AND THEIR INTEGRATIVE PROPERTIES

Although the cat spinal cord lumbar motoneuron is one of the best studied neurons electrophysiologically, relatively little is known directly about the function of its dendrites. One reason is that intracellular recordings are usually somatic or presumed so, and an adequate motoneuron slice preparation permitting localization of electrode impalement in the dendritic tree has not yet been successfully established. In this chapter, we will concentrate on data from adult cat lumbar motoneurons, and we will attempt to integrate the results of morphologic, electrical modeling, and electrophysiologic studies as applied to dendritic function. Biochemical and developmental studies of dendrites will not be covered. For excellent reviews of relevant aspects of motoneuron dendritic function see Llínas (1), Lux and Schubert (2), and Redman (3).

In the late 1950s some interpretations of intracellular motoneuronal recordings suggested that although the dendritic tree was large, the synaptic input on the tree was electrotonically remote and its input was relatively insignificant at the soma where postsynaptic potential integration occurs (4). However, Rall (5,6) challenged this view, and showed that the specific membrane resistance was

*Present affiliation: University of Manitoba, Winnipeg, Manitoba, Canada
†Present affiliation: Case Western Reserve University, Cleveland, Ohio

not as low as previously thought, and he suggested that even distal synapses can contribute effectively to somatic depolarization (7). Thus, the large motoneuronal dendritic tree became recognized as being functionally important for somatic integration.

II. MORPHOLOGY

The most important recent advance in single-cell anatomic techniques has been the staining of individual neurons by intracellular injection of the horseradish peroxidase (HRP) enzyme complex (8–10). An advantage of this technique is to allow electrophysiologic recording before injection. Such a stained neuron can be reconstructed from several serial sections using a drawing tube; Figure 1 shows the appearance of a typical adult cat lumbar motoneuron reconstructed from transverse sections. Note the enormous dendritic tree, the large irregular-shaped soma.

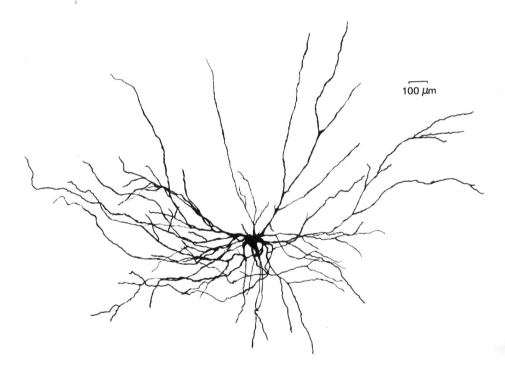

100 μm

Figure 1 Camera lucida drawings of 50-μm thick transverse sections of the adult cat lumbar spinal cord were used to reconstruct this motoneuron supplying the medical gastrocnemius muscle. This cell was stained with HRP by passing 120 nA·min depolarizing current through the electrode. The animal was perfused and the tissue was frozen sectioned and processed using diaminobenzidine. (Unpublished results courtesy of W. T. Tatton and D. A. McCrea, Playfair Neuroscience Unit, Toronto Western Hospital, University of Toronto, Canada.)

Because of the irregular soma shape many authors prefer to report the mean cell body diameter [(major elliptical axis + minor elliptical axis)/2]. Values from 35 to 75 μm, with an average of 50-60 μm (11,12) or slightly lower (13), have been reported for adult cat lumbar motoneurons stained with HRP. Motoneurons give rise to a single axon which leaves the soma unmyelinated (the initial segment, mean diameter 3.5 μm), becomes myelinated after 20-35 μm, and continues out the ventral root (14). The significance of these observations is that the entire axon system should be of relatively high electrical impedance, and thus it only contributes a small electrical "load" to potentials generated in the soma and dendrites.

The motoneuron's dendritic tree obviously accounts for the vast majority of the surface area (see Fig. 1) (15-17). Lux et al. (18) estimated that the dendritic surface area was 20 times that of the soma. Emanating from the soma are between seven and 20 primary dendrites [mean = 11 or 12 (11-13)], which themselves give rise to extensive arborizations, although Golgi studies (15) show on the average fewer primary dendrites than those reported using HRP (e.g., 11), Procion yellow (1,20), or tritiated glycine (18). The primary dendrites (stem dendrites) have diameters ranging from ~1 to more than 20 μm, with a mean of 8.0 μm in the HRP material of Ulfhake and Kellerth (12), and 4.7 μm in the predominantly Procion material of Zwaagstra and Kernell (13). There seems to be a weak relationship between somal size and the combined diameter of the primary dendrites, but there is none between the soma and the range of primary dendritic diameters (12). In order to analyze the combined variations in primary dendrite number and size, Zwaagstra and Kernell (13) calculated the "sum of dendritic holes," which is the sum of the cross-sectional area of all the primary dendrites, and found a strong correlation between this parameter and soma size ($r = 0.83$). Of great importance for motoneuron models which reduce the entire dendritic tree to an equivalent electrical cylinder is the assumption that when branching occurs there is a relationship between the diameters of the mother (D_m) and daughter (D_b) branches, such that $D_m^{3/2} = \Sigma\ D_b^{3/2}$. Lux (21), Brown and Fyffe (11), and Ulfhake and Kellerth (12) have made detailed analyses and they have found that the branching point equation was closely verified, showing that the ratio of $D_m^{3/2}/\Sigma D_b^{3/2}$ was on average close to 1. This meant that the reduction to an equivalent electrical cylinder was a reasonable assumption, but because of the wide range of this ratio (0.67:1.7) (11) for some dendritic branches this may not be true. When this 3/2 power relation is not followed, then the neuron cannot be modeled by an equivalent cylinder and the potential distribution along the dendritic tree must be calculated for each dendrite (e.g., 19).

The common cable equations as applied to motoneurons also assume that the surface of the dendrites is not covered with spines (which would increase surface area estimates), and the data obtained using HRP in the adult cat show very few spines (11,12). The fine dendrites, however, often terminate in thin beadlike structures which are difficult to quantify at the light microscopic level [e.g., Fig. 2b in Cullheim and Keller (14) Fig. 5b in Ulfhake and Kellerth (12)]. The exact effect that these nonregular geometries have on determining the impedance of the dendrite is difficult to assess, but one would predict high impedances and, therefore, higher local potentials for the same synaptic current. To date, no one has made a systematic search for synapses on these final distal dendrites. Such distal synapses could have important consequences for dendritic integration, since the potential inside the dendrite could markedly change the driving force for other nearby postsynaptic potentials.

The presence of dendritic spines is mentioned by Brown and Fyffe (11) and by Ulfhake and Kellerth (12), but their number is small. Ulfhake and Kellerth (12), however, refer to their unpublished data on kittens which show large numbers of spines. In addition, Rose and Richmond (22) reported a significant number of spines in Golgi and HRP material in cat adult cervical cord motoneurons. These motoneurons also had dendrites which projected to the contralateral spinal gray matter, a feature not reported for lumbar motoneurons. Zwaagstra and Kernell (13) point out differences in both the size and number of stem dendrites of motoneurons innervating different muscle groups in the lumbar spinal cord. Tatton et al. (13a), using HRP injections, showed that in young kitten motoneurons, most dendritic processes were less than 2 μm in diameter, whereas adult motoneurons had significantly larger dendrites. Thus any generalizations about motoneuron anatomy should be qualified by information about the neuronal species and stage of development of the animal.

Even the early Golgi studies showed that the spread of cat lumbar motoneuron dendritic trees is quite extensive with many dendrites extending into the white matter (e.g., 23). The results using HRP are even more dramatic and show that in the adult cat the tip to tip dendritic spread may be on the order of 1 to 3 mm (e.g., see Fig. 1). Ulfhake and Kellerth (12) calculated a mean length of 4.7 mm for the combined length of the branches of a single dendrite, of which a motoneuron has on average 12. These authors (12) also gave mean values of 1.1 mm for the distance from the soma to the tip of a single dendrite. Their finding that the diameter of the first-order (stem) dendrite was highly correlated with the combined dendritic length is suggestive of an orderly manner of dendritic branching, as is their data indicating that the total surface area of a dendrite can be predicted by the diameter of that first-order dendrite.

Motoneuron dendrites usually branch up to the fourth or sixth order, with bifurcations being much more frequent than trifurcations (11); and as mentioned previously, the 3/2 power law is on the average obeyed at the branch points. Of great importance for neuronal modeling is whether the dendritic branches taper between branch points. A synapse ending on a tapering dendrite would see a different impedance at different points along the dendrite, since the ratio of axial resistance to surface area would vary. Barrett and Crill (19) reported considerable tapering in their Procion-stained material between 0 and 300 μm from the soma, but Brown and Fyffe (11) and Ulfhake and

Kellerth (12), both of whom used HRP, disagree with this finding. When the Swedish investigators (12) excluded end branches, they saw little tapering, but the end branches were markedly tapered. Brown and Fyffe (11) came to similar conclusions and state that there was little tapering up to 800 μm from the soma. The presence of both taper and the beaded structures in the fine distal dendrite terminations may have physiologic importance for synapses at these sites and just proximal to these endpoints.

If one wishes to discuss dendritic integration, it becomes important to ascertain the physical location of the synapses involved (23). Soon after the introduction of intracellular recording from motoneurons came the postulate that the synapses mediating the disynaptic inhibitory postsynaptic potential (IPSP) from group Ia muscle spindle afferents were situated more proximally than those mediating the monosynaptic excitatory postsynaptic potential (EPSP) (24). Based on the assumption that the diffusion of Cl⁻ ions to distal synapses would take longer than to more proximal synapses, Burke et al. (25) concluded that the synapses responsible for Renshaw cell inhibition of motoneurons were farther away from the soma than those for the Ia inhibitory postsynaptic potential, and Llínas and Terzuolo (26) similarly concluded that inhibitory postsynaptic potentials resulting from reticular formation stimulation are generated distally. Recently, HRP injections of single interneurons mediating this Ia inhibition have shown that many of the responsible synapses end directly on the soma as well as on the proximal dendrites (27). In contrast, HRP injection of Ia afferents (11, 27a,28) reveal that the Ia fibers terminate considerably more distally (e.g., 20–820 μm). In addition, Brown and Fyffe (11) report that even if an axon makes contact with several dendrites of a motoneuron, they tend to occur at about the same distance from the soma. The available evidence thus supports the idea that there may be distinct organization of the synaptic endings on the dendritic tree. One might expect that other factors being equal, a unitary postsynaptic potential generated by one of the systems ending more distally may be of smaller amplitude than one coming from a "proximal" system (29), but recent findings by Redman and coworkers suggest that the situation is more complex (30).

The amplitude of a postsynaptic potential (PSP) which reaches the soma is determined by many factors: the number of synaptic endings involved; postsynaptic receptor density and sensitivity; driving potential (difference between the reversal potential for the postsynaptic potential and the "resting" membrane potential); the amount of transmitter released from the presynaptic ending; the electric impedance of the postsynaptic area; the duration of transmitter action (i.e., the duration of conductance change produced by the transmitter); the distance over which the PSP must propagate before reaching the soma; and, finally, the geometry of more proximal neuronal structures which could attenuate the potential by impedance mismatching. Redman and Walmsley (30) recorded from and stained pairs of Ia afferents and motoneurons and examined the effect of synaptic location on the rise time of the unitary excitatory postsynaptic potential. Since they could later reconstruct both the afferent and the target cell, they were able to test directly the theoretic assumption that the rise time of a PSP is a reliable index of its electrotonic distance from the soma. Faster rise times and shorter half-widths are noted in modeled excitatory postsynaptic potentials which are closer to the soma (29,31,32). Their results fully supported this assumption concerning rise time and location and were used in a subsequent study which examined the relationship between synaptic location (i.e., rise time) and amplitude of unitary excitatory postsynaptic potentials (33). Unexpectedly, the distal excitatory postsynaptic potentials with slower rise times were not smaller than the proximal excitatory postsynaptic potentials. They suggested that postsynaptic factors act to maintain the postsynaptic potential amplitude to a constant value, in direct opposition to earlier views (e.g., 4) that distal synapses may be less "important" than proximal ones. Any theoretic treatment of the subject of dendritic integration would be simplified greatly if one could assume that for any particular physiologic system the amplitude of the postsynaptic potential was independent of location. Such an assumption is unjustified until more data on other systems becomes available, which may take some time because of the difficulty in labeling pairs of pre- and postsynaptic neurons.

III. PASSIVE ELECTRICAL MOTONEURONAL MODELING

The measurement of the passive electrotonic properties of motor neurons is crucial to the understanding of their capabilities for neuronal integration. Neuronal integration is a concept dealing with the effectiveness of synaptic inputs at various locations on the dendritic tree and their summated postsynaptic potential amplitude at the soma. The local potential change produced at the synaptic site by a postsynaptic potential is believed to spread passively along the dendritic branches toward an area with low threshold for spike initiation, the soma or the axon hillock.

A. Cable Models

Electrotonic propagation along a cylindrical cable (34) was first described mathematically by Weber (35; cited in 36), and extensively applied to neuronal dendrites by Rall (5-7,29,36–40). The cable or core model of nerve cells is based on the geometry and the electrical properties of the membrane and cytoplasm. Therefore, one must know both the physiologic and morphologic properties of a particular neuron in order to assess its electrotonic parameters (e.g., 36). However, it was not until the early 1970s that intracellular recordings were combined with dye injection, enabling morphologic analysis of single motoneurons (18,19,41). These experiments confirmed that the electrotonic length of motoneurons lies between 1 and 2 (21,42) and pointed to a lower bound value of 1800 $\Omega \cdot$cm for the specific membrane resistance (R_m), allowing estimation of the current and voltage distribution in the dendritic trees. The current leakage across the dendritic membrane is determined by the cable properties of the dendrites. Therefore, in order to assess the relative effectiveness of synapses it is necessary to estimate the specific membrane resistance, capacitance (C_m), and the specific axoplasmic resistance (R_i). These estimates can be performed using an electrical neuronal model described in the following paragraphs, wherein the individual dendrites are replaced by a single electrically equivalent dendrite (Fig. 2A). This model is applicable to neurons whose dendrites follow the 3/2 power law (37,38), as discussed in Sec. II.

Provided that all dendrites have the same electrotonic length, L, (l/λ; see Sec. III.B.2), and the same boundary conditions (discussed below), the whole dendritic tree can then be modeled by a single equivalent cable (Fig. 2B). Lux et al. (18) found a 20% variation in the electrotonic lengths of major dendritic branches from the same neuron, but lumping 10 or more such dendrites together to form an equivalent cylinder with a single L is unlikely to cause a significant error (3). Because of its simplicity a single cable equivalent cylinder model is very useful and provides a good approximation of more exact motoneuron models wherein the dendritic tree is specifically represented by many small segments (e.g., 43).

This model then consists of an equivalent cable for the dendrites and an equivalent impedance for the soma. Another assumption has to be made for the type of boundary condition or the effective impedance at the end of the dendrites. Iansek and Redman (44) combined both theoretic models and experimental recordings from spinal cord neurons to provide evidence for mainly "sealed"-end (high-impedance or open-circuit) terminations, at least in deeply anesthetized preparations. The beadlike structures seen at many motoneuron dendrite terminations would likely contribute to a sealed-end boundary condition. Tonic distal dendritic synaptic activity associated with postsynaptic conductance increase would tend to make the dendritic terminations "leaky." The most significant parameters of the finite single cable model are detailed in Figure 2.

Other assumptions underlying such a dendritic model as described previously should be emphasized, as they can be very restrictive. The core resistance, R_m, and the R_i are assumed to be constant, linear, and passive throughout the dendritic tree and soma. However, active responses have been noted in dendrites (45), and there is evidence suggesting that the somatic R_m may be lower than the dendritic R_m (44). Estimates of R_m are made when the cell is assumed to be in a resting state, but it is clear that factors such as anesthesia may greatly alter background synaptic activity, thus changing R_m but not necessarily invalidating the model. However, if this activity causes differential changes in dendritic and

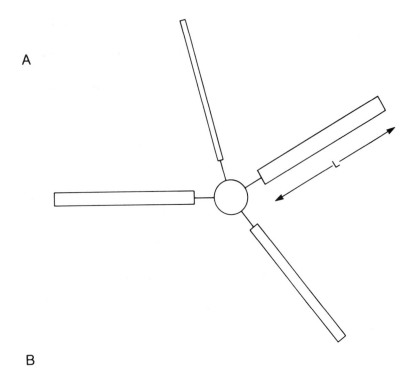

B

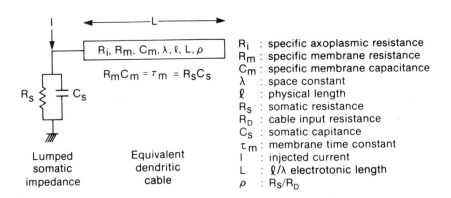

Lumped	R_i : specific axoplasmic resistance
somatic	R_m : specific membrane resistance
impedance	C_m : specific membrane capacitance

R_i : specific axoplasmic resistance
R_m : specific membrane resistance
C_m : specific membrane capacitance
λ : space constant
ℓ : physical length
R_S : somatic resistance
R_D : cable input resistance
C_S : somatic capitance
τ_m : membrane time constant
I : injected current
L : ℓ/λ electrotonic length
ρ : R_S/R_D

Lumped somatic impedance   Equivalent dendritic cable

Figure 2 A: Equivalent cable model of a motoneuron: When the dendritic branch points follow the 3/2 power law (see text) the dendritic tree of each primary dendrite is collapsed into a single equivalent cable. The diameter of this cable is equal to the diameter of the corresponding primary dendrite and its length calculated to give the same membrane surface area as the original tree.

somatic resistance, then R_m is neither constant nor homogeneous. In most models, the extracellular surface of the neurons is assumed to be isopotential with negligible resistance of the extracellular space. The soma is also assumed to be isopotential and is usually modeled by a single impedance, but this assumption has only been verified in large snail neurons (46). The soma is the origin of all dendrites and the voltage distribution is assumed continuous between the soma and dendrites and at dendritic branching points. The axon which is classically modeled by core conductors (47,48) can be considered infinite in length compared to the dendrites, but is small in diameter and is neglected in most models. Calculations comparing a neuronal model with and without an infinite axonal cable show that the addition of this infinite cable does not affect the final neuronal time constant (49).

B. Passive Electrotonic Parameters

1. Time Constant (τ)

Following a brief injection of current, the membrane capacitance will decay with what at first was thought to be an exponential function. However, as suggested by Rall (5,6), the current injected at the soma also flows into the dendritic tree in a fashion described by the core model, and therefore the exponential function underestimates the value of the membrane time constant. After an initially fast decay due to current spread into the dendrites, the voltage along the dendritic tree is distributed equally and then the voltage decay becomes exponential. The currently accepted method for estimating the membrane time constants is to measure the decay of the final or equalization phase of the voltage response to a constant current pulse injection (42,49). For methodologic considerations see Jack et al. (31), Carlen and Durand (32), and Durand (50).

2. Electrotonic Length (L), Dendritic Dominance (ρ), and Transmission Coefficient (T)

L is very commonly used to predict voltage attenuation along dendritic cables. However, as explained later, this method can be misleading. L is defined as the

---

The separate cables, each corresponding to a primary dendrite (only a few are represented here for the neuron in Fig. 1) are attached to a spherical soma. B: The cables of different diameters but identical electrotonic length are then collapsed into a single equivalent cable with the same electrotonic length (L) and diameter (D) given by:

$$D = (\Sigma \, d_i^{3/2})^{2/3}$$

where d_i are the diameters of the primary dendrites. The single equivalent cable is attached to a soma modeled by a single lumped impedance.

ratio of the physical length to the space constant (l/λ). L is very useful for solving the partial differential cable equation, which describes the passive spread of current along a cable, since L represents the distance normalized to λ. The space constant, λ, is defined as the rate of voltage decay/unit length along an *infinite* cable. In a *finite* cable model, L cannot by itself be used to predict voltage decay. However, the cable theory applied to a finite cable allows the calculation of a transmission coefficient (T) along the cable. This transmission coefficient is defined as the ratio of the measured voltage at the end of the cable (V_L) to the voltage measured at the soma (V_O) from a constant current injection. In a cable with sealed ends and electrotonic length, L,

$$T = \frac{V_L}{V_O} = \frac{1}{\cosh L}$$

With an average value for L of approximately 1.5 in adult cat motoneurons, as estimated by many authors (19,21,41,42,44,51,52), according to the equation, 42.5% of the voltage generated at one end is transmitted to the other end. When a soma is present at one end of the cable, this relatively high transmission ratio can only be applied from soma to dendrites (T_{SD}). In the other direction, the efficacy of transmission is reduced because of the load represented by the soma and other dendrites. However, the neuron can overcome low transmission ratios by larger distal input resistances producing higher postsynaptic voltages or by increasing the synaptic current distally, for example, by increased receptor density.

The importance of the soma for determining transmission coefficients is characterized by the ratio of the input conductance of the dendritic tree to the conductance of the soma.

$$\rho = G_D/G_S$$

The smaller the value of ρ, the larger the electrical load placed by the soma on the dendrites. The transmission coefficient from the dendritic terminal points to the soma (T_{DS}) can then be expressed as a function of T_{SD} and ρ by:

$$T_{DS} = \frac{T_{SD}}{1 + \dfrac{1 - T_{SD}^2}{\rho}}$$

This expression, derived from the modeling equation in Rall (36) for a single equivalent cable in neurons obeying the 3/2 power law, shows that T_{DS} is always lower than or equal to T_{SD}, as illustrated in Figure 3. For motoneurons, however, the values of ρ vary between 4 to 35 (18,19,44,51). These high values of ρ mean that the soma itself does not represent a significant electrical load to the dendritic tree. However, the transmission coefficients along a dendrite

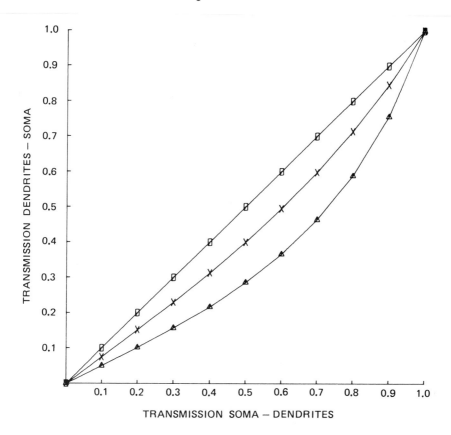

Figure 3 The transmission of D.C. potentials from dendrites to soma is plotted as a function of transmission from soma to dendrites for three values of ρ in a single equivalent cylinder: $\rho = \infty$ ($\square$), $\rho = 3$ ($\times$), and $\rho = 1$ ($\triangle$). Note that for the ranges of values of ρ for motoneurons this transmission is initially identical in the two directions.

toward the soma will be markedly reduced by the load created by the other dendrites. This problem was treated by Rall and Rinzel (40), where they showed that voltages are markedly attenuated in distal branches when traveling toward the soma, but that they hardly affected when traveling away from it. This has interesting consequences for neuronal integration of synaptic input as discussed in Sec. III.C.

C. Synaptic Efficiency

The introduction of cable models to study the neuronal integrative properties has shown that even distal synapses can play a significant role in the total function of the neuron. Synaptic efficiency, or the ability of a synaptic input to depolarize the low-threshold somatic region, can be separated into synaptic charge injection and transmission from the synaptic site. The transmission is influenced by the specific membrane parameters and the electrical load at the soma as outlined previously. The high values calculated for the membrane specific resistance, 1800–8000 $\Omega \cdot cm^2$ (19), are directly responsible for the low loss transmission along the dendrites. However, the factors modulating the charge injection at the synaptic site are varied and difficult to assess experimentally. Some of these factors, such as nonlinear summation, will be explained in Sec. IV. The effects of background synaptic activity, synaptic conductance change, and membrane parameters on synaptic efficacy have been reviewed by Barrett (41a). Other authors have also discussed aspects of attenuation of potentials generated in dendrites and measured in the soma (20,29,40,53–55).

We will mention here only one aspect of synaptic modulation; that is, reduction of the synaptic driving potential distally to the synaptic input. The flow of ionic current across the subsynaptic membrane can be described by the equation:

$$I_s = g_s(t) (V_{rev} - V(t))$$

where I_s is the net current flow, $g_s(t)$ the conductance change, and $(V_{rev} - V(t))$ the driving force or difference between the reversal potential of I_s and the membrane voltage $V(t)$. Barrett and Crill (20) calculated that an excitatory postsynaptic potential generated in the distal dendrites from one "quantum" of synaptic current would be as large as 16–20mV, and compared this to 100–160 μV for the amplitude product by a similar current originating at the soma (56). Although the peak amplitude of these potentials would be quickly attenuated toward the soma, the high transmission coefficient in the distal direction would lead to marked distal dendritic depolarization, and therefore significantly reduce the driving force for all distally located excitatory postsynaptic potentials on the same dendritic branch. Rall's calculations also show very little attenuation of potentials in adjacent sister branches (40). This factor has been largely underestimated and is an important element in the distributed memory model of Cooper (57). The dissymmetry of the transmission coefficients from synapses to soma and synapses to terminal points also creates some interesting weighting functions that could play a significant role in complex neuronal integration. A large depolarizing synaptic potential in a distal dendrite would then significantly attenuate nearby excitatory synaptic potentials with depolarizing reversal potentials, concomitantly enhancing nearby inhibitory postsynaptic potentials.

IV. POSTSYNAPTIC POTENTIAL INTERACTIONS

It is presently understood that neuronal integration in motoneurons occurs at the soma. Excitatory and inhibitory postsynaptic potentials summate at the soma, and if the membrane is sufficiently depolarized, an action potential is generated in the axon initial segment. When the presynaptic element releases transmitter, a postsynaptic conductance change occurs, and if the membrane potential is not at the equilibrium potential a voltage change is produced. Post-synaptic potentials can interact in terms of both potential and conductance and, thus, the time course and magnitude of conductances as well as voltage ampli-tudes are necessary to describe the interactions between two postsynaptic poten-tials. As an example, the conductance increase underlying an inhibitory post-synaptic potential can decrease the amplitude of an excitatory postsynaptic potentials. When the conductance changes are over, the postsynaptic potential amplitudes will summate algebraically. In vivo motoneuronal recordings show that there is relatively little nonlinear summation of different Ia excitatory postsynaptic potentials (58), suggesting little electrotonic or spatial overlap of the generating conductances. On the other hand, presynaptic inhibition may be in part an interaction between the Ia excitatory postsynaptic potential and a distally located long-lasting conductance increase (52). The after-hyperpolariza-tion following an action potential is another example of a long-lasting conduc-tance change in spinal motoneurons (59). In an attempt to understand post-synaptic potential interactions along motoneuronal dendrites, neural modeling techniques have been applied. Carlen and Durand (32) used a simple analog passive electrical model of the motoneuron (modified from [60]) and examined the effects of a focal tonic conductance increase (simulating a long-lasting inhibitory postsynaptic potential with a reversal potential equal to the resting membrane potential) on an "electrical EPSP" generated by a short constant current pulse without a conductance change. In a model with the soma and the recording electrode at one end, the closer the tonic conductance was located to the soma, the greater was the relative decrease in the excitatory postsynaptic potential height, except in the case where the excitatory postsynaptic potential was generated in the most distal dendritic compartment. However, when the soma was situated in the center of the analog neuronal model, the excitatory postsynaptic potential was most decreased by a tonic conductance placed at its point of origin, as also demonstrated by Jack et al. (31). Further modeling of the effects of tonic shunts on postsynaptic potentials generated by conductance changes with different reversal potentials and dendritic location should be done as well as the interactions of postsynaptic potentials caused by conductance decreasing mechanisms with those caused by conductance increasing mechanisms and their respective dendritic locations. Changes in neuronal membrane capaci-tance are relatively more difficult to measure, and little is known about the interactions between focal or diffuse neuronal capacitance changes, postsynaptic potentials, and dendritic location.

An attempt was made to localize focal dendritic tonic conductance increases by analyzing the interaction between these shunts, and the amplitude and time

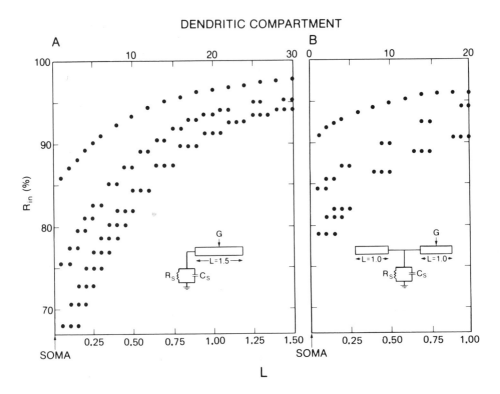

Figure 4 The effect of shunt magnitude and location on input resistance measured in the soma from short or long somatic constant current pulses. R_{in} estimations using short pulse (integrating the area under the curve) and long pulse (measuring the peak saturation voltage) were superimposable. Each point represents a shunt and its location is indicated on the abscissa. The top curve of points represents the decrease in R_{in} (as % of maximum R_{in} without any shunt) from a single shunt on the cable, the middle curve from two shunts, each in adjacent compartments (two points), and the bottom curve from three adjacent shunts (three points). A: The model with L = 1.5 is used. B: the model with two dendritic branches, each with and L = 1.0 is used. The shunts are placed in one dendritic tree. (From Ref. 32.)

course of voltage transients resulting from somatic constant current phase injection (32). This was a simulation of the in vivo or in vitro experimental situation wherein the intracellular recording and current-passing electrode(s) is usually situated in the neuronal soma. As intuitively expected, the closer a tonic conductance increase was to the soma, the greater the measured decrease in the measured input resistance (R_{in}) (Fig. 4). When R_{in} is decreased one expects the membrane time constant (τ_0) to decrease as well. τ_0 can be estimated from the

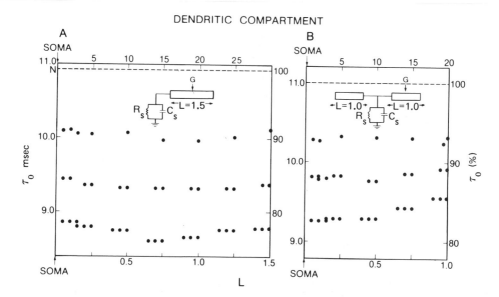

Figure 5 Effects of shunt magnitude and location on estimated τ_0's. The top row of points are the τ_0's from one shunt, the middle row from two shunts, each in adjacent dendritic segments (two points), and the lowest row from three adjacent shunts (three points). A: The model with L = 1.5 was used. Shunts were placed in various compartments along the cable and the corresponding τ_0's were estimated. B: The model with L = 1.0 was used. Shunts were placed at various locations in one of the two equivalent dendritic cables and the corresponding τ_0 was estimated. (From Ref. 32.)

voltage decay following a short or long current pulse or from the charging curve of a long pulse. τ_0 decreased proportionately to the magnitude of the tonic conductance regardless of its location on the motoneuronal cable model (Fig. 5), that is, whether a shunt was placed in the most distal or most proximal dendritic compartment, the final voltage decay as measured by τ_0 was essentially the same. Hence, changes in τ_0 can be used to estimate the magnitude of a tonic shunt regardless of its location(s) in the neuron.

A. Putative Dendrodendritic and Dendroaxonic Interactions

It has been assumed that neuronal signals flow in one direction (61). However, as mentioned earlier, important voltage interactions could occur in distal dendrites that would not be easily seen by an intrasomatic recording electrode. There is also evidence for short latency antidromic motoneuronal activation of cat dorsal root afferents (62). Whether this effect is mediated by extracellular field potentials, interneuronal synaptic connections, or direct electrotonic current flow between cat motoneuron dendrites and primary afferents is unknown. In amphibian motoneurons evidence for a combined electrical-chemical synapse on motoneurons from dorsal root fibers has been noted (63,64). However, when an amphibian motoneuron was directly stimulated by an intracellular electrode only long latency polysynaptic potentials were measured intracellularly in a dorsal root fiber innervating that recorded motoneuron (65).

The Scheibels (66) have shown that motoneuronal dendrites can run in tightly packed bundles wherein the dendrites are often directly opposed. Brown and Fyffe (11), however, point out that the flexor muscle motoneurons in their material had dendritic trees with a predominant rostral-caudal orientation, whereas those innervating ankle extensors had dendrites in all directions. The reader is also referred to Figure 18 in Burke (67) for an example of dendritic organizations between motoneurons. Zieglgansberger and Reiter (68) showed that intracellular injection of Procion yellow into a cat spinal motoneuron was associated with uptake of the dye into some, but not all adjacent motoneurons. They attributed this finding to direct dendrodendritic connections, but this finding has not been confirmed using HRP (11,12). When recording intracellularly from a lumbar motoneuron and stimulating the ventral root containing its axon, but subthreshold for eliciting an antidromic spike, often small depolarizing potentials are seen at the time delay as expected for the antidromic spike (69,70). These potentials are thought to result from direct electrical interactions between motoneurons, or synaptically via recurrent axon collateral terminals (71). Magherini et al. (72) showed that in frog spinal motoneurons this recurrent excitation is transmitted electrotonically between the soma-dendritic regions of nearby motoneurons.

B. Inhibitory Postsynaptic Potentials (IPSPs)

From electrophysiologic evidence, different postsynaptic potentials are known to be generated at the soma and proximal dendrites as discussed previously. Long-lasting inhibitory postsynaptic potentials (few hundred msec) which were relatively insensitive to intracellular injection of Cl^- ions, suggesting a remote dendritic origin (73), have been demonstrated in extensor lumbar motoneurons following conditioning from hamstring afferents (74). These electrotonically remote inhibitory postsynaptic potentials may in part explain "presynaptic inhibition" (52), since a subtle conductance increase was noted following just suprathreshold conditioning stimuli appropriate for the generation of presynaptic inhibition. Also, when the baseline following these conditioning stimuli was averaged often a small inhibitory postsynaptic potential became apparent. The previous does not rule out presynaptic inhibitory mechanisms, which are discussed in detail by Burke and Rudomín (75), Levy (76), Nicoll and Alger (77), and Davidoff and Hackman (78). In the majority of central nervous system neurons studied to date, most inhibitory postsynaptic potentials seem to be generated perisomatically and little evidence is available for distal dendritic inhibitory postsynaptic potentials.

C. Excitatory Postsynaptic Potentials (EPSPs)

The best studied motoneuronal postsynaptic potential is the excitatory postsynaptic potential, resulting from the stimulation of Ia muscle spindle afferents (Ia excitatory presynaptic potential). Different unitary Ia excitatory postsynaptic potentials on a motoneuron generated by stimulation of a single afferent have been carefully studied regarding their rise times and half-widths and their sensitivity to intracellular current injection. Slower rise times and half-widths imply a more distal dendritic input (29). If the Ia excitatory postsynaptic potential is generated by a conductance-increasing postsynaptic mechanism with a single reversal potential, then those excitatory postsynaptic potentials generated closer to the soma should be more sensitive to intracellular current injection (79). However, no relationship has been seen between the estimated distance of the Ia excitatory postsynaptic potential from the soma and the sensitivity to current injection (39,80–82). The actual mechanism of the Ia excitatory postsynaptic potential is unclear, since some authors are unable to reverse it clearly, particularly the earliest portion (39,80–82), whereas others (83,84), using two intracellular electrodes, have been able to show complete reversals of nonunitary Ia excitatory postsynaptic potentials. This anomalous behavior may be due in part to the fact that L-glutamate, the putative Ia excitatory postsynaptic potential neurotransmitter, has both conductance-increasing and -decreasing effects when iontophoresed on motoneurons (85,86), which is discussed at length by Puil (87,88). Interestingly, microiontophoretic application of L-glutamate to predominantly dendritic sites caused a more rapid onset of depolarization than application to more somatic sites, without measurably increased conductance in the former case (86), suggesting the possibility of specific glutamate receptors in the more distal part of the dendritic tree. These findings for the excitatory postsynaptic potential are in contrast to the Ia inhibitory postsynaptic potential (89) or other non-Ia excitatory postsynaptic potentials (82), which are relatively easy to reverse with current injection.

V. IONIC CONDUCTANCES

The data in Sec. IV raise the issue of localization of transmitter receptors and ionophores in the dendritic tree. For passive electrical modeling purposes, it is usually assumed that the dendritic and somatic membrane properties are uniform. Intradendritic recordings from other neuronal types (90,91) suggest that ionic conductances are not distributed uniformly, and it also seems reasonable to expect a heterogeneity in neurotransmitter receptor distribution. Traub and Llínas (92) have modeled the spatial distribution of ionic conductances in normal and axotomized motoneurons to explain differences in both the firing rates produced by injected current and the spikelike partial responses seen in axotomized motoneurons. Their conclusions included the following:

1. A major part of the slow potassium conductance (gK) causing the spike after-hyperpolarization is localized to the proximal dendrites.
2. There is at least some g_{Na} in the proximal dendrites of normal motoneurons.
3. To explain partial spikelike responses in axotomized motoneurons, "hot spots" of high g_{Na} should exist at least 0.4 λ away from the soma. Also, their model included g_{Ca} extending into the proximal dendrites.

These data suggest a lower perisomatic R_m, which is necessary postulate to explain the exponential decays from constant current pulse injections and the difficulties in estimation of ρ in some cat motoneurons (2,19,44) and other neurons [e.g., hippocampal cells, [50]). Nonlinearities of membrane resistance are observed in many motoneurons in response to hyper- and depolarizing current injection. Lux and Schubert (2) reasonably suggest that these nonlinearities measured in the soma are most likely occurring in the dendrites as well as the somatic membrane. Thus, it is reasonable to expect nonuniformity of ionic conductances, and possibly R_m, in the dendritic tree.

VI. ACTION POTENTIALS IN DENDRITES

It is usually assumed that dendrites are passive electrical cables that transmit charge to the soma, where neuronal integration and spike generation occurs. However, it is not known how far up the dendritic tree spikes can be actively generated or passively decay. Pottala et al. (93) model the spread of a simulated action potential into the distal dendritic tree, showing some depolarization of distal dendrites and marked attenuation of the spike after-hyperpolarization. As mentioned in Sec. IV.A, Decima and Goldberg (62) demonstrated very short latency activation of dorsal root afferents by antidromic motoneuronal stimulation. This raises the possibility of significant dendritic depolarization beside primary afferent terminations. Antidromic spike invasion into dendrites could have an erasing action on dendritic integrative activity for a few milliseconds (1). In chromatolyzed motoneurons (following axotomy) Kuno and Llínas (45) showed that a given neuron may generate a few distinct all-or-none potentials following afferent fiber stimulation. They concluded that separate dendrites may generate an action potential that is conducted in a decremental manner to the soma, with the soma itself being the site of summation of spikes coming from different dendritic segments. Evidence strongly suggesting that action potentials do invade dendrites antidromically, at least in axotomized motoneurons, was provided by Kuno and Llínas (45), who showed that orthodromic dendritic spikes have a refractory period of approximately 6 msec following either antidromic invasion or spike initiation from direct stimulation through the recording intrasomatic microelectrode (1).

VII. CONCLUSIONS

Although most of the innervation and surface area of the motoneuron is localized to its vast dendritic tree, much remains to be learned about dendritic function. This review has covered certain electrophysiologic aspects of motoneuron dendrites and their integrative properties, and has not discussed biochemical or developmental factors. Except for axotomized motoneurons, virtually no pathophysiologic investigations of motoneuronal dendritic function have been undertaken. One could predict potentially significant dendritic changes such as morphologic plasticity and altered synaptic effectiveness in such disease states as amyotrophic lateral sclerosis or spasticity. Also, systemic drug administration would be expected to affect motoneuronal function more through the voluminous dendritic tree and its massive innervation than the soma.

ACKNOWLEDGMENTS

This work was supported in part by The National Institute of Health (grant No. R01 NS16660-02 to P.L.C., a Medical Research Council of Canada grant to P.L.C. and D.A.M., and a Canadian Society for Multiple Sclerosis grant to P.L.C.

REFERENCES

1. Llínas, R. (1975). Electroresponsive properties of dendrites in central neurons. In *Advances in Neurology*, vol. 12, W. Kreutzberg (Ed.), Raven, New York, pp. 1–13.
2. Lux, H. D., and Schubert, P. (1975). Some aspects of the electroanatomy of dendrites. In *Advances in Neurology*, vol. 12, W. Kreutzberg (Ed.), Raven, New York, pp. 29–44.
3. Redman, S. J. (1976). A quantitative approach to integrative function of dendrites. In *Neurophysiology II*, vol. 10, R. Porter (Ed.), University Park Press, Baltimore, pp. 17–35.
4. Eccles, J. C. (1957). *The Physiology of Nerve Cells*, John Hopkins Press, Baltimore.
5. Rall. W. (1957). Membrane time constant of motoneurons. *Science 126*: 454.
6. Rall, W. (1960). Membrane potential transients and membrane time constant of motoneurons. *Exp. Neurol. 1*:491–527.

7. Rall, W. (1959). Branching dendritic trees and motoneuron membrane resistivity. *Exp. Neurol. 1*:491–527.

8. Jankowska, E., Rastad, J., and Westman, J. (1976). Intracellular application of horseradish peroxidase and its light and electron microscopical appearance in spinocervial tract cells. *Brain Res. 105*:557–562.

9. Cullheim, S., and Kellerth, J. O. (1976). Combined light and electron microscopic tracing of neurons, including axons and synaptic terminals, after intracellular injection of horseradish peroxidase. *Neurosci. Lett. 2*:307–313.

10. Snow, P. J., Brown, A., and Rose, P. K. (1976). Tracing axons and axon collaterals of spinal neurons using intracellular injection of horseradish peroxidase. *Science 191*:312–313.

11. Brown, A. G., and Fyffe, R. E. W. (1981). Direct observations on the contacts made between Ia efferent fibres and α-motoneurons in the cat's lumbosacral spinal cord. *J. Physiol (Lond.) 313*:121–140.

12. Ulfhake, B., and Kellerth, J. O. (1981). A quantitative light microscopic study of the dendrites of cat spinal α-motoneurons after intracellular staining with horseradish peroxidase. *J. Comp. Neurol. 202*:571–583.

13. Zwaagstra, B., and Kernell, D. (1981). Sizes of soma and stem dendrites in intracellularly labelled α-motoneurons of the cat. *Brain Res. 204*:295–309.

13a. Tatton, W. G., Hay, M., McCrea, D., and Bruce, I. C. (1983). Postnatal dendritic development in motoneurons: evaluation by a Monte Carlo technique. *Exp. Brain Res. 52*:461–465.

14. Cullheim, S., and Kellerth, J. O. (1978). A morphological study of the axons and recurrent axon collaterals of cat sciatic α-motoneurons after intracellular staining with horseradish peroxidase. *J. Comp. Neurol. 178*:537–558.

15. Aitken, J. T., and Bridger, J. E. (1961). Neuron size and population density in lumbosacral region of the cat's spinal cord. *J. Anat. 95*:38–53.

16. Schadé, J. P. (1964). On the volume and surface area of spinal neurons. *Prog. Brain Res. 11*:261–277.

17. Gelfan, S., Kao, G., and Ruchkin, D. S. (1970). The dendritic tree of spinal neurons. *J. Comp. Neurol. 139*:385–411.

18. Lux, H. D., Schubert, P., and Kreutzberg, G. W. (1970). Direct matching of morphological and electrophysiological data in cat spinal motoneurons. In *Excitatory Synaptic Mechanisms*, P. Andersen and J. K. S. Jansen (Eds.), Universitetsforlaget, Oslo, pp. 189–198.

19. Barrett, J. N., and Crill, W. E. (1974). Specific membrane properties of cat motoneurons. *J. Physiol. (Lond.) 239*:301–324.

20. Barrett, J. N., and Crill, W. E. (1974). Influence of dendritic location and membrane properties on the effectiveness of synapses on cat motoneurons. *J. Physiol. (Lond.) 239*:325–345.

21. Lux, H. D. (1967). Eigenschaften eines Neuron-Modells mit Dendriten begrenzter Lange. *Pflugers Arch. 297*:238–255.

22. Rose, P. K., and Richmond, F. J. R. (1981). White-matter dendrites in the upper cervical spinal cord of the adult cat: A light and electron microscopic study. *J. Comp. Neurol. 199*:191–203.

23. Sprague, J. M., and Ha, H. (1964). The terminal fields of dorsal root fibres in the lumbosacral spinal cord of the cat, and the dendritic organization of the motor nuclei. *Prog. Brain Res. 11*:261–277.

24. Curtis, D. R., and Eccles, J. C. (1959). The time courses of excitatory and inhibitory synaptic actions. *J. Physiol. (Lond.) 145*:529–546.

25. Burke, R. E., Fedina, L., and Lundberg, A. (1971). Spatial synaptic distribution of recurrent and group Ia inhibitory systems in cat spinal motoneurons. *J. Physiol. (Lond.) 214*:305–326.

26. Llínas, R., and Terzuolo, C. A. (1965). Mechanisms of supraspinal actions upon spinal cord activities. Reticular inhibitory mechanisms upon flexor motoneurons. *J. Neurophysiol. 28*:413–422.

27. Rastad, J. (1981). Ultrastructural morphology of axon terminals of an inhibitory spinal interneuron in the cat. *Brain Res. 223*:397–401.

27a. Burke, R. E., Walmsley, B., and Hodgson, J. A. (1979). HRP anatomy of group Ia afferent contacts on alpha motoneurons. *Brain Res. 160*:347–352.

28. Burke, R. E., Walmsley, B., and Hodgson, J. A. (1979). Structural-functional relations in monosynaptic action on spinal motoneurons. In *Integration in the Nervous System,* H. Asanuma and V. J. Wilson (Eds.), Igaku-Shoin, Tokyo, pp. 27–46.

29. Rall, W. (1967). Distinguishing theoretical synaptic potentials computed for different soma-dendritic distributions of synaptic input. *J. Neurophysiol. 30*:1138–1168.

30. Redman, S. H., and Walmsley, B. (1981). The synaptic basis of the monosynaptic stretch reflex. *Trends in Neurosci. 4*:248–250.

31. Jack, J. J. B., Noble, D., and Tsien, R. W. (1975). *Electric Current Flow in Excitable Cells.* Clarendon Press, Oxford, pp. 1–502.

32. Carlen, P. L., and Durand, D. (1981). Modeling the postsynaptic location and magnitude of tonic conductance changes resulting from neurotransmitter or drugs. *Neurosci. 6(5)*:839–846.

33. Jack, J. J. B., Redman, S. J., and Wong, K. (1981). The components of synaptic potentials evoked in cat spinal motoneurons by impulses in single group Ia afferents. *J. Physiol. (Lond.) 321*:65–96.

34. Hodgkin, A. L., and Rushton, W. A. H. (1946). The electrical constant of a nerve fiber. *Proc. Roy. Soc. (Lond.) (Biol.) 133*:444–479.

35. Weber, H. (1873). Veber die stationaren stromunger der Ele Klucitat in Cylindern. *J. Reine Angewandte Math. 70*:281–288.

36. Rall, W. (1977). Core conductor theory and cable properties of neurons. In *Handbook of Physiology*, vol. I, J. M. Brookhart and V. B. Mountcastle (Eds.), American Physiological Society, Bethesda, Maryland, pp. 39–97.

37. Rall, W. (1962). Electrophysiology of a dendritic neuron model. *Biophys. J. 2*:145–167.

38. Rall, W. (1964). Theoretical significance of dendritic trees for neuronal input-output relations. In *Neural Theory and Modelling*, R. Reiss (Ed.), Stanford University Press, Stanford California, pp. 73–97.

39. Rall, W., Burke, R. E., Smith, T. G., and Frank, K. (1967). Dendritic location of synapses and possible mechanisms for the monosynaptic epsp in motoneurons. *J. Neurophysiol.* 30:1169–1193.

40. Rall, W., and Rinzel, J. (1973). Branch input resistance and steady attenuation for input to one branch of a dendritic neuron model. *Biophys. J.* 13:648–688.

41. Barrett, J. N., and Crill, W. E. (1971). Specific membrane properties resistance of dye injected cat motoneurons. *Brain Res.* 28:556–561.

41a. Barrett, J. N. (1975). Motoneuron dendrites: role in synaptic integration. *Fed. Proc.* 34:1398–1407.

42. Burke, R. E., and ten Bruggenate, G. (1971). Electrotonic characteristics of alpha motoneurons of varying size. *J. Physiol. (Lond.)* 212:1–20.

43. Kurchavy, G. G., Motorina, M. V., and Shapovalov, A. I. (1973). Investigation of distribution of synaptic inputs on analogous model of motoneurons. *Neurophysiologica* 5:289–297.

44. Iansek, R., and Redman, S. J. (1973). An analysis of the cable properties of spinal motoneurons using a brief intracellular current pulse. *J. Physiol. (Lond.)* 234:613–636.

45. Kuno, M., and Llínas, R. (1970). Enhancement of synaptic transmission by dendritic potentials in chromatolysed motoneurons of the cat. *J. Physiol. (Lond.)* 210:807–821.

46. Roberge, F. A., Jacob, R., Gulzajani, R. M., and Mathieu, P. A. (1977). A study of soma isopotentiality in *Aplysia* neurons. *Can. J. Physiol. Pharmacol.* 55:1162–1169.

47. Hodgkin, A. L. (1947). The membrane resistance of a non-medullated nerve fibre. *J. Physiol. (Lond.)* 106:305–318.

48. Katz, B. (1966). *Nerve, Muscle, and Synapse.* McGraw-Hill, New York.

49. Jack, J. J. B., and Redman, S. J. (1971). An electrical description of the motoneuron and its application to the analysis of synaptic potentials. *J. Physiol. (Lond.)* 215:321–352.

50. Durand, D. (1982). "Alcohol Induced Brain Damage: Morphology and Physiology in the Hippocampus In-vitro," Ph.D. dissertation, University of Toronto, Canada.

51. Nelson, P. G., and Lux, H. D. (1970). Some electrical measurements of motoneuron parameters. *Biophysi. J.* 10:55–73.

52. Carlen, P. L., Werman, R., and Yaari, Y. (1980). Post-synaptic conductance increase associated with presynaptic inhibition in cat lumbar motoneurons. *J. Physiol. (Lond.)* 298:539–556.

53. Redman, S. J. (1973). The attenuation of passively propagating dendritic potentials in a motoneuron cable model. *J. Physiol. (Lond.)* 234:637–664.

54. Rinzel, J., and Rall, W. (1974). Transient response in a dendritic neuron model for current injected at one branch. *Biophysic. J.* 14:759–790.

55. Rinzel, J. (1975). Voltage transients in neuronal dendritic trees. *Fed. Proc.* 34:1350–1356.

56. Kuno, M., and Miyahara, J. T. (1969). Analysis of synaptic efficacy in spinal motoneurons from "quantum" aspects. *J. Physiol. (Lond.)* 201:479–493.

57. Cooper, L. N. (1980). Distributed memory in the central nervous system: Possible test of assumptions in the visual cortex. The organization of the cerebral cortex. MIT Press, Cambridge, Massachusetts, pp. 479–503.

58. Burke, R. E. (1967). Composite nature of the monosynaptic excitatory postsynaptic potential. *J. Neurophysiol. 30*:1114–1136.

59. Baldissera, F., and Gustafsson, B. (1974). Afterhyperpolarization conductance time course in lumbar motoneurons of the cat. *Acta Physiol. Scand. 91*:512–527.

60. Walmsley, B. (1975). "An Analysis of Unitary Ia Excitatory Post-synaptic Potentials Evoked in Cat Spinal Motoneurons," Ph.D. dissertation, Monash University, Victoria, Australia.

61. Sherrington, C. S. (1906). *The Integrative Action of the Nervous System*. Yale University Press, New Haven, Connecticut.

62. Decima, E. E., and Goldberg, L. J. (1970). Centrifugal dorsal root discharges induced by motoneuron activation. *J. Physiol. (Lond.) 207*:103–118.

63. Shapovalov, A. I., and Shiriaev, B. I. (1979). Single-fibre EPSPs in amphibian motoneurons. *Brain Res. 160*:519–523.

64. Shapovalov, A. I., and Shiriaev, B. I. (1980). Dual mode of junctional transmission at synapses between single primary afferent fibres and amphibian motoneurons. *J. Physiol. (Lond.) 306*:1–15.

65. Shapovalov, A. I., and Shiriaev, B. I. (1980). Recurrent interactions between individual motoneurons and dorsal root fibres in the frog. *Exp. Brain Res. 38*:115–116.

66. Schiebel, M. E., and Schiebel, A. B. (1970). Organization of spinal motoneuron dendrites in bundles. *Exp. Neurol. 28*:106–112.

67. Burke, R. E. (1981). Motor units: Anatomy, physiology, and functional organization. In *Handbook of Physiology,* vol. II, J. M. Brookhart and V. B. Mountcastle (Eds.), American Physiological Society, Bethesda, Maryland, pp. 345–422.

68. Zieglgänsberger, W., and Reiter, C. H. (1974). Intraneuronal movement of Procion yellow in cat spinal neurons. *Exp. Brain Res. 20*:527–530.

69. Nelson, P. G. (1966). Interaction between spinal motoneurons of the cat. *J. Neurophysiol. 29*:275–287.

70. Gogan, P., Gueritaud, J. P., Horcholle-Bossavit, G., and Tyc-Dumont, S. (1977). Direct excitatory interactions between spinal motoneurons of the cat. *J. Physiol. (Lond.) 272*:755–767.

71. Cullheim, S., Kellerth, J. O., and Conradi, S. (1977). Evidence for direct synaptic intraconnections between cat spinal alpha-motoneurons via the recurrent axon collaterals: A morphological study using intracellular injection of horseradish peroxidase. *Brain Res. 132*:1–10.

72. Magherini, P. C., Precht, W., and Schwindt, P. C. (1976). Evidence of electrotonic coupling between frog motoneurons in the situ spinal cord. *J. Neurophysiol. 39(3)*:474–483.

73. Cook, A., and Cangiano, A. (1972). Presynaptic and postsynaptic inhibition of spinal motoneurons. *J. Neurophysiol. 35*:389–403.

74. Kellerth, J. O., and Szumski, A. J. (1966). Effects of picrotoxin on stretch activated–post-synaptic inhibition in spinal motoneurons. *Acta Physiol. Scand. 66*:146–156.

75. Burke, R. E., and Rudomín, P. (1977). Spinal neurons and synapses. In *Handbook of Physiology*, vol. I, J. M. Brookhart and V. B. Mountcastle (Eds.), American Physiological Society, Bethesda, Maryland, pp. 877–944.

76. Levy, R. A. (1980). Presynaptic control of input to the central nervous system. *Can. J. Physiol. Pharmacol. 58*:751–766.

77. Nicoll, R. A., and Alger, B. E. (1979). Presynaptic inhibition: Transmitter and ionic mechanisms. *Int. Rev. Neurobiol. 21*:217–258.

78. Davidoff, R. A., and Hackman, J. C. (1984). Spinal inhibition. In *Handbook of the Spinal Cord*, vols. 2 and 3, R. A. Davidoff (Ed.), Marcel Dekker, New York.

79. Calvin, W. H. (1969). Dendritic synapses and reveral potentials: Theoretical implications of the view from the soma. *Exp. Neurol. 24*:248–264.

80. Shapovalov, A. I., and Kurchavyi, G. C. (1974). Effects of transmembrane polarization and TEA injection on monosynaptic actions from motor cortex red nucleus and group Ia afferent on lumbar motoneurons in the monkey. *Brain Res. 82*:49–67.

81. Edwards, F. R., Redman, S. J., and Walmsley, B. (1976). The effect of polarizing currents on unitary Ia excitatory post-synaptic potentials evoked in spinal motoneurons. *J. Physiol. (Lond.) 259*:705–723.

82. Werman, R., and Carlen, P. L. (1976). Unusual behavior of the Ia E.P.S.P. in cat spinal motoneurons. *Brain Res. 112*:395–401.

83. Coombs, J. S., Eccles, J. C., and Fatt, P. (1955). Excitatory synaptic action in motoneurons. *J. Physiol. (Lond.) 130*:374–395.

84. Engberg, I., and Marshall, K. C. (1979). Reversal potential for Ia excitatory postsynaptic potentials in spinal motoneurons of cats. *Neuroscience 4*:1583–1591.

85. Engberg, I., Flatman, J. A., and Lambert, J. D. (1979). The actions of excitatory amino acids on motoneurons in the feline spinal cord. *J. Physiol. (Lond.) 288*:227–261.

86. Zieglgänsberger, W., and Champagnat, J. (1979). Cat spinal motoneurons exhibit topographic sensitivity to glutamate and glycine. *Brain Res. 160*:95–104.

87. Puil, E. (1981). S-Glutamate: Its interactions with spinal motoneurons. *Brain Res. Rev. 3*:229–322.

88. Puil, E. (1983). Actions and interactions of S-glutamate in the spinal cord. In *Handbook of the Spinal Cord*, vol. 1, R. A. Davidoff (Ed.). Marcel Dekker, New York, pp. 105–169.

89. Eccles, J. C. (1964). *The Physiology of Synapses*. Springer, Berlin, 1964.

90. Llínas, R., and Sugimori, M. (1980). Electrophysiological properties of in-vitro Purkinje cell dendrites in mammalian cerebellar slices. *J. Physiol. (Lond.) 305*:197–213.

91. Wong, R. K. S., Prince, D. A., and Basbaum, A. I. (1979). Intradendritic recordings from hippocampal neurons. *Proc. Natl. Acad. Sci. U.S.A. 76*: 986–990.

92. Traub, R. D., and Llínas, R. (1977). The spatial distribution of ionic conductances in normal and axotomized motoneurons. *Neuroscience 2*:829–849.

93. Pottala, E. W., Colburn, T. R., and Humphrey, D. R. (1973). A dendritic compartment model neuron. *I.E.E.E. Trans. Biomed. Eng. 20(2)*:132–139.

8

MAMMALIAN MOTOR UNITS

Donald M. Lewis   *The Medical School, University of Bristol, Bristol,*
England

I. INTRODUCTION

The term motor unit was introduced by Liddell and Sherrington (1) in 1925 and
defined as the "motoneurone axon and its adjunct muscle fibres." A later paper
by Sherrington (2) extended the definition to include: "The muscle-fibres
innervated by the unit and the whole axon of the motoneurone from its hillock
on the perikaryon down to its terminals in the muscle." The concept of a motor
unit was understood much earlier; for example, Mines (3) demonstrated that
increasing the intensity of a stimulus applied to a muscle nerve caused stepwise
increases in muscle twitch contractions, the steps being much larger than those
elicited by stimulating the same muscle directly after application of curare
(Fig. 1). The formal introduction of the idea of a motor unit was important
because, at that time, measurement of muscle tension was the method of
assessing quantitatively the motor output of the central nervous system. The
motor unit is the smallest element of the muscle which can be excited by
nervous action. Indeed, with hindsight, Sherrington's definition (2) of the motor
unit was precisely correct as the action potential starts in the axon hillock of the
motoneuron, so the motor unit as defined previously behaves in an all-or-none
manner through all its elements. In contrast, the motoneuron soma integrates
the excitatory and inhibitory inputs. Although this chapter will not analyze this

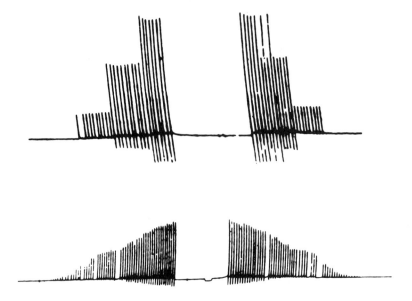

Figure 1 Early evidence about motor units in frog sartorius muscle (3). In both records the stimulus strength was increased and then decreased with a rest period between. Upper: The stimuli were applied to the nerve, and all-or-none motor unit twitches are seen. Lower: The muscle was curarized and stimulated directly, and the steps are individual muscle fibers.

function of the soma, it will be necessary to consider later their resultant rates of discharge in order to understand motoneuronal control of muscle.

Typically, in the normal adult mammal motor units are separate because each skeletal muscle fiber is innervated by only one motoneuron. This is not true of lower vertebrates, in which muscle fibers may be innervated by several axons, and motor units overlap because axons share muscle fibers. This condition of polyneuronal innervation also occurs in mammals when the muscle fibers first receive their innervation in utero and for a time after birth. Polyneuronal innervation also recurs in adults if a motor nerve is sectioned and allowed to reinnervate a muscle.

Two exceptions are found to this rule of discreteness of motor units in normal adult mammals. The first is found in certain muscles innervated by cranial nerves: the extrinsic muscles of the eye (4) and the small muscles acting on the ossicles of the inner ear (5). These muscles contain many fibers which are similar to the tonic muscles in lower vertebrates which have polyneuronal innervation. It is known that these fibers do not show all-or-none action potentials but are excited by local end-plate (junction) potentials from multiple endings all along the fibers; the resulting contraction is slow. The other exception is more widespread and involves the intrinsic muscle fibers of muscle spindles. There are a variety of types involved here with innervation which is both discrete, as in the extrafusal fibers, and diffuse, as in the tonic fibers. Again, intrafusal fibers are innervated by several axons which may be of a small diameter (Aγ axons derived from a special group of small motoneurons), or may they be branches of the large-diameter Aα axons that innervate the extrafusal fibers. These were called β fibers by Bessou et al. (40), although they do not fall outside the range of sizes of those Aα axons which exclusively innervate extrafusal muscle. With these two groups of muscle fibers, polyneuronal innervation prevents the occurrence of discrete, individually acting, all-or-none motor units, and they will not be considered further in this chapter.

II. THE MOTONEURON

Motoneurons are found in the ventral (anterior) horn of the spinal cord. As indicated earlier, the population is bimodal with respect to soma size, and it is the group of larger, more numerous cells which innervates the extrafusal muscle fibers. These large motoneurons show a twofold range of diameters (6), and the largest (up to 75 μm in diameter) innervate a class of motor units different from those supplied by the smallest ones (40 μm and upward); the differences between these two groups of motor units are important and are described in the following paragraphs.

It is possible to trace the motoneurons innervating a particular muscle. This has been done in patients in whom a limited number of muscles had been affected by poliomyelitis, a disease which destroys motoneurons (7). Chromatolysis of the motoneuron soma follows nerve transection, and has been used as a tracer in animals. Recently, good quantitative results have been obtained by exposing motoneuron axons of selected muscles to the protein horseradish peroxidase (HRP). This substance is taken up by nerve endings or cut nerves and transported retrogradely to accumulate in the cell body. Histologic sections of the spinal cord can then be stained to reveal the motoneuron somata corresponding to the treated nerve. Burke et al. (6) have used this method, which is illustrated in Figure 2. It is found that a single anatomic muscle has motoneurons arranged in a column which extends over one or two spinal segments and is limited in transverse section to part of the ventral horn. The motoneuron columns occupy consistent positions in individuals of one species, and there are similarities when comparing species. There is probably a somatotopic organization within the columns as well as between them. The number of motoneurons in a column and, therefore, the number of motor units increases directly (but not linearly) with the size and tension capability of the muscle. This holds true between species, so that the number of innervating a given muscle in the cat is intermediate between the values for the mouse and for man.

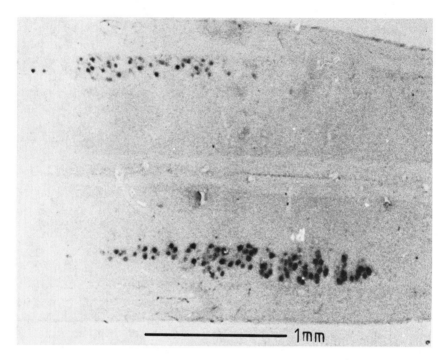

Figure 2 Motoneurons of mouse spinal cord labeled with HRP injected into muscle groups and transported retrogradely in the axons to the somata. The longitudinal section of the lumbar region shows motoneurons innervating anterior and lateral (above) and posterior (below) muscles of the lower leg. (Courtesy of S. McHanwell, University College, London.)

The number of motor units may also be estimated from the number of axons in a muscle nerve. This may be done reasonably accurately because the difference between large and small motoneurons is represented as clearly in axon diameter as in soma size. Figure 3 shows the bimodal distribution of A fibers in a muscle nerve (corresponding to α and γ axons; see Sec. I). Figure 3 also illustrates the fact that the Aα axons innervating one muscle (soleus) have a range different from those innervating another (medial gastrocnemius). The two classes of Aα axons correspond to the two types of large motoneurons referred to previously. The histograms of Figure 3 were obtained after removal of spinal dorsal root ganglia and subsequent degeneration of sensory fibers in the muscle nerve. Application of axon counts to assessing motor unit number in man (11) involves guesses about the number of sensory fibers (about half). Another

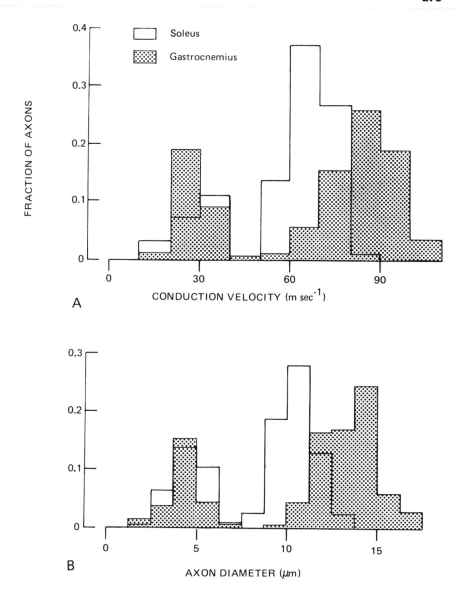

Figure 3 Physiologic (A) and anatomic (B) properties of axons innervating gastrocnemius (shaded: fast-twitch) and soleus (plain: slow-twitch) muscles. (A from Refs. 8 and 9; B from Ref. 10.)

substantial problem is that motor axons branch well before they reach the muscle. Eccles and Sherrington (10) dissected the nerve to the medial gastrocnemius (a calf muscle) to the point in the upper thigh where it mingled with other muscle nerves, a distance of 60 mm in the cat. They found that there was an increase of about one quarter in the number of axons over this length of nerve, an increase caused by branching of motor axons. Sherrington and Eccles reported that branching was more common in large axons than in small. In some cases motor axon branches may go to anatomically distinct muscles, for example, adjacent lumbrical muscles of the cat foot (12).

Indirect methods of estimating the number of motor units depend upon recording from representative samples of motor units and comparing the mean motor unit response with that of the whole muscle. If motor unit tetanic tension is used for such a comparison, good agreement has been reached with anatomic methods (13,14). If twitch tension is used in larger muscles, it is found that motor units sum in a nonlinear manner to give a large overestimate of the number of motor units (15). In smaller, more uniform muscles, such as those of the mouse, estimates from twitches do not differ from those derived from tetanic contractions (16). Such methods have been applied to man for analysis of the relative importance of axonal loss in various types of neuromuscular diseases where, despite limitations in accuracy, it is necessary to obtain some indication of the nature of the pathologic process. Sica and McComas (17) were aware of the problem of using twitch tension for estimating mean motor unit number because of an earlier demonstration of nonlinear summation of submaximal muscle twitches (18). These workers developed a technique which used the electromyogram of single motor units and the whole muscle (19), which they used for investigation of neuromuscular disease [see (20)]. The method can be applied only to a limited number of accessible muscles, and it suffers from two problems. First, the sample of motor units must be small and also consists of those with low nerve thresholds, which may have properties different from the true average. Second, the assumption of linear summation of electromyographic motor unit potentials has been doubted (21). Despite this, the method gives reasonable agreement when compared with the more rigorous methods available for other mammals (22).

Within the muscle extensive branching occurs, either within a limited territory in larger mammals (cat: 15; man: 23), or over the muscle in smaller ones (rat: 24). The finer terminal branches end in single motor end-plates, often in a fairly discrete end-plate zone.

III. THE MUSCLE ELEMENTS

The muscle fibers of a single motor unit may be identified by a technique developed by Edström and Kugelberg (24). The motor unit is stimulated for long periods until its muscle fibers are depleted of glycogen. Subsequently, histologic sections of the muscle may be stained for glycogen to reveal the glycogen fibers of the motor unit (Fig. 4). Interpretation of the data from such experiments is not unambiguous (see Sec. IV.G), but it is clear that the fibers of a motor unit are scattered reasonably uniformly over the territory of that unit. This conclusion had been anticipated by earlier electrophysiologic work (e.g., 25). A certain number of fibers of a motor unit are adjacent, forming pairs and triplets, but it is possible that such contiguous fibers are less frequent than would occur by chance, indicating the operation of mechanisms reducing the innervation of adjacent muscle fibers by the same nerve axon. There is one interesting exception to this rule in that rosettes of similar fibers (presumably from one motor unit) develop and expand during postnatal development of the pig (26). Similar observations have been made in human foot muscles (27), but there are suggestions that such findings may be related to subclinical pathologic changes in the muscle nerves (effects of reinnervation are discussed in Sec. IV.J).

The number of muscle fibers innervated by a single axon (the innervation ratio) has been a subject of investigation for many years. The earliest work involved estimation of the mean innervation ratio from measurements of the number of motor axons [Eccles and Sherrington (10): note that they included γ axons in their numbers] and of muscle fibers (28). Such methods are the only anatomic ones available in man (11). Within one species mean innervation ratio varies from one muscle to another, although it is reasonably consistent for one muscle compared between individuals. As might be expected the innervation ratio is larger for larger muscles: In human gastrocnemius muscle there are nearly 2000 fibers per axon and in the small muscles of the hand the ratio is about 100. When the range of muscle sizes is considered, however, this variation in motor unit size is relatively small. The extrinsic eye muscles have even smaller ratios, for example, Björkman and Wöhlfart (29) gave a value of 10 for external rectus, but these estimates are much less certain because nerves can only be examined near the muscle where extensive branching may have occurred. Further, the presence of tonic muscle fibers must add uncertainty to the data. An equally important factor in determining the size of a muscle is the number of motor units. This is necessary because it seems that there is some limitation to the number of fibers an axon can innervate [discussed in Sec. IV.J (101)]. Thus, a small muscle has a smaller number of motor units than a large muscle. In addition, its motor units are smaller. As a result a small muscle has a relatively high level of innervation and the capability of finer control.

Comparisons can be made between species, and it may be concluded that a small animal has fewer motor units and that these are of smaller size. The human medial gastrocnemius, for example, has about 580 motor units and the cat about 270, while their innervation ratios are about 1970 and 590, respectively.

Estimates of mean innervation ratios give only limited information. Although glycogen depletion methods directly estimate the number of fibers in a motor unit, the technique can only give an answer for one motor unit in a particular

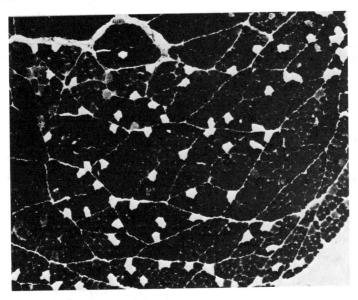

A

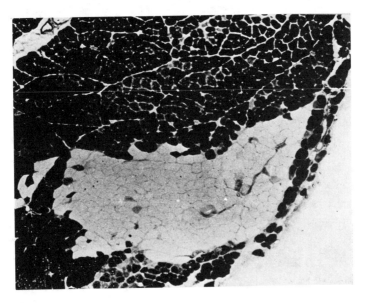

B

├────────────┤ 1mm

muscle and the total number of such studies reported in the literature is very small. Motor unit sizes in the rat appear to be relatively uniform (24). In cat gastrocnemius Burke and Tsairis (30) found clear evidence of motor units that contained from 440 to 750 fibers. They found smaller numbers in other units (down to about 15), but considered that the counts were erroneously low because of difficulties in depleting glycogen in some types of motor units (see Secs. IV.F and H).

Indirect methods of estimating innervation ratios are available but these methods depend upon knowing the range of motor unit tensions and making assumptions about the tension output of muscle fibers. The tension of a fiber depends upon the area of the fiber, which can be measured directly, and on the tension output per unit area, which can only be guessed at (unless the original problem of the number of fibers per motor unit is solved). On these bases, Burke and Tsairis (30) estimated that the smallest motor units in the gastro-cnemius may have had as few as 50 fibers; if their estimates of tension output per fiber are too low (see Sec. IV.H), then the number may be as low as 18—a value in agreement with direct, glycogen-depletion methods. The size of the smallest motor units must, therefore, be regarded as unsettled at present.

IV. PHYSIOLOGIC PROPERTIES

This section will consider the electrical properties of the motor unit and the con-tractile and metabolic properties of its muscle fibers. In order to understand some of the limitations of the conclusions it is necessary to consider briefly the methods by which single motor units have been functionally "isolated," that is, how the response of one motor unit can be recorded in the presence of anatomically contiguous motor units.

A. Methods of Study

In general, two methods have been used to study the motor unit. One is to study more or less physiologic activation of a muscle and to pick out unitary responses. The other involves artificial stimulation of a unit. The first method has been most commonly applied to the electromyographic recording of motor units with fine needle electrodes introduced acutely or with wires implanted chronically. Such information is of direct value in understanding the electrical properties of

---

Figure 4 Cross section of rat tibialis anterior muscles. A: A normal muscle. B: A muscle reinnervated after nerve transection. A single motor unit has been tetanized repeatedly and its muscle fibers depleted of glycogen so that they do not stain with the periodic acid–Schiff preparation. (Courtesy of E. Kugelberg, Karolinska Institute, Stockholm.)

muscle fibers and neuromuscular transmission (e.g., 31), and with the use of multielectrode arrays the extent of motor unit territories (32). More importantly, single unit electromyographic recording allows investigation of the ways in which motor units are used in normal activity. This method has been employed more frequently in man than in other mammals, but the ability of recording needles to survive activity (and vice versa) limits the range of movement which can be studied.

Natural activity has also been used to study contractile properties. Gordon and Holbourn (33) used phonographic pick-ups to record the movement of localized, presumed unitary, contractions in minimal reflexes. More recently, Stein et al. (34) recorded single-unit electromyographic and twitch tension in human muscles. The unit potentials were used to trigger an averager so that after several thousands samples the tension of the single unit could be built up and distinguished from the random discharge of other units. The method has been applied to other species and extended to allow examination of axonal properties (35).

Although the methods briefly described previously have the enormously important advantages of allowing study of motor units in conscious individuals with normally activated muscles and also of following the time course of changes in individual animals, they do suffer from inherent problems. For example, the sample obtained will not be an unbiased set of the whole population. There are two reasons for this. One is that the chances of selecting a single motor unit depend upon the amplitude of the electromyograph and on the extent of its territory. In the cat it has been shown that both properties are directly related to the tension of the motor unit. Those units which develop large tensions have larger territories and higher amplitude-evoked electromyographic potentials (36). As a consequence, they would be more likely to be within the field of an electrode and, once within recording distance, to be detected against other activity. The second bias arises from the fact that it becomes more and more difficult to distinguish individual motor units as a greater fraction of the muscle becomes active. As there is good evidence that those motor units recruited in a weak contraction differ from those recruited at higher levels of force (see Sec. V), the inability to distinguish motor units at even quite moderate levels of activity must introduce considerable bias. A further problem for the spike-triggered averaging technique for motor unit tension is that synchronization (not necessarily precisely in time) of other motor units will distort the records and, unless tests are made to detect synchronous activity (in the electromyogram, for example), it may be difficult to interpret data.

The second general method of "isolation" is to stimulate single axons. An early method of cutting down the muscle nerve was wasteful, producing only a few units per muscle (10). The other simple, early method, which is illustrated in Figure 1, involved stimulating the motor nerve with gradually increasing voltage.

The method is satisfactory when only a few motor units are present and when these are similar in properties. As described earlier, the method has been used in man, but it is necessary to depend upon samples because many motor units are involved, and once the sample has reached more than about 10 it becomes difficult to measure accurately the motor units recruited on top of the summed response of all the lower threshold ones. Moreover, it may be impossible to distinguish small motor units from noise even when only a small number of motor units have been recruited. The possibility of bias also exists because excitability is higher for large axons than for small ones. Fortunately, excitability also depends upon the position in the nerve relative to the stimulating electrodes. The position factor is not related to the physiology of the motor unit and is also strong so that the bias introduced by differences in intrinsic excitability of axons seems to be small. An alternative method of stimulating axons is in the muscle via a needle electrode (37). This has been of great use in recording properties of human motor units and comparing these with data obtained in other mammals (38). Again, it may not be suitable for making statements about populations because of selectivity. The method seems to depend upon stimulation of an axonal branch with antidromic and orthodromic invasion of all other branches of the motor unit. The chance of stimulating a particular motor unit will depend upon the number of branches, and this will favor motor units with a high innervation ratio (discussed in Sec. III).

The methods which have yielded most results in terms of mechanical properties of motor units have been ones which depend upon isolating motoneurons in a region remote from the muscle, either by penetrating the motoneuron with a microelectrode or by mechanically subdividing the nerve or the ventral (motor) root near the spinal cord (a site favored because of the lack of tough connective tissue which impedes separation of nerve filaments from each other). Both methods give excellent electrical isolation—the motor unit may be stimulated up to 10 times threshold without recruiting other axons. In addition, stable preparations are obtained which allow recordings to be made for several hours if necessary. Ventral root splitting does involve extensive surgery, especially as the ventral root "motor unit" is not a single axon; the other axons innervate other muscles which have to be denervated to prevent mechanical interference (Fig. 5). Moreover, very careful testing of the ventral root filament must be performed if one is to be certain that only one motor unit is present. (Annoyingly, a pair often seems to have very similar electrical thresholds so that many trials have to be made to be sure that the response is all-or-none at constant stimulus strength, as in Figure 5.) In contrast, penetration of a single motoneuron is clear and unambiguous.

The first report of the use of ventral root filaments to systematically investigate motor units was by Denslow and Gutensohn (39), but the method was not exploited fully for more than a decade when a full study by Bessou et al. (39a)

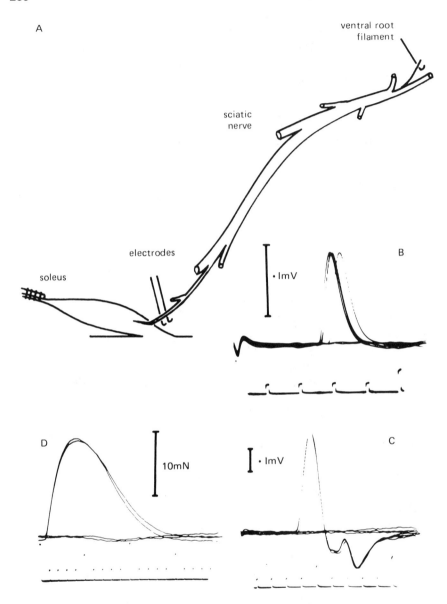

Figure 5 Isolation of motor units by splitting ventral root filaments (A). The filament is judged to be functionally single by all-or-none behavior of the antidromic nerve action potential (B), the muscle EMG (C), and twitch (D). (Courtesy of J. Bagust, University of Bristol, England, Ph.D. dissertation, 1971.)

and preliminary reports by Henneman et al. (41,8,9) were published at about the same time. The microelectrode technique was first shown to be useful by Devanandan et al. (42), but it has been most fully utilized by Burke and his colleagues (43).

Neither the method of ventral root splitting nor that of motoneuron penetration is free of possible selectivity. Some ventral root filaments may consist only of branches of a motor unit, and although the data of Eccles and Sherrington (10) show that branching only occurs relatively near to the muscle in a peripheral nerve, it could occur within the spinal cord. There is no evidence of spinal branches other than those going to Renshaw cells, but investigations have not been directed specifically at this question. The other problem is that small axons are more likely to be damaged by the splitting procedure, and the sample biased toward larger ones. There is no direct solution to this problem, but isolated examples have been reported which show that the proportion of γ to α fibers in ventral root filaments is not too far from the ratio obtained histologically, even in kitten roots where small size should make selectivity worse (44). The microelectrode searches of motoneuron pools ought also to introduce bias against small motoneurons; presumably, the chance of a microelectrode touching a cell is proportional to the area presented by that cell, and as Burke et al. (6) have shown, the smallest alpha motoneurons innervating extrafusal fibers have half the diameter of the largest (a fourfold difference in area). The chances of stably penetrating a small motoneuron may well be even smaller because it will be more likely to be damaged. So a more realistic estimate of bias between the chances of selecting the largest against the smallest motoneuron may be at least five to one, but it is very difficult to be sure of these figures. (It is certainly known that it is difficult to penetrate and hold gamma motoneurons that innervate intrafusal fibers, but these are a factor of two smaller still.) A comparison of the data obtained by the two methods should give some idea of their relative bias. Devanandan et al. (42) obtained almost no small motor units (corresponding to small alpha motoneurons), but later data with improved techniques do not show such extreme bias.

B. Variety of Muscles

It has been known for more than a century that different types of skeletal muscles exist in all mammals. A broad division was originally made into fast white and slow red muscles (but see Sec. IV.C) on the basis of speed of contraction and of histologic characteristics. This division derives from early descriptions by Ranvier (45). Differences between the twitch contractions of three muscles are illustrated in Figure 6, which has been reconstructed from records of Cooper and Eccles (46), and shows the classic fast- and slow-twitch muscle. The third set of contractions is from an extrinsic eye muscle and the twitch is seen to be even

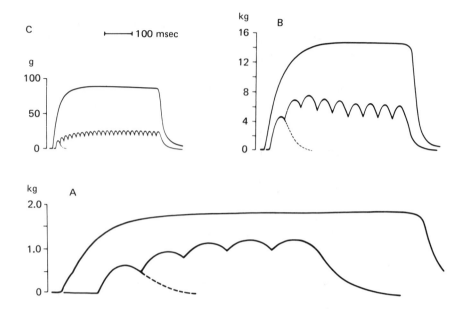

Figure 6 Isometric myograms of slow-twitch (A), fast-twitch limb (B), and extrinsic eye (C) muscles, all scaled to the same time base. Each panel shows a twitch and an unfused and a fused tetanus. (From Ref. 46.)

briefer than that of a fast-twitch limb muscle. More recently, Close and Luff (47) demonstrated that, in contrast to the isometric twitch illustrated in Figure 6, the isotonic shortening velocity of the eye muscle was almost identical with that of a fast-twitch muscle of a limb. The faster eye muscle twitch is a consequence of a briefer activation within the fibers (presumably a briefer intracellular calcium transient), so that the contraction is maintained for a shorter period and is smaller in relation to full tetanic tension. This difference between two types of fast-twitch muscle is emphasized because it makes the point that investigations of the properties of motor units must be less complete than is possible with whole muscles (or single fibers), and that some care must be taken in interpreting the limited data.

C. Variety of Motor Units

Gross inspection of muscles reveals that many are not uniform in color, the deeper layers often being redder than the superficial layer of fibers. Gordon and Phillips (48) sliced a muscle longitudinally to demonstrate that the visually distinguishable parts of a muscle have different twitch contraction times. It was also clear early on from the work of Eccles and Sherrington (10) that motor

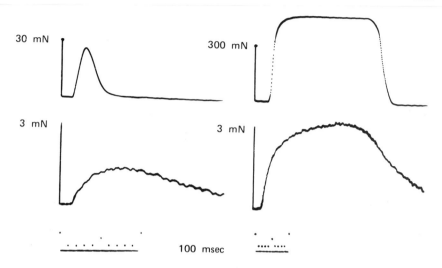

Figure 7 Isometric twitch and tetanus myograms of large, fast (above) and small, slow (below) motor units from cat flexor digitorum longus muscle. (From Ref. 13.)

axons ranged over a twofold range of diameters and that the axons innervating fast-twitch muscles (gastrocnemius in Fig. 3) were larger than those of slow-twitch muscle. It was later shown by the first motor unit studies that there was a corresponding range of axonal conduction velocities with differences between muscle types, the fast muscle having fast conducting axons (see Fig. 3).

These studies also revealed a wide range of contractile properties in the motor units, which were not uniform either in tension or in twitch contraction and relaxation time, the differences being especially pronounced in fast-twitch muscle (Fig. 7). There was, however, order within this variation in that axonal conduction velocity, tension, and contraction time were interrelated. This was most clearly seen in the small lumbrical muscles intrinsic to the cat foot investigated by Emonet-Denand and colleagues (39a,49) and illustrated in Figure 8. It was shown that in larger hindlimb muscles the same general pattern was present— those motor units with fast-conducting axons developed the largest tension and had the briefest twitches (50). In the larger muscles, however, there was often much more scatter (Fig. 9). The slow-twitch cat soleus muscle had the same pattern, although the range of tension was much smaller. Fast-twitch muscles contain a few large motor units that develop up to 5% of the total muscle tension, although a majority of the motor units are small ones—as little as one thousandth of the tension of the largest (cf. Fig. 17, top row). The slow motor units in cat fast-twitch muscle have many characteristics in common with the motor units of

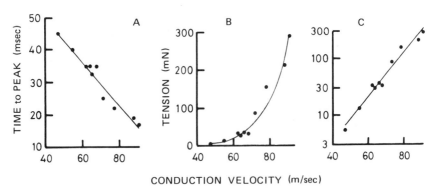

Figure 8 Relationship between axonal conduction velocity and twitch time to peak (A) and tetanic tension: on a linear (B) and logarithmic (C) ordinate. Motor units of lumbrical muscle of cat foot. (From Ref. 49.)

slow-twitch muscle (see Sec. IV.F), but in many muscles they have much smaller tension. A fair comparison can be made between the fast flexor digitorum longus and the slow soleus (13,14) (Figs. 17 and 18) because in the cat these two muscles develop approximately the same tetanic tension (51) and have about equal number of alpha motoneurons (52). The tensions of flexor digitorum longus motor units range from 820 to 3 mN, with the slow subgroup mainly occupying the range from ~70 to 3mN. In contrast, soleus slow motor units vary between 250 and 20 mN, some three to seven times larger (the values apply to muscles in animals weighing 2-3 kg). There is a smaller discrepancy in tension if the soleus is compared with the much larger medial gastrocnemius, which shows a total motor tension range of 20-1,350 mN, with slow motor units developing between 20 and 360 mN (53). These figures reinforce the conclusions drawn previously from mean innervation ratios—the mean motor unit tension is larger for larger muscles and this difference exists at both the top and bottom ends of the range. It may again be noted that the differences between motor unit tensions account for part of the differences between muscles; for example, the largest motor unit tensions are 1,350, 750, and 300 mN in the gastrocnemius, flexor digitorum longus, and lumbrical muscles, respectively, while the tetanic tensions of these three whole muscles are about 100, 25, and 1 N. Thus, there is less than a fivefold range of maximum motor unit tensions in muscles with a 100-fold range of total tensions.

The time course of twitches of motor units also show a wide range of variation, both in the contraction time and the relaxation time. Contraction and relaxation are very closely related and only the former will be discussed. As seen in Figure 18, in the cat the range of contraction times is wider in the soleus than in the flexor digitorum longus or medial gastrocnemius (although the relative

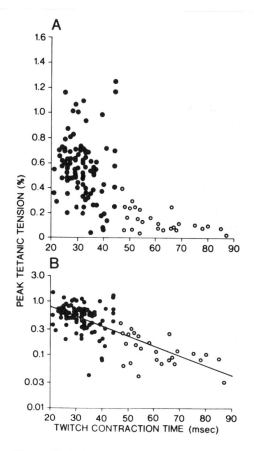

Figure 9 Relationship between twitch times-to-peak and tetanic tension on a linear (A) and logarithmic (B) ordinate. Motor units from gastrocnemius muscle of the cat. Open circles, slow-twitch; closed circles, fast-twitch motor units. (From Ref. 50.)

range, i.e., range divided by mean, is smaller in the soleus). A further difference is that the distribution in the soleus is symmetrical, whereas that of all fast muscles is skewed to large values; another reflection of the two groups of fast and slow motor units in the latter.

The differences in twitch characteristics parallel the differences in the biochemical activity of muscle fibers revealed by histochemistry, especially for adenosine triphosphatase (ATPase) activity (54), and by immunohistochemistry (55). This topic will be considered in more detail in Sec. IV.F, but briefly, fast and slow fibers can be distinguished as dark and light staining, respectively, with

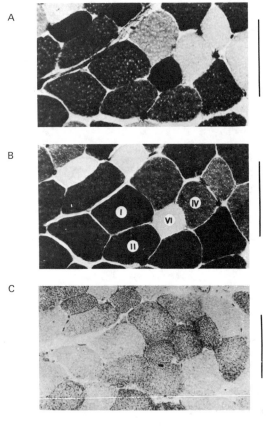

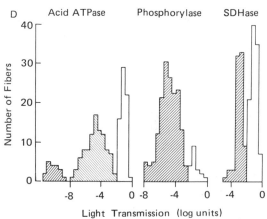

Acid ATPase   Phosphorylase   SDHase

Light Transmission (log units)

ATPase reactions preceded by alkaline preincubation (Fig. 10) or by antibodies specific to fast or slow muscle myosin. As shown in Sec. IV.D, these histologic distinctions can be experimentally related to individual motor units. On the basis of this evidence, whole muscle histochemistry allows reasonable inferences to be made about the range of motor units in the absence of direct evidence.

The examples quoted previously have all been taken from the cat, which histochemically has a pure soleus muscle composed only of type I fibers (staining weakly for ATPase after alkaline preincubation) which react with antibody to slow muscle myosin. Most fast muscles consist of a mixture of type I and type II fibers (dark staining after alkaline preincubated ATPase). Jaw muscles have the highest proportion of type II fibers, although they do not react with antibody prepared against the fast myosin of limb fast muscles (and vice versa). Intrafusal fibers may resemble either type I or II; tonic muscle fibers are closer to type I.

D. Species Variation

If species other than the cat are compared, then there is a tendency for larger animals to have a higher proportion of type I fibers. For example, man has more type I fibers in the gastrocnemius than the cat; small rodents and the rabbit have type II fibers in the soleus (about half in the mouse) and fewer type I in fast muscles (none in most mouse muslces). These are only very general rules—guinea pig soleus is pure type I as in the cat. There are also strain differences—greyhounds and racehorses have a higher proportion of type II fibers than less highly specialized individuals of their species, and there is some evidence that comparable differences occur in human sprinters.

Differences in fiber type composition and, presumably, in the proportion of fast and slow motor units account partly for differences in the speed of contraction of muscles. There are, however, other factors which make the contractions of muscles of small mammals faster than those of large ones. This second factor is shown by motor unit recording which has demonstrated that the twitch contraction of an average fast motor unit of a mouse (16) is faster than that of the fast motor unit of a rat (57), which, in turn, is faster than that of the cat, with the fast motor unit in man being the slowest in this series. Corresponding

---

Figure 10 Histochemistry of cat flexor digitorum longus muscle. Serial sections have been stained for ATPase after acid (A) or alkaline (B) preincubation and for SDH (C). Fiber (I) is type IIB, (IV) is IIA and (VI) is I; (II) has ATPase characteristics of type IIB, but has strong SDH activity. Calibrations 100 μm. The histograms (D) show semiquantitative estimates of staining density of about 120 fibers. (From Ref. 56.)

species differences have been found for slow motor units. It should be noted that these differences in contraction speeds are not reflected in muscle histochemistry (although biochemical reaction speeds parallel twitch characteristics (58) and that antibodies to fast and slow myosin react strongly across species.

There are other differences between species. For example, the range of motor unit contraction times are much narrower in the rat than in the cat, not only in absolute terms, but also relatively, so that the fast and slow motor units in slow and in fast muscle form distinct populations (Fig. 11) rather than the

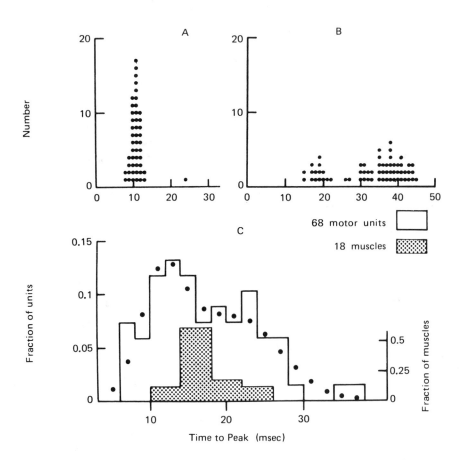

Figure 11 Distribution of twitch times-to-peak of motor units from rat extensor digitorum longus (A) and soleus (B) muscles, compared with mouse soleus (C: open columns). (Shaded columns show data from the muscles from which the motor units were isolated; the dots are a fitted double normal distribution.) (From Refs. 57 and 16.)

skewed, continuous distribution in the cat, which is the result of overlap in properties between the two types. This is not, however, a reflection of animal size because in mouse soleus fast and slow motor units overlap extensively (Fig. 11), whereas baboon extensor digitorum communis (a forearm muscle; 59) has a rather limited range. It is safe, however, to generalize that tension range is very limited in the simpler animals; there is a 10:1 range in the mouse and 100:1 in the rat compared with more than 1000:1 in the cat. But again, there may be exceptionally small ranges in the baboon muscle (mentioned previously) and in man (although selectivity might well exclude the smallest motor units given the methods used in both these species).

E. Recording Conditions

In comparing results from different laboratories, or even at different periods of time from the same laboratory, it is necessary to consider the environment in which the recordings are made. Differences may be trivial, but occasionally large effects are produced which make direct comparisons impossible. Some factors are listed in the following paragraphs.

Strain differences within a species have been referred to and often are responsible for small variation. Males and females are also different—the twitch of the female rat muscle is about 10% briefer than that of the male, mainly owing to different proportions of fast and slow motor units. Age is so important that it is discussed separately later, but even with mature adults changes occur. Many mammals continue to grow during adult life with a parallel increase in muscle and motor unit force (there is no change in the number of motor units except in old age). Growth also increases nerve lengths, but since conduction time remains constant after early postnatal life (60), conduction velocity also increases with age, altering the relationship between conduction velocity and motor unit twitch time (16). Also affecting this relationship is the fact that the mean conduction velocity differs between species—the cat has the fastest axons, man and the rabbit slower, and the rat and mouse the slowest. Moreover, conduction slows peripherally, hence differences between values for axons supplying cat lumbricals and cat gastrocnemius.

Temperature has a very large effect on twitch times (decrease with increasing temperature, with a Q_{10} of about 2.2) and on twitch tension (fast muscle decreases and slow muscle increases with temperature increase). Some investigators (Lewis, Burke) maintain fluid around the muscles at 37°C; others (Close) at 35°C. Others only maintain the animal temperature (Henneman, Proske), and muscle temperature may be as low as 33°C. In man, normally no control is exercised, and muscle temperature is known to vary between 31 and 41°C, depending upon room temperature and time after exercise.

Twitch tension and time course depend upon muscle length (e.g., 51). The muscle may be set at the length at which twitch tension is maximal or set for

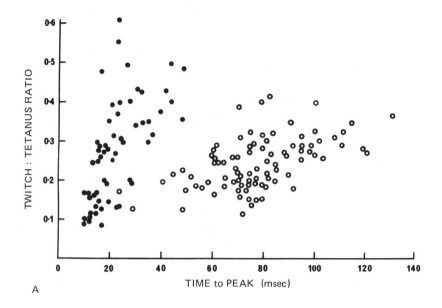

A

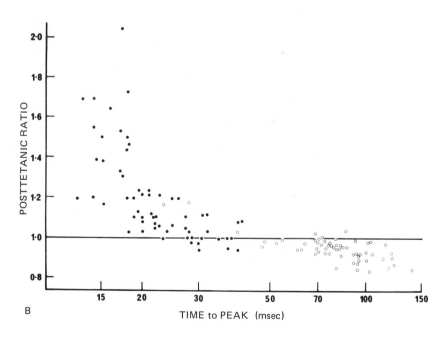

B

maximum tetanic tension; both procedures standardize the data, but the former (twitch optimum) is longer by about 10% of fiber length than tetanus optimum. Other authors use a constant passive tension on the muscle, and since the relationship between passive tension and muscle length depends upon muscle type and size, this method introduces small variations within a set of data as well as differences from other workers.

The force generated by a motor unit is sometimes quoted in terms of twitch tension rather than tetanic tension, particularly in human experiments when techniques limit measurements to the twitch. The ratio of twitch tension to tetanic tension (the twitch:tension ratio) has been shown to depend upon twitch contraction time in some series of experiments (Fig. 12), so motor unit tension using twitches may be impossible to compare with those using tetanic contractions.

The human "twitches" may be even less comparable when they have been derived by spike-triggered averaging because motoneurons fire at rates which result in unfused tetanic contractions rather than discrete twitches. The oscillations of the unfused tetanic contractions will be briefer and probably smaller than true twitches. Even a true, discrete twitch is not a constant entity. The "staircase effect" is an increase in twitch tension with increasing frequency of stimulation, and there may be a 30% increase in the tension of fast motor unit twitch when stimulated at say five per second compared with one per 50 seconds (with no great change in time course). In contrast, twitch tension and time course decrease as stimulation rate is increased for a slow motor unit. Most authors stimulate once per five to 20 seconds, and this results in little difference. In recent papers, however, Burke's laboratory has reported data from "potentiated twitches" (61). These are not the twitches recorded shortly after a short tetanus which most authors refer to as posttetanic potentiation or depression (53,62,63). Burke and his colleagues measure twitches recorded after a series of tetanic contractions which produces a long-lasting increase in twitch tension (two- or threefold) and prolongation of the rising phase and, more markedly, the falling phase of the twitch. The twitch data of Burke and his colleagues is, therefore, very different from that of others. Both methods are internally consistent, neither is right in that neither represents a "physiologic state" of the motor unit (if there were such a state). It is important, however, to remember

---

Figure 12 A: Relationship between twitch:tetanus ratio and twitch times-to-peak for motor units of cat flexor digitorum longus (closed circles) and soleus (open circles). B: Extent of posttetanic potentiation and depression related to twitch times-to-peak for the same set of motor units used in A. (From Refs. 14, 13, and 63.)

that there are big differences between the sets of data recorded by the two methods which may be unrelated to real differences between the properties of the motor units in the two sets.

F. Classification of Motor Units

The description of the motor unit, so far has referred to fast and slow motor units without evidence for different types. Are the fast and slow motor units simply opposite ends of a continuous range of variation? This is not so for the rat, which shows clear bimodal distributions (Fig. 11). Moreover, in all species histochemistry shows three quite separate groups of fibers which have distinct peaks in the distribution when staining reactions are estimated semiquantitatively (Fig. 10). A similar separation of motor units into three clear groups began to evolve as more tests were applied.

The first suggestion that small fast motor units were of a different type from the large fast ones was made by Olson and Swett (64) working in Henneman's laboratory; but a sound division only became possible with the use of ATPase histochemistry (54), and the introduction of the technique of glycogen depletion by which fibers of a motor unit are tagged by fatiguing them with repeated tetanic contractions (Fig. 4; 24). Burke added two tests of motor unit function which finally allowed a clear distinction into types (43). One of these is the sag test: If an unfused tetanus of the motor unit is elicited with a train of pulses with an interval equal to 125% of the contraction time of the twitch, then fast motor units show a sag in the tetanus; the oscillations rise to an early peak and then decrease in amplitude. In contrast, slow motor units show a progressively increasing tension (cf. Fig. 6). Burke has used this sag test as an absolute distinction between fast and slow motor units (although no quantitative justification has been presented in the literature). The second test is of fatigue: Tetanic contractions are repeated every second and the fall of tension noted; at a critical time it is possible to distinguish easily fatigued motor units in which tension falls more than 75% from fatigue resistant ones with less than 25% fall. The results of all these tests are illustrated in the multidimensional graph of Figure 13 (this has essentially four dimensions, since the all-or-none sag behavior is indicated by the presence or absence of shading on the data spheres). Figure 13 separates three groups of motor units. The first group is of large-tension, fast-twitch, and easily fatigued motor units which show sag in unfused tetani; these are called FF (fast-fatiguable) units by Burke (65). The second group is composed of small, fast, and slowly fatiguing motor units with sag: FR (fast-resistant to fatigue). The third group comprises the small, slow, and almost nonfatiguing motor units: type S (slow). The transition group with intermediate values of fatigue resistance is small, but it is found consistently and has been termed F(int) units. By applying these tests, therefore, it is possible to separate FF from FR by fatigue

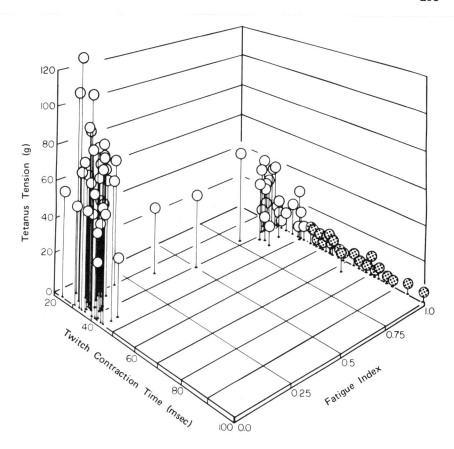

Figure 13 Three-dimensional representation of relationships between three characteristics for cat gastrocnemius motor units. Shading indicates motor units with no sag in an unfused tetanus. (From Ref. 65.)

resistance, although their twitch times overlap; or FR from S by the presence or absence of sag in an unfused tetanus, although fatigue indices and tensions overlap and twitch times-to-peak show no discontinuity. Although grouping is convenient, Burke has emphasized the caution necessary because of overlap. This is particularly important in modified muscles (Sec. IV.J) in which boundaries might move.

Fibers of motor units can be tagged by glycogen depletion, and then histochemically examined in serial sections. This technique shows that S motor units are composed of type I fibers which, in addition to the slow myosin, have a high mitochondrial content with correspondingly strong succinic dehydrogenase

(SDH) and other oxidative enzyme reactions (originally called B fibers on the basis of SDH reactions by Stein and Padykula [66]). The FR motor units are composed of type IIA fibers which have fast myosin with high levels of glycogen and phosphorylase but also high oxidative enzyme levels [C-fibers, distinguished from B by Stein and Padykula (66) on the basis of the distribution of SDH within the fiber cross section]. The FF motor units have type IIB fibers with a fast myosin (which can be distinguished from that of IIA fibers by preincubation at pH 4.6–4.3) and low levels of oxidative enzymes [A fibers; Stein and Padykula (66)], but they have large levels of glycogen and phosphorylase. The F(int) motor units resemble FF fibers, but they have moderate levels of oxidative enzymes (possibly fiber II in Figure 10B), which correlate well over the range of motor unit types with fatigue resistant units. Correspondingly, duration of twitch contraction is related to ATPase activity, although there are no gross differences between the twitches of FF and FR units to match the different histochemistry.

G. Homogeneity of Motor Units

Histochemists have described more complex subdivisions of motor unit fibers, for example, a type IIC fiber is generally recognized and type I fibers have been subdivided. These divisions are based on different pH values of preincubation at which ATPase reaction is inhibited, but no quantitative evidence has been presented that these are discrete groups rather than artificial divisions of a continuum. Kugelberg (67) presents the intermediate forms as transitions from one to another of the definitive types; transition being associated with some inhomogeneity within the motor units. Other cases have been reported of inhomogeneity with a small admixture of different types within a motor unit (24), but if a motor unit contained fibers, some of which could not be depleted of glycogen, gross inhomogeneities could exist without detection.

Small mechanical differences have been described by Emonet-Dénand et al. (12), who studied axons which sent branches to two adjacent lumbrical muscles—the two half units did not always have identical twitch contraction times. Ridge (68) demonstrated that the twitches of component single fibers of a motor unit (elicited by intracellular stimulation) were not always identical or even similar. This study was done in a snake muscle which was structurally suitable for such a study and which has a range of motor units similar to that in the mammal.

Similar quantitative comparisons of the histochemistry of fibers within a motor unit is not often possible because measurements of reaction intensity are not normally made. Measurements have been made for fibers of the whole muscle (56,69), and although the subjective classification into types has been justified for any one enzyme system, it seems that the hard and fast correlation of different enzyme systems implicit in the I, IIA, and IIB (or A, C. B) classification is not justified. Both Spurway (69) and Edjtehadi and Lewis (56) believe that ATPase activity and SDH level may be determined independently for any fiber; the implications for motor units have not yet been considered. There is one notable example of quantification of motor unit biochemistry. Nemeth et al. measured the lactic dehydrogenase activity of dissected single fibers of a motor unit using glycogen depletion and a microbiochemical technique. They found very close uniformity between fibers of a motor unit, despite large differences between motor units. As mentioned previously, this technique assumes that all fibers are depleted of glycogen, that is, it starts with an assumption of reasonable homogeneity as regards glycogen stores and utilization.

H. Other Motor Unit Properties

Fiber areas have also been measured for motor units. Within cat fast muscles fiber areas are directly related to fatigue resistance, with those of the most resistant (S motor units) being smallest. This correlation is not consistent—the areas of fibers in cat soleus are moderately large despite its being composed of slow motor units. Also, in species in which soleus muscles are mixed the type II fibers are slightly smaller than type I.

Conduction velocities of fibers of a motor unit vary between 1 and 6 m/sec (36), the slowest being in the slow motor units. This might be expected from differences in fiber diameter, but soleus muscle fibers also have slow conduction velocities (71).

The genesis of tetanus has been studied in motor units, and as might be expected, the fusion frequency is a function of twitch duration—the fastest motor units requiring the highest stimulation rate. The frequency necessary to generate half maximal tension is almost linearly proportional to the reciprocal of twitch contraction time. The rate of tension development in a tetanus is also frequency dependent, and fast motor units develop tetanic tension at the highest rate (although they require higher rates of stimulation to achieve maximal effects).

Irregular stimulation has also been studied, and a short or long stimulus interval interposed in an otherwise regular, unfused tetanus produces a potentiation or depression respectively of the tension. The modification lasts for several hundred milliseconds after the immediate effect on the fusion of the contractions (72). This phenomenon may be important in the control of muscle tension, as many contractions are initiated by a pair of impulses at an interval much shorter than the rest of the train, potentiating the initial tension of the muscle when most force is needed to accelerate limbs or to shorten delays. This effect is seen in all types of motor units.

Variation of the twitch:tetanus ratio with twitch contraction time has been described (Fig. 12), and the correlation is different for fast and slow motor units.

Many authors have failed to elicit this correlation, which may depend upon very precisely controlled recording conditions or may reflect a particular state of the animal. It may be possible to explain the correlation of twitch:tetanus ratio and twitch contraction time of motor units in terms of systematic differences in the intracellular calcium transient during the twitch without changes in contractile proteins (as seen between eye and limb fast muscles, discussed previously). The degree of posttetanic potentiation or depression is also a function of twitch duration as discussed earlier (Fig. 12).

Motor units differ in their sensitivity to drugs. Epinephrine (adrenaline) potentiates fast units and depresses slow; the sensitivity of the latter to the drug is higher. Slow motor units are also more sensitive to neuromuscular blocking agents of the competitive type (such as curare), whereas the fast motor units are more readily blocked by depolarizing agents (decamethonium).

The tension developed by motor units depends upon the total area of contractile material (the thick and thin filaments of the 1-μm diameter myofibrils) in parallel. The total area of myofibrils is a function of the number of fibers in the unit, of their mean cross-sectional area, and the number of myofibrils per fiber (much space within the fiber is taken up by other structures, such as sarcoplasmic reticulum, mitochondria, and nuclei; see Fig. 14). In many species there is little difference between the force development of motor units (rat: 57; mouse: 16). In fast muscles of some species there is wide variation; there is controversy about the reason. The slow motor units of cat gastrocnemius develop less force than the fast ones (cf. Fig. 13). Burke and Tsairis (30) considered that the small force was due in part to the small areas of fibers and in part to a very low specific tension of the fibers (0.06 N/mm^2). Specific tension is the tension per unit area and depends upon myofibrillar density (and degree of activation, although it is unlikely that myofibrils are not fully activated in a tetanus). They concluded that the innervation ratio was only slightly smaller for the slow motor units. Edjtehadi and Lewis (56) in cat flexor digitorum longus agreed on the smaller area of slow fibers, but thought that the specific tension was about 0.3 N/mm^2. Therefore, the largest factor in the low tension of slow motor units was a very small innervation ratio. There may be differences between the muscles used by the two groups, or the differences may be due to classification discrepancies, since Edjtehadi and Lewis (56) used only twitch contraction time and tetanic tension to distinguish between fast and slow motor units, criteria which might lead to different boundaries. Another possibility is that Burke and Tsairis' (30) technique of isolation of motor units (microelectrode penetration of motoneurons) may be biased against small motor units and may underestimate their number. This would lead to overestimation of innervation ratio and to low values for specific tension. Certainly, electron microscopists have not reported very low myofibrillar densities which should accompany a low specific tension. In addition, slow motor units with a very small number of fibers were

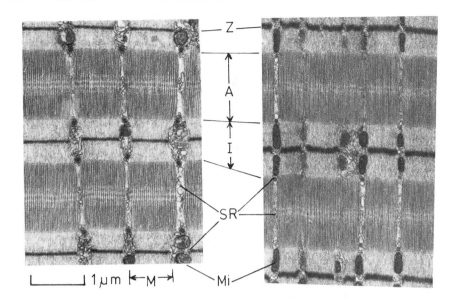

Figure 14 Electron micrographs of longitudinal sections of fast- (Left) and slow-twitch fibers (Right) of mouse muscles. A, I, and Z bands and myofilaments (M) are indicated; Mi, mitochondria; SR, sarcoplasmic reticulum. (Courtesy of L. W. Duchen, The National Hospital, London.)

found by Burke and Tsairis, but they were dismissed because of the possibility that other fibers within these units may not have been depleted of glycogen. Experiments need to be designed to examine this problem directly.

I. Development of Motor Units

Several processes occur in muscles after birth which affect motor unit properties. One has already been referred to, that is, polyneuronal innervation. The presence of multiple endings on a fiber was demonstrated by Redfern (73), who recorded intracellularly from young rat diaphragm muscle. He found that increasing the strength of a stimulus to the motor nerve caused several discrete increments of the end-plate potential (Fig. 15), showing the presence of multiple innervation of end-plates. These could have been branches of single axons, but later Bagust et al. (44) found that if they stimulated two ventral root subdivisions, either separately or together (Fig. 15), there was evidence of overlap. That is, the sum of the two individual tensions was greater than the whole muscle response, indicating that some fibers were innervated by axons in each ventral root

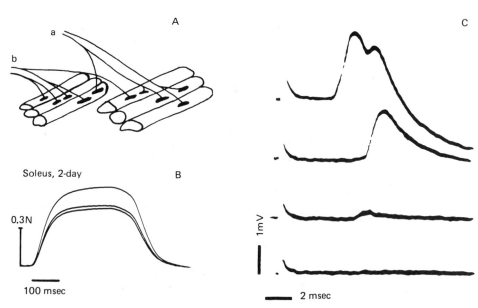

Figure 15 A: diagram illustrating polyneuronal innervation of neonatal muscle fibers from two ventral roots. B: Isometric tetanic myograms of two-day kitten soleus muscle. The smaller pair of myograms were elicited by stimulation of each of the ventral roots (a, b) individually, the largest myogram by stimulation of both together. C: Intracellular records from the end-plate region of a mouse fiber of 12-day rat diaphragm while applying stimuli to the phrenic nerve at increasing strengths. (From Refs. 44 and 73.)

filament (Fig. 15). The amount of overlap was higher in slow muscle than fast, and was found to be greater still in rats, which are very immature at birth (74). In the rat, polyneuronal innervation seems to be at one end-plate region (75,76). This has also been claimed for the kitten (77), but Westerman et al. (78) found fibers with two end-plates several millimeters apart, and the evidence of the interaction of two stimuli on muscle contractions also indicates separate end-plates (44).

The loss of polyneuronal innervation which occurs over two to six weeks is not accompanied by motoneuron death as in amphibia and birds; indeed, axon growth is incomplete at birth, and nerve fiber counts may increase by a quarter in this period (79). Loss of terminal branches is the important process, and there is evidence that the rate of loss of extra synapses slows during inactivity (80) and is accelerated by artificial stimulation (81). There is an increase in the number of fibers in rat muscles over the first week or two (82).

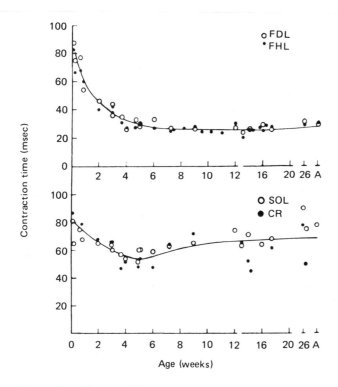

Figure 16 Changes of twitch time-to-peak with age in kitten slow (soleus and crureus, below) and fast (flexor digitorum longus and flexor hallucis longus, above) muscles. (From Ref. 83.)

The second type of change influencing motor units after birth is seen as the modification of twitch contraction (83) and isotonic shortening velocity (84), since at birth all types of muscle are slow. Over six to eight weeks (depending upon species) the speed of fast muscle increases to its adult value. Over the same period slow muscles initially become a little faster and then slow to their adult state (Fig. 16). There are accompanying changes in histochemistry, the secondary slowing of slow muscle being accompanied by a conversion of type II to type I fibers. The picture is complicated by the presence of a fetal myosin which has specific biochemical characteristics and which has much in common biochemically with fast muscle myosin, although it results in a slow contraction.

The result of changes in polyneuronal innervation is a reduction in the average size and range of motor unit tensions (expressed as a percentage of total muscle tension to normalize for muscle growth). However, the characteristic shapes of the tension distributions seem to be maintained through all stages (Fig. 17, left). These changes are related to motoneuron properties as tension is related to axonal conduction velocity at all ages studied (Fig. 17, right). Similar statements may be made about the twitch speed of motor units at different ages (Fig. 18). It should be noted that both fast and slow motor units in cat fast muscle become faster during postnatal development; in contrast, slow muscle motor units become progressively slower (measurements were made after the initial dip in the soleus development curve). It may also be said that the range of motor unit times increases greatly, especially in the soleus in late development.

Kugelberg (67) showed that transformation of motor units could occur very late, well into adult life in the rat. There was a transformation of fast to slow motor units, accompanied by fiber type transformation (discussed in Sec. IV.G), and transitional states were observed. Gutmann and Hanzlíková (85) have suggested that in senile rats motor units become slower and smaller owing to loss of nerve terminals and more easily fatigued with loss of oxidative enzymes, but there is no direct motor unit evidence for these changes.

Prenatally, motor units have not been observed, although interesting deductions can be made from immunohistochemical studies of whole muscles. Muscle fibers are formed from the fusion of myotubes, which are single cells. A group of larger primary myotubes is present at the time of initial innervation, which are immunohistochemically shown to contain the slow type of myosin (86,87). Later, secondary myotubes form around the primary ones and these contain fast-type myosin. This organization must be remodeled to reach the postnatal checkerboard pattern of muscle fiber types (Fig. 4). Polyneuronal innervation provides a mechanism for this remodeling. Soon after birth many fibers contain both types of myosin (55), indicating transition from one fiber type to another.

J. Plasticity of Adult Motor Units

Buller et al. (88) showed that reinnervation of a fast-twitch muscle by the nerve which had innervated a slow-twitch muscle resulted in a conversion of the fast muscle to slow. The reverse is also true, although Buller et al. found this conversion to be complete. Subsequent experiments have shown that cross-reinnervation produced changes in structural, biochemical, and physiologic aspects of the muscle. In 1969, artificially stimulated fast muscle at a rate of 10 pulses per second (which was supposed to mimic discharge patterns of slow motoneurons) and produced a transformation at least as complete as cross-reinnervation (89). Later Lømo et al. (90) stimulated denervated slow muscle with bursts of pulses at 100 Hz for two thirds of a second, about once per 100 seconds (to mimic assumed discharge patterns of fast motoneurons) and again observed transformation. Although the second series of experiments have not been extended to many aspects of muscle properties, it is clear that activity of the

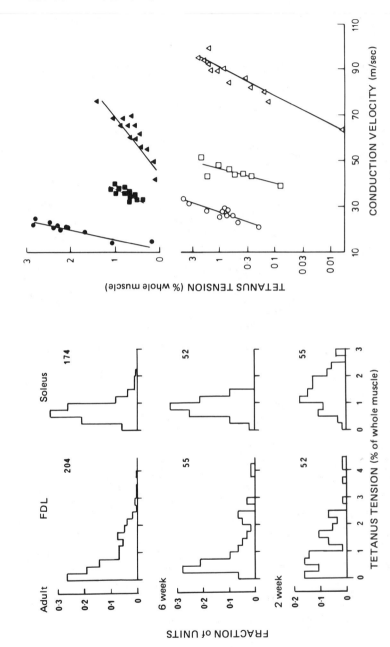

Figure 17 Left: Distribution of motor unit tensions at three different ages from cat soleus and flexor digitorum longus (numbers of motor units shown to right of each histogram). Right: Relationships between twitch tension and axonal conduction velocity of motor units from individual animals: slow muscles, filled symbols; fast muscles, open symbols; circles, two weeks; squares, six weeks; triangles, adult. (From Refs. 14, 13, 61, and Finol, H. J., Lewis, D. M., and Webb, S. N., unpublished data.)

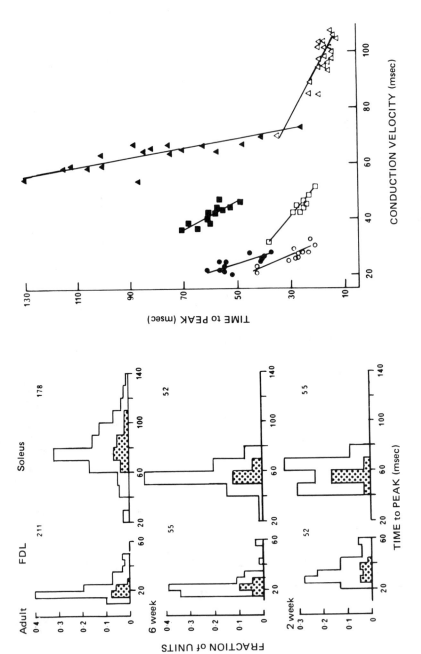

Figure 18 Similar to Figure 17 but illustrating twitch times-to-peak rather than tetanic tension of the motor units. Different individuals used to illustrate regressions. Shaded histograms are of whole muscle contractions (on a smaller ordinate).

muscle plays a major, direct part in the determination of muscle biochemistry and physiology. The relationship between twitch contraction time and axonal conduction velocity indicates that motoneuronal influence on muscle operates at the motor unit level. The uncertainty about the low tension of slow motor units in fast muscle are important here: If the low tension is due to low specific tension of fibers, then this is another example of motoneuronal influence on muscle; if low tension is a consequence of low innervation ratios, then the control factor would operate on perinatal innervation rather than continuously modulating muscle properties.

Reinnervation after nerve transection produces abnormal motor units in which the component fibers tend to be packed together in a limited region (Fig. 4). The first motor units to be examined after reinnervation were in cat lumbricals. Bessou et al. (91) found that normal nerve and muscle interrelations were restored but with greater scatter than normal. Bagust and Lewis (92) in larger limb muscles found much more disruption of motor unit patterns after reinnervation, with possible reversal in some cases. One obvious difference was the presence of motor units that developed much higher tensions and others with very low tensions. More recently, in conscious cats, Gordon and Stein (35) using implanted transducers and electrodes have been able to follow the time course of changes in motor units (nerve and muscle elements) during and after reinnervation. Gordon and Stein claim normal motor-unit properties are restored, but the method may not be able to detect very small motor units. There is also a problem of definition. Bagust and Lewis (92) in fact agree with Gordon and Stein (35) in that the tensions (in N) of the largest motor units in reinnervated muscle are similar to those occurring normally. This, however, does not take into account animal and motor unit growth, and normalized tensions [motor unit tension divided by whole muscle tension (Fig. 17)] in the two groups are different. It is important to consider these details if correct conclusions are to be drawn; whether absolute or normalized tension is important depends upon the nature of the question being asked.

Cross-reinnervation of fast muscle seems to produce the changes in motor units expected from whole muscle responses, but the opposite cross has raised a number of problems. Cross-reinnervated (slow) soleus is only partially converted, and histochemical studies have suggested that most of the fibers remain type I (93). Motor unit contractions after up to six months of cross-reinnervation showed a range of times-to-peak similar to that in normal fast muscle, but there was no correlation with tension, so that the overall muscle response is slower than that of fast muscle (94,95). In an examination of motor units in soleus muscles cross-reinnervated for more than three years, Lewis et al. (96) have clarified the problem. At this time, there appear to be two groups of motor units, one having twitches as fast as in normal fast muscle and the other as slow as in the original soleus. In contrast to normal fast or slow muscle, however, the slow motor units developed more than 10 times the tension of the fast ones (Fig. 19). This fits with histochemical observations, if it is assumed that the twitch

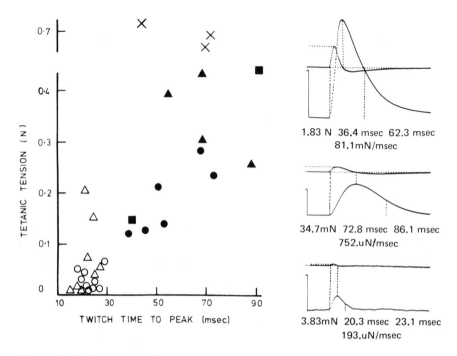

Figure 19 Left: Relationship between tetanic tension and twitch times-to-peak for motor units of soleus muscle cross-reinnervated by the nerve to flexor hallucis longus three years previously (triangles and circles) or soleus nerve (crosses). Right: Myograms of whole muscle response (above) and two motor units (below). Numbers are peak tension, times-to-peak, and half relaxation and maximum rate of rise of tension. (From Ref. 96.)

characteristics of motor units are more labile than fiber typing, and the latter stabilizes earlier.

This interpretation introduces a further problem of explaining why slow axons can capture a much larger share of fibers in adult reinnervation than they do in postnatal development. It should be recalled that prenatal innervation occurs first to slow fibers, and it is only later that the fast motor units expand and establish the normal adult pattern; this second stage seems to be missing in adult reinnervation.

Reinnervation has effects on the motoneuron. Nerve transection modifies the properties of the soma, with reversal occurring as soon as the regenerating axons make anatomic contact with the muscle (97). The axonal conduction velocity falls even above the site of the lesion and recovery is slow, probably never complete. Cross-reinnervation may modify this recovery process and soleus axons reinnervating a fast muscle have a higher mean conduction velocity than ones reinnervating their own muscle (98). When reinnervation first occurs polyneuronal innervation is present, although to a lesser extent than in the neonate (99). The polyneuronal innervation fades over six months, and minor remodeling may occur later by loss of axonal branches that supply large motor units as the maximum motor unit tension falls after three years of self-reinnervation in soleus (100). Preterminal and terminal sprouting occurs in the remaining axons if a muscle is partially denervated, so that motor units expand to take over all the fibers, provided that at least one third of the axons are retained (101). Shrinkage of these enlarged motor units' territories occurs if regeneration of the other axons is allowed, but not back to normal.

Although cross-reinnervation and chronic stimulation brings about large changes in motor units organization, other more physiologic procedures have only limited effects. If a muscle is overused (denervation of synergists) or underused (by immobilization or tenotomy) there seems to be uniform hypertrophy or atrophy of motor units, respectively (102,103). Similarly, when slow muscle twitches are made faster by tenotomy of rabbit soleus (103) or by spinal transection soon after birth in cats (104) the changes seem to be uniform in all units. From histochemical and whole muscle studies it would be expected that physiologic levels of exercise would only produce changes in fatigue properties of motor units (interconversion of FF and FR types), but none in the speed of contraction.

Recently, very large and interesting effects have been explored in responses to altered hormone levels. Thyroidectomy slowed rat soleus motor unit twitch contraction time and transformed fast fatigue-resistant into slow motor units (105). Administration of thyroid hormone, conversely, produced shortening of fast and slow motor units in rat soleus. This change was partly a transformation of type I to type IIA fibers, but it was partly a shift of the twitch time course within each group (106). Experimental diabetes produces changes which are selective between fast and slow motor units (105).

V. USE OF MOTOR UNITS

The central nervous system increases the tension or shortening of a muscle by an increase in the firing rate of individual motor units and by the recruitment of new units (107). The activity of motor units is largely asynchronous, so that the contraction is smooth. Recent work has investigated how the variety of motor units is made use of in the regulation of muscle response. Clues about this came from the work of Gordon and Holbourne (33), who showed that the motor units of deep layers of cat tibialis anterior muscle, which were slow contracting, had low thresholds compared with superficial ones. The idea grew that there were tonic and phasic motor units (108). The tonic units were active for longer periods and, partly as a consequence of a longer after-hyperpolarization of their motoneurons (109), discharged at lower frequencies. The tonic motoneurons are those with slow-conducting axons (110), and so correspond to slow-contracting motor units. The tonic motoneurons had higher input resistances (later correlated with smaller soma size and dentritic tree [6]) which made them more sensitive to currents applied through an intracellular electrode or to normal synaptic input. These ideas were gathered together by Henneman et al. (111) and backed by experiments on triceps surae motor units of decerebrate cats. They studied pairs of motor units in ventral root filaments and found that the smaller units (the ones with the smaller action potentials) were recruited earlier when the muscle tension was reflexly increased by progressive stretch. The "size principle" was proposed whereby excitability and recruitment order were inversely determined by motoneuron size—the slow motor units are recruited earliest in reflexes. This recruitment order has an advantage in the coordination of activity, in that the quantal steps in the smallest contractions would also be small because of the low tensions of the slow motor units, and accuracy of control would be kept approximately constant over a full range of tension. These observations were extended by studies in man, where it is possible to use voluntary contractions rather than reflexes elicited under artificial conditions. Tanji and Kato (112) and Milner-Brown et al. (113) examined electromyograms during progressively increasing tension. Milner-Brown et al. (114) also examined motor unit "twitches" (see Sec. IV.E) revealed by spike-triggered averaging from the electromyogram. As seen in Figure 20, they found that the twitch tension of a motor unit was directly proportional to the total muscle tension at which the unit was recruited over a wide range of forces up to about a quarter of maximum effort (single units could not be distinguished at higher forces). The low threshold motor units had slow twitches. Milner-Brown et al. (114) also calculated that recruitment was more important in increasing muscle tension at lower forces, whereas increasing frequency of discharge of motor units was dominant near maximum force. Desmedt and Godaux (115) extended the observations to ballistic (twitchlike) voluntary contractions and found that, although the tension threshold of a motor unit was lower in a ballistic movement than during a progressive slow increase in force, the order of recruitment was preserved.

Thus, the size principle holds over a wide range of contractions, but not for all contractions. It has been shown that cutaneous stimulation can upset the recruitment order described previously, so that large, fast motor units may be brought in first. This is true in decerebrate cats (116,117) and in man (118). The stimuli necessary to reverse recruitment order in man were not painful but were "like the finger being gripped firmly by a pair of pliers." These cannot be considered physiologic conditions, but the experiments certainly show that synaptic organization can be as important as the size of the motoneuron. Presumably, the

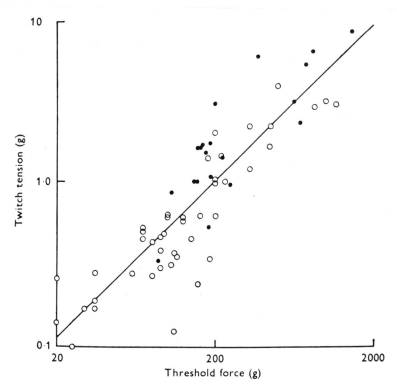

Figure 20 Recruitment of motor units in man. Twitch tension is plotted against muscle force at which it was recruited during a progressively increasing voluntary contraction. (From Ref. 114.)

mechanism operating depends upon the type of activity. A possible picture is that motoneuron size is important in regulating output in stereotyped, planned movements, but with unexpected, particularly cutaneous stimuli large motor units would be recruited by strong synaptic activation. Such a scheme would make best use of motor units of different properties. A voluntary contraction would use small slow motor units for small contractions, only recruiting larger, easily fatigued ones when greater force is needed. In an emergency, large fast motor units would be preferentially recruited for rapid strong but, possibly, less well coordinated responses. The mechanisms of control require further work, and the two described mechanisms are not likely to be the only ones. It is clear, however, that whatever the mechanisms finally described, the relationships between mononeuron and muscle components which are established during postnatal development and modulated during adult life are made use of in optimizing muscle responses.

REFERENCES

1.   Liddell, E. G. T., and Sherrington, C. S. (1925). Recruitment and some other factors of reflex inhibition. *Proc. Roy. Soc. (Lond.) (Biol.) 97*: 488–518.

2.   Sherrington, C. S. (1925). Remarks on some aspects of reflex inhibition. *Proc. Roy. Soc. (Lond.) (Biol.) 97*:519–545.

3.   Mines, G. R. (1913). On the summation of contractions. *J. Physiol. (Lond.) 46*:1–27.

4.   Hess, A., and Pilar, G. (1963). Slow fibres in the extra-ocular muscles of the cat. *J. Physiol. (Lond.) 169*:780–798.

5.   Erulkar, S. D., Shelanskl, M. L., Whitsel, B. L., and Ogle, P. (1969). Studies of muscle fibers of the tensor tympani of the cat. *Anat. Rec. 149*: 279–298.

6.   Burke, R. E., Strick, P. L., Kanda, K., Kim, C. C., and Walmsley, B. (1977). Anatomy of medial gastrocnemius and soleus motor nuclei in cat spinal cord. *J. Neurophysiol. 40*:667–680.

7.   Sharrard, W. J. W. (1955). The distribution of the permanent paralysis in the lower limb in poliomyelitis. *J. Bone Joint Surg. 37B*:540–558.

8.   McPhedran, A. M., Wuerker, R. B., and Henneman, E. (1965). Properties of motor units in a homogeneous red muscle (soleus) of the cat. *J. Neurophysiol. 28*:71–84.

9.   Wuerker, R. B., McPhedran, A. M., and Henneman, E. (1965). Properties of motor units in a heterogeneous pale muscle (m gastrocnemius) of the cat. *J. Neurophysiol. 28*:85–99.

10. Eccles, J. C., and Sherrington, O. M. (1930). Numbers and contraction values of individual motor-units examined in some muscles of the limb. *Proc. Roy. Soc. (Lond.) (Biol.) 106*:326–357.

11. Feinstein, B., Lindegård, B., Nyman, E., and Wohlfart, G. (1955). Morphologic studies of motor units in normal human muscles. *Acta Anat. 23*: 127–142.

12. Emonet-Dénand, F., Laporte, Y., and Proske, U. (1971). Contraction of muscle fibres in two adjacent muscles innervated by branches of the same axon. *J. Neurophysiol. 34*:132–138.

13. Bagust, J., Knott, S., Lewis, D. M., Luck, J. C., and Westerman, R. A. (1973). Isometric contractions of motor units in a fast twitch muscle of the cat. *J. Physiol. (Lond.) 231*:87–104.

14. Bagust, J. (1974). Relationships between motor nerve conduction velocities and motor unit contraction characteristics in a slow twitch muscle of the cat. *J. Physiol. (Lond.) 238*:269–278.

15. Lewis, D. M., Luck, J. C., and Knott, S. (1972). A comparison of isometric contractions of the whole muscle with those of motor units in a fast-twitch muscle in the cat. *Exp. Neurol. 37*:68–85.

16. Lewis, D. M., Parry, D. J., and Rowlerson, A. (1982). Isometric contractions of motor units and immunohistochemistry of mouse soleus muscle. *J. Physiol. (Lond.) 325*:393–401.

17. Sica, R. E. P., and McComas, A. J. (1971). Fast and slow twitch units in a human muscle. *J. Neurol. Neurosurg. Psychiatry 34*:113–120.
18. Brown, M. C., and Matthews, P. B. C. (1960). An investigation into the possible existence of polyneuronal innervation of individual skeletal muscle fibres in certain hind-limb muscles of the cat. *J. Physiol. 151*: 436–457.
19. McComas, A. J., Fawcett, P. R. W., Campbell, M. J., and Sica, R. E. P. (1971). Electrophysiological estimation of the numbers of motor units within a human muscle. *J. Neurol. Neurosurg. Psychiatry 34*:121–131.
20. McComas, A. J., Sica, R. E. P., and Campbell, M. J. (1973). Numbers and sizes of human motor units in health and disease. In *New Developments in Electromyography and Clinical Neurophysiology*, vol. 1, J. E. Desmedt (Ed.), Karger, Basel, pp. 55–63.
21. Parry, D. J., Mainwood, G. W., and Chan, T. (1977). The relationship between surface potentials and the number of active motor units. *J. Neurol. Sci. 33*:283–296.
22. Peyronnard, J. M., and Lamarre, Y. (1977). Electrophysiological and anatomical estimation of the number of motor units in the monkey extensor digitorum brevis muscle. *J. Neurol. Neurosurg. Psychiatry 40*:756–764.
23. Stålberg, E., and Thiele, B. (1975). Motor unit fibre density in the extensor digitorum communis muscle. *J. Neurol. Neurosurg. Psychiatry 38*: 874–880.
24. Edström, L., and Kugelberg, E. (1968). Histochemical composition, distribution of fibres and fatiguability of single motor units. Anterior tibial mucle of the rat. *J. Neurol. Neurosurg. Psychiatry 31*:424–433.
25. Krnjević, K., and Miledi, R. (1958). Motor units in the rat diaphragm. *J. Physiol. (Lond.) 140*:427–439.
26. Davies, A. S. (1972). Postnatal changes in the histochemical fibre types of porcine skeletal muscle. *J. Anat. 113*:213–240.
27. Jennekens, F. G., Tomlinson, B. E., and Walton, J. N. (1971). The sizes of the two main histochemical fibre types in five limb muscles in man. An autopsy study. *J. Neurol. Sci. 13*:281–292.
28. Clarke, D. A. (1931). Muscle counts of motor units: A study in innervation ratios. *Am. J. Physiol. (Lond.) 96*:296–304.
29. Björkman, A., and Wöhlfart, G. (1936). Faseranalyse der Nn. uculomotorius, trochlearis und abduceus des Menschem und des N. abducens verchiedener Tiere. *Z. Mikrosk. Anat. Forsch. 39*:631–647.
30. Burke, R. E., and Tsairis, P. (1973). Anatomy and innervation ratios in motor units of cat gastrocnemius. *J. Physiol. (Lond.) 234*:749–765.
31. Thiele, B., and Stålberg, E. (1974). The bimodal jitter: A single fibre electromyographic finding. *J. Neurol. Neurosurg. Psychiatry 37*:403–411.
32. Buchthal, F., Guld, C., and Rosenfalck, P. (1957). Multielectrode study of the territory of a motor unit. *Acta Physiol. Scand. 39*:83–104.
33. Gordon, G., and Holbourn, A. H. S. (1949). The mechanical activity of single motor units in reflex contractions of skeletal muscle. *J. Physiol. (Lond.) 110*:26–35.

34. Stein, R. B., French, A. S., Mannard, A., and Yemm, R. (1972). New methods for analyzing motor unit function in man and animals. *Brain Res.* 40:187–192.

35. Gordon, T., and Stein, R. B. (1982). Time course and extent of recovery in reinnervated motor units of cat triceps surae muscles. *J. Physiol.* 323: 307–324.

36. Knott, S., Lewis, D. M., and Luck, J. C. (1971). Motor unit areas in a cat limb muscles. *J. Exp. Neurol.* 30:475–483.

37. Buchthal, F., and Schmalbruch, H. (1970). Contraction times and fibre types in intact human muscle. *Acta Physiol. Scand.* 79:435–452.

38. Garnett, R. A. F., O'Donovan, M. J., Stephens, J. A., and Taylor, A. (1979). Motor unit organization of human medial gastrocnemius. *J. Physiol. (Lond.)* 287:33–43.

39. Denslow, J. S., and Gutensohn, O. R. (1950). Distribution of muscle fibres in a single motor unit. *Fed. Proc.* 9:31.

39a. Bessou, P., Emonet-Dénand, F., and Laporte, Y. (1963). Relation entre la vitesse de conduction des fibres neurveuses motrices et le temps de contraction de leurs unités motrices. *C. R. Acad. Sci. (Paris) D 256*:5625–5627.

40. Bessou, P., Emonet-Dénand, F., and Laporte, Y. (1965). Motor fibres innervating extrafusal and intrafusal muscle fibres in the cat. *J. Physiol. (Lond.) 180*:649–672.

41. Henneman, E., McPhedran, A. M., and Wuerker, R. B. (1963). Tensions of single motor units in cat muscle. *Fed. Proc.* 22:279.

42. Devanandan, M. S., Eccles, R. M., and Westerman, R. A. (1965). Single motor units of mammalian muscle. *J. Physiol. (Lond.) 178*:359–367.

43. Burke, R. E., Levine, D. N., Zajac, F. E., III, Tsairis, P., and Engel, W. K. (1971). Mammalian motor units: Physiological-histochemical correlation in three types in cat gastrocnemius. *Science 174*:709–712.

44. Bagust, J., Lewis, D. M., and Westerman, R. A. (1973). Polyneuronal innervation of kitten skeletal muscle. *J. Physiol. (Lond.) 229*:241–255.

45. Ranvier, L. (1873). Properties et structures differentes des muscles rouges et des muscles blanc chez les lapins et chez les raies. *C. R. Seances Acad. Sci.* 77:1030–1043.

46. Cooper, S., and Eccles, J. C. (1930). The isometric responses of mammalian muscles. *J. Physiol. (Lond.)* 69:377–385.

47. Close, R., and Luff, A. R. (1974). Dynamic properties of inferior rectus muscle of the rat. *J. Physiol. (Lond.) 236*:259–270.

48. Gordon, G., and Phillips, C. G. (1953). Slow and rapid components in a flexor muscle. *Q. J. Exp. Physiol. 38*:35–45.

49. Appelberg, B., and Emonet-Dénand, F. (1967). Motor units of the first superficial lumbrical muscle of the cat. *J. Neurophysiol.* 30:154–160.

50. Stephens, J. A., and Stuart, D. G. (1975). The motor units of cat medial gastrocnemius: Speed-size relations and their significance for the recruitment order of motor units. *Brain Res.* 91:177–195.

51. Buller, A. J., and Lewis, D. M. (1963). Factors affecting the differentiation of mammalian fast and slow muscle fibres. In *The Effect of Use and Disuse*

on *Neuromuscular Functions*, E. Gutmann and P. Hnik, (Eds.), Czecho-slovak Academy of Science, Prague, pp. 149-159.

52. Boyd, I. A., and Davey, M. R. (1968). *Composition of Peripheral Nerve*, Livingstone, Edinburgh.

53. Proske, U., and Waite, P. M. E. (1976). The relation between tension and axonal conduction velocity for motor units in the medial gastrocnemius muscle of the cat. *Exp. Brain Res. 26*:325-328.

54. Guth, L., and Samaha, F. J. (1969). Qualitative differences between actomy-osin ATPase of slow and fast mammalian muscle. *Exp. Neurol. 25*:138-152.

55. Gauthier, G. F., Lowey, S., and Hobbs, A. W. (1978). Fast and slow myosin in developing muscle fibers. *Nature 274*:25-29.

56. Edjtehadi, G. D., and Lewis, D. M. (1979). Histochemical reactions of fibres in a fast twitch muscle of the cat. *J. Physiol. (Lond.) 287*:439-453.

57. Close, R. (1967). Properties of motor units in fast and slow skeletal muscles of the rat. *J. Physiol. (Lond.) 193*:45-55.

58. Bárány, M. (1967). ATPase activity of myosin correlated with speed of muscle shortening. *J. Gen. Physiol. 50*:197-218.

59. Eccles, R. M., Phillips, C. G., and Chien-Ping, W. U. (1968). Motor inner-vation, motor unit organization and afferent innervation of m. extensor digitorum communis of the baboon's forearm. *J. Physiol. (Lond.) 198*: 179-192.

60. Ridge, R. M. A. P. (1967). The differentiation of conduction velocities of slow twitch and fast twitch muscle motor innervation in kittens and cats. *Q. J. Exp. Physiol. 52*:293-304.

61. Mayer, R. F., Burke, R. E., Toop, J., Walmsley, B., and Hodgson, J. A. (1984). The effect of spinal cord transection on motor units in cat medial gastrocnemius muscles. *Muscle and Nerve 7*:23-31.

62. Olson, C. B., and Swett, C. P. (1971). The effect of prior activity on prop-erties of different types of motor units. *J. Neurophysiol. 34*:1-16.

63. Bagust, J., Lewis, D. M., and Luck, J. G. (1974). Post-tetanic effects of motor units of fast and slow twitch muscle of the cat. *J. Physiol. (Lond.) 237*:115-121.

64. Olson, C., and Swett, C. P. (1966). A functional and histochemical charac-terization of motor units in a heterogeneous muscle (flexor digitorum longus) of the cat. *J. Comp. Neurol. 128*:475-498.

65. Burke, R. E., Levine, D. N., Tsairis, P., and Zajac, F. E., III (1973). Physio-logical types and histochemical profiles in motor units of the cat gastro-cnemius. *J. Physiol. (Lond.) 234*:723-748.

66. Stein, J. M., and Padykula, H. A. (1962). Histochemical classification of individual skeletal muscle fibers of the rat. *Am. J. Anat. 110*:103-124.

67. Kugelberg, E. (1976). Adaptive transformation of rat soleus motor units during growth. *J. Neurol. Sci. 27*:269-289.

68. Ridge, R. M. A. P. (1980). Contraction times of single muscle fibres in motor units and muscles of garter snakes. *J. Physiol. (Lond.) 308*:102P.

69. Spurway, N. C. (1978). Objective typing of mouse ankle-extensor muscle fibres based on histochemical photometry. *J. Physiol. (Lond.) 277*:47-48P.

70. Nemeth, P. M., Pette, D., and Vrbová, G. (1981). Comparison of enzyme activities among single muscle fibres within defined motor units. *J. Physiol. (Lond.) 311*:489–496.

71. Buller, A. J., Lewis, D. M., and Ridge, R. M. A. P. (1965). Some electrical characteristics of fast twitch and slow twitch skeletal muscle fibres in the cat. *J. Physiol. (Lond.) 180*:29–30P.

72. Burke, R. E., Rudomín, P., and Zajac, F. E. (1976). The effect of activation history on tension production by individual muscle units. *Brain Res. 109*:515–529.

73. Redfern, P. A. (1970). Neuromuscular transmission in new-born rats. *J. Physiol. (Lond.) 209*:701–709.

74. Brown, M. C., Jansen, J. K. S., and Van Essen, D. (1976). Polyneuronal innervation of skeletal muscles in new-born rats and its elimination during maturation. *J. Physiol. (Lond.) 261*:387–422.

75. Bennett, M. R., and Pettigrew, A. G. (1974). The formation of synapses in striated muscle during development. *J. Physiol. (Lond.) 241*:515–545.

76. Riley, D. A. (1977). Spontaneous elimination of nerve terminals from the endplates of developing skeletal myofibers. *Brain Res. 134*:279–285.

77. Riley, D. A. (1976). Multiple axon branches innervating single endplates of kitten soleus muscle. *Brain Res. 110*:158–161.

78. Westerman, R. A., Lewis, D. M., Bagust, J., Edjtehadi, G., and Pallot, D. (1974). Communication between nerves and muscles: Postnatal development in kitten hindlimb fast and slow twitch muscle. In *Memory and Transfer of Information*, H. P. Zippel (Ed.), Plenum, New York, pp. 255–291.

79. Nyström, B. (1968). Fibre diameter increase in nerves to 'slow-red' and 'fast-white' cat muscles during postnatal development. *Acta Neurol. Scand. 44*:265–294.

80. Benoit, P., and Changeux, J. P. (1975). Consequences of tenotomy in the evolution of multi-innervation in developing rat soleus muscle. *Brain Res. 99*:354–358.

81. O'Brien, R. A. D., Östberg, A. J. C., and Vrbová, G. (1978). Observations on the elimination of polyneuronal innervation in developing mammalian skeletal muscle. *J. Physiol. (Lond.) 282*:571–582.

82. Betz, W. J., Caldwell, J. H., and Ribchester, R. B. (1979). The size of motor units during post natal development of rat lumbrical muscles. *J. Physiol. (Lond.) 297*:463–478.

83. Buller, A. J., Eccles, J. C., and Eccles, R. M. (1960). Differentiation of fast and slow muscles in the cat hind limb. *J. Physiol. (Lond.) 150*:399–416.

84. Close, R. (1964). Dynamic properties of fast and slow skeletal muscles of the rat during development. *J. Physiol. (Lond.) 173*:74–95.

85. Gutmann, E., and Hanzlíková, V. (1976). Fast and slow motor units in aging. *Gerontology 22*:280–300.

86. Rowlerson, A. (1980). Differentiation of muscle fibres in fetal and young rats studied with a labelled antibody of slow myosin. *J. Physiol. (Lond.) 301*:19P.

87. Rubinstein, N. A., and Kelly, A. M. (1981). Development of muscle fibre specialization in the rat hind limb. *J. Cell Biol. 90*:128–144.

88. Buller, A. J., Eccles, J. C., and Eccles, R. M. (1960). Interaction between motoneurones and muscles in respect of the characteristic speeds of their responses. *J. Physiol. (Lond.) 150*:417–439.

89. Salmons, S., and Vrbová, G. (1969). The influence of activity on some contractile characteristics of mammalian fast and slow muscles. *J. Physiol. (Lond.) 201*:535–549.

90. Lømo, T., Westgaard, R. H., and Dahl, H. A. (1974). Contractile properties of muscle: Control by pattern of muscle activity in the rat. *Proc. Roy. Soc. (Lond.) (Biol.) 187*:99–103.

91. Bessou, P., Laporte, Y., and Pagés, B. (1966). Etude de la relation entre le temps de contraction d'unités motrices et la vitesse de conduction de leurs fibres motrices dans les muscles réinnervés. *C. R. Acad. Sci. (D) 263*:1486–1489.

92. Bagust, J., and Lewis, D. M. (1974). Isometric contractions of motor units in self-reinnervated fast and slow twitch muscles of the cat. *J. Physiol. (Lond.) 237*:91–102.

93. Edgerton, V. R., Goslow, G. E., Rasmussen, S. A., and Spector, S. A. (1980). Is resistance to muscle fatigue controlled by its motor neuron? *Nature 285*:589–590.

94. Bagust, J., Lewis, D. M., and Westerman, R. A. (1981). Motor units in cross-reinnervated fast and slow twitch muscle of the cat. *J. Physiol. (Lond.) 313*:223–235.

95. Burke, R. E., Dum, M. J., O'Donovan, M. J., Toop, J., and Tsairis, P. (1979). Properties of soleus muscle and of individual soleus motor units after cross-innervation by FDL motoneurons. *Neurosci. Abstr. 5*:765.

96. Lewis, D. M., Rowlerson, A., and Webb, S. N. (1982). Motor units and immunohistochemistry of cat soleus muscle after long periods of cross-reinnervation. *J. Physiol. (Lond.) 325*:403–418.

97. Kuno, M., Miyata, Y., and Muños-Martinez, E. J. (1974). Properties of fast and slow alpha motoneurones following motor reinnervation. *J. Physiol. (Lond.) 242*:273–288.

98. Lewis, D. M., Bagust, J., Webb, S. N., Westerman, R. A., and Finol, H. J. (1977). Axon conduction velocity modified by reinnervation of mammalian muscle. *Nature 270*:745–746.

99. Guth, L. (1962). Regeneration of interrupted nerve fibers into partially denervated muscle. *Exp. Neurol. 6*:129–141.

100. Lewis, D. M., and Owens, R. (1979). Motor units in mammalian skeletal muscle after long periods of reinnervation. *J. Physiol. (Lond.) 296*:111P.

101. Brown, M. C., and Ironton, R. (1978). Sprouting and regression of neuromuscular synapses in partially denervated mammalian muscle. *J. Physiol. (Lond.) 278*:325–348.

102. Walsh, J. V., Burke, R. E., Rymer, W. A., and Tsairis, P. (1978). Effect of compensatory hypertrophy studied in individual motor units in medial gastrocnemius of the cat. *J. Neurophysiol. (Lond.) 41*:496–508.

103. Bagust, J. (1979). The effects of tenotomy upon the contraction characteristics of motor units in rabbit soleus muscle. *J. Physiol. (Lond.) 290*: 1–10.

104. Edgerton, V. R., Smith, L. A., Eldred, T. C., Cope, T. C., and Mendell, L. M. (1980). Muscle and motor unit properties of exercised and non-exercised chronic spinal cats. In *Plasticity of Muscle*, D. Pette (Ed.), Walter de Gruyter, New York, pp. 355–371.

105. Ashton, J. A. (1982). "Effects of Experimental Diabetes on Motor Units of the Rat." Ph.D. dissertation, University of Liverpool.

106. Montgomery, A., and Webb, S. N. (1982). Motor unit characteristics of hyperthyroid rat slow-twitch muscle. *J. Physiol. (Lond.) 325*:29–30P.

107. Adrian, E. D., and Bronk, D. W. (1929). The discharge of impulses in motor nerve fibres. II. The frequency of discharge in reflex and voluntary contraction. *J. Physiol. (Lond.) 67*:119–151.

108. Granit, R., Henatsch, H. D., and Steg, G. (1956). Tonic and phasic ventral horn cells differentiated by post-tetanic potentiation in cat extensors. *Acta Physiol. Scand. 37*:114–126.

109. Eccles, J. C., Eccles, R. M., and Lundberg, A. (1958). The action potentials of the alpha motoneurones supplying fast and slow muscles. *J. Physiol. (Lond.) 142*:275–291.

110. Kuno, M. (1959). Excitability following antidromic activation in spinal motoneurones supplying red muscles. *J. Physiol. (Lond.) 149*:374–393.

111. Henneman, E., Somjen, G., and Carpenter, D. O. (1965). Functional significance of cell size in spinal motoneurones. *J. Neurophysiol. 28*:560–580.

112. Tanji, J., and Kato, M. (1973). Recruitment of motor units in voluntary contraction of finger muscle in man. *Exp. Neurol. 40*:759–770.

113. Milner-Brown, H. S., Stein, R. B., and Yemm, R. (1973). The contractile properties of human motor units during voluntary isometric contractions. *J. Physiol. (Lond.) 228*:285–306.

114. Milner-Brown, H. S., Stein, R. B., and Yemm, R. (1973). The orderly recruitment of human motor units during voluntary isometric contractions. *J. Physiol. 230*:359–370.

115. Desmedt, J. E., and Godaux, E. (1977). Ballistic contractions in man: Characteristic recruitment pattern of single motor units of the tibialis anterior muscle. *J. Physiol. (Lond.) 264*:673–693.

116. Wyman, R. J., Waldron, I., and Wachtel, G. M. (1974). Lack of fixed order of recruitment in cat motoneuron pools. *Exp. Brain Res. 20*:101–114.

117. Kanda, K., Burke, R. E., and Walmsley, B. (1977). Differential control of fast and slow twitch motor units in the decerebrate cat. *Exp. Brain Res. 29*:57–74.

118. Garnett, R., and Stephens, J. A. (1981). Changes in the recruitment threshold of motor units produced by cutaneous stimulation. *J. Physiol. (Lond.) 311*:463–474.

9
EXCITATORY SYNAPSES

George W. Sypert   *University of Florida, College of Medicine, and Veterans Administration Medical Center, Gainesville, Florida*

John B. Munson   *University of Florida, College of Medicine, Gainesville, Florida*

I. INTRODUCTION

This chapter deals largely with excitatory junctional transmission from muscle spindle afferents (group Ia and group II) to spinal motoneurons in the spinal cord of the cat.

Excitatory synapses function as a major communications link between spinal neurons. In this role, excitatory synapses serve primarily to process information coded as nerve impulses. An excitatory synapse accomplishes this function by depolarizing a postsynaptic neuron, producing an excitatory postsynaptic potential (EPSP) which increases the probability of nerve impulse generation by the postsynaptic neuron.

The excitatory synapses in the spinal cord can be grouped into three categories: (1) group Ia-motoneuron synapses, (2) spindle group II-motoneuron synapses, and (3) other synapses. Each of these categories is considered separately, with the major emphasis given to group Ia-motoneuron synapses as these synapses have received the greatest investigative effort and have provided the basis for much of what is known about excitatory junctional transmission in the vertebrate central nervous system. The term "motoneuron," as used in this chapter, refers exclusively to the alpha motoneuron.

II. GROUP Ia–MOTONEURON SYNAPSES

The group Ia afferents project monosynaptically to motoneurons of the same muscle from which they arise (homonymous connections), and also to motoneurons of synergistic muscles which have a similar action at the same joint (heteronymous connections). This direct projection of group Ia fibers to motoneurons forms the monosynaptic reflex loop which is the basis of the stretch reflex.

A. Morphology

Group Ia afferent fibers arise from single muscle spindles, which are among the largest peripheral nerve axons, ranging in diameter from 20 to 12 μm, with conduction velocities between 120 and 72 m/sec (1). Early histologic studies of the intramedullary trajectories and terminations of primary afferent fibers used Golgi's method (2-4) and degeneration methods (5-10). More recent experiments using cobaltous chloride (11) and horseradish peroxidase (HRP) (12,13) to fill primary afferent fibers by application of these substances to the cut ends of transected dorsal rootlets have added further important information regarding the central trajectories of these elements. However, interpretations of these elegant morphologic studies have been complicated by demonstrations that spindle group II afferent fibers project into the motor nuclei (14-16) and make monosynaptic excitatory connections with spinal motoneurons (17-21).

1. Branching and Terminations of Group Ia Afferents

The recently developed techniques of intracellular staining of neurons, including their distal dendritic tree and axons, and of primary afferent fibers, including their terminal arborizations (22-27), opened now possibilities for detailed examinations of physiologically identified neurons and afferent fibers at both the light microscopic and ultrastructural levels. The most detailed anatomic descriptions of the intramedullary trajectories and terminations of group Ia afferents have been accomplished by injecting single identified Ia stem axons in the dorsal funiculus with HRP (22-27). The results of these studies are in essential agreement and will be summarized for medial gastrocnemius (MG) Ia afferents. Medial gastrocnemius Ia afferent fibers branch upon entering the spinal cord and rostral and caudal stem axons ascend and descend in the dorsal funiculus. These stem axons give off about six to eight major collateral branches (range 5-11) over about the 8-12 mm rostral-caudal extent of the homonymous and heteronymous motoneuron pools. The major collateral branch spacing is ~100-3000 μm (mean 1000 μm). The major collateral branches descend directly to lamina IV or V, where they branch medially to innervate neurons of lamina VI and ventrolaterally at about 45 degrees toward the region of the triceps surae motor nucleus. The terminal arborizations of these major collateral branches ramify rostrally and caudally, forming synaptic contacts with neurons in laminae VI, VII, and IX. Terminal branches innervating triceps surae motoneurons spread rostrocaudally up to 1000 μm (mean 400-500 μm) in lamina IX. The minor collateral branches in these terminal arborizations often consist of long very fine axons of 1.0 μm (11). Unfortunately, it is not possible to determine where myelin sheaths end in the fine group Ia terminal arborization using light microscopy to study axons filled with cobalt or HRP. In an ultrastructural study, Conradi (28-30) found that the majority of preterminal axons were myelinated to within 25 μm of the synaptic bouton. This is consistent with the observation that central nervous system axons with diameters of 0.5 μm can be myelinated (31).

The typical group Ia synaptic structures terminating on the motoneuron soma-dendritic membrane consist of single-terminal and *en passant* boutons, or more commonly multiple synaptic contacts (11,22-27). The multiple synaptic contact arrangements may consist of either a series of *en passant* contacts that end as a terminal bouton or a branched terminal axon with small clusters of boutons.

Alpha motoneuron cell bodies (somata) give rise to a single axon via the axon hillock and an extensive dendritic network. From four to 22 primary dendritic trunks arise from the soma. These dendrites may extend well over 100 μm from the soma (27,32-34), repeatedly dividing into daughter branches which are smaller than the parent branches. This tapering may be from ~10-15 μm where the stem dendrite emerges from the soma to < 1 μm diameter distally (27,32). Motoneurons have medium to large cell bodies (30-70 μm, soma diameter) and an extensive surface area. The soma and dendrites constitute the major receptive surface area of the motoneuron. Based on the investigations of Procion dye-filled motoneurons, Barrett and Crill (32,35) have estimated the soma-dendritic surface area to range from 79,000 μm^2 to 250,000 μm^2. The ratio of dendritic to somatic surface area has been estimated to range from 10 to 20 (33,36,37). The distribution of receptive surface area as a function of distance from the soma remains unresolved; some investigators (33,38,39) suggest that the distribution is uniform, while others (32) have found evidence that the receptive area tapers off in an exponential fashion with distance from the soma. The details of dendritic branching, taper, and surface area are important to the development of mathematic models of dendritic function (40). Motoneuron dendrites arborize both cross-sectionally and rostrocaudally, but a rostrocaudal (or longitudinal) orientation predominates. The entire soma-dendritic surface appears to be covered with both presynaptic terminals (boutons) of afferent fibers and glial appendages. There are no regions devoid of synapses (41-42). About 15-20 synaptic boutons per 100 μm^2 have been found on the motoneuron's surface, irrespective of location (29,41,42). Hence, a single alpha motoneuron may receive from 4000 to 12,000 synaptic contacts. Although some order has been described for the terminations of some presynaptic systems on motoneurons (43,44), motoneurons do not appear to receive highly topographic, layered series of synaptic terminations.

Estimates of how many Ia synaptic contacts are made on a given motoneuron by a single Ia afferent fiber have been made recently by direct counts of functionally identified and HRP-labeled single-fiber Ia synapses impinging on a similarly stained and physiologically identified motoneuron (24,25,27). Since these investigations used light microscopy, there is uncertainty regarding the completeness of afferent staining and an inability to demonstrate unequivocally the presence of a true synaptic contact, demonstration of the latter requires ultrastructural methodology. Given this limitation, Brown and Fyffe (27) found 34 contacts in 10 pairs of Ia afferent-motoneuron combinations, with a range of 2 to 5. Since the presence of somatic contacts could not be determined by their technique, they concluded that a single Ia afferent fiber makes between 2 and 6 synaptic contacts with an individual motoneuron. These data are in excellent agreement with the recent studies from Burke's laboratory (24,25). However, Burke et al. (25) have found that a single Ia afferent may make up to 20 synaptic contacts with a single motoneuron.

In studies involving HRP injection of single Ia afferents combined with counter staining of spinal cord sections, Brown and Fyffe (27) demonstrated that up to 5 (mean, 2.05) Ia synaptic boutons were in close apposition to the soma and proximal dendrites out to a distance of 30 μm. Ishizuka et al. (26) used similar techniques and reported a mean of 3.3 somatic and proximal dendritic contacts per motoneurons. These latter investigators were able to examine the proximal dendrites out to a distance of 100 μm. In an earlier study of primary afferent axons filled via dorsal rootlets with cobalt, Iles (11) also found up to 6 synaptic contacts (mean, 1.85) on the motoneuron soma and proximal dendrites.

Even though a motoneuron's dendrites extend long distances rostrocaudally (up to 1600 μm from the soma), Brown and Fyffe (27) reported that in 10 pairs of HRP-filled Ia afferent–motoneuron combinations the vast majority of synaptic contacts are made on the proximal half of the dendritic tree (within 600 μm of the soma). Only 9% of the Ia synaptic contacts appeared to terminate on a motoneuron's soma or proximal dendritic trunk. They observed a strong tendency for synaptic contacts to be clustered at about the same geometric distance from the soma, even when on different dendrites. Although multiple major collaterals from the same stem axon may pass through the dendritic tree of a given motoneuron, only one of the collaterals was observed to make synaptic contact with that motoneuron. These results are largely consistent with previous reports of Burke and his colleages (24,25). These latter investigators, however, clearly demonstrated that some Ia single-fiber synaptic contacts include terminals at widely different geometric and, hence, electrotonic, distances from the soma (Fig. 1).

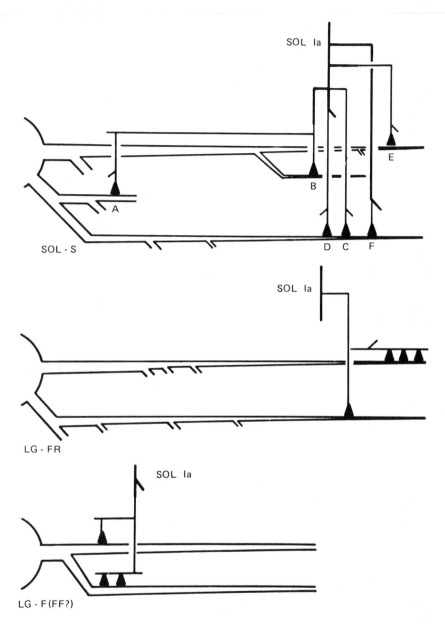

Figure 1 "Wiring diagram" of three reconstructed contact systems between HRP-filled single Ia afferents and HRP-filled alpha motoneurons. (From Ref. 25.)

2. Ultrastructure of Group Ia Synaptic Contacts

There is little ultrastructural data about group Ia synaptic terminations on motoneurons. During the first week after homolateral dorsal root section, Conradi
(30) observed that largely (M-type (monosynaptic) boutons characteristically
disappear. These boutons have large profiles (4–7 μm in length) and contain
spherical synaptic vesicles (30–50 nm in diameter). Large synaptic complexes of
irregular shape, in which the entire postsynaptic membrane is covered by a
20–30 nm thick layer of contrast-rich material and postsynaptic dense bodies,
are formed by these synapses. Small P-type (presynaptic) boutons containing
small, irregularly shaped synaptic vesicles (25–40 nm in diameter) are regularly
apposed to the convex side of the M-boutons. Although it is now known that
spindle group II afferents make monosynaptic connections with alpha motoneurons (16–21,193), the majority of these M-boutons must arise from group Ia
afferents (see Sec. III).

Consistent with both electrophysiologic (40,46,47) and light microscopic
(22–27) data, M-boutons have been found to be very scarce on the motoneuron's
somatic and distal dendritic membrane (28–30). Even on the proximal dendrites
of the motoneuron, Conradi (28) found the density of M-boutons to be only
$1/1000$ μm^2. This is to be compared to a total bouton density of about
$200/1000$ μm^2. McLaughlin (48) also found that type M-boutons were primarily
concentrated on the proximal dendrites. On the soma, Conradi (28) found the
density of M-boutons to be $0.05/1000$ μm^2, whereas McLaughlin (48) failed to
observe any M-boutons. Conradi estimated that type M-boutons make up about
0.5% of the total presynaptic terminations that end on the motoneuron.

B. Physiology

Several types of excitatory postsynaptic potentials in spinal neurons may be
recorded or computed and, hence, require definition. In this chapter, we shall
apply the following definitions.

A *quantal excitatory postsynaptic potential* is generated in a neuron by the
action of one packet, or quantum, of transmitter liberated by an afferent
terminal.

A *single-terminal excitatory postsynaptic potential* is generated by the activation of a single synaptic terminal, or bouton, which arises from the terminations of a single parent excitatory afferent fiber on that neuron. Most afferent
fibers ending on spinal neurons appear to terminate with multiple presynaptic
elements on a given neuron.

A *single-fiber excitatory postsynaptic potential* is the postsynaptic potential
generated by a nerve impulse in a single excitatory afferent fiber which makes
synaptic contact with that neuron. Various terminologies have been used in the
literature to refer to single-fiber excitatory postsynaptic potentials: miniature

(49), individual (50), minimal (51), and unitary (52). Group Ia single-fiber excitatory postsynaptic potentials appear to be composed of smaller excitatory postsynaptic potentials that occur in an all-or-none fashion resembling quantal end-plate potentials observed at the neuromuscular junction (49,53). This smaller minimal excitatory postsynaptic potential is termed a *unit excitatory postsynaptic potential*.

A *composite excitatory postsynaptic potential* is generated by action potentials arriving more or less synchronously in the terminations of two or more presynaptic excitatory afferent fibers which make synaptic contact with a neuron.

A *computed maximal composite excitatory postsynaptic potential* is an estimated amplitude of a maximal composite excitatory postsynaptic potential for a defined afferent system. It is calculated by multiplying the mean single-fiber excitatory postsynaptic potential amplitude by the mean number of afferent fibers connecting with the target neuron.

It is now generally accepted that the stretch reflex is mediated by group Ia afferent fibers which synapse monosynaptically on motoneurons innervating the same (homonymous) and functionally synergistic (heteronymous) muscles. Each group Ia afferent fiber arises from a single muscle spindle (54). Group Ia fibers are the largest sensory fibers in muscle nerves with high conduction velocities (72–120 m/sec) and were shown by Lloyd (55–57) to mediate the stretch reflex.

Using intracellular recording techniques, the synchronous discharge of Ia afferents evoked by electrical stimulation of a given muscle nerve produces a characteristic depolarizing potential with a rapid rising phase and slower decay (an excitatory postsynaptic potential) (58–62) in the motoneurons of homonymous and heteronymous muscles. Such a *composite* excitatory postsynaptic potential evoked in a motoneuron by impulses arriving more or less synchronously in two or more afferent fibers can also be produced by simultaneous activation of muscle spindle primary afferents by sudden muscle stretch (1,63,64). Although much of the early development of information about the group Ia–motoneuron excitatory synapses was based on the study of composite excitatory postsynaptic potentials, recent technical advances have permitted the investigation of excitatory postsynaptic potentials produced in a motoneuron by activity in a single group Ia afferent fiber. Such *single-fiber* Ia excitatory postsynaptic potentials can be recorded in some motoneurons during small amplitude, maintained stretch of muscle spindles (65,66). Using the technique of spike-triggered averaging (STA), dissected dorsal root filaments, and natural stimulation of the muscle spindle by stretch it is possible to accurately and reliably record single-fiber excitatory postsynaptic potentials in most motoneurons to which the single Ia fiber projects (Fig. 2) (50,67). These single-fiber excitatory postsynaptic potentials appear to be, in turn, composed of smaller, all-or-none components (49,68–71) which may be termed *unit excitatory*

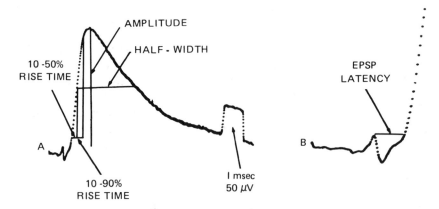

Figure 2 Averaged MG group Ia afferent single-fiber EPSP recorded in a MG motoneuron in normal cat lumbosacral spinal cord. This example illustrates the method of computing the EPSP shape indices: amplitude, latency, rise time (10–50%), rise time (10–90%), and half-width. Slope, 10–50% and 10–90%, is computed from the expression dVm/dt, where Vm represents the potential difference across the membrane (inside potential minus the outside potential) and t time. Normalized amplitude, v, may be expressed as $v = (Vm - E_r)/E_\epsilon - E_r$, where E_r represents resting potential and E the theoretic reversal potential of the EPSP. Normalized latency, rise time, and half-width are defined as t/τ, where τ represents the passive membrane time constant. Normalized slope can be computed from the expression $(dV/dt) = \tau(dV/dt)$. Normalization allows comparison of EPSPs from motoneurons with different passive membrane properties. Note calibration is 50 μV and 1 msec in all cases.

postsynaptic potentials. It is not known whether these unit excitatory postsynaptic potentials are *terminal* or *quantal* excitatory postsynaptic potentials. Hence, there is a hierarchy of Ia excitatory postsynaptic potentials. Electrical stimulation of dissected dorsal root filaments has also been used to evoke single-fiber excitatory postsynaptic potentials (68–72). This latter method as used by some investigators does not, however, rigorously assure that only a "single" afferent fiber is activated.

1. Electrical Potentials Generated by Ia Afferents

The electrical potentials and excitatory postsynaptic potentials generated by single Ia afferent fibers are exceedingly small. The development of the spike-triggered signal averaging technique (67) has made it possible to extract these very low-amplitude signals from electronic and biologic noise, that is, the moment-to-moment fluctuations in net extracellular and intracellular current flow produced by the asynchronous activity of many thousands of synapses

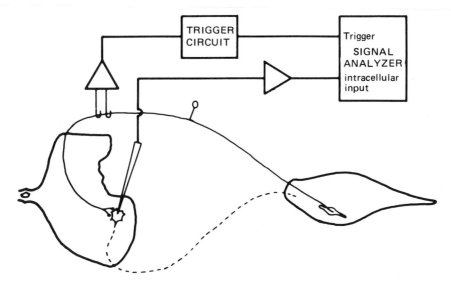

Figure 3 Schematic of the experimental design used in our laboratory for spike-triggered computer averaging of single-fiber potentials.

(67,73–75). This technique is illustrated in Figure 3. It was first used by Mendell and Henneman (50,67), who triggered an averaging computer with impulses from a single Ia fiber in a dorsal root filament. Subsequently, methods were devised to ensure that the Ia afferent was conducting centrally and was not injured by the dissection or recording electrodes (19,121). More recently, Harrison and Taylor (75a) used the spike-triggered averaging technique to elicit Ia single-fiber excitatory postsynaptic potentials in motoneurons by triggering from single Ia afferent fibers recorded in the dorsal columns with an extracellular tungsten microelectrode. Collins and Mendell (75b) have further modified the spike-triggered averaging technique by eliciting excitatory postsynaptic potentials in motoneurons using an intra-axonal microelectrode in a dorsal root filament to electrically stimulate identified Ia afferent fibers. Similarly, Willis and coworkers electrically stimulated individual dorsal root ganglion cells to activate single Ia afferents in isolation (119).

Four types of electrical potentials evoked by single group Ia or group II spindle afferent fibers can be recorded in the spinal cord using the spike-triggered averaging technique (73–75). These potentials are illustrated in Figure 4. The electrophysiologic properties of these potentials are discussed in the following paragraphs.

Single-fiber axonal potentials (APs) are negative or triphasic positive-negative-positive potentials recorded in the extracellular space in the spinal cord

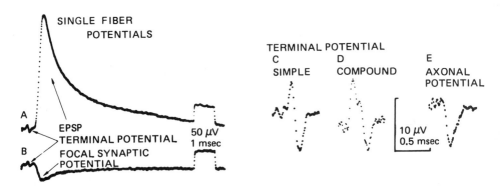

Figure 4 Averaged potentials generated by single MG Ia fibers in cat lumbosacral spinal cord. A: EPSP with TP. B: TP and FSP recorded immediately extracellular to motoneuron in A. C and D: Simple and compound TPs recorded in the MG motor nucleus. E: AP recorded in lamina IV. Calibration shown for C–E. (From Ref. 160.)

gray or white matter outside pools of target cells (Fig. 4E). When recorded with low-impedance (3–5 MΩ) beveled electrolyte-filled micropipette electrodes, single-fiber axonal potentials are of small amplitude (10 μV) and brief duration (300 μsec) and have a very limited spatial extent over which they may be recorded within the dorsal column and dorsal gray matter. Available evidence is consistent with the conclusion that single-fiber axonal potentials are generated by the stem axon in the dorsal funiculus or by single major collateral branches of the Ia afferent, spaced at mean intervals of about 1000 μm (22,26,74). Recording of single-fiber axonal potentials is thus particularly dependent upon the location of the microelectrode tip. When the microelectrode tip is close to an axon *en passant*, a triphasic potential is recorded with the negative potential dominant. The predominant negative polarity is in accord with the earlier theoretic discussion and experimental findings of Renshaw et al. (76), Brooks and Eccles (77), Lorente de No (78), and Katz and Miledi (79). Inward current flow at the active axonal site is responsible for the large negativity. To the extent that the recording site is a current source for the approaching or departing nerve impulse, there will also be positive potentials before and after the predominant negative potential, in proportion to the current density at the microelectrode tip. Our observation that there is an orderly increase in latency of axonal potentials progressing from caudal to rostral in the dorsal funiculus and from dorsomedial to ventrolateral across the spinal cord is consistent with this interpretation (74).

Single-fiber *terminal potentials (TPs)* are recorded in regions of synaptic contact between the Ia afferent and its target cells (e.g., laminae VI, VII, and IX).

The field potentials are readily recorded with the microelectrode tip placed in the extracellular space in the target neuronal pool (Fig. 4B) or inside an alpha motoneuron (Fig. 4A). The amplitude of terminal potentials may be as large as 50 μV, but generally ranges from 5 to 20 μV. No significant difference is found in the amplitude of terminal potentials recorded intra- or just extracellularly. The amplitude of terminal potentials produced by medial gastrocnemius Ia afferents in medial gastrocnemius motoneurons or lateral gastrocnemius–soleus (LG/S) motoneurons also does not differ. Interestingly, the amplitude of medial gastrocnemius Ia single-fiber terminal potentials does differ among physiological characterized medical gastrocnemius motoneurons (80). The mean amplitude of terminal potentials (and excitatory postsynaptic potentials) recorded in motoneurons innervating slow-twitch motor units is larger than those innervating fast-twitch muscles (P < 0.01). This difference may relate to the previous observation that terminal potential amplitude is directly related to the single-fiber excitatory postsynaptic potential amplitude (73,75). However, the amplitude of Ia single-fiber terminal potentials is significantly larger than spindle group II single-fiber terminal potentials even when populations of excitatory postsynaptic potentials matched for amplitude are compared (21). Group Ia terminal potentials have been classified as *simple* Fig. 4C) or *compound* (Fig. 4D). Simple terminal potentials generally consist of a single positive-negative wave (Fig. 4A, B, and C). Compound terminal potentials typically exhibit two positive peaks (Fig. 4D), and appear to be composed of two (or occasionally more) simple terminal potentials, each with a different latency from the trigger point. Rise times of simple terminal potentials are 60–80 μsec; time from positive peak to negative peak is 80–100 μsec; total duration is about 400 μsec. The time course of compound terminal potentials is longer and more variable.

The configuration (simple vs. compound) of the intracellularly recorded single-fiber terminal potential is related to the shape indices of the single-fiber excitatory postsynaptic potential. Terminal potentials with "simple" configurations tend to occur in conjunction with excitatory postsynaptic potentials generated at localized electrotonic distances from the soma (81–85), whereas terminal potentials with "compound" configurations tend to occur in conjunction with excitatory postsynaptic potentials generated at multiple electrotonic distances from the soma (Fig. 5) (74). Rostral-caudal mapping of medial gastrocnemius Ia single-fiber terminal potentials in the triceps surae motoneuron pool demonstrates that the smaller "compound" terminal potentials tend to occur between areas where the larger "simple" terminal potentials are recorded. Presumably, the latter terminal potentials are generated at sites of maximal terminal arborization by the major collaterals.

The relatively large amplitude of Ia single-fiber terminal potentials compared to axonal potentials indicates that there is a large expansion of Ia membrane that is invaded by the impulse. The terminal boutons of the Ia fiber in the

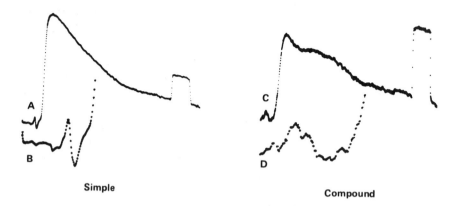

Figure 5 Intracellular recordings of MG Ia single-fiber TPs and EPSPs in two triceps surae motoneurons. A: Example of single TP with typical EPSP having rising and falling phases consistent with a postsynaptic current generated in a single electrotonic compartment. C: Example of a compound TP with an EPSP that demonstrates a break in the rising phase and a late peak in the falling phase. Such a TP and FSP could be generated by synaptic currents in two different soma-dendritic compartments, each arising from a different major collateral branch of the afferent fiber. B and D: Same as A and C, respectively, at 4× gain and sweep speed. (From Ref. 75.)

target motoneuron nucleus represent such an expansion of membrane (11,22–30,48). The large number and relatively large size of the terminal boutons compared to the smaller minor collateral axons, if actively invaded, would result in a greater current density and increase the probability of recording from the vicinity of one or several terminals. In fact, it is difficult to conceive how the fine preterminal minor collateral axons could generate the relatively large and brief "simple" terminal potentials recorded in the target motoneuron pool. In addition, the amplitude of Ia single-fiber terminal potentials is directly correlated with Ia single-fiber excitatory postsynaptic potential amplitude, strongly inversely correlated with normalized rise time, and not correlated with Ia afferent diameter estimated by measurements of conduction velocity (86). The latency from the terminal potential to the onset of the single-fiber excitatory postsynaptic potential also varies predictably (based on estimates of electrotonic distance) with the shape indices of the excitatory postsynaptic potential (73,75). Although any of these various lines of evidence are open to individual interpretation, taken in sum, the evidence is inconsistent with the interpretation that the diphasic terminal potential is a composite field potential made up of action currents in the minor collaterals and/or major collateral branches and/or spread of action currents from other distant terminal arborizations. On the other hand, when recorded intracellularly in conjunction with an excitatory postsynaptic potential, terminal potentials appear to represent electrical activity primarily in the afferent terminals generating the excitatory postsynaptic potential (160).

Single-fiber *focal synaptic potentials (FSPs)* are slow potentials of negative polarity recorded when a microelectrode tip is located within a pool of target neurons of the Ia afferent (i.e., laminae VI, VII, and IX). They tend to occur in conjunction with a terminal potential. They often appear as the attenuated mirror image of a single-fiber excitatory postsynaptic potential recorded in the immediate vicinity, that is, their time course is the same as that of the excitatory postsynaptic potential and not that of the current transient generating the excitatory postsynaptic potential (Fig. 4B). While focal synaptic potentials are usually recorded with the microelectrode tip in the extracellular space, it is occasionally possible to record negative slow potentials from within moto-neurons that do not receive functional connections from the Ia afferent. These potentials are distinguishable from inhibitory postsynaptic potentials (IPSPs) by the observations that they do not reverse polarity with hyperpolarizing current injection or following chloride injection. Presumably, this intracellularly recorded negative slow potential represents an excitatory postsynaptic potential generated by an adjacent motoneuron. Focal synaptic potentials were originally identified as the extracellular concomitants of composite excitatory post-synaptic potentials by Eccles et al. (87) and by Fu et al. (14), who showed their distribution (following muscle nerve electrical stimulation) was limited to spinal cord laminae VI, VII, and IX, that is, the loci of Ia target neurons (7).

a. Electroanatomy of Central Ia Afferents. Based on a recent electro-physiologic analysis of the temporal progression of these group Ia single-fiber potentials through the spinal cord, Munson and Sypert (74) described the central anatomic structure of medial gastrocnemius group Ia afferents in the cat and calculated conduction velocities in dorsal funiculus stem axons, in major collateral branches, and in terminal branches. A composite picture of a single central Ia afferent is illustrated in Figure 6. Upon entering the spinal cord, the Ia afferent fiber bifurcates rostrally and caudally in the dorsal funiculus. The rostrally directed stem axon in the dorsal funiculus conducts action potentials at ~50-60 m/sec as far as the L3 segment, where it slows to about one third that rate through the L1 segment. Major collateral branches (usually nine or fewer) descend into the spinal gray matter at about 1-mm intervals over the ~1-cm rostrocaudal extent of the triceps surae motoneuron pool at spinal cord levels L7 and S1. The conduction velocity in these major collateral branches is in the range of 8-19 m/sec. Three distinct loci of synaptic activation exist: laminae VI, VII, and IX. Terminal branches in the motoneuron pool extend for several hundreds of micrometers laterally, rostrally, and caudally from the major collateral branch. Action potential conduction velocity in these terminal branches is 0.2-1.0 m/sec. These data, derived from the use of the spike-triggered

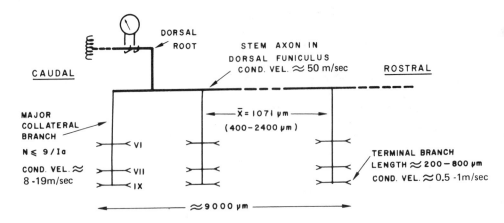

Figure 6 Morphology of single central MG Ia afferent fibers projecting to moto-neurons in cat lumbosacral spinal cord, based on electrophysiologic data. (Details in text.) (From Ref. 74.)

averaging technique, are in excellent agreement with recent anatomic (11,22–27) and previous classic electrophysiologic investigations (15,55,76,86,88).

2. Group Ia-Motoneuron Excitatory Postsynaptic Potentials

Utilizing intracellular recording techniques, Brock et al. (58) found that electrical stimulation of the dorsal roots or peripheral nerves sufficiently intense to activate group Ia afferent fibers evoked monosynaptic group Ia composite excitatory postsynaptic potentials in motoneurons. These Ia composit excitatory postsynaptic potentials were found to be depolarizing potentials having a rapid rise time (~1-2 msec) and a slower approximately exponential decay with a total duration of about 20 msec. The peak amplitude of the composite excitatory postsynaptic potential was shown to be proportional to the intensity of the electrical stimulation until saturation is reached when the stimulus is supramaximal for all Ia afferents that converge on the motoneuron studied. Hence, the amplitude of the Ia composite excitatory postsynaptic potential was directly related to the number of simultaneously activated group Ia fibers terminating on the motoneuron. Depending on the motoneuron and the rate of rise of the Ia composite excitatory postsynaptic potential, a motoneuron action potential was evoked when the excitatory postsynaptic potential depolarization reached a level of somewhere between 6 and 14 mV.

Eccles and his colleagues (89,90) made the first detailed studies of the convergence of group Ia inputs on spinal motoneurons in different motoneuron pools (Table 1). Electrical stimulation of given muscle nerves at a strength

Table 1 Motoneurons Supplying Popliteal Nerve in Cat Nerves Stimulated for Testing Volleys

Moto-neurons	Resting potential[a]	MG[b]	LG[c]	S[d]	P[e]	FDB[f]	FDL[g]	Quad[h]
MG	61 (18)	6.2 (20)	1.05 (15)	1.5 (20)	0.05 (19)	–	0.02 (12)	0 (20)
LG	58 (6)	3.0 (10)	3.0 (10)	1.85 (10)	1.1 (10)	0 (2)	0 (4)	0.05 (6)
S	59 (8)	2.3[h] (9)	1.7[h] (6)	5.6[h] (9)	1.3 (9)	–	0 (6)	0.95 (13)
P	57 (31)		0.4 (22)		5.05 (33)	1.49 (17)	0.5 (26)	– (6)
FDB	51 (7)		0.1 (3)		0.45 (8)	2.4 (9)	0.1 (5)	–
FDL	66 (29)		0.1 (26)		0.3 (29)	0.3 (3)	5.8 (31)	0 (5)

[a]Mean resting membrane potentials and mean voltages of maximum monosynaptic EPSPs (mV) (numbers of motoneurons investigated in parentheses).
[b]Medial gastrocnemius.
[c]Lateral gastrocnemius.
[d]Soleus.
[e]Plantaris.
[f]Flexor digitorum brevis.
[g]Flexor digitorum longus.
[h]Quadriceps.
[i]The large brace signifies that the three nerves were used conjointly.
Source: Data from Ref. 90.

sufficient to simultaneously activate all group Ia fibers was found to generally evoke larger Ia maximal composite excitatory postsynaptic potentials in homonymous motoneurons than in heteronymous motoneurons (66,89,90). Moreover, such Ia maximal composite excitatory postsynaptic potentials were usually of greater amplitude in heteronymous motoneurons supplying close synergists than in motoneurons innervating distant synergists. These investigators also found that the average amplitude of Ia maximal composite excitatory postsynaptic potentials produced by homonymous stimulation was larger in motoneurons innervating slowly contracting ("slow-twitch") muscles (e.g., soleus) than in motoneurons supplying innervating rapidly contracting ("fast-twitch") muscles (.eg., gastrocnemius) (90). Furthermore, a direct correlation was found to exist between the amplitude of either homonymous or heteronymous maximal composite excitatory postsynaptic potentials and the input resistance, R_N, of motoneurons within a single motoneuron pool (66,91,92). These data indicate that there is an inverse correlation between Ia maximal composite excitatory postsynaptic potential and anatomic cell size (Secs. II.B.3, II.C). It is evident that each alpha motoneuron and the skeletal muscle cells it innervates (the "motor unit") can be grouped into one of at least two or three major types based on certain parameters (38,93-97). Available data indicate that small motoneurons, innervating muscles with slow-twitch contraction times, have larger average amplitude Ia maximal composite excitatory postsynaptic potentials and lower thresholds to natural stimulation than do large motoneurons innervating fast-twitch contracting muscle fibers (see 98-100).

Eccles et al. (90) found little difference in the time course of Ia maximal composite excitatory postsynaptic potentials whether of homonymous or heteronymous origin or of large or small amplitude. Based on studies of extracellular field potentials elicited by Ia composite excitatory postsynaptic potentials, Fatt (101) indicated that the Ia composite excitatory postsynaptic potential was predominantly generated in motoneuron dendrites. One early study of the electrical properties of the motoneuron estimated that the specific membrane resistance of the motoneuron's membrane was so low (600 Ω cm^2) as to indicate that most of the current generated at distal dendritic synapses would leak out through the dendrites and never reach the soma. Hence, Eccles (59) suggested that only synapses adjacent to the soma, that is, proximal dendritic synapses, could have a substantial effect on the motoneuron's membrane potential. However, in an important series of investigations of Ia excitatory postsynaptic potentials in cat spinal motoneurons (49,81,102-104) convincing evidence was presented that more distal dendritic synapses could be very effective. This evidence received strong theoretic support from the mathematic predictions of Rall (40,81,104-109). Rall developed a powerful model of the motoneuron, based on the assumption that the motoneuron soma and dendritic tree can be mathematically represented as an electrotonic equivalent cylinder with the soma at one end. The subsequent studies of Barrett and Crill (32,35) and of Lux et al. (39) which allowed comparisons of electrophysiologic measurements with morphologic measurements from the same alpha motoneurons further confirmed the applicability of the equivalent cylinder model to alpha motoneurons. Additional empirical support for this quantitative model has been derived in the recent studies of the effects of impulses in single Ia afferent fibers on individual motoneurons (see subsequent sections). The Rall model of the motoneuron predicts that the greater the distance that a synapse eliciting an excitatory postsynaptic potential is from the soma (the presumed site of microelectrode penetration, since only the soma and proximal dendrites are large enough to maintain a stable microelectrode penetration), the longer the time course (e.g., rise time and half-width) and the greater the decrement in amplitude of the excitatory postsynaptic potential. This is due to passive decay along the dendritic branches toward the soma, since a brief current transient such as that which generates an excitatory postsynaptic potential initially disturbs the voltage only locally and is not distributed with spatial uniformity. This passive spread of potential along the relatively inexcitable dendritic branches is termed electrotonic propagation (110), and is described using concepts and equations originally applied to undersea cables (111). Hence, the dendrites of the motoneuron have been treated as core conductors, and the passive resistive and capacitative properties of the motoneuronal membrane and cytoplasm are termed cable properties.

   a. Electrotonic Properties of Alpha Motoneurons. Only a fraction of the excitatory synaptic current (or charge) injected at a somatic or dendritic location will reach the site of impulse initiation and thereby have an effect on motoneuronal output. The current transient elicited by activation of a Ia synaptic terminal is very brief, such that its efficacy in altering the transmembrane potential is highly dependent upon the *input impedance* of the motoneuron at the synaptic site (57,86,112,113). Moreover, the current leaks out through the intervening motoneuronal soma-dendritic membrane. The motoneuronal cable properties and geometry determine the "effective" fraction of the synaptic current generated at a particular site on the motoneuron's surface. For instance, the lower the cytoplasmic resistivity (R_I), the higher the specific membrane resistance (R_M), and the more proximal the synaptic site, the greater the efficacy of a given synapse. Hence, in order to estimate the relative efficacy of various synapses, it is requisite to measure $(R_I, R_M,$ the specific membrane capacitance (C_M), the effective membrane time constant (τ), the electrotonic length of the equivalent dendritic cylinder (L), the ratio of the steady-state input conductance of the dendritic tree to the steady-state conductance of the soma (dendritic-to-somatic conductance ratio, ρ), and the geometry of the motoneuron. Presently, the cat spinal motoneuron is the only vertebrate neuron which has been extensively investigated both mathematically and experimentally. Accordingly, reasonably accurate estimates of these parameters have been obtained, permitting rigorous testing of theoretic predictions derived from the Rall model (40) of the motoneuron.

   Most investigations of the electrotonic properties of alpha motoneurons have been accomplished by injecting small current steps (relative to threshold) into the soma via intracellular micropipette electrodes. This current initially charges and flows across the membrane isopotential with the anatomic soma (and probably the proximal dendritic trunks). Furthermore, the injected current flows out into the dendritic trees and across the dendritic membrane until a steady-state distribution of transmembrane voltage is established. The voltage transient produced by this injected current can be dissected ("peeled") into components with different time constants, the longest of which is the τ. The measured values of τ in cat alpha motoneurons range from 2 to 12 msec, with a mean value of about 5 msec (35,39,51,74,84,94,112). Since

$$\tau = R \times C$$

estimation of R_M and the experimentally measured τ should permit an estimate of C_M, provided that the specific membrane properties of the motoneuron are uniform over the entire cell surface.

Estimation of R_M for a given motoneuron requires morphologic measurements of the neuron's geometry (membrane area) and electrophysiologic measurement of its input resistance, R_N. The R_N measured with a microelectrode in the soma is calculated by measuring the slope of the relation between the steady-state change in soma-dendritic voltage produced by injection of a subthreshold current step into the soma, and the magnitude of that current. The R_N depends upon the R_M, the area of the cell's surface, and the electronic properties of the dendritic arborizations. Utilizing the Rall model (40) of the motoneuron, these relationships may be expressed as

$$R_N = L/A_N (R_M/\tanh L)$$
or
$$R_N = R_M \frac{1}{[1 (\rho + 1)A_S}$$

where A_N is the total membrane area of the cell and A_S is the area of isopotential membrane (soma and proximal dendrites) (40,105). In cat alpha motoneurons, the experimentally measured values of R_N range from 0.3 MΩ to about 6.0 MΩ, with most values falling between 0.4 and 2.0 MΩ (35,38,39,59,66,80, 112,114,136,137). Assuming uniform passive membrane properties throughout the motoneuron, theoretic treatment of the current distribution in dendrites, and experimental measurements of R_N and cell surface area, estimates of R_M have been calculated. Studies that combine both electrophysiologic and morphologic measurements in the same motoneuron indicate that the values of R_M range between 1200 and 3500 Ω cm^2 (averaging about 2000 Ω cm^2), depending upon whether the terminal dendrites are assumed to be sealed (infinite resistance, closed-end conditions) or leaky (infinite conductance, open-end conditions) (32,35,39). If sealed terminations are assumed, R_M values near the lower end of the range are applicable. Although Lux et al. (39) have suggested that open-end conditions may be caused by tonic synaptic activity in the fine terminal dendrites, detailed analysis of the voltage response to brief intracellular current pulses (84) and to brief, localized, synaptic currents (51,82) indicate that closed-end conditions apply to cat alpha motoneurons under deep anesthesia (105).

Given the experimentally observed range of τ and the calculated range of R_M, the C_M of the alpha motoneuron has been estimated to be between 2 and 3 $\mu F/cm^2$ (35). This C_M value is higher than the value of 1 $\mu F/cm^2$ found in most biologic membranes. Some highly convoluted membranes appear to have high C_M values (115), but ultrastructural studies demonstrate that the motoneuron membrane is not substantially convoluted.

Utilizing equations derived by Rall (108) to calculate λ from the time course of a voltage transient produced by a step of current injected at the soma, Nelson and Lux (112) and Burke and ten Bruggencate (94) estimated that the motoneuron dendrites, in aggregate, are relatively short in electrotonic length, ranging between 1 and 2 length constants (1–2 λ). Studies of group Ia excitatory postsynaptic potentials (51,104) and combined electrophysiologic-morphologic investigations in identified motoneurons (35,39) have confirmed these estimates of λ. Moreover, the value of λ appears to be unrelated to size of alpha motoneurons measured by either input resistance (R_N) or by anatomic study of injected motoneurons (35,39,94,116). These data thus suggest that despite the fewer and smaller dendritic trees of small motoneurons, the dimensions and properties of the dendritic arborizations appear to be scaled in a fashion to preserve a similar electrotonic length among motoneurons with wide ranges in size (38,46,117). Furthermore, the number of stem dendrites appears to be large (5 to 15, generally >10) in both large and small motoneurons (32,35,42, 51,84). Taken in sum, these data strongly suggest that the decrement in amplitude of an excitatory postsynaptic potential generated in a distal dendrite will be minimal. For single-fiber excitatory postsynaptic potentials which produce subthreshold voltage changes the fraction of the injected synaptic charge that reaches the soma from a given dendritic site is independent of the time course of the charge (or current) injection because the motoneuron may be considered to approximate a linear system between resting potential and threshold (32,25, 51,83,105,118). Utilizing cable equations applied to segments of a detailed core conductor model of the motoneuron (105), Barrett and Crill (35,118) demonstrated that most of the current injected at dendritic synapses reaches the soma (Fig. 7). Therefore, current injected into even the most distal dendritic synapses will be at least 20–50% as effective in depolarizing the soma as current injected directly into the soma. Experimental data from studies of Ia single-fiber excitatory postsynaptic potentials are all consistent with this conclusion (51,52,70).

The assumption of uniform electrotonic properties (R_M, C_M) of the membrane of the alpha motoneuron remains unproven. How much of the motoneuron membrane is effectively involved in passive current flows such as that generated by a subthreshold current injection via either a synapse or microelectrode has not been resolved. Although synapses appear to cover greater than 50% of the motoneuron's surface (30), it is not known whether or not the

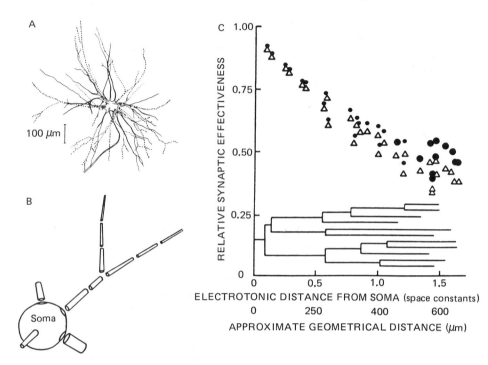

Figure 7 A: Reconstruction of cat lumbar alpha motoneuron with Procion yellow dye. This neuron has 19 primary dendrites and a total membrane surface area of 180,000 μm^2. Dendrites with dashed line project behind the plane of the soma. R_N was 1.5 MΩ. B: Schematic diagram of the soma and a dendritic branch, illustrating how dendrite reconstructed as in A was approximated as a series of interconnected cylinders to facilitate calculation of membrane properties and synaptic efficacy. C: Relative synaptic efficacy as a function of distance from the soma, calculated for a reconstructed dendrite (A and B) in a resting motoneuron (R_M = 2000 Ω cm^2). Filled circles indicate the fraction of injected charge reaching the soma from each site, larger circles represent values calculated for terminal dendritic branches. Open triangles plot the relative effectiveness of quantal excitatory synaptic conductance changes in contributing to the net depolarization of the soma. For a given dendritic site, the difference between the circle and triangle reflects reduced charge injection due to the reduction in synaptic driving potential that occurs during the synaptic conductance change (nonlinear summation). (From Ref. 118.)

motoneuron's subsynaptic membrane participates in passive current flow. More-over, Iansek and Redman (84) have found some evidence for higher membrane resistivity in the dendrites than the soma. With respect to this possibility, they point out that it is difficult to sort out the effect of a lower soma R_M from the effect of microelectrode damage at the soma. The high calculated C_M value further suggests that R_M may not be uniform over the resting alpha motoneuron. In fact, within experimental error, the calculations of Barrett (118) indicate that the transient voltage response to the current step injected into the soma can be fit as well by assuming a very high dendritic R_M (8000 Ω cm^2), a low soma R_M (250 Ω cm^2), and a "standard" C_M (1 μF/cm^2) as by assuming a uniform R_M of 2000 Ω cm^2 and a higher uniform C_M (2.5 μF/cm^2). Hence, it is possible that the resting value of motoneuronal R_M may be considerably higher than 2000 Ω cm^2, and even the soma may have a higher R_M when it has not been injured by microelectrode penetration. A higher distal dendritic R_M should further enhance the efficacy of distal dendritic synapses by reducing the loss of synaptic current across the dendritic membrane during passive propagation to the soma.

  b. Group Ia Single-Fiber Excitatory Postsynaptic Potentials. Group Ia single-fiber excitatory postsynaptic potentials in cat alpha motoneurons were first studied by Kuno (68). This was accomplished by electrical stimulation of a fine filament of a muscle nerve that was dissected until it appeared to contain only a single Ia afferent fiber. In 1966, Burke and Nelson (65) studied rhythmically occurring excitatory postsynaptic potentials recorded in moto-neurons during stretch of the homonymous muscle. These excitatory postsynap-tic potentials were identified as being elicited by activation of a single Ia afferent by the use of such criteria as regular discharge during sustained muscle stretch, increased firing rate with increasing muscle stretch, and silence during muscle contraction. Such excitatory postsynaptic potentials were observed in only about 10% of motoneurons investigated. Ia single-fiber excitatory postsynaptic potentials elicited by intracellular electrical stimulation of Ia somata in a dorsal root ganglion were examined by Willis et al. (119). Jack and Redman and their colleagues (51,52,71,72,82-85,116,120) have used small dorsal root filaments containing one or only a few Ia afferent fibers and electrical stimulation adjusted in order to apparently activate a single Ia afferent. Signal averaging techniques were required to resolve these small excitatory postsynaptic potentials from biologic and electronic noise. A more useful and reliable technique for record-ing Ia single-fiber excitatory postsynaptic potentials is spike-triggered averaging (see Sec. II.B.1).

  Under deep barbiturate anesthesia, Ia single-fiber excitatory postsynaptic potentials recorded in cat alpha motoneurons using the spike-triggered averaging technique are small (5-650 μV) depolarizing transients having a brief time course (rise time: 0.1-3.0 msec; half-width: 0.5-10.0 msec), as illustrated in Figure 2

Table 2 Triceps Surae Homonymous and Heteronymous Medial Gastrocnemius Ia Single-Fiber EPSP Parameters[a]

	Medial gastrocnemius	Lateral gastrocnemius/ soleus	P
Connectivity (%)	85 64–100[c] (293)	60 24–80[c] (163)	<0.001[b]
Amplitude (μV)	91 ± 6 5–464 (206)	73 ± 7 6–331 (78)	<0.1[b]
Rise time 10–50 (msec)	0.23 ± 0.01 0.04–0.71 (201)	0.31 ± 0.02 0.07–1.02 (75)	<0.001[b]
Rise time 10–90 (msec)	0.60 ± 0.03 0.11–2.83 (201)	0.78 ± 0.06 0.11–2.30 (75)	<0.005[b]
Slope 10–50 (dv/dt) (μV/msec)	235 ± 20 4–1808 (201)	155 ± 25 6–1326 (75)	<0.05[b]
Half-width (msec) (msec)	3.96 ± 0.17 0.69–10.00 (182)	4.28 ± 0.34 0.53–9.67 (62)	<0.4[b]

[a]The range is given below the mean values. Numbers in parentheses give the sample size. (In a few cases, accurate EPSP parameters were not available.)
[b]Two-tailed t test.
[c]Based on samples of 10 or more motoneurons.

(19,21,50,67,70,75,75a,75b,80,122). Table 2 is a typical sample of Ia single-fiber excitatory postsynaptic potential data derived from the effect of single Ia afferent fibers on 554 triceps surae motoneurons: 359 homonymous (medial gastrocnemius) motoneurons and 195 heteronymous (lateral gastrocnemius/ soleus) motoneurons.

   c. Connectivity of Ia Single-Fiber Excitatory Postsynaptic Potentials. The spike-triggered avearing technique is especially valuable for the investigation of the percentage of motoneurons in a given motoneuron pool which receives a functional projection from a single identified primary afferent fiber. In the early experiments of Mendell and Henneman (50,67), single medial gastrocnemius Ia afferents were observed to generate single-fiber excitatory postsynaptic potentials in almost all (94%) of the medial gastrocnemius motoneurons examined. They suggested that each of the approximately 60 medial gastrocnemius Ia afferents (123,124) make synaptic connections with each of the 300 homonymous alpha motoneurons (125) innervating this muscle. Kuno and Miyahara (69) found a much lower percentage (44%) of medial gastrocnemius Ia single-fiber excitatory postsynaptic potentials in homonymous motoneurons. They suggested that this difference was caused by their inability to detect very small single-fiber excitatory postsynaptic potentials as they utilized single sweeps instead of averaging techniques. Hence, caution must be exercised in the interpretation of functional connectivity data, since failure to resolve small excitatory postsynaptic potentials may lead to an underestimation of the total afferent projection. However, more recent studies using techniques with the capacity to detect Ia single-fiber excitatory postsynaptic potentials as small as 1-5 μV did not substantially increase the estimate of functional connectivity of single Ia afferents with homonymous motoneurons (19,75; see also 135). Thus, it appears, at least under the experimental conditions of deep general anesthesia and an intact spinal cord (but see 19), that the average functional connectivity of single Ia afferents to homonymous motoneurons ranges from 78% to 85% (19,20,21, 50,67,70,75,75a,121,122; however, see later, and Sec. II.B.2.f). Some Ia afferents, often having slow conduction velocities (<98 m/sec), have been observed to have a relatively low functional connectivity to homonymous motoneurons (65%) (21,74,121,122). These Ia afferents have been arbitrarily termed "type Y" by Scott and Mendell (122). The majority of Ia afferents, which have functional connections with more than 80% of homonymous motoneurons, have been termed "type X" fibers. The functional connectivity of single Ia fibers to both homonymous and heteronymous motoneurons is directly related to the conduction velocity, and, hence, to the size of the afferent fiber (21,100). Interestingly, the mean conduction velocity of the axons of medial gastrocnemius motoneurons receiving connections from fast Ia afferents was found to be significantly higher than the mean conduction velocity of motoneurons receiving connections from slow Ia afferents. Furthermore, Fleshman et al. (80) and Harrison and Taylor (75a) observed that the functional connectivity of Ia afferents was significantly higher in fatigue-resistant (motor unit types S and FR) than in fatigue-sensitive (motor unit type FF) medial gastrocnemius motoneurons.

Group Ia afferent fibers make functional synaptic connections with both homonymous and heteronymous motoneurons (Fig. 8). The functional connectivity is greater, however, with homonymous than with heteronymous motoneurons (19,21,50,67,69,75,75a,122-126). With respect to the early intracellular studies demonstrating that the monosynaptic excitatory input from Ia

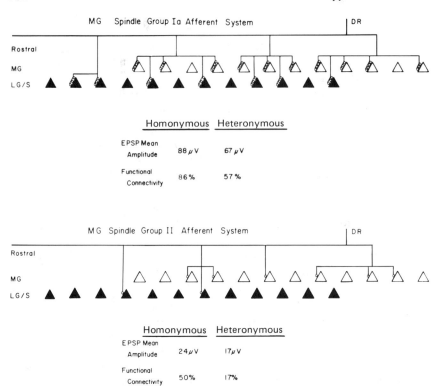

Figure 8 A schematic model of the functional organization of the overall projections of single MG group Ia fibers (above) and single MG spindle group II fibers (below) to homonymous and heteronymous motoneurons. Open triangles represent homonymous motoneurons, and filled triangles heteronymous motoneurons. The relative density of active terminals (open circles) is estimated, based on the mean amplitude of single-fiber EPSPs. (From Ref. 21.)

fibers is stronger in homonymous than in heteronymous motoneurons (89,90; Table 1), these data indicate that the larger Ia maximal composite excitatory postsynaptic potential in homonymous motoneurons results in part from greater spatial summation owing to the higher functional connectivity of Ia fibers with homonymous than with heteronymous motoneurons.

In a recent study performed in barbiturate-anesthetized cats, Nelson et al. (127) reported that the functional connectivity of single Ia afferents to triceps surae motoneurons increased immediately after acute spinal cord transection at either T13 or L5. With respect to medial gastrocnemius Ia afferent homonymous projection frequency, the functional connectivity increased from the 85% found in intact preparations to virtually 100% after spinal cord transection. Furthermore, the heteronymous functional connectivity of medial gastrocnemius Ia afferents was reported to increase to 85% compared to normal values of 60%. Since these changes occurred immediately after spinal cord transection, these authors (127) have suggested that this increase in functional connectivity results from the activation of previously inactive Ia synapses rather than from the growth of new connections. Moreover, this increase in functional connectivity can occur in spinal cord transection preparations exhibiting normal Ia single-fiber excitatory postsynaptic potential amplitudes, a finding which indicates that an improvement in the resolution of small excitatory postsynaptic potentials is an unlikely explanation for the finding of an increased projection frequency. Although the mechamism remains unknown, it has been suggested that acute spinal cord transection eliminates descending presynaptic inhibitory input. In turn, this results in a presynaptic disinhibition and Ia terminals previously inactive because of this descending inhibitory input now become responsive to impulses in their parent axons (100). This study emphasizes the importance of critical evaluation of any morphologic interpretations based on electrophysiologic data, since estimates of connectivity obtained physiologically may underestimate the anatomic projection of a presynaptic afferent system.

   d. Spatial Distribution of Group Ia–Motoneuron Boutons. The wide range of the time course (i.e., shape indices: rise time and half-width) of Ia single-fiber excitatory postsynaptic potentials recorded in alpha motoneurons indicates that Ia boutons have a wide spatial termination on the motoneuron soma-dendritic surface (Figs. 2 and 9). Group Ia single-fiber excitatory postsynaptic potentials generated in motoneurons vary from very brief transients with rise time of 0.1 msec and half-width of 0.5 msec to quite prolonged potentials with rise times up to 3.0 msec and half-widths up to 10.0 msec (19,20,49,50,51,70,72–75,81,121, 122). These differences in time courses has been shown to be the case for single-fiber excitatory postsynaptic potentials evoked by the same Ia fiber in a number of different motoneurons and also for single-fiber excitatory postsynaptic potentials evoked in the same motoneuron by different Ia afferents (70). Temporal dispersion of impulses invading the terminal arborization of a single group Ia afferent can account for only part of the observed variation in the time course of the single-fiber excitatory postsynaptic potential (49–50,74,75). In addition, there is no correlation between the Ia single-fiber excitatory postsynaptic potential time course and the conduction velocity of the parent Ia axon (50,72,75). Hence, these various observations lend strong support to an argument that the factor(s) responsible for the Ia single-fiber excitatory postsynaptic potential time course variation are not inherent in the presynaptic Ia afferents, assuming that there is no substantial variation in the time course of the subsynaptic current. This assumption is very reasonable, since available evidence indicates that the duration of the subsynaptic current elicited by a single Ia bouton is very brief

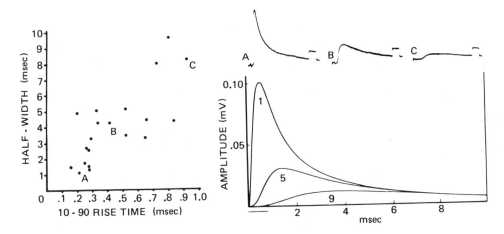

Figure 9 Left: Scatter plot of the 10–90% rise time (abscissa) vs. the half-width (ordinate) for single-fiber EPSPs evoked in 20 different MG motoneurons by impulses in the same MG group Ia afferent fiber. Above right: A, B, and C are examples taken from the population of single-fiber EPSPs in the scatter plot. Below right: Computed EPSP for input distributed to three different parts of the motoneuron's soma-dendritic membrane using a theoretic compartmental model (40). The three curves represent EPSPs produced by inputs limited to the soma (1), proximal dendrites (2), and distal dendrites (3). (Additional details in text.)

(<0.3 msec), and there is no evidence for residual transmitter activity (49,51, 128; see Sec. II.C). Another factor that may influence the time course of a Ia single-fiber excitatory postsynaptic potential is the electrotonic properties of the alpha motoneuron (i.e., L,ρ). The electrotonic architecture of alpha motoneurons appears, however, to be relatively constant from cell to cell (Sec. II.B.2.a). Moreover, two Ia afferents converging on the same motoneuron can evoke single-fiber excitatory postsynaptic potentials with markedly different time courses (70). Taken in sum, these data indicate that different spatial locations of the active Ia terminals on the motoneuronal membrane surface are a major factor in the time course of Ia single-fiber excitatory postsynaptic potentials.

The wide variation in the time course of Ia single-fiber excitatory postsynaptic potentials, the fact that impulses in two Ia afferents can elicit single-fiber excitatory postsynaptic potentials with different time courses, and, conversely, that the same Ia afferent elicits single-fiber excitatory postsynaptic potentials with very different time courses in different motoneurons are all consistent with the Rall model (50,51,70,73,75,104,113,121,122). Furthermore, as predicted by this theory (40), Ia single-fiber excitatory postsynaptic potential rise time and half-width (21,50,51,70,73,75,104,114,121,122) and latency and rise time

(73,75) are all positively correlated, whereas Ia single-fiber excitatory post-synaptic potential rise time and amplitude or rise time and latency are substantially more weakly related than predicted by Rall's theoretic work. However, the smaller differences observed between the amplitudes of dendritic and somatic Ia single-fiber excitatory postsynaptic potentials do not necessarily weaken the Rall model of the motoneuron.

Mathematic models developed by Rall (40,81) and by Jack and Redman (82,83) have given a quantitative description of the spatial distribution of the functional connections of single Ia on alpha motoneurons. The models are based upon analysis of the time course of Ia single-fiber excitatory postsynaptic potentials recorded at the soma, coupled with independent measurements of the electrotonic properties of the motoneuron. In order to calculate accurately the distance between the active boutons and the soma from the Ia single-fiber excitatory postsynaptic potential time course, the following factors must be specified: (1) τ, (2) λ, (3) ρ, (4) boundary conditions at dendritic terminations, and (5) time course of the subsynaptic current. There are two basic assumptions of these models: (1) the subsynaptic current is brief (in comparison with λ) and (2) all of the synaptic terminations of a single Ia afferent are at the same electrotonic distance from the soma. Although the subsynaptic current time course has never been directly measured, available evidence indicates that it is sufficiently brief to not substantially interfere with estimates of synaptic location. Moreover, electrophysiologic (50,51,70,73,75,84,104,114,121,122) and morphologic (24,25,27) data indicate that the majority of the synaptic contacts of a single Ia afferent on the motoneuron's surface are located at about the same geometric distance from the soma.

Comparisons of observations made of actual Ia single-fiber excitatory postsynaptic potentials with results derived from mathematic neuron models support the conclusion that the terminations of different Ia afferents are widely distributed over the entire soma-dendritic receptive surface of alpha motoneurons (51,104). Jack et al. (51) and Iansek and Redman (84) found that Ia functional connections were denser on the proximal half than on the distal half of motoneuron dendrites. The largest concentration was located in the range of 0.2–0.8 λ from the soma. Although some Ia afferents appear to terminate on the soma and distal dendrites, these occur relatively infrequently (51,52,75,82,85). This distribution computed electrophysiologically is in excellent agreement with morphologic data (27,28,48). It must be considered that these electrophysiologic investigations of Ia single-fiber excitatory postsynaptic potentials are largely limited to excitatory postsynaptic potentials exhibiting simple time courses consistent with their terminations being spatially distributed to a single electrotonic compartment, hence biasing any interpretations. In fact, available data indicate that 40% of Ia single-fiber excitatory postsynaptic potentials may be generated by multiple electrotonically distinct synaptic sites on alpha motoneurons (74,75).

Investigations of cat triceps surae motoneurons have indicated that the rise times of homonymous Ia single-fiber excitatory postsynaptic potentials are significantly shorter than the rise times of heteronymous excitatory postsynaptic potentials (73,122). This homonymous-heteronymous difference appears to be related to differences in time constants of the recorded motoneurons rather than to differences in synaptic location (122). This conclusion has been supported by the report that there was no significant difference between homonymous and heteronymous Ia single-fiber excitatory postsynaptic potential normalized rise times and half-widths (75). The rise times of Ia single-fiber excitatory postsynaptic potentials (122) and composite excitatory postsynaptic potentials (94) are also briefer in large than in small motoneurons (122). Since larger motoneurons tend to have shorter τ than smaller motoneurons, and a shorter τ would shorten the time course of excitatory postsynaptic potentials irrespective of spatial distribution of the terminals, these data are difficult to interpret. Interesting, Jack et al. (72) reported data that suggest a tendency for Ia terminations to be located more distally on small than on large motoneurons. In this latter study, the effect of τ was accounted for by normalization of the temporal parameters of the Ia single-fiber excitatory postsynaptic potentials. These investigators also reported that there were no spatial differences in the terminations of Ia afferents with different conduction velocities.

    e. Amplitude of Group Ia–Motoneuron Excitatory Postsynaptic Potentials. Group Ia single-fiber excitatory postsynaptic potentials recorded in cat alpha motoneurons do not appear to have a fixed amplitude, but vary in size from presynaptic impulse to presynaptic impulse (65,68,70,75b,120,148). The mechanisms responsible for this amplitude variability remain to be elucidated. Irrespective of the mechanism(s) involved, meaningful amplitude comparisons can only be made between averaged excitatory postsynaptic potentials.

    Even when limiting amplitude comparisons to averaged Ia single-fiber excitatory postsynaptic potentials, substantial disparities exist among the values reported for mean amplitudes by various investigators. Although sampling error undoubtedly contributes to some of the reported disparities, a major source of the variation in mean Ia single-fiber excitatory postsynaptic potential amplitude appears to be the result of different experimental protocols and techniques used in different studies. A variety of anesthetic agents have been used in different investigations. Anesthetics have been shown to significantly affect the size of group Ia-motoneuron excitatory postsynaptic potentials (129). Mendell and Henneman (50) also found that the mean amplitude of excitatory postsynaptic potentials recorded in unanesthetized high spinal cats was twice that of excitatory postsynaptic potentials recorded in anesthetized preparations with intact spinal cords. Moreover, Nelson et al. (127) reported that mean amplitude of Ia single-fiber excitatory postsynaptic potentials increased after either T13 or L5 acute spinal cord transection in barbiturate-anesthetized cats. However, single-fiber group Ia excitatory postsynaptic potentials recorded in chloralose-anesthetized cats with acutely transected spinal cords (126,193) were no larger than in barbiturate-anesthetized animals with intact spinal cords (21,50,67,75, 75a,80,122). Another source of disparity is that in some studies electric stimulation of Ia afferents was used to evoke presumed single-fiber excitatory postsynaptic potentials instead of natural stimulation as used with the spike-triggered averaging technique.

Group Ia single-fiber excitatory postsynaptic potentials elicited by electrical stimulation methods (51,114,130) are, on the average, much larger than those obtained by spike-triggered averaging methods (21,50,70,75,75a,80,121,122, 126,193). Furthermore, a substantial difference in the amplitude distributions of Ia single-fiber excitatory postsynaptic potentials exists for the two techniques. In studies using electrical stimulation, Ia single-fiber excitatory postsynaptic potentials are reported to range in amplitude up to 2 mV or greater and few are reported <100 μV in amplitude. In contrast, spike-triggered averaging studies in barbiturate-anesthetized cats with intact spinal cords report that more than half of Ia single-fiber excitatory postsynaptic potentials are <100 μV in amplitude, with no excitatory postsynaptic potentials >700 μV (Table 2). Moreover, the results of investigations using spike-triggered methods are remarkably reproducible from laboratory to laboratory.

A number of factors may contribute to the disparity in amplitude between Ia single-fiber excitatory postsynaptic potentials elicited by electrical stimulation and spike-triggered averaging techniques. It is possible that in some cases electrical stimulation of more than one Ia afferent fiber evoked composite excitatory postsynaptic potentials which were categorized as single-fiber excitatory postsynaptic potentials, since a criterion used in studies with electrical stimulation for identifying single-fiber excitatory postsynaptic potentials was that the rising phase of the excitatory postsynaptic potential exhibit no discontinuities suggestive of the action of more than one Ia afferent. However, this would not be a reasonable explanation of why so few excitatory postsynaptic potentials of less than 100 μV were recorded under these conditions. Since this technique selects Ia fibers with the lowest electrical threshold (fastest conducting fibers) and the fastest conducting Ia afferents elicit the largest excitatory postsynaptic potentials (21,50), this sampling error would lead to larger excitatory postsynaptic potentials. In addition, it is possible that the relatively greater concurrent synaptic activity observed with spike-triggered averaging, than with electrical stimulation, may act as a shunt, reducing the amplitude of Ia single-fiber excitatory postsynaptic potentials recorded by spike-triggered averaging methods. It should be kept in mind, however, that the spike-triggered averaging technique is the only method that ensures that an excitatory postsynaptic potential is generated by a presynaptic impulse in a single Ia afferent.

In spite of the reported disparities in single-fiber excitatory postsynaptic potential amplitudes, all investigators are in general agreement that the majority of Ia single-fiber excitatory postsynaptic potentials recorded in motoneurons are small (<300 μV). While Ia single-fiber excitatory postsynaptic potentials range from 5 to 700 μV in lumbar spinal motoneurons of cats with intact spinal cords, the average amplitude in homonymous motoneurons is $\sim$100 μV. This small amplitude implies that considerable convergence of Ia afferents is required to discharge an alpha motoneuron monosynaptically.

Despite the fact that Ia afferents with fast conduction velocities preferentially connect with fast-conducting motoneurons, presumed to have low R_N (21), fast Ia afferents generate larger single-fiber excitatory postsynaptic potentials than do slow Ia afferents (21,50). Luscher et al. (131) also showed that there was a positive correlation between the conduction velocity of medial gastrocnemius Ia afferent fibers and the amplitude of the spike-triggered averaging–elicited postsynaptic population potential recorded from ventral roots perfused with sucrose. These data indicate that larger Ia afferents have greater synaptic efficacy than smaller afferents, presumably as a result of giving off more terminals. Interestingly, Mendell and colleagues have reported that lateral gastrocnemius Ia afferents evoke larger Ia single-fiber excitatory postsynaptic potential in alpha motoneurons, on the average than do medial gastrocnemius or soleus Ia afferents (122) or semitendinosis Ia afferents (121) despite similar conduction velocities.

On the average, Ia single-fiber excitatory postsynaptic potentials are larger in homonymous than heteronymous motoneurons (21,50,73,75,75a,121,122, 126,130,193). One possible mechanism responsible for this amplitude difference could be a tendency for Ia synapses to have a more proximal location on the soma-dendritic membrane of homonymous motoneurons. Although Ia single-fiber excitatory postsynaptic potentials recorded in homonymous motoneurons have a slightly briefer rise time—a finding consistent with this hypothesis (73,75, 121,122,130)—Mendell and colleagues (121,122) have convincingly demonstrated that this rise time difference is largely related to differences in τ. Hence, it appears that factors other than systematic differences in the location of Ia terminals on the motoneuron soma-dendritic membrane must account for this amplitude difference. A reasonable hypothesis is that Ia afferents give off larger arborizations and more terminations, on the average, to homonymous than to heteronymous motoneurons (21,122; Fig. 8). This simple hypothesis requires that the Ia terminals function identically so that their number is the variable determining synaptic efficacy. However, it is also possible that the Ia terminations on homonymous motoneurons may be qualitatively different from those ending on heteronymous motoneurons, for example, larger Ia boutons that release more transmitter end on homonymous motoneurons or homonymous motoneurons have greater postsynaptic ionophore density or longer duration of synaptic current. At present, there is no evidence for a systematic variation in Ia bouton size, ionophore density, or current duration among alpha motoneurons. On the other hand, available morphologic (24-26) and physiologic (74-75) data are consistent with the aforementioned hypothesis.

Not only is the mean amplitude of the Ia single-fiber excitatory postsynaptic potential larger in homonymous than in heteronymous motoneurons, but the functional connectivity of single Ia afferents is significantly greater in homonymous motoneurons. Hence, it is apparent that the previous findings (90) that maximal composite excitatory postsynaptic potentials are larger in homonymous than in heteronymous motoneurons can be attributed to both a larger homonymous mean Ia single-fiber excitatory postsynaptic potential amplitude as well as to a larger homonymous functional connectivity.

One important factor that could account for the variability in Ia excitatory postsynaptic potential amplitude is the R_N (or size) of the alpha motoneuron (38). Combined morphologic and electrophysiologic investigations have demonstrated that R_N is an excellent correlate of motoneuron size (32). The concept that Ia excitatory postsynaptic potential amplitude is causally related to R_N *per se* (50,93)—a concept analogous to a conclusion based on observations at the neuromuscular junction (132)—appeared to be supported by the direct correlation between composite Ia excitatory postsynaptic potential amplitude and motoneuronal R_N (66). Moreover, Ia single-fiber excitatory postsynaptic potentials are larger, on the average, in small motoneurons than in large motoneurons with smaller R_N (50,69,80,122). However, Burke et al. (134) showed that Ia composite excitatory postsynaptic potential amplitudes are more closely correlated with motor unit type in the cat medial gastrocnemius motoneuron pool than with indices of R_N such as motoneuronal axonal conduction velocity. Hence, these findings indicate that other factors must be involved. In an attempt to examine more rigorously the synaptic organization of Ia afferents to a single motoneuron pool, Fleshman et al. (80) investigated the distribution of Ia single-fiber excitatory postsynaptic potentials to type-identified cat medial gastrocnemius motoneurons. Mean Ia single-fiber excitatory postsynaptic potentials amplitude and variance were found to differ significantly among motor unit types, increasing in the order: fast-twitch, fast-fatiguing (FF) fast-twitch, fatigue-resistant (FR), slow-twitch, fatigue-resistant (S). Excitatory postsynaptic potentials in S units ranged from <50 μV to >500 μV, whereas no excitatory postsynaptic potentials >300 μV were found in FF units. Fatigue-resistant units (FR and S) received monosynaptic connections from a larger proportion of Ia fibers than did fatigue-sensitive units (FF). R_N decreased in the same order as Ia single-fiber excitatory postsynaptic potential amplitude (S > FR > FF), despite the fact that the axonal conduction velocities of FF and FR units were equal. An analysis of covariance revealed that after adjusting for any linear effect of R_N motor unit type *per se* had a significant effect on excitatory postsynaptic potential amplitude. Within a given unit type there was no correlation between motoneuronal R_N and Ia single-fiber excitatory postsynaptic potential amplitude, despite a threefold within-group range of R_N. Moreover, the FF < FR < S ordering of Ia excitatory postsynaptic potential amplitude is preserved among motoneurons of different unit type that have a similar R_N. Hence, it is not possible to explain the distribution of excitatory postsynaptic potential amplitudes on the basis of differences in R_N (i.e., cell size) among unit type. Fleshman and coworkers (80) concluded that mean Ia single-fiber excitatory postsynaptic potential amplitudes differ among motor unit types reflecting a motor unit-specific organization of group Ia synaptic efficacy. This conclusion was further supported by using the values for mean connectivity and mean Ia single-fiber excitatory postsynaptic potential amplitude to compute an estimate of the maximal composite excitatory postsynaptic potential. The computed maximal composite excitatory postsynaptic potential values for each motor unit type were in excellent agreement with the experimentally obtained values reported by Burke et al. (134).

Again, the factors responsible for this alpha motoneuron–specific organization of Ia synaptic efficacy are uncertain. It is apparent that R_N *per se* does not play a dominant role in determining the amplitude of Ia excitatory postsynaptic potentials. In addition, the monosynaptic group II single-fiber excitatory postsynaptic potential amplitude in medial gastrocnemius alpha motoneurons does not vary systematically over the fivefold range of motoneuron R_N (135; see Sec. III). Similar to Ia excitatory postsynaptic potentials, composite recurrent inhibitory postsynaptic potentials differed systematically with unit type such that mean inhibitory postsynaptic potential amplitude increased in the order FF < FR < S (136). Furthermore, within a unit type, there was no relation to R_N, despite a threefold range in motoneuron R_N. Taken in sum, these data strongly indicate that postsynaptic processes are not likely determinants of systematic differences in the synaptic efficacy of terminations on alpha motoneurons (see also 70). One simple explanation for the systematic difference in Ia excitatory postsynaptic potential amplitudes in motoneurons is schematized in Figure 10. Based upon measures of motoneuron R_N, which increases in the order FF < FR < S, the size of motoneurons increases in the order S < FR < FF (32,80,135-137). Anatomic investigations (99) support these findings. Accordingly, the size differences among motoneurons are depicted: S < FR < FF. These anatomic size differences may be less than suggested by the respective differences in R_N, since specific membrane resistance may differ between motoneurons with rapidly or slowly conducting axons (138). The fact that Ia single-fiber excitatory postsynaptic potential amplitude varies systematically with unit type indicates that, on the average, the density of Ia synapses increases in the order FF < FR < S. Hence, the smaller S-type motoneurons receive a greater

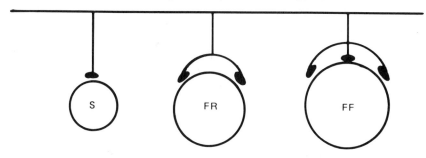

Group Ia - Motoneuron Terminations

Spindle Group II - Motoneuron Terminations

Figure 10 Above: Hypothetic relationships between the efficacy of Ia afferent input and homonymous motoneuron size for principal motor unit types. Type-S motoneurons appear to receive a disproportionately large number of Ia synaptic boutons relative to their cell size. Below: Hypothetic relationship between the efficacy of spindle group II afferent input and homonymous motoneuron size for principal motor unit types. In the spindle group II–motoneuron system, homonymous motoneurons appear to receive an equal density of functional synapses despite size and type differences of the motoneurons comprising the pool.

number of functional Ia boutons per unit of membrane surface area (assuming equal efficacy of terminals).

The preceding conclusion assumes that the amplitude of an excitatory post-synaptic potential is a simple function of the synaptic current and R_N of the motoneuron (e.g., 139). However, the relationship is not quite so simple because other factors must be considered which include R_M and C_M (the electrotonic properties of the motoneuron) and the frequency spectrum of the synaptic current. In muscle fibers, Gage and McBurney (140) found that the amplitude of individual end-plate potentials relates more to characteristic impedance than to steady-state R_N. Accordingly the absence of a relationship between postsynaptic potential amplitude and R_N (80,113,135) may merely signify that the characteristic impedance of a motoneuron to a synaptic current transient is not closely related to that motoneuron's steady-state R_N (141; see also 51,81).

As mentioned previously in Section II.B.2.c, the experimentally observed values of Ia single-fiber excitatory postsynaptic potential amplitude reveal remarkably little attenuation with increasingly distal dendritic sites of excitatory postsynaptic potential generation (49,50,67,70,75,142,143). As expected, a negative correlation between Ia single-fiber excitatory postsynaptic potential amplitude and rise time does exist, but it is much weaker than originally computed from mathematic models of alpha motoneurons (35,113; see Fig. 7). The mechanisms responsible for the observed enhanced synaptic efficacy of distally generated dendritic excitatory postsynaptic potentials are not known. A variety of hypotheses have been suggested. These include: increased receptor sensitivity at dendritic synapses (52,70); enhanced dendritic R_M compared to that of the soma (84,101,144); an increased area of distal synaptic contacts (145), which increases the magnitude and duration of the postsynaptic current (or charge) injected (145); and a regional specialization of dendritic membrane, resulting in greater separation of the membrane potential from the excitatory postsynaptic potential reversal potential, which could result in a greater driving potential and reduced nonlinear summation (145). Although presently available evidence does not lend support to any of these hypotheses, some evidence exists which favors exclusion of some of these possibilities. For instance, Iansek and Redman (52) found no evidence for a longer duration of synaptic currents at increasing electrotonic distances from the soma. Furthermore, the size of Ia boutons is uniform over the motoneuronal soma-dendritic surface (11,28) and the density of Ia terminals does not appear to increase on the distal dendrites (11,145). Although the fundamental basis remains uncertain, Ia synapses on distal dendrites are not spatially disadvantaged in their ability to influence the somatic membrane potential. In fact, if as suggested by Barrett and Crill (35) the synaptic efficacy is defined as the time integral of the soma-recorded Ia excitatory postsynaptic potential, then the synaptic efficacy of motoneuronal dendritic Ia excitatory postsynaptic potentials is even greater than that indicated by measurements of amplitude (the time course of dendritic excitatory postsynaptic potentials is prolonged compared to proximally generated owing to the cell's electrotonic properties). This latter concept is consistent with observations that the mean current depolarizing the soma (and the nearby axon hillock) is the major determinant of motoneuronal firing rate (146), and that the peak amplitude of Ia single-fiber excitatory postsynaptic potentials is very small, well below threshold values and substantial spatial summation of many Ia fibers required to reach threshold.

Group Ia–motoneuronal excitatory postsynaptic potentials have been shown to exhibit nonlinear summation (49,104,130). This observation is expected if chemical synaptic sites are located sufficiently close to one another (in electrotonic terms) to permit mutual interaction of conductance increases (shunting) and voltage changes (reduction in driving potential as membrane potential approximates the reversal potential). The finding that computed maximal composite Ia excitatory postsynaptic potentials (80,121,122) are larger than the experimentally observed values (89,90,134) has been attributed to nonlinear summation. Interestingly, it appears that nonlinear summation among Ia single-fiber excitatory postsynaptic potentials (130) may be substantially greater than that observed between composite excitatory postsynaptic poteticals elicited by volleys in two different muscle nerves (49). This effect has been attributed to the greater likelihood of the terminals of a single Ia fiber to cluster in proximity on the motoneuronal surface than the terminals of Ia fibers from different muscle nerves (100).

f. Amplitude Fluctuations of Group Ia Single-Fiber Excitatory Postsynaptic Potentials. Ia single-fiber excitatory postsynaptic potentials recorded in alpha motoneurons have been shown to fluctuate in amplitude from presynaptic impulse to presynaptic impulse (49,53,68–71,75,120,147,148). These amplitude fluctuations were first investigated by Kuno (68), who suggested that Ia single-fiber excitatory postsynaptic potentials (or small composite excitatory postsynaptic potentials) are composed of discrete all-or-none components, and that some afferent impulses fail to generate excitatory postsynaptic potentials. When the distribution of amplitudes of presumed Ia single-fiber excitatory postsynaptic potentials was plotted, he found that the amplitude histograms could be fitted to predictions based upon simple statistical models, primarily the Poisson model and, in some cases, binomial models. Subsequent similar studies of Ia single-fiber excitatory postsynaptic potentials have supported these observations (46,65,69,70). Depending upon the statistical model used to fit the experimentally observed excitatory postsynaptic potential amplitude distributions, the quantal content values (mean number of quanta of transmitter released by a single presynaptic impulse, M) range from <1 to >5. The percentage of failures decreases as M increases (68,69). Although M values were generally found to be <5, occasionally, single Ia afferent–motoneuron combinations were estimated to have rather large (10–25) M values (65,68,69). Large M values were found to occur in association with relatively large peak amplitude of averaged Ia excitatory postsynaptic potentials. These results, which suggested the existence of "unit" Ia excitatory postsynaptic potentials, have been used to infer that the mechanisms of chemical transmitter liberation at Ia–motoneuron synapses are "quantitized" in a manner similar to that observed at the neuromuscular junction (149). In the acquisition, analysis, and interpretation of such data, however, investigators must consider a number of serious difficulties. These difficulties include the degree of electrotonic attenuation and distortion of the Ia single-fiber excitatory postsynaptic potentials produced at varying distances from the motoneuron soma, nonlinear summation of unit excitatory postsynaptic potentials generated at dendritic sites (69), and finally, poor signal-to-noise conditions. Spontaneous biologic (synaptic) and electronic (recording) noise combine to provide a noise level that frequently exceeds the amplitude of Ia single-fiber excitatory postsynaptic potentials such that failures may be missed and peak amplitudes of individual Ia single-fiber excitatory postsynaptic potentials are difficult to determine accurately.

Because of the aforementioned difficulties, Edwards et al. (71) recently used another approach which has even more recently been refined by Jack et al. (148). Edwards et al. (71) used charge transfer (time integral of the voltage recorded at the soma) and Jack et al. (148) used peak amplitude of Ia single-fiber excitatory postsynaptic potentials in their respective studies. In these studies, a statistical procedure was used to estimate the background noise obscuring Ia excitatory postsynaptic potentials. This was then used to separate the excitatory postsynaptic potential from the noise in order to estimate the amplitude fluctuations of a given Ia single-fiber excitatory postsynaptic potential. In about one third of the Ia single-fiber excitatory postsynaptic potentials examined a single peak amplitude which did not fluctuate in amplitude was observed (71,148). The majority of Ia single-fiber excitatory postsynaptic potentials were found, however, to fluctuate between a number of discrete amplitudes which had no detectable variability. Peaks corresponding to failures, which were common in previous investigations, were observed only rarely in these latter studies. The incremental or unit voltage was about 100 μV, a value similar to that estimated by Kuno (68). Occasionally, these investigators (68,69) found that the time course of the Ia excitatory postsynaptic potential was different when certain discrete amplitudes occurred. In addition, the amplitude of averaged Ia single-fiber excitatory postsynaptic potentials could be increased by a prior tetanus (150), or by the systemic administration of 4-aminopyridine (151). Finally, the peak amplitude distributions could not be described using either Poisson or binomial statistical models. These investigators suggest that at each bouton, impulse invasion results in either a failure to release transmitter, or the release of sufficient transmitter to saturate all available postsynaptic receptors and that the various boutons or terminations of a single Ia afferent ending on a single motoneuron can have different probabilities of failure to release. This hypothesis is consistent with the suggestions of Burke and Rudomín (46) that the unit Ia excitatory postsynaptic potentials can in fact only represent events that occur at individual synaptic contacts and that their existence does not imply a particular release mechanism. A recent report by Redman and Walmsley (147) combines anatomic (HRP filling of Ia afferents and single motoneurons) and electrophysiologic data (Ia single-fiber excitatory postsynaptic potential peak amplitudes) to provide additional support for the aforementioned hypothesis. The mechanisms responsible for this hypothetic failure of an invaded bouton to release transmitter are not known. One possibility is that the failure follows inadequate terminal depolarization by the presynaptic afferent impulse (147,148). Another possibility is that the failure of occurrence of unit Ia excitatory postsynaptic potentials may depend in part upon a process of failure of impulse invasion into terminal branches of the afferent arborization caused by a decreased safety factor for impulse conduction through branch points (31, 152–155). This latter hypothesis has been rejected by Redman and colleagues (147,148), since they were unable to detect any significant latency variations in the onset time of the Ia single-fiber excitatory postsynaptic potential (however, see 74,156–158, and Sec. II.B.2.g).

At present, it is not possible to resolve the differences between these two approaches to the amplitude fluctuations of Ia single-fiber excitatory postsynaptic potentials recorded in alpha motoneurons. The results and conclusions are obviously quite different. It is not certain that statistical methods can be used to resolve these issues. No readily apparent solution to this problem is evident unless techniques become available for the study of Ia single-fiber excitatory postsynaptic potentials under conditions of reduced biologic and electronic noise, combined with the acquisition of microanatomic data.

g. *Synaptic Delay*. "Synaptic latency" is a term broadly applied to the interval of time required for neural activity to traverse a synapse, whether that synapse be electrical or chemical (159). Synaptic delay at an electrical synapse is very brief (<0.05 msec) and consists of the time required for the presynaptic action current to charge the postsynaptic C_M to a measurable voltage plus any time required for passive propagation of the synaptic current from the synapse to the site of recording (e.g., dendrite to soma). These latter delays are referred to as "electrotonic delays" because they result from the passive electrotonic cable properties (R_M, C_M, L) of the postsynaptic cell. At electrical synapses, electrotonic delay is synaptic latency.

Chemical synapses depend upon the action of a chemical neurotransmitter to mediate the transfer of activity from the pre- to the postsynaptic cell. This requires time for the mobilization and release of the neurotransmitter from the presynaptic terminals, diffusion of the neurotransmitter across the synaptic cleft, and the reaction of the neurotransmitter with the postsynaptic membrane to initiate a synaptic current in the postsynaptic cell. For purposes of this section, the time interval required for these latter specific processes is termed "synaptic delay." In addition to synaptic delay, chemical synapses also demonstrate electrotonic delay, since the postsynaptic current must passively propagate to the recording site as well as charge the C_M to a measurable voltage. At a chemical synapse, therefore, synaptic latency is synaptic delay plus electrotonic delay.

Until recently, direct measurement of synaptic delay at a single synapse in the mammalian central nervous system was not possible. An early attempt at measurement for the monosynaptic reflex arc was made by Brooks and Eccles (77). They electrically stimulated group Ia afferents and, using an extracellular microelectrode in the homonymous motoneuron pool, recorded a complex evoked response made up of the composite volley generated by impulses in the intraspinal group I afferent branches and terminals and a composite focal synaptic potential generated by monosynaptic composite excitatory postsynaptic potentials in motoneurons. Based on measurements of the interval between the afferent potential and the focal synaptic potential, they estimated that the synaptic delay was ~0.3-0.45 msec.

More recently, spike-triggered averaging techniques have permitted direct measurements of synaptic latency at single-fiber Ia-motoneuron synapses (73, 75,160). Munson and Sypert (75) measured the Ia–motoneuron single-fiber excitatory postsynaptic potential latency as the time interval between the positive peak of the terminal potential and the onset of the excitatory postsynaptic potential. The positive peak was chosen, since it most probably signals the maximum rate of rise of the action potential invading the presynaptic terminal (78,79,162), and thus the beginning of the processes leading to transmitter release (161). Assuming active invasion of the terminal boutons, such measurements of excitatory postsynaptic potential latency would be the sum of two values: synaptic delay and electrotonic delay. For measurements of excitatory postsynaptic potential latency, Ia single-fiber excitatory postsynaptic potentials preceded by simple terminal potentials were used, since such excitatory postsynaptic potentials are largely generated in a restricted synaptic compartment of the motoneuron's soma-dendritic membrane (75). Five excitatory postsynaptic potentials had normalized rise times and half-widths, which indicated that they originated very close to the microelectrode tip (Fig. 11). The excitatory postsynaptic potential latency for the five averaged excitatory postsynaptic potentials in which electrotonic delay should be minimal range from 0.26 msec to 1.09 msec. In order to determine a value for a minimum averaged synaptic delay,

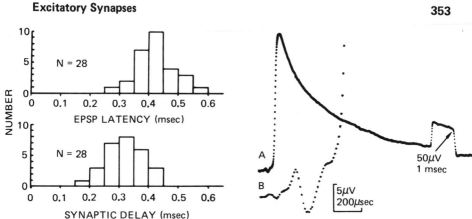

Figure 11 Left: Histograms of EPSP latency (above) and synaptic delay (below for 32 EPSPs for which electrotonic delay could be estimated. Synaptic delay (below) was calculated by subtracting the electrotonic delay from the EPSP latency. Right: MG Ia–motoneuron single-fiber EPSP with briefest measured EPSP latency (0.26 msec) and briefest calculated synaptic delay (0.17 msec). (From Ref. 75.)

the normalized rise times and half-widths values were plotted on a nomogram computed by Iles (163) which allowed calculation of the electrotonic delay for each excitatory postsynaptic potential. After subtracting the electrotonic delay from each individual excitatory postsynaptic potential latency, a mean synaptic delay of 0.30 msec (range 0.17-0.44 msec) was computed. Hence, this study directly demonstrated the existence of a "true" synaptic delay, that is, a finite time interval between pre- and postsynaptic potential changes in the Ia-motoneuron synapse. Previously, there was some doubt whether such a synaptic delay existed owing to the uncertainty as to how much time could be attributed to intramedullary conduction and to electronic delay for a synaptic input which is spatially distributed over the motoneuron surface. The briefest averaged synaptic delay (0.17 msec) is very close to the mean averaged synaptic delay of 0.22 msec recorded at the rat neuromuscular junction (164), a known chemical synapse.

h. Ia Single-Fiber Excitatory Postsynaptic Potential Latency Fluctuations. Synaptic latency at a given Ia-motoneuron synaptic ensemble (single group Ia fiber to a motoneuron) does not appear to be constant, but has been observed to fluctuate from individual excitatory postsynaptic potential to individual excitatory postsynaptic potential (74,156-158). This variability in synaptic latency has been localized to the synapse, since the latency of the terminal potential is constant, unlike the fluctuations in latency observed in the subsequent Ia single-fiber excitatory postsynaptic potentials (156–158). The distribution of these latency fluctuations is unimodal in all cases examined and varied in duration from ~220 to 600 μsec (157). The excitatory postsynaptic potentials with shorter latencies have similar time courses to those with longer latencies, indicating that they are generated by Ia terminals located on the same electrotonic regions of the motoneuron (40). Cope and Mendell (157) also reported that excitatory postsynaptic potential amplitude and rise time are negatively correlated with latency. Since Barrett and Stevens (165) observed similar correlations in amplitude and latency of synaptic potentials at the frog neuromuscular junction, Cope and Mendell (157) have reached similar conclusions, that is, the origin of the fluctuations in these excitatory postsynaptic potential parameters is presynaptic and results from the stochastic nature of transmitter release rather than from variability in axonal conduction or bouton invasion. Further support for these conclusions comes from the observations of Shapovalov and Shiriaev (166) on synaptic transmission between dorsal root afferents and motoneurons. This system appears to involve both electrical and chemical processes in the frog spinal cord. They found that the chemical component fluctuates in spite of constancy of the electrical component.

Cope and Mendell (157) specifically attempted to evaluate the effect of noise on the latency fluctuations and the variability of amplitude and rise time as a function of latency. They concluded that these fluctuations and relationships could not be accounted for entirely by noise. However, Jack et al. (148) recently reported that analysis of their data failed to reveal any evidence that latency fluctuations in Ia single-fiber excitatory postsynaptic potential onset occur. Resolution of these major differences will require further investigation.

   i. Time Course of Synaptic Current. Owing to technical limitations, the time course and magnitude of synaptic current generating a Ia single-fiber excitatory postsynaptic potential in an alpha motoneuron has not been measured. Using the time course of averaged Ia single-fiber excitatory postsynaptic potentials and the measured electrotonic properties of the respective motoneurons, the time-to-peak current has been calculated in the range of 120–125 μsec (51) and 50–390 μsec (114). It is quite likely that this wide range of values is related to conduction time differences in the fine terminal branches of single Ia fibers, spatial dispersion of the terminals of a single Ia fiber on the motoneuron surface, and possibly fluctuations in the onset of individual excitatory postsynaptic potentials making up the average (see Sec. II.B.2.h). It is not known whether the time course of synaptic current at an individual bouton is constant. In an attempt to achieve a more accurate estimate of the time course at a single Ia synapse, Ia single-fiber excitatory postsynaptic potentials with time courses consistent with highly localized spatial distributions in electrotonically measured motoneurons were analyzed using a mathematic neuron model (128). Based on this analysis, it was concluded that: (1) the time course of the synaptic current transient at the Ia–motoneuron synapse is very brief (time-to-peak, 0.05 msec; half-width, 0.123 msec), (2) the time course of the synaptic current transient is the same at proximal and distal locations, and (3) the time course of the synaptic current is too brief to be produced directly by presynaptic action currents (electrical transmission).

The exceedingly brief time course of synaptic currents generated by single Ia–motoneurons synapses has major consequences for the synaptic efficacy of this synapse. For instance, alterations in cell size and hence, R_N, will have very little influence on the amplitude of an excitatory postsynaptic potential generated by a very brief synaptic current transient, whereas the specific membrane properties, such as C_M, will have considerable effect in excitatory postsynaptic potential amplitude (51,81,140,141). Furthermore, this brief synaptic current transient will also reduce the nonlinear interactions of Ia boutons consistent with experimental observations (49,130).

j. Reversal Potential. A synaptic potential generated by a conductance change in series with an ionic transmembrane potential should have a reversal potential at which no net transmembrane synaptic current flows and, hence, at which no voltage change is recorded (62). If the transmembrane potential is polarized beyond this reversal potential, the synaptically generated voltage transient is reversed in polarity. Coombs et al. (59) performed the first extensive attempts to determine the presence of a reversal potential at the Ia–motoneuron synapse. During the intracellular injection of large depolarizing currents in cat alpha motoneurons, the composite Ia excitatory postsynaptic potential was observed to reverse, on a few occasions, at a transmembrane potential of ~0 mV. Subsequent attempts by various investigators to determine a reversal potential for Ia–motoneuron excitatory postsynaptic potentials were, however, largely unsuccessful. Smith et al. (102) reported that the initial phase of the composite Ia excitatory postsynaptic potential could rarely be reversed. Werman and Carlen (167) were also unable to reverse the initial phase of the composite Ia excitatory postsynaptic potential, despite the demonstration of a reversal potential for excitatory postsynaptic potentials generated in the same motoneurons from other inputs. Shapovalov and Kurchavyi (168) were unable to reverse composite Ia excitatory postsynaptic potentials in primate lumbar alpha motoneurons. Recently, Edwards et al. (85) and Sypert et al. (160) reported that they were unable to directly demonstrate a reversal of the rising or falling phase of Ia–motoneuron single-fiber excitatory postsynaptic potentials that have

a time course indicative of a somatic site of generation. Furthermore, attempts
to arrive at a reversal potential by extrapolation were also unsuccessful. However, Engberg and Marshall (169) more recently used a technique which permits
the introduction of two microelectrodes into cat alpha motoneurons. One electrode was used for passage of large depolarizing currents and the other for
recording continuous measurements of membrane potential. They reported a
reversal potential between 0 and +10mV for composite Ia excitatory postsynaptic potentials. Moreover, Flatman and Lambert (170) were also able
to demonstrate a reversal potential for Ia–motoneuron composite excitatory
postsynaptic potential using two microelectrodes with the intracellular injection of QX222 (a local anesthetic which blocks sodium channels and prevents
spike activity) and depolarizing current via one electrode. These latter studies
thus provide compelling evidence to confirm the existence of a reversal potential for Ia–motoneuron synapses as originally observed by Coombs et al. (59).
It is likely that the large decrease in R_M that accompanies depolarizing
currents often prevents determination of an excitatory postsynaptic potential reversal potential in alpha motoneurons, since equal increments of depolarizing current do not cause equal increments of membrane potential depolarization, particularly if the principal ionic conductance increase is for potassium
ions.

3. Historical Effects of Group Ia-Motoneuron Synaptic Activity

The synaptic efficacy of most synapses, whether it be peripheral or central,
depends upon the immediate history of proceeding activations. It has been
demonstrated that when a chemically mediated synapse is stimulated repetitively
the synaptic efficacy (postsynaptic potential amplitude) with each presynaptic
impulse is not constant but varies as a function of the previous frequency and
duration of the presynaptic stimulation (e.g., 171-173). Depending upon the
experimental conditions, repetitive stimulation can lead to either an increase or
to a decrease in synaptic efficacy by each presynaptic impulse.

Changes in synaptic efficacy by previous synaptic activation have been
described at the Ia–motoneuron synapse. Depression and posttetanic potentiation (PTP) at the Ia–motoneuron synapse in the cat spinal cord were first
described by Lloyd (57), who demonstrated that following tetanic stimulation
of the medial gastrocnemius muscle nerve the response recorded from the ventral
root was first decreased, then increased, reaching a maximum value after a delay
of ~10-40 msec. Lloyd also demonstrated that increasing the number of conditioning presynaptic impulses resulted in an increase in both the magnitude and
time course of potentiation. Moreover, Lloyd found that potentiation and
depression did not result from a change in the postsynaptic excitability of the

motoneurons. Stimulation of one group of monosynaptic afferent fibers did not alter the synaptic efficacy of another (unstimulated) group of monosynaptic afferents. Hence, these experiments indicated that the potentiation and depression in this monosynaptic system is homosynaptic; that is, it is restricted to the stimulated synaptic connections and results from a change in the efficacy of the synapse itself. Subsequently, these effects of repetitive stimulation have been directly verified in studies of Ia composite excitatory postsynaptic potentials using intracellular recording in cat alpha motoneurons (174,175).

In addition to the slowly decaying potentiation and a slowly recovering depression, a more rapidly decaying component of enhanced synaptic efficacy (facilitation) has also been observed for Ia composite excitatory postsynaptic potentials following one or a few presynaptic impulses. Curtis and Eccles (174) found that following electrical activation of Ia afferents, the Ia composite excitatory postsynaptic potential produced by a second stimulus is facilitated at short interstimulus intervals (5-40 msec) and depressed at longer intervals (40-2000 msec). Continuous activation of Ia afferents at a wide range of frequencies (2-200 Hz) was observed to result in a depression of Ia composite excitatory postsynaptic potentials. Kuno (175) applied quantal analysis to the fluctuations of small Ia excitatory postsynaptic potentials elicited by one or a few fibers before and after conditioning stimuli. Assuming that the fluctuations followed the Poisson model, his analysis indicated that double stimulation of a limited number of Ia afferents at varying time intervals produces analogous enhancement and depression in the probability of generation of unit excitatory postsynaptic potentials (M) with appreciable changes in the size of unit excitatory postsynaptic potentials. Kuno (175) also performed a similar analysis of the fluctuations of Ia excitatory postsynaptic potentials generated by a small number of afferents during posttetanic potentiation. Following the conditioning tetanus, he reported that the unit excitatory postsynaptic potential size remained constant, but that the M values increased with a time course similar to that of posttetanic potentiation in Ia composite excitatory postsynaptic potentials—findings which indicate that posttetanic potentiation also results from an increased probability of occurrence of unit excitatory postsynaptic potentials. Recently, Hirsch et al. (150) investigated facilitation and posttetanic potentiation of presumed Ia single-fiber excitatory postsynaptic potentials elicited by electrical stimulation in cat alpha motoneurons. In this study, the statistical techniques described by Jack et al. (148) were used to separate excitatory postsynaptic potential fluctuations from the noise. They found that the averaged peak amplitude of some Ia single-fiber excitatory postsynaptic potentials was increased by a single conditioning impulse. Furthermore, the ability of excitatory postsynaptic potentials to potentiate following a conditioning tetanus was correlated with their ability to facilitate following a single conditioning stimulus. Similar to the previous report of Edwards et al. (85), who used analogous analytic techniques, some excitatory postsynaptic potentials were found that failed to potentiate following a conditioning tetanus. When posttetanic potentiation was maximal for a given Ia single-fiber excitatory postsynaptic potential, facilitation was found to be abolished. Based on previously proposed mechanisms for Ia single-fiber excitatory postsynaptic potentials amplitude fluctuations (148; see Sec. II.B.2.e), Hirst et al. (150) suggested that both facilitation and potentiation in single-fiber Ia–motoneuron synapses result from a reduction in the probability of failure of a terminal to release transmitter following conditioning stimuli.

Recently, several investigators have suggested that the mechanism underlying depression and potentiation at Ia–motoneuron synapses may involve blocking and unblocking, respectively, of impulse transmission at sites of low safety factor in the Ia afferent arborization (85,176; see Sec. II.B.2.e). In a study of posttetanic potential in cat medial gastrocnemius motoneurons, Luscher et al. (176) reported that motoneurons with high R_N values have larger Ia composite excitatory postsynaptic potentials and less posttetanic potentiation that result from homonymous conditioning tetanic stimulation than cells with low R_N. Since R_N is inversely related to cell size, they concluded that Ia terminals innervating larger motoneurons were potentiated more than those innervating small motoneurons. To explain this phenomenon, they suggested that Ia afferent axons may undergo more branching in their terminal arborizations as they approach large motoneurons, and that this augmented branching could result in a greater probability of conduction failures at branch points. If this were the case, then anything that would enhance invasion of Ia terminals and activate more synaptic endings should lead to larger excitatory postsynaptic potentials. Because of the postulated greater branching of Ia afferents that innervate large motoneurons, any enhancement should be greater in large than in small motoneurons. On the basis of these arguments, Luscher et al. (176) proposed that the posttetanic potentiation at the Ia–motoneuron synapse is caused by the activation of previously silent synapses through the invasion of axonal branches which otherwise would have remained blocked. A more recent study (177), however, failed to find evidence for a failure of action potential invasion following conditioning stimulation, and instead suggested that the differences in the amount of posttetanic potentiation of Ia composite excitatory postsynaptic potentials seen in different sized motoneurons could be attributed to differences in nonlinear summation, which would be inversely related to cell size (see also Sec. II.B.2.d).

4. Extracellular Ionic Concentration Changes

Alterations in the concentrations of a variety of ions in the solutions bathing peripheral synapse preparations have been exceedingly useful in elucidating the mechanisms of junctional transmissions at these synapses. Unfortunately, reliable alterations in either the extracellular or intracellular ionic concentrations are not possible in the intact spinal cord with available techniques, such as close arterial injection, topical application, or iontophoresis. This is especially true for attempts to alter the ionic concentration at relevant sites such as the terminal boutons or immediately subsynaptic regions. Another problem encountered with attempts to alter extracellular ionic concentrations is that any measured change in synaptic transmission may be caused by alterations in the impulse invasion of the presynaptic afferent arborization, rather than by a direct effect on the presynaptic terminals.

In the intact cat spinal cord, Decima (178) reported that monosynaptic and polysynaptic reflexes were largely absent in acute hypocalcemic preparations. Moreover, the intra-arterial injection of calcium ions to induce spinal cord hypercalcemia was reported to prolong the time course of the posttetanic potentiation. Decima concluded that these data supported the hypothesis that Ia–motoneuron synapses are chemically mediated.

Alterations in the extracellular concentrations of a variety of divalent cations have been used in the isolated frog spinal cord to determine the effect of changes in these ions on synaptic transmission. Attempts to reduce intraspinal extracellular calcium concentration by using calcium-free Ringer's solution (with egtazic acid [EGTA]) resulted in a reduced synaptic transmission in response to stimulation of the lateral column and dorsal root afferents (179). Subsequently, Barrett and Barrett (180) reported that dorsal root-elicited composite excitatory postsynaptic potentials could be completely blocked following perfusion with low calcium Ringer's solutions. Alvarez–Leefmans et al. (181) also found that removal of calcium and its replacement by strontium or barium blocked synaptic potentials in motoneurons elicited by dorsal root stimulation. Although Shapovalov et al. (182) reported that the late monosynaptic component of the dorsal root–evoked excitatory postsynaptic potential in motoneurons is abolished by perfusion with 2 mM magnesium, they observed that a brief latency component of the dorsal-evoked monosynaptic excitatory postsynaptic potential remained. In addition, this brief latency component was unaltered by reduced extracellular calcium or raised extracellular magnesium concentrations (183). Because of the observations that this brief latency excitatory postsynaptic potential could not be reversed (184) and that gap junctions are present on motoneurons (185), there appear to be both chemical and electrical junctional transmission between some primary afferent fibers and frog spinal motoneurons (186).

In a study of synaptic transmission in the isolated perfused spinal cord of the kitten, Shapovalov et al. (187) reported that both the monosynaptic and polysynaptic responses recorded in motoneurons in response to dorsal root stimulation were completely lost when calcium was removed and magnesium was added to the perfusion medium. The observed effect was reversible. Moreover, they observed no effect of changes in the perfusion medium on the presynaptic spike. Hence, these authors concluded that primary afferent-elicited synaptic transmission in feline spinal cord is mediated exclusively by chemical transmission.

Recently, Krnjević et al. (188) investigated the effect of divalent cations extracellularly applied by iontophoresis on Ia composite excitatory postsynaptic potentials recorded in cat alpha motoneurons. They reported that manganese and cobalt ions consistently depressed the Ia composite excitatory postsynaptic potential peak amplitude and rise time and half-width values. Moreover, the terminal potential was not depressed in amplitude, but an increase in synaptic latency was observed. Hence, these investigators also concluded that the Ia-motoneuron excitatory postsynaptic potential in the mammalian spinal cord is mediated by chemical transmission.

C. Chemical Transmission

With the advent of intracellular micropipette recording techniques, the group Ia-motoneuron excitatory postsynaptic potentials at first appeared to have the properties characteristic of chemically mediated synaptic transmission. Coombs et al. (59) reported that some Ia-motoneuron composite excitatory postsynaptic potentials were depressed or even reversed by depolarization and that they were associated with an increase in membrane conductance. Subsequently, Kuno (68) reported that the amplitude fluctuations of Ia-motoneuron single-fiber excitatory postsynaptic potentials could be described by classic quantal analysis. Hence, these authors concluded that the mechanism of junctional transmission was similar to that at a known chemical synapse, the neuromuscular junction. In subsequent investigations, serious questions were raised about whether the Ia-motoneuron synapse was a conventional chemical synapse. For instance, conductance changes could be shown in only a minority of excitatory postsynaptic potentials (102). Furthermore, various investigators were unable to demonstrate convincingly that Ia-motoneuron composite excitatory postsynaptic potentials have a reversal potential (104,167,168,189). Single-fiber excitatory postsynaptic potentials that have a time course indicative of a somatic site of generation also could not be reversed by large depolarizing currents (103,186). It has not been possible to demonstrate that the current generating the excitatory postsynaptic potential is ion-specific. Moreover, a neurotransmitter at this synapse has not been unequivocally identified. Finally, recent investigations indicate the possibility that transmission at a single Ia–motoneuron synapse may be all-or-none (71,148). Therefore, serious consideration has been given to the possibility that the Ia–motoneuron excitatory postsynaptic potential is mediated by electrical coupling, either alone or jointly, with chemical transmission.

However, accumulated evidence has provided convincing support for the hypothesis that junctional transmission at the Ia–motoneuron synapse is chemical. Engberg and Marshall (169) were able to demonstrate clearly a reversal potential using a double micropipette technique. In an investigation of synaptic latency, Munson and Sypert (75) directly demonstrated the existence of a "true" synaptic delay at the Ia–motoneuron synapse. Moreover, Krnjević et al. (188) demonstrated that the peak of the Ia–motoneuron excitatory postsynaptic potential was depressed and its rate of rise decreased when manganese and cobalt ions were electrophoretically applied outside alpha motoneurons. Since an electrical component would normally contribute to the rising phase of the excitatory postsynaptic potential, it should not be affected by these divalent cations. In isolated immature cat spinal cord, Shapovalov et al. (182) have also shown that the monosynaptic excitatory postsynaptic potential could be reversably abolished by perfusion with calcium-deficient, manganese-containing solutions. Furthermore, it has been shown that an unrealistically low value of resistivity of the synaptic cleft and subsynaptic membrane is required for significant electrical coupling to occur at the Ia–motoneuron synapse (47,104). Finally, all ultrastructural data indicate that the Ia–motoneuron synapse is a chemical synapse (30,48).

D. Functional Role of Group Ia–Motoneuron Synapse

The Ia–motoneuron synapse is the junctional mechanism for the powerful monosynaptic stretch reflex. Most theories have generally regarded the stretch reflex as part of a system for the servocontrol of limb position through which a discrepancy between the actual limb position (e.g., muscle length, muscle stiffness) and an intended position generates feedback activity that minimizes this error. However, it is an interesting fact that the function of this, the best known and most extensively studied of all reflex pathways involved in motor control, remains a subject of debate and much controversy (189,190).

III. SPINDLE GROUP II–MOTONEURON SYNAPSE

The secondary endings of muscle spindles are innervated by axons with conduction velocities in the group II range (191), that is, 24–72 m/sec. These axons have a peripheral diameter of 4–12 μm. Although there is some overlap between the conduction velocities of very rapidly conducting spindle group II afferents with very slowly conducting Ia afferents, spindle afferents conducting at less than 65 m/sec almost always innervate secondary endings (54). Conduction velocity is unreliable for spindle afferent classification in the range of ~65–85 m/sec.

The central actions of spindle group II afferents have been poorly understood, primarily because of the difficulty in activating them selectively using electrical stimulation and blocking techniques (1,191,192). In 1974, Fu et al. (14) and Fu and Schomburg (15) provided the first detailed electrophysiologic evidence of the location of the segmental terminals of spindle group II afferents in cat lumbosacral spinal cord. They used extracellular recording and microstimulation techniques to demonstrate that the major collateral branches of spindle group II afferents had slower conduction velocities than the parent axons and the major collateral branches of Ia afferents. Moreover, they reported that spindle group II afferents terminated in the dorsal horn and lamina IX (the motor nuclei). Nonetheless, it was not until the development of the spike-triggered averaging technique that the monosynaptic connections of spindle group II afferents with alpha motoneurons could be identified unequivocally.

Kirkwood and Sears (17,18) were the first to report the presence of a spindle group II monosynaptic projection to cat spinal alpha motoneurons. Stauffer et al. (193) confirmed this result and made the first quantitative investigation of the monosynaptic connections of medial gastrocnemius spindle group II afferents to triceps surae motoneurons. More recently, Munson and Sypert and associates (20,21,135) have greatly expanded the knowledge of the electrophysiology of the spindle group II-motoneuron synapses. Furthermore, Fyffe (16,194) has recently described the central segmental morphology of three cat triceps surae spindle group II afferents stained with HRP.

A. Functional Morphology

The only morphologic description of the intramedullary trajectories and terminations of spindle group II afferents has been recently accomplished by Fyffe (16,194), who injected three single identified triceps surae spindle group II stem axons in the dorsal funiculus with HRP. On entering the cat lumbosacral spinal cord, all three afferents bifurcated into ascending and descending stem axons. These stem axons give off about six major collaterals (4–5 μm, diameter) at the levels of the homonymous and heteronymous motoneuron pools. The branch spacing of the major collaterals is approximately 1 mm. Remarkably similar estimates of major collateral branch spacing were also obtained in recent electrophysiologic studies of spindle group II afferents (20; Fig. 8). The major collaterals descend directly to lamina IV before branching to innervate neurons in laminae IV and V. A second region of terminal arborization is developed in laminae VI and VII. Finally, a single axonal branch (0.8–1.2 μm, diameter) that is a continuation of the major collateral descends into the homonymous and heteronymous motoneuron pools. This latter branch to the motor nuclei is not always present and sometimes there are two branches descending to the motor nuclei. Unfortunately, the terminations in the ventral horn were too faint to permit a description of the synaptic boutons.

Spindle group II-motoneurons synaptic boutons have not been identified ultrastructurally. Conradi (30) has shown that two types of presynaptic boutons that terminate on alpha motoneurons disappear following dorsal rhizotomy in cats: type M-boutons and a subclass of S-boutons, which are characterized by their relatively large size and by the apposition of P-boutons. Recent electro-physiologic studies (20,21,135) have demonstrated substantial functional differences between group Ia–motoneuron and spindle group II–motoneuron synapses. These physiologic data, in light of Conradi's ultrastructural studies (30), are consistent with a hypothesis that Ia afferents may terminate on motoneurons as M-boutons and spindle group II afferents may terminate as the less numerous and smaller S-boutons. Critical testing of this hypothesis must ultimately depend on ultrastructural examination of identified and labeled Ia and spindle group II synaptic boutons in contact with alpha motoneurons.

B. Spindle Group II-Motoneuron Excitatory Postsynaptic Potentials

For many years, the generally accepted role for spindle group II afferents in segmental motor control was that of reflex excitation of flexor muscles with concurrent inhibition of extensors (195). This concept was based on the observations that stimulation of muscle nerves at group II strength generally resulted in a facilitation of the monosynaptic test reflex or as excitatory postsynaptic potential in flexor motoneurons and inhibitory postsynaptic potentials in extensor motoneurons (58,195,196). Hence, spindle group II afferents have been included in a wide range of afferents from muscle and other structures in a system termed flexor reflex afferents (FRA) (197). However, stimulation of muscle nerves has been also shown to elicit flexor inhibition and extensor excitation (196–198). More recently, Matthews (45) has suggested that the role of spindle group II afferents is autogenic excitation; that is, excitation of homonymous and heteronymous motoneurons via polysynaptic reflex pathways. Such widely divergent hypotheses have resulted from the inability to stimulate spindle group II afferents in isolation from either Ia afferents or other muscle afferents. With the advent of the spike-triggered averaging technique it became feasible to study monosynaptic action of single-spindle group II fibers on alpha motoneurons.

1. Monosynaptic Junctional Transmission

Recent studies of the central projections of single-spindle group II afferent fibers have led to the concept that transmission from spindle group II afferents to alpha motoneurons contains a monosynaptic component: the brief latency of spindle group II–motoneuron excitatory postsynaptic potentials (20,193), the persistence of spindle group II–motoneuron excitatory postsynaptic potentials in barbiturate-anesthetized animals (20) in which the activity of interneurons is depressed, the fact that spindle group II afferents may be antidromically activated by microstimulation in the motoneuron pool (15), and the recent demonstration that HRP-filled spindle group II fibers extend into the ventral horn motor nuclei (16,194). Moreover, Munson et al. (20) have demonstrated that single-trace spindle group II–motoneuron excitatory postsynaptic potentials are similar in amplitude, that is, the summed potential is not the result of occasional large-amplitude excitatory postsynaptic potentials summed with numerous failures, as would be expected if spindle group II–motoneuron transmission required an interneuron (Fig. 12). Unfortunately, the signal-to-noise ratio does not permit a detailed analysis of these excitatory postsynaptic potentials for either amplitude or latency fluctuations as has been attempted with Ia–motoneuron excitatory postsynaptic potentials.

2. Connectivity

Similar to group Ia afferents, single medial gastrocnemius spindle group II afferents have greater functional connections with homonymous (50%) than with heteronymous (17%) motoneurons (20,193; Table 3). Furthermore, the functional connectivity is based on afferent conduction velocity (20,21,135; Fig. 13). Faster conducting spindle group II afferents project to more motoneurons than do slowly conducting afferents. However, unlike Ia afferents (80), spindle group II afferents failed to demonstrate any specificity in connectivity for motor unit types (135). Maps of the location of homonymous motoneurons having functional connections with spindle group II afferents indicate that major collateral branches descend into the motoneuron pool at 1–1.5 mm intervals (20). The terminal arborization appears to be greater for rapidly conducting than for slowly conducting afferents.

3. Temporal Parameters

The temporal characteristics of single-fiber excitatory postsynaptic potentials generated in triceps surae motoneurons by spindle group II afferents are similar to Ia–motoneuron excitatory postsynaptic potentials (21; Fig. 12). These temporal parameters include: rise time and half-width and latencies of amplitude-matched single-fiber excitatory postsynaptic potential samples (Table 3). Since rise time, half-widths, and latency can be used to estimate the electrotonic

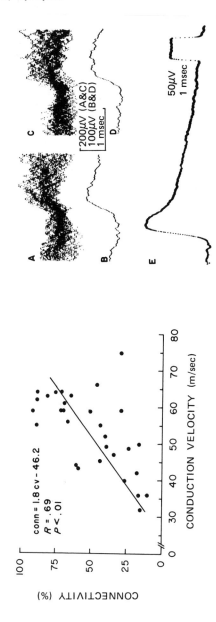

Figure 12 Left: Scatter plot of relationship of spindle group II afferent fiber conduction velocity to cat MG spindle group II-motoneuron connectivity. Right (A–E): superimposed single-trace averaged MG spindle group II single-fiber EPSPs recorded in an MG motoneuron. A,C, superimpositions of 25 single-trace EPSPs; B,D, algebraic sums of potentials of A and C, respectively; E, summation of 1024 sweeps for same afferent-motoneuron combination as A–D above. (Additional details in text.)

Table 3 Parameters of EPSPs Generated by Single MG Spindle Group II Afferents in MG and LG/S Motoneurons[a]

	MG[b] motoneurons	LG/S[c] motoneurons	P
Functional connectivity (%)	50.4 10–91 (196/389)	17.1 0.75 (22/129)	<0.005
EPSP amplitude (μV)	24.3 ± 1.6 3–136 (164)	17.0 ± 3.9 3–84 (22)	NS[d]
10–90% rise time (msec)	0.65 ± 0.04 0.13–2.42 (160)	0.72 ± 0.10 0.12–1.72 (22)	NS
Half-width (msec)	3.88 ± 0.24 0.49–14.04 (143)	2.76 ± 0.51 0.44–7.60 (16)	NS
EPSP latency (msec)	0.58 ± 0.02 0.26–1.52 (86)	0.49 ± 0.07 0.20–0.99 (10)	NS

[a]Values are means ±SE for fast and slow afferents combined. The range is given below the mean values. Numbers in parentheses give the sample size. (In a few cases, accurate EPSP parameters could not be determined.)
[b]Medial gastrocnemius.
[c]Lateral gastrocnemius/soleus.
[d]Not significant.

location of presynaptic terminals, it appears that the active terminals of spindle group II and Ia afferent fibers are similarly distributed over the motoneuron soma-dendritic membrane. The size or conduction velocity of spindle afferent fibers also does not appear to influence the location of their terminations on motoneurons.

4. Amplitude

Virtually all medial gastrocnemius spindle group II single-fiber excitatory post-synaptic potentials are <70 μV (Table 3), whereas only about one half of medial gastrocnemius group Ia single-fiber excitatory postsynaptic potentials are <70 μV (Table 2). Similar to Ia afferents, the mean amplitude of medial gastrocnemius spindle group II excitatory postsynaptic potentials is > (24 μV) in homonymous than in heteronymous (17 μV) motoneurons (20,193). However, in contrast with Ia-motoneuron single-fiber excitatory postsynaptic potentials, the mean amplitude of excitatory postsynaptic potentials elicited by single-spindle group II afferents was not related to afferent conduction velocity (20). Furthermore, the amplitude of medial gastrocnemius spindle group II-moto-neuron excitatory postsynaptic potentials was found to have no significant relationship to motoneuron conduction velocity, motoneuron R_N, motoneuron rheobase, motor unit type, or the maximum tetanic tension of the motor unit (20,135). Hence, it appears that the amplitude of a single-spindle group II excitatory postsynaptic potentials does not relate to the size, excitability, or muscle unit strength of the motoneuron in which it is generated.

The observation that spindle group II single-fiber excitatory postsynaptic potential amplitude does not vary systematically over the fivefold range of motoneuron R_N (135) suggests that, on the average, an equal density of spindle group II terminals exists on all motoneurons regardless of size or type (Fig. 10). The increasing number of terminals on larger cells provides proportionately greater synaptic current, offsetting the reduced R_N and producing excitatory postsynaptic potentials of equal size (assuming equal distribution and efficacy of terminals; however, see Sec. II.B.2.d). In contrast, the density of group Ia-motoneuron synapses is apparently greater on small cells, as judged by their larger excitatory postsynaptic potentials (80,91,199; Fig. 10). This hypothesis represents an interesting problem for synaptogenesis as well as a striking difference in the organization of spindle group Ia and group II synaptic input to motoneurons.

C. Functional Role of Spindle Group II-Motoneuron Synapse

Present data support the hypothesis that like the segmental role of the Ia afferent system, one segmental role of the spindle group II afferent system is autogenous excitation (45). However, major differences have been observed between the homonymous projections of group Ia and group II spindle afferents. First, group Ia afferents project to greater numbers of fatigue-resistant than to fatigue-sensitive motor units (80,75a). Second, Ia afferents generate single-fiber excitatory postsynaptic potentials which are larger in S than in FR units and larger in FR than in FF units (80,75a), while spindle group II afferents generate single-fiber excitatory postsynaptic potentials of equal amplitude in motoneurons of all motor unit types (135). Third, while larger Ia afferents generate larger homonymous excitatory postsynaptic potentials than do smaller Ia afferents (50,21), large and small spindle group II afferents generate homonymous single fiber excitatory postsynaptic potentials of equal amplitude (20). These observations indicate that the differences in synaptic organization between group Ia and II spindle afferents are substantial. It appears that the monosynaptic Ia system functions most powerfully in segmental motor control by recruiting motor units capable of frequent or sustained activity (the S and FR units), whereas the monosynaptic spindle group II system serves a more subtle and diffuse biasing function (135).

IV. OTHER EXCITATORY SYNAPSES

Because of formidable technical difficulties of either intracellular recording from identified spinal interneurons and/or eliciting pure monosynaptic inputs to these neurons from a given input, there is much less detailed information about spinal excitatory synapses other than the monosynaptic input to alpha motoneurons from the spindle afferents. As an organizing framework, the excitatory synapses will be grouped on the basis of the destination of the presynaptic elements.

From a quantitative standpoint, most of the excitatory synapses on alpha motoneurons are derived from "last-order interneurons." As mentioned previously, the spindle afferents (group Ia and group II) are the only primary afferent fibers to terminate on motoneurons. Relatively few excitatory synapses on motoneurons arise from descending long-axon systems. However, all of the primary afferent systems, and a majority of suprasegmental descending systems elicit excitatory postsynaptic potentials in neurons on which they terminate (46,62). A simplified schematic representation of this organization of spinal cord excitatory transmission to alpha motoneurons is present in Figure 13.

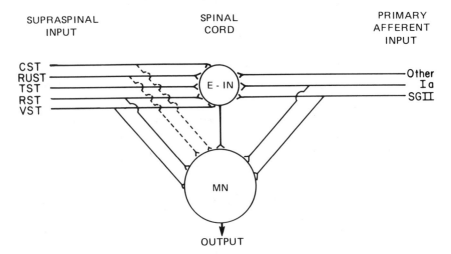

Figure 13 Simplified schematic diagram of excitatory synaptic circuitry in the spinal cord. In this scheme the single excitatory interneuron illustrated represents both single interneurons and chains of excitatory interneurons. (Additional details in text.)

A. Interneuronal Input

All species of primary afferents and descending systems having any relation to motor control project to alpha motoneurons via segmental interneurons (46,62, 90,200). Most primary afferents having excitatory effects on motoneurons, with the exception of the spindle afferents, appear to project through at least two interneurons (i.e., a minimum trisynaptic linkage). Moreover, electrical activation of diverse species of afferent fibers in peripheral nerves or supraspinal elements generally elicit complex admixtures of excitatory postsynaptic potentials and inhibitory postsynaptic potentials. Thus, the results of such studies depend critically upon experimental conditions and are exceedingly difficult to interpret.

One fruitful line of investigation of this complex interneuronal circuitry has been directed to identification and examination of interneurons that terminate directly on alpha motoneurons. These interneurons have been termed last-order interneurons (201). For example, Kuno and Weakly (202) reported that monosynaptic excitatory postsynaptic potentials elicited in motoneurons by microstimulation of local interneurons have a reversal potential more negative ($\sim$ -30 mV) than that of Ia composite excitatory postsynaptic potentials (59,169). Furthermore, they found that interneuronal excitatory postsynaptic potentials have more prominent frequency potentiation than Ia excitatory postsynaptic potentials, with a relative enhancement of the probability of unit excitatory postsynaptic potential occurrence. Since interneurons have a tendency to fire in high-frequency bursts of impulses, such facilitation should have functional significance (202).

B. Supraspinal Input

Five major suprasegmental systems related to motor control project to the spinal cord via long descending axons: the vestibulospinal (VST), the reticulospinal (RST), the tectospinal (TST), the rubrospinal (RuST), and the corticospinal (CST) tracts (203). The reticulospinal, vestibulospinal, and tectospinal tracts are largely uncrossed, whereas the rubrospinal and corticospinal tracts are largely crossed pathways. Of these systems, all except the tectospinal tract appear to have some fibers that yield monosynaptic excitatory terminations on some motoneurons in some mammalian species (204).

The vestibulospinal tract system contains two distinct descending subdivisions: the lateral (LVST) and the medial (MVST) pathways. The lateral vestibulospinal tract originates in Deiter's nucleus and gives rise to fast-conducting axons (90-140 m/sec) that descend in the ipsilateral ventral funiculus to reach all levels of the spinal cord (205,206). Electrophysiologic investigations indicate that lateral vestibulospinal tract axons produce monosynaptic excitatory postsynaptic potential in the neck and back and hindlimb extensor, but not in the forelimb motoneurons of the cat (206,207). Maximal monosynaptic composite excitatory postsynaptic potentials elicited by lateral vestibulospinal tract stimulation are small (usually <2 mV) and exhibit little enhancement or depression with repetitive stimulation compared to Ia-motoneuron excitatory postsynaptic potentials (207). The time course of lateral vestibulospinal tract composite excitatory postsynaptic potentials is the same or slightly briefer than Ia-motoneuron excitatory postsynaptic potentials, indicating that lateral vestibulospinal tract terminations are largely on the proximal half of the motoneuron dendrites (207).

The cat medial vestibulospinal tract originates largely in the medial vestibular nucleus, which gives rise to rapidly conducting axons that descend in the medial longitudinal fusciculus (MLF) to terminate predominantly in the cervical and upper thoracic spinal cord (205). Stimulation of the medial vestibulospinal tract has been reported to produce some monosynaptic excitatory postsynaptic potentials in some back and neck motoneurons (206).

The pontine and bulbar reticular formation gives rise to axons that descend to all levels of the cat spinal cord via the medial tegmentum or medial longitudinal funiculus (205). Activation of these reticulospinal tract axons have been reported to elicit small monosynaptic composite excitatory postsynaptic potentials in the neck and back and forelimb flexor and extensor and hindlimb flexor motoneurons (206-209).

The red nucleus gives rise to rubrospinal tract axons that cross in the pontomesencephalic brainstem to descend in the contralateral dorsolateral funiculus to terminate at all levels of the spinal cord (205). Although rubrospinal tract monosynaptic projections to alpha motoneurons are rare in the cat, very small amplitude rubrospinal tract–motoneuron excitatory postsynaptic potentials have been reported in primate distal hindlimb motoneurons (210).

The corticospinal tract originates from the somatosensory cortex and descends predominantly via the ipsilateral ventral funiculus to reach all levels of the spinal cord (205). Analogous to the rubrospinal tract, the corticospinal tract makes some monosynaptic excitatory connections with alpha motoneurons in primates but not in the cat (211,212).

V. COMMENTS

This chapter has dealt primarily with a very large and growing literature on the functional properties of excitatory synapses in the mammalian spinal cord. The organizational scheme of this chapter used firstly the postsynaptic element, then secondly the origin of the presynaptic element to categorize excitatory synapses. The emphasis on intracellular recording techniques and cellular neurophysiology was requisite as this approach has generated the most systematic analysis of spinal cord excitatory synapses. Moreover, the concentrated attention devoted to the group Ia-motoneuron synapse is consistent with the fact that more is known regarding this excitatory synapse than any other central synapse. Notwithstanding the considerable contributions that convention electrophysiologic and morphologic techniques have made toward understanding central junctional transmission, there remain numerous important unresolved issues. These unresolved problems result in part from the formidable difficulties that are encountered by such investigations in the intact spinal cord. Progress in the development of spinal cord slice preparations and tissue culture preparations of spinal cord cells and should overcome some of the obstacles encountered in vivo. However, it remains quite likely that the final answers about the basic mechanisms of central synaptic transmission will still have to come from in vivo studies of the intact, functioning spinal cord. Hence, the resolution of many critical questions, such as the nature of the unit excitatory postsynaptic potentials, the invasion of terminals by presynaptic impulses, and the factors determining synaptic efficacy, will require the development of new research strategies and methods.

ACKNOWLEDGMENTS

This work was supported by the Veterans Administration MRS (821-103) and RERDS (822-124) and the National Institute of Neurological and Communicative Disorders and Stroke (NS 15913).

REFERENCES

1. Matthews, P. B. C. (1972). *Mammalian Muscle Receptors and Their Central Actions*. Williams & Wilkins, Baltimore.
2. Ramon y Cajal, S. (1909). *Histologie du Système de l'Homme et des Vertébrés*. Maloine, Paris.
3. Scheibel, M. E., and Scheibel A. B. (1969). Terminal patterns in cat spinal cord. III. Primary afferent collaterals. *Brain Res. 13*:417–443.
4. Scheibel, M. E., and Scheibel, A. B. (1970). Organization of spinal motoneuron dendrites in bundles. *Exp. Neurol. 38*:106–112.
5. Szentágothai, J. (1958). The anatomical basis of synaptic transmission of excitation and inhibition of motoneurons. *Acta Morphol. Acad. Sci. Hung. 8*:287–309.
6. Sprague, J. M. (1958). The distribution of dorsal root fibers on motor cells in lumbosacral spinal cord of the cat and the site of excitatory and inhibitory terminals in monosynaptic pathways. *Proc. R. Soc. Lond. (Biol.) 149*:534–556.
7. Szentágothai, J. (1967). Synaptic architecture of the spinal motoneuron pool. In *Recent Advances in Clinical Neurophysiology*, L. Widen (Ed.), Elsevier, Amsterdam, pp. 4–19.

8. Szentágothai, J. (1964). Neuronal and synaptic arrrangement in the substantia gelatinosa Rolandi. *J. Comp. Neurol. 122*:219–239.

9. Sterling, P., and Kuypers, H. G. J. M. (1967). Anatomical organization of the brachial spinal cord of the cat. II. The motoneuron plexus. *Brain Res. 4*:16–32.

10. Sprague, J. M. (1958). The distribution of dorsal root fibres on motor cells in the lumbosacral spinal cord of the cat, and the site of excitatory and inhibitory terminals in monosynaptic pathways. *Proc. R. Soc. Lond. (Biol.) 149*:534–556.

11. Iles, J. F. (1976). Central terminations of muscle afferents on motoneurons in the cat spinal cord. *J. Physiol. (Lond.) 262*:91–117.

12. Proshansky, E., and Egger, M. D. (1977). Staining of the dorsal root projection to the cat's dorsal horn by anterograde movement of horseradish peroxidase. *Neurosci. Lett. 5*:103–110.

13. Redman, S., and Walmsley, B. (1980). A combined electrophysiological and anatomical location of single group Ia fibre connections with cat spinal motoneurones. *J. Physiol. (Lond.) 308*:99P.

14. Fu, T. C., Santini, M., and Schomberg, E. D. (1974). Characteristics and distribution of spinal focal synaptic potentials generated by group II muscle afferents. *Acta Physiol. Scand. 91*:298–313.

15. Fu, T. C., and Schomberg, E. G. (1974). Electrophysiological investigation of the projection of secondary muscle spindle afferents in the cat spinal cord. *Acta Physiol. Scand. 91*:314–329.

16. Fyffe, R. E. W. (1979). The morphology of group II muscle afferent fibre collaterals. *J. Physiol. (Lond.) 296*:39–40P.

17. Kirkwood, P. A., and Sears, T. A. (1974). Monosynaptic excitation of motoneurons from secondary endings of muscle spindles. *Nature 252*:243–244.

18. Kirkwood, P. A., and Sears, T. A. (1975). Monosynaptic excitation of motoneurons from muscle spindle secondary endings of intercostal and triceps surae muscles in the cat. *J. Physiol. (Lond.) 245*:64–66P.

19. Watt, D. G. D., Stauffer, E. K. Taylor, A., Reinking, R. M., and Stuart, D. G. (1976). Analysis of muscle receptor connections by spike-triggering averaging. I. Spindle primary and tendon organ afferents. *J. Neurophysiol. 38*:1375–1392.

20. Munson, J. B., Fleshman, J. W., and Sypert, G. W. (1980). Properties of single fiber spindle group II EPSPs in triceps surae motoneurons. *J. Neurophysiol. 44*:713–725.

21. Sypert, G. W., Fleshman, J. W., and Munson, J. B. (1980). Comparison of monosynaptic actions of medial gastrocnemius group Ia and group II muscle spindle afferents on triceps surae motoneurons. *J. Neurophysiol. 44*:726–738.

22. Brown, A. G., and Fyffe, R. E. W. (1978). The morphology of group Ia afferent fibre collaterals in the spinal cord of the cat. *J. Physiol. (Lond.) 174*:111–127.

23. Hongo, T., Ishizuka, N., Mannen, H., and Sasaki, S. (1978). Axonal trajectory of single group Ia and Ib fibers in the cat spinal cord. *Neurosci. Lett.* 8:321–328.
24. Burke, R. E., Walmsley, B., and Hodgson, J. A. (1979). HRP anatomy of group Ia afferent contacts on alpha motoneurons. *Brain Res.* 160:347–352.
25. Burke, R. E., Walmsley, B., and Hodgson, J. A. (1979). Structural-functional relations in monosynaptic action on spinal motoneurons. In *Integration in the Nervous System*, H. Asanuma and V. J. Wilson (Eds.), Igaku-Shoin, Tokyo, pp. 27–45.
26. Ishizuka, N., Mannen, H. Hongo, T., and Sasaki, S. (1979). Trajectory of group Ia afferent fibers stained with horseradish peroxidase in the lumbosacral spinal cord of the cat: Three dimensional reconstructions from serial sections. *J. Comp. Neurol.* 186:189–212.
27. Brown, A. G., and Fyffe, R. E. W. (1981). Direct observations on the contacts made between Ia afferent fibres and α-motoneurones in cat's lumbosacral spinal cord. *J. Physiol. (Lond.)* 313:121–140.
28. Conradi, S. (1969). Ultrastructure and distribution of neuronal and glial elements on the motoneuron surface in the lumbosacral spinal cord of the adult cat. *Acta Physiol. Scand.* (Suppl.) 332:5–48.
29. Conradi, S. (1969). Ultrastructure and distribution of neuronal and glial elements on the surface of the proximal part of a motoneuron dendrite, as analyzed by serial sections. *Acta Physiol. Scand.* (Suppl.) 332:49–64.
30. Conradi, S. (1969). Ultrastructure of dorsal root boutons on lumbosacral motoneurons of the adult cat. *Acta Physiol. Scand.* (Suppl.) 332:85–115.
31. Waxman, S. G., and Bennett, M. V. L. (1972). Relative conduction velocities of small myelinated and non-myelinated fibres in the central nervous system. *Nature New Biol.* 238:217–219.
32. Barrett, J. N., and Crill, W. E. (1974). Specific membrane properties of cat motoneurones. *J. Physiol. (Lond.)* 239:301–324.
33. Aitken, J. T., and Bridger, J. E. (1962). Neuron size and neuron population density in the lumbosacral region of the cat's spinal cord. *J. Anat.* 95:38–53.
34. Gelfan, S., Kao, G., and Ruchkin, D. S. (1970). The dendritic tree of spinal neurons. *J. Comp. Neurol.* 139:385–411.
35. Barrett, J. N., and Crill, W. E. (1974). Influence of dendritic location and membrane properties on the effectiveness of synapses in cat motoneurones. *J. Physiol. (Lond.)* 239:325–345.
36. Young, J. Z. (1958). Anatomical considerations. *Electroencephalogr. Clin. Neurophysiol.* (Suppl.) 10:9–11.
37. Romanes, G. J. (1951). The motor cell columns of the lumbo-sacral spinal cord of the cat. *J. Comp. Neurol.* 94:313–363.
38. Kernell, D. (1966). Input resistance, electrical excitability, and size of ventral horn cells in cat spinal cord. *Science* 152:1627–1640.

39. Lux, H. D., Schubert, P., and Kreutzberg, G. W. (1970). Direct matching of morphological and electrophysiological data in cat spinal motoneurons. In *Excitatory Synaptic Mechanisms*, P. Anderson and J. K. S. Jansen (Eds.), Universitetsforlaget, Oslo, pp. 189–198.

40. Rall, W. (1977). Core conductor theory and cable properties of neurons. In *Handbook of Physiology*, vol. I, E. R. Kandel (Ed.), American Physiological Society, Bethesda, Maryland, pp. 39–97.

41. Gelfan, S., and Rapisarda, A. G. (1964). Synaptic density on spinal neurons of normal dogs and dogs with experimental hindlimb rigidity. *J. Comp. Neurol. 123*:73–95.

42. Wyckoff, R. W. G., and Young, J. Z. (1955). The motor neuron surface. *Proc. R. Soc. Lond. (Biol.) 144*:440–450.

43. Kuno, M., and Llínas, R. (1970). Enhancement of synaptic transmission by dendritic potentials in chromatolyzed motoneurones of the cat. *J. Physiol. (Lond.) 210*:807–821.

44. Kuno, M., and Llínas, R. (1970). Alterations of synaptic action in chromatolysed motoneurones of the cat. *J. Physiol. (Lond.) 210*:823–383.

45. Matthews, P. B. C. (1969). Evidence that the secondary as well as the primary endings of the muscle spindles may be responsible for the tonic stretch reflex of the decerebrate cat. *J. Physiol. (Lond.) 204*:365–393.

46. Burke, R. E., and Rudomín, P. (1977). Spinal neurons and synapses. In *Handbook of Physiology*, vol. I, E. R. Kandel (Ed.), American Physiological Society, Bethesda, Maryland, pp. 877–944.

47. Redman, S. J. (1979). Junctional mechanisms at group Ia synapses. *Prog. Neurobiol. 12*:33–83.

48. McLaughlin, B. J. (1972). Dorsal root projections to the motor nuclei in the cat spinal cord. *J. Comp. Neurol. 144*:461–474.

49. Burke, R. E. (1967). Composite nature of the monosynaptic excitatory post-synaptic potential. *J. Neurophysiol. 30*:1114–1126.

50. Mendell, L. M., and Henneman, E. (1971). Terminals of single Ia fibers: Location, density, and distribution within a pool of 300 homonymous motoneurons. *J. Neurophysiol. 34*:171–187.

51. Jack, J. J. B., Miller, S., Porter, R., and Redman, S. J. (1971). The time course of minimal excitatory post-synaptic potentials evoked in spinal motorneurones by group Ia afferent fibers. *J. Physiol. (Lond.) 215*:353–380.

52. Iansek, R., and Redman, S. J. (1973). The amplitude, time course and charge of unitary excitatory post-synaptic potentials evoked in spinal motoneuron dendrites. *J. Physiol. (Lond.) 234*:665–688.

53. Kuno, M. (1964). Mechanism of facilitation and depression of the excitatory synaptic potential in spinal motoneurons. *J. Physiol. (Lond.) 175*: 100–112.

54. Matthews, B. H. C. (1933). Nerve endings in mammalian muscle. *J. Physiol. (Lond.) 78*:1–53.

55. Lloyd, D. P. C., and McIntyre, A. K. (1949). On the origin of dorsal root potentials. *J. Gen. Physiol. 32*:409–443.

56. Lloyd, D. P. C. (1943). Reflex action in relation to pattern and peripheral source of afferent stimulation. *J. Neurophysiol.* 6:111–120.
57. Lloyd, D. P. C. (1949). Post-tetanic potentiation of response in monosynaptic reflex pathways of the spinal cord. *J. Gen. Physiol.* 33:147–170.
58. Brock, L. G., Coombs, J. S., and Eccles, J. C. (1952). The recording of potentials from motoneurons with an intracellular electrode. *J. Physiol. (Lond.) 117*:431–460.
59. Coombs, J. S., Eccles, J. C., and Fatt, P. (1955). The electrical properties of the motoneurone membrane. *J. Physiol. (Lond.) 130*:291–325.
60. Eccles, J. C. (1957). *The Physiology of Nerve Cells*, Johns Hopkins Press, Baltimore.
61. Eccles, J. C. (1961). Membrane time constants of cat motoneurons and time courses of synaptic actions. *Exp. Neurol.* 4:1–22.
62. Eccles, J. C. (1964). *The Physiology of Synapses*. Academic Press, New York.
63. Lundberg, A., and Winsbury, G. (1960). Selective adequate activation of large afferents from muscle spindles and Golgi tendon organs. *Acta Physiol. Scand.* 49:155–164.
64. Stuart, D. G., Willis, W. J., and Reinking, R. M. (1971). Stretch-evoked excitatory postsynaptic potentials in motoneurons. *Brain Res. 33*:115–125.
65. Burke, R. E., and Nelson, P. G. (1966). Synaptic activity in motoneurons during natural stimulation of muscle spindles. *Science 151*:1088–1091.
66. Burke, R. E. (1968). Group Ia synaptic input to fast and slow twitch motor units of cat triceps surae. *J. Physiol. (Lond.) 196*:605–630.
67. Mendell, L. M., and Henneman, E. (1968). Terminals of single Ia fibers: Distribution within a pool of 300 homonymous motor neurons. *Science 160*:96–98.
68. Kuno, M. (1964). Quantal components of excitatory synaptic potentials in spinal motoneurones. *J. Physiol. (Lond.) 175*:81–99.
69. Kuno, M., and Miyahara, J. T. (1969). Analysis of synaptic efficacy in spinal motoneurones from "quantum" aspects. *J. Physiol. (Lond.) 201*:479–493.
70. Mendell, L. M., and Weiner, R. (1976). Analysis of pairs of individual Ia–EPSPs in single motoneurones. *J. Physiol. (Lond.) 255*:81–104.
71. Edwards, F. R., Redman, S. J., and Walmsley, B. (1976). Statistical fluctuations in charge transfer at Ia synapses on spinal motoneurones. *J. Physiol. (Lond.) 259*:665–688.
72. Jack, J. J. B., Miller, S., Porter, R., and Redman, S. J. (1970). The distribution of group Ia synapses on lumbrosacral spinal motoneurones in the cat. In *Excitatory Synaptic Mechanisms*, P. Anderson and J. K. S. Jansen (Eds.), Universitetsforlaget, Oslo, pp. 199–205.
73. Munson, J. B., and Sypert, G. W. (1978). Latency-rise time relationship in unitary postsynaptic potentials. *Brain Res. 151*:404–408.
74. Munson, J. B., and Sypert, G. W. (1979). Properties of single central Ia fibers projecting to motoneurones. *J. Physiol. (Lond.) 296*:315–328.

75.   Munson, J. B., and Sypert, G. W. (1979). Properties of single fiber excitatory post-synaptic potentials in triceps surae motoneurones. *J. Physiol. (Lond.) 296*:329-342.

75a. Harrison, P. J., and Taylor, A. (1981). Individual excitatory post-synaptic potentials due to muscle spindle Ia afferents in cat triceps surae motoneurones. *J. Physiol. (Lond.) 312*:455-470.

75b. Collins, W. F., III, and Mendell, L. M. (1981). Frequency dependence of Ia-motoneuron EPSPs. *Soc. Neursoci. Abstr. 7*:438.

76.   Renshaw, B., Forbes, A., and Morison, B. R. (1940). Activity of isocortex and hippocampus: Electrical studies with microelectrodes. *J. Neurophysiol. 3*:74-105.

77.   Brooks, C. Mc.C., and Eccles, J. C. (1947). Electrical investigation of the monosynaptic pathway through the spinal cord. *J. Neurophysiol. 10*: 251-274.

78.   Lorente de No, R. (1947). A study of nerve physiology. Studies from the Rockefeller Institute for Medical Research, vol. 132, New York, pp. 384-471.

79.   Katz, B., and Miledi, R. (1965). Propagation of electric activity in motor nerve terminals. *Proc. R. Soc. Lond. (Biol.) 161*:453-482.

80.   Fleshman, J. W., Munson, J. B., and Sypert, G. W. (1981). Homonymous projection of individual group Ia-fibers to physiologically characterized medial gastrocnemius motoneurons in the cat. *J. Neurophysiol. 46*:1339-1348.

81.   Rall, W. (1967). Distinguishing theoretical synaptic potentials computed for different soma-dendritic distributions of synaptic input. *J. Neurophysiol. 30*:1138-1168.

82.   Jack, J. J. B., and Redman, S. J. (1971). The propagation of transient potentials in some linear cable structures. *J. Physiol. (Lond.) 215*:283-320.

83.   Jack, J. J. B., and Redman, S. J. (1971). An electrical description of the motoneurone, and its application to the analysis of synaptic potentials. *J. Physiol. (Lond.) 215*:321-352.

84.   Iansek, R., and Redman, S. J. (1973). An analysis of the cable properties of spinal motoneurones using a brief intracellular current pulse. *J. Physiol. (Lond.) 234*:613-636.

85.   Edwards, F. R., Redman, S. J., and Walmsley, B. (1976). The effect of polarizing currents on unitary Ia excitatory postsynaptic potentials evoked in spinal motoneurones. *J. Physiol. (Lond.) 259*:705-723.

86.   Hursh, J. B. (1939). Conduction velocity and diameter of nerve fibers. *Am. J. Physiol. 127*:131-139.

87.   Eccles, J. C., Fatt, P., Landgren, S., and Winsbury, G. J. (1954). Spinal cord potentials generated by volley in the large muscle afferents. *J. Physiol. (Lond.) 125*:590-606.

88.   Wall, P. D., and Werman, R. (1976). The physiology and anatomy of long ranging afferent fibres within the spinal cord. *J. Physiol. (Lond.) 255*: 321-334.

89. Eccles, R. M., and Lundberg, A. (1958). Integrative pattern of Ia synaptic actions of motoneurones of hip and knee muscles. *J. Physiol. (Lond.) 144*: 271-298.

90. Eccles, J. C., Eccles, R. M., and Lundberg, A. (1957). The convergence of monosynaptic excitatory afferents onto many different species of alpha motoneurones. *J. Physiol. (Lond.) 137*:22-50.

91. Burke, R. E. (1968). Firing patterns of gastrocnemius motor units in the decerebrate cat. *J. Physiol. (Lond.) 196*:631-654.

92. Zengle, J. E., Reid, S. A., Sypert, G. W., and Munson, J. B. (1983). Presynaptic inhibition, EPSP amplitude and motor unit type in triceps surae motoneurons. *J. Neurophysiol. 49*:922-931.

93. Henneman, E., Somjen, G., and Carpenter, D. O. (1965). Excitability and inhibitibility of motoneurons of different sizes. *J. Neurophysiol. 28*:599-620.

94. Burke, R. E., and ten Bruggencate, G. (1971). Electrotonic characteristics of alpha motoneurones of varying size. *J. Physiol. (Lond.) 212*:1-20.

95. Burke, R. E., Levine, D. N., Salcman, M., and Tsairis, P. (1974). Motor units in cat soleus muscle: Physiological, histochemical and morphological characteristics. *J. Physiol. (Lond.) 238*:503-514.

96. Burke, R. E., Levine, D. N., Zajac, F. E., Tsairis, P., and Engel, W. K. (1971). Mammalian motor units: Physiological-histochemical correlation in three types in cat gastrocnemius. *Science 174*:709-712.

97. Burke, R. E., Levine, D. N., Tsairis, P., and Zajac, F. E., III. (1973). Physiological types and histochemical profiles in motor units of the cat gastrocnemius. *J. Physiol. (Lond.) 234*:723-748.

98. Sypert, G. W., and Munson, J. B. (1981). Basis of segmental motor control: Motoneuron size or motor unit type? *Neurosurgery 8*:608-621.

99. Burke, R. E. (1981). Motor units: Anatomy, physiology, and functional organization. In *Handbook of Physiology*, vol. II, J. M. Brookhart and V. B. Mountcastle (Eds.), American Physiological Society, Bethesda, Maryland, pp. 345-422.

100. Henneman, E., and Mendell, L. M. (1981). Functional organization of motoneuron pool and its inputs. In *Handbook of Physiology*, vol. II, J. M. Brookhart and V. B. Mountcastle (Eds.), American Physiological Society, Bethesda, Maryland, pp. 423-507.

101. Fatt, P. (1957). Sequence of events in synaptic activation of a motoneurone. *J. Neurophysiol. 20*:61-80.

102. Smith, T. G., Wuerker, R. B., and Frank, K. (1967). Membrane impedance changes during synaptic transmission in cat spinal motoneurons. *J. Neurophysiol. 30*:1072-1096.

103. Nelson, P. G., and Frank, K. (1967). Anomalous rectification in cat spinal motoneurons and effect of polarizing currents on excitatory postsynaptic potentials. *J. Neurophysiol. 30*:1097-1113.

104. Rall, W., Burke, R. E., Smith, R. G., Nelson, P. G., and Frank, K. (1967). Dendritic location of synapses and possible mechanisms for the monosynaptic EPSP in motoneurons. *J. Neurophysiol. 30*:1169-1193.

105. Rall, W. (1959). Branching dendritic trees and motoneuron membrane resistivity. *Exp. Neurol. 1*:491-527.

106. Rall, W. (1960). Membrane potential transients and membrane time constant of motoneurons. *Exp. Neurol.* 2:503–532.
107. Rall, W. (1962). Theory of physiological properties of dendrites. *Ann. N.Y. Acad. Sci.* 96:1071–1092.
108. Rall, W. (1969). Time constants and electric length of membrane cylinders and neurons. *Biophys. J.* 9:1483–1508.
109. Rall, W., and Rinzel, J. (1973). Branch input resistance and steady attenuation for input to one branch of a dendritic neuron model. *Biophys. J.* 13:648–688.
110. Hodgkin, A. A., and Huxley, A. F. (1952). A quantitative description of membrane current and its application to conduction and excitation in nerve. *J. Physiol. (Lond.)* 117:500–544.
111. Cole, K. C. (1968). *Membranes, Ions and Impulses*, University of California Press, Berkeley.
112. Nelson, P. G., and Lux, H.-D. (1970). Some electrical measurements of motoneuron parameters. *Biophys. J.* 10:55–73.
113. Redman, S. J. (1973). The attenuation of passively propagating dendritic potentials in a motoneurone cable model. *J. Physiol. (Lond.)* 234:637–664.
114. Frank, K., and Fuortes, M. G. F. (1956). Stimulation of spinal motoneurones with intracellular electrodes. *J. Physiol. (Lond.)* 134:451–470.
115. Gorman, A. L. F., and Mirolli, M. (1972). The geometrical factors determining the electrotonic properties of a molluscan neurone. *J. Physiol. (Lond.)* 222:227–249.
116. Iansek, R., and Redman, S. J. (1973). The amplitude, time course and charge of unitary excitatory post-synaptic potentials evoked in spinal motoneurone dendrites. *J. Physiol. (Lond.)* 234:665–688.
117. Zucker, R. S. (1973). Theoretical implications of the size principle of motoneuron recruitment. *J. Theor. Biol.* 38:587–596.
118. Barrett, J. N. (1975). Motoneuron dendrites: Role in synaptic integration. *Fed. Proc.* 34:1398–1407.
119. Willis, W. D., Letbetter, W. D., and Thompson, W. M. (1968). A system of neurons in the mammalian spinal cord. *Brain Res.* 9:152–155.
120. Edwards, F. R., Redman, S. J., and Walmsley, B. (1976). Non-quantal fluctuations and transmission failures in charge transfer at Ia synapses on spinal motoneurones. *J. Physiol. (Lond.)* 259:689–704.
121. Nelson, S. G., and Mendell, L. M. (1978). Projection of single knee flexor Ia fibers to homonymous and heteronymous motoneurons. *J. Neurophysiol.* 41:778–787.
122. Scott, J. G., and Mendell, L. M. (1976). Individual EPSPs produced by single triceps surae Ia afferent fibers in homonymous and heteronymous motoneurons. *J. Neurophysiol.* 39:679–692.
123. Chin, N. K., Cope, M., and Pang, M. (1962). Number and distribution of spindle capsules in seven hindlimb muscles of the cat. In *Symposium on Muscle Receptors*, D. Barker (Ed.), Hong Kong University Press, pp. 241–248.

124. Boyd, A. I., and Davey, M. R. (1968). *Composition of Peripheral Nerves*, Edinburgh, Livingston.
125. Burke, R. E., Strick, P. L., Kanda, K., Kim, C. C., and Walmsley, B. (1977). Anatomy of medial gastrocnemius and soleus motor nuclei in cat spinal cord. *J. Neurophysiol. 40*:667–680.
126. Taylor, A., Watt, D. G. D., Stauffer, E. R., Reinking, R. M., and Stuart, D. G. (1976). Use of afferent triggered averaging to study the central connections of muscle spindle afferents. *Prog. Brain Res. 44*:171–183.
127. Nelson, S. G., Collatos, T. C., Niechaj, A., and Mendell, L. M. (1979). Immediate increase in Ia-motoneuron synaptic transmission caudal to spinal cord transection. *J. Neurophysiol. 42*:655–664.
128. Sypert, G. W., Munson, J. B., and Rall, W. (1982). Time course of group Ia synaptic current transients in alpha motoneurons. *Soc. Neurosci. Abstr. 8*:726.
129. Weakly, J. N. (1969). Effect of barbiturates on "quantal" synaptic transmission in spinal neurones. *J. Physiol. (Lond.) 204*:63–77.
130. Kuno, M., and Miyahara, J. T. (1969). Non-linear summation of unit synaptic potentials in spinal motoneurones of the cat. *J. Physiol. (Lond.) 201*:465–477.
131. Luscher, H.-R., Ruenzel, P., Fetz, E., and Henneman, E. (1979). Postsynaptic population potentials recorded from ventral roots perfused with isotonic sucrose: Connections of groups Ia and II spindle afferent fibers with large populations of motoneurons. *J. Neurophysiol. 42*:1146–1164.
132. Katz, B., and Thesleff, S. (1957). On the factors which determine the amplitude of the miniature end plate potential. *J. Physiol. (Lond.) 137*:267–278.
133. Burke, R. E., Rymer, W. Z., and Walsh, J. V. (1973). Functional specialization in the motor unit population of cat medial gastrocnemius muscle. In *Control of Posture and Locomotion*, R. B. Stein, K. G. Pearson, R. S. Smith, and J. B. Redford (Eds.), Plenum, New York, pp. 29–44.
134. Burke, R. E., Rymer, W. Z., and Walsh, J. V., Jr. (1976). Relative strength of synaptic input from short-latency pathways to motor units of defined type in cat medial gastrocnemius. *J. Neurophysiol. 39*:447–458.
135. Munson, J. B., Sypert, G. W., Zengel, J. E., Lofton, S. A., and Fleshman, J. W. (1982). Monosynaptic projections of individual spindle group II afferents to type-identified medial gastrocnemius motoneurons in the cat. *J. Neurophysiol. 48*:1164–1174.
136. Friedman, W. A., Sypert, G. W., Munson, J. B., and Fleshman, J. W. (1981). Recurrent inhibition of type-identified motoneurons. *J. Neurophysiol. 46*:1349–1359.
137. Fleshman, J. W., Munson, J. B., Sypert, G. W., and Friedman, W. A. (1981). Rheobase, input resistance, and motor-unit type in medial gastrocnemius motoneurons in the cat. *J. Neurophysiol. 46*:1326–1338.
138. Kernell, D., and Zwaagstra, B. (1981). Input conductance, axonal conduction velocity and cell size among hindlimb α-motoneurones of the cat. *Brain Res. 204*:311–326.

139. Kuno, M. (1974). Factors in efficacy of central synapses. In *Synaptic Transmission and Neuronal Interaction*, M. V. L. Bennett (Ed.), Raven, New York, pp. 79–85.

140. Gage, P. W., and McBurney, R. N. (1973). An analysis of the relationship between the current and potential generated by a quantum of acetylcholine in muscle fibers without transverse tubules. *J. Membrane Biol. 12*: 247–272.

141. Gage, P. W. (1976). Generation of end-plate potentials. *Physiol. Rev. 56*: 177–247.

142. Burke, R. E. (1967). Motor unit types of cat triceps surae muscle. *J. Physiol. (Lond.) 193*:141–160.

143. Blankenship, J. E., and Kuno, M. (1968). Analysis of spontaneous subthreshold activity in spinal motoneurons of the cat. *J. Neurophysiol. 31*: 195–209.

144. Katz, B., and Miledi, R. (1963). A study of spontaneous miniature potentials in spinal motoneurones. *J. Physiol. (Lond.) 168*:389–422.

145. Redman, S. J. (1976). A quantitative approach to the integrative function of dendrites. In *International Review of Physiology: Neurophysiology II*, vol. 10, R. Porter (Ed.). University Park Press, Baltimore, pp. 1–36.

146. Granit, R., Kernell, D., and Lamarre, Y. (1966). Algebraic summation in synaptic activation of motoneurones firing within the "primary range" to injected currents. *J. Physiol. (Lond.) 187*:379–399.

147. Redman, S., and Walmsley, B. (1981). The synaptic basis of the monosynaptic stretch reflex. *Trends in Neuroscience 4*:248–251.

148. Jack, J. J. B., Redman, S. F., and Wong, K. (1981). The components of synaptic potentials evoked in cat spinal motoneurones by impulses in single group Ia afferents. *J. Physiol. (Lond.) 321*:65–96.

149. DelCastillo, J., and Katz, B. (1954). Quantal components of the end-plate potential. *J. Physiol. (Lond.) 124*:560–573.

150. Hirst, G. D. S., Redman, S. J., and Wong, K. (1981). Post-tetanic potentiation and facilitation of synaptic potentials evoked in cat spinal motoneurones. *J. Physiol. (Lond.) 321*:97–109.

151. Jack, J. J. B., Redman, S. J., and Wong, K. (1981). Modifications to synaptic transmission at group Ia synapses on cat spinal motoneurones by 4-aminopyridine. *J. Physiol. (Lond.) 321*:111–126.

152. Krnjević, K., and Miledi, R. J. (1958). Failure of neuromuscular propagation in rats. *J. Physiol. (Lond.) 140*:440–461.

153. Barron, D. H., and Matthews, B. H. C. (1939). Intermittent conduction in the spinal cord. *J. Physiol. (Lond.) 85*:73–103.

154. Howland, B., Lettvin, J. Y., McCulloch, W. S., Pitts, W., and Wall, P. D. (1955). Reflex inhibition by dorsal root interaction. *J. Neurophysiol. 18*:1–17.

155. Parnas, I. (1972). Differential block at high frequency of branches of a single axon innervating two muscles. *J. Neurophysiol. 35*:903–914.

156. Collatos, T. C., Niechaj, A., Nelson, S. J., and Mendell, L. M. (1979). Fluctuations in time of onset of Ia–motoneuron EPSPs in the cat. *Brain Res.* *160*:514-518.

157. Cope, T. C., and Mendell, L. M. (1982). Parallel fluctuations of EPSP amplitude and rise time with latency at single Ia-fiber-motoneuron synapses in the cat. *J. Neurophysiol. 47*:455-468.

158. Cope, T. C., and Mendell, L. M. (1982). Distribution of EPSP latency at different group Ia-fiber-α-motoneuron connections. *J. Neurophysiol. 47*: 469-478.

159. Bennett, M. V. L. (1979). Electrical transmission: A functional analysis and comparison to chemical transmission. In *Handbook of Physiology*, vol. I, E. R. Kandel (Ed.), American Physiological Society, Bethesda, Maryland, pp. 357-416.

160. Sypert, G. W., Munson, J. B., and Fleshman, J. W. (1981). Terminal potentials, synaptic delay and presynaptic inhibition in the spinal monosynaptic reflex pathway. In *Advances in Physiological Science*, vol. I, *Regulator Functions of the CNS. Motion and Organization Principles*, J. Szentágothai, M. and Palkovits, and J. Jamois (Eds.), Permagon, Budapest, pp. 73-81.

161. Llínas, R., Steinberg, I. A., and Walton, K. (1976). Presynaptic calcium currents and their relation to synaptic transmission: Voltage clamp study in squid giant synapse and theoretical model for calcium gate. *Proc. Natl. Acad. Sci. U.S.A. 73*:2918-2922.

162. Takeuchi, A., and Takeuchi, N. (1962). Electrical changes in the presynaptic and postsynaptic axons of the giant synapse of Loligo. *J. Gen. Physiol. 45*:1181-1193.

163. Iles, J. F. (1977). The speed of passive dendritic conduction of synaptic potentials in a model motoneurone. *Proc. R. Soc. Lond. (Biol.) 197*:225-229.

164. Hubbard, J. I., and Schmidt, R. F. (1963). An electrophysiological investigation of mammalian nerve terminals. *J. Physiol. (Lond.) 166*:145-167.

165. Barrett, E. R., and Stevens, C. F. (1972). Quantal independence and uniformity of presynaptic release kinetics at the frog neuromuscular junction. *J. Physiol. (Lond.) 227*:665-689.

166. Shapovalov, A. I., and Shiriaev, V. I. (1979). Spontaneous miniature potentials in primary afferent fibres. *Experientia 35*:348-349.

167. Werman, R., and Carlen, P. L. (1976). Unusual behavior of the Ia EPSP in cat spinal motoneurones. *Brain Res. 112*:395-401.

168. Shapovalov, A. I., and Kurchavyi, G. G. (1974). Effects of transmembrane polarization and TEA injection on monosynaptic actions from motor cortex, red nucleus and group Ia afferents on lumbar motoneurons in the monkey. *Brain Res. 82*:49-67.

169. Engberg, I., and Marshall, K. C. (1979). Reversal potential for Ia excitatory post-synaptic potentials in spinal motoneurons of cats. *Neuroscience 4*:1583-1591.

170. Flatman, J. A., and Lambert, J. D. C. (1979). The use of intracellular QX222 as a tool in neurophysiological experiments on cat spinal motoneurones. *J. Physiol. (Lond.) 295*:7-8P.
171. Feng, T. P. (1941). Studies on the neuromuscular junction XXIV. The changes of the end-plate potential during and after prolonged stimulation. *Chin. J. Physiol. 16*:341-372.
172. del Castillo, J., and Katz, B. (1954). Statistical factors involved in neuromuscular facilitation and depression. *J. Physiol. (Lond.) 124*:574-585.
173. Liley, A. W. (1956). The quantal components of the mammalian end-plate potential. *J. Physiol. (Lond.) 133*:571-587.
174. Curtis, D. R., and Eccles, J. C. (1960). Synaptic action during and after repetitive stimulation. *J. Physiol. (Lond.) 150*:374-398.
175. Kuno, M. (1964). Mechanism of facilitation and depression of the excitatory synaptic potential in spinal motoneurones. *J. Physiol. (Lond.). 175*:100-112.
176. Luscher, H.-R., Ruenzel, P., and Henneman, E. (1979). How the size of motoneurons determines their susceptibility to discharge. *Nature 282*:859-861.
177. Lev-Tov, A., Pinter, M. J., and Burke, R. E. (1981). Post-tetanic potentiation of Ia EPSPs: Differential distribution and possible mechanisms. *Soc. Neurosci. Abstr. 8*:438.
178. Decima, E. E. (1972). Effects of blood calcium changes on spinal reflex activity. *Exp. Neurol. 1*:14-34.
179. Dambach, G. E., and Erulkar, S. D. (1973). The action of calcium at spinal neurones of the frog. *J. Physiol. (Lond.) 228*:799-817.
180. Barrett, E. F., and Barrett, J. N. (1976). Separation of two voltage-sensitive potassium currents and demonstration of a tetrodotoxin-resistant calcium current in frog motoneurones. *J. Physiol. (Lond.) 255*:734.
181. Alvarez-Leefmans, F. J., de Santis, A., and Miledi, R. (1978). Effects of removal of calcium and its replacement by strontium and barium ions on synaptic transmission in frog spinal motoneurones. *J. Physiol. (Lond.) 278*:10P.
182. Shapovalov, A. I., Shiriaev, B. I., and Velumian, A. A. (1978). Mechanisms of postsynaptic excitation in amphibian motoneurones. *J. Physiol. (Lond.) 179*:437-455.
183. Velumian, A., and Shapovalov, A. I. (1975). Unequal sensitivity of different synaptic inputs of amphibian motoneurones to the deficiency of calcium ions and to magnesium ions. *Dokl. Akad. Nauk. S.S.S.R. 225*:466-469.
184. Shapovalov, A. I. (1977). Interneuronal synapses with electrical and chemical mode of transmission and evolution of the central nervous system. *J. Evol. Biochem. Physiol. 13*:621-633.
185. Motorina, M. (1978). Ultrastructure of synapses of gap junction type in the motor nuclei of the frog spinal cord. *Arch. Anat. Histol. Embryol. 75*:27-34.

186. Shapovalov, A. I. (1980). Interneuronal synapses with electrical, dual and chemical modes of transmission in vertebrates. *Neuroscience 5*:1113–1124.

187. Shapovalov, A. I., Shiriaev, B. I., and Tamarova, Z. A. (1979). Synaptic activity in motoneurones of the immature cat spinal cord in vitro. Effects of manganese and tetrodotoxin. *Brain Res. 160*:524–528.

188. Krnjević, K., Lamour, Y., MacDonald, J. F., and Nistri, A. (1979). Depression of monosynaptic excitatory postsynaptic potentials by Mn^{2+} and Co^{2+} in cat spinal cord. *Neuroscience 4*:1331–1339.

189. Houk, J. C., and Rymer, W. Z. (1981). Neural control of muscle length and tension. In *Handbook of Physiology*, vol. II, J. M. Brookhart and V. B. Mountcastle (Eds.), American Physiological Society, Bethesda, Maryland, pp. 257–323.

190. Taylor, A., and Prochazka, A. (1981). *Muscle Receptors and Movement*, Oxford University Press, New York.

191. Hunt, C. C. (1955). Monosynaptic reflex response of spinal motoneurons to graded afferent stimulation. *J. Gen. Physiol. 38*:813–832.

192. Somjen, G., Carpenter, D. O., and Henneman, E. (1965). Responses of motoneurons of different sizes to graded stimulation of supraspinal centers of the brain. *J. Neurophysiol. 28*:958–965.

193. Stauffer, E. K., Watt, D. G. D., Taylor, A., Reinking, R. M., and Stuart, D. G. (1976). Analysis of muscle receptor connections by spike triggered averaging. 2. Spindle group II afferents. *J. Neurophysiol. 39*:1393–1402.

194. Brown, A. G. (1981). *Organization in the Spinal Cord*, Springer-Verlag, Berlin.

195. Lloyd, D. P. C. (1946). Integrative pattern of excitation and inhibition in two-neuron flex arcs. *J. Neurophysiol. 9*:439–444.

196. Eccles, R. M., and Lundberg, A. (1959). Supraspinal control of interneurones mediating spinal reflexes. *J. Physiol. (Lond.) 147*:565–584.

197. Holmquist, B., and Lundberg, A. (1961). Differential supraspinal control of synaptic actions evoked by volleys in the flexor reflex afferents in motoneurones. *Acta Physiol. Scand.* (Suppl.) *186*:1–51.

198. Eccles, R. M., and Lundberg, A. (1959). Synaptic actions in motoneurones by afferents which may evoke the flexion reflex. *Arch. Ital. Biol. 97*:199–221.

199. Dum, R. P., and Kennedy, T. T. (1980). Synaptic organization of defined motor-unit types in cat tibialis anterior. *J. Neurophysiol. 43*:1631–1644.

200. Lundberg, A. (1969). Convergence of excitatory and inhibitory action on interneurones in the spinal cord. In *UCLA Forum in Medical Sciences. The Interneuron*, vol. 11, M. A. B. Brazier (Ed.), University of California Press, Los Angeles, pp. 231–265.

201. Baldissera, F., ten Bruggencate, G., and Lundberg, A. (1971). Rubrospinal monosynaptic connexion with last order interneurones of polysynaptic reflex pathways. *Brain Res. 27*:390–392.

202. Kuno, M., and Weakley, J. N. (1972). Quantal components of the inhibitory synaptic potential in spinal motoneurones of the cat. *J. Physiol. (Lond.) 224*:287–303.

203. Kuypers, H. G. J. M. (1964). The descending pathways to the spinal cord, their anatomy and function. In *Progress in Brain Research. Organization of the Spinal Cord*, vol. 11, J. C. Eccles and J. P. Schade (Eds.), Elsevier, Amsterdam, pp. 178-200.

204. Anderson, M. E., Yoshida, M., and Wilson, V. J. (1972). Tectal and tegmental influences on cat forelimb and hindlimb. *J. Neurophysiol. 35*: 462-470.

205. Petras, J. M. (1967). Cortical, Tectal and tegmental fiber connections in the spinal cord of the cat. *Brain Res. 6*:275-324.

206. Wilson, V. J., and Yoshida, M. (1969). Comparison of effects of stimulation of Deiter's nucleus and medial longitudinal fasciculus on neck, forelimb and hindlimb motoneurons. *J. Neurophysiol. 32*:743-758.

207. Grillner, S., Hongo, T., and Lund, S. (1970). The vestibulospinal tract. Effects on alpha-motoneurons in the lumbosacral spinal cord in the cat. *Exp. Brain Res. 10*:94-120.

208. Grillner, S., Hongo, T., and Lund, S. (1971). Convergent effects on alpha motoneurons from the vestibulospinal tract and a pathway descending in the medial longitudinal fasciculus. *Exp. Brain Res. 12*:457-479.

209. Lund, S., and Pompeiano, O. (1968). Monosynaptic excitation of alpha motoneurons from supraspinal structures in the cat. *Acta Physiol. Scand. 73*:1-21.

210. Shapovalov, A. I., Karamyan, O. A., Kurchavyi, G. G., and Repina, Z. A. (1971). Synaptic actions evoked from the red nucleus on the spinal alpha-motoneurons in the Rhesus monkey. *Brain Res. 32*:325-348.

211. Stewart, D. H., and Preston, J. B. (1967). Functional coupling between the pyramidal tract and segmental motoneurons in cat and primate. *J. Neurophysiol. 30*:453-465.

212. Landgren, S., Phillips, C. G., and Porter, R. (1962). Minimal synaptic actions of pyramidal impulses on some alpha motoneurones of the baboon's hand and forearm. *J. Physiol. (Lond.) 161*:91-111.

10
SPINAL INHIBITION

Robert A. Davidoff and John C. Hackman   *University of Miami School of Medicine, and Veterans Administration Medical Center, Miami, Florida*

I. INTRODUCTION

The first definitive evidence for neural inhibition by stimulation of an appropriate nerve was obtained in 1845 by the Weber brothers. Their classic demonstration of the action of the vagus nerve on the heart (1) was followed in succeeding decades by other examples of peripheral inhibition, but it was the observations of Sechenov (2) that first indicated that inhibition existed in the central nervous system. It remained for Sherrington (3) to demonstrate that inhibition is an active process, and not merely the absence of excitation. He developed the concept of "reciprocal innervation" as a basic part of the normal reflex process. These seminal observations were developed further by Eccles and his colleagues (4). Intracellular recordings from spinal motoneurons showed that at least one major form of spinal inhibition was associated with a hyperpolarization of the motoneuronal membrane. Other work—first sketched out by Frank and Fuortes (5)—has since demonstrated that inhibition may also affect spinal function by affecting the release of excitatory transmitter from afferent fibers.

It was the purpose of this chapter to discuss these two forms of spinal inhibition from a variety of points of view—morphologic, biophysical, and functional. Much of this material has been reviewed elsewhere (4,6-11).

II. POSTSYNAPTIC INHIBITION

It is now completely accepted that as well as producing excitation of interneurons and motoneurons, activation of inputs to the spinal cord can result in
inhibition of neurons by altering the conductance of their postsynaptic
membranes.

A. Structure of Inhibitory Synapses

The mammalian spinal motoneuron is the termination of a variety of morphologically distinct types of synaptic knobs, or boutons, identifiable in electron
micrographs. These boutons have been studied extensively from an ultrastructural point of view (6,12-28) and at least six different types have been distinguished in the motoneuron neuropile. Although descriptions of the various types
have differed somewhat, two major types have been repeatedly recognized on
the basis of the shape of the contained synaptic vesicles. These are the S-type,
containing spheroid vesicles, and the F-type, containing flattened vesicles
(Fig. 1).

It has been suggested that typing of boutons into S- and F-types is of
physiologic significance (6,13,20). It is believed that S-type synapses are predominantly excitatory and that F-types release inhibitory transmitter, but this
hypothesis has been the subject of debate (cf. 21,29,30). However, particularly
convincing evidence that F-type synapses are inhibitory is supplied by the observations that this type is the sole one found on the crayfish abdominal stretch
receptor neuron—a cell that is known to receive only inhibitory inputs (31). In
addition, it appears that F-type boutons on spinal neurons preferentially
transport tritiated glycine (32), the major inhibitory spinal transmitter.

F-type boutons are mostly 0.5-3.0 μm in diameter (6,30,33). Following
aldehyde fixation they contain ellipsoidal, elongated, agranular vesicles that may
be 100-300 Å wide and 300-600 Å long (6,20,30). The entire synaptic complex
is flattened with a narrow synaptic cleft and only a thin layer of postsynaptic
dense material.

Figure 1 Excitatory and inhibitory spinal synapses. A, S-type synaptic bouton
with spheroid vesicles. To the right is seen an F-type bouton with ovoid vesicles.
Note the thin rim of postsynaptic material. B, F-type of presynaptic terminal.
The bouton is surrounded by a thin astrocytic lamella (arrow). To the left, a
desmosomelike junction (DE) is seen between the terminal and the postsynaptic
dendrite. C, Semischematic representation of motoneuron soma and proximal
dendrities made from a montage of several electron micrographs. E, excitatory
terminal; I, inhibitory terminal; N, motoneuron nucleus. The ratio of inhibitory
to excitatory synapses was about 3:2. (A and B from Ref. 6; C from Ref. 13.)

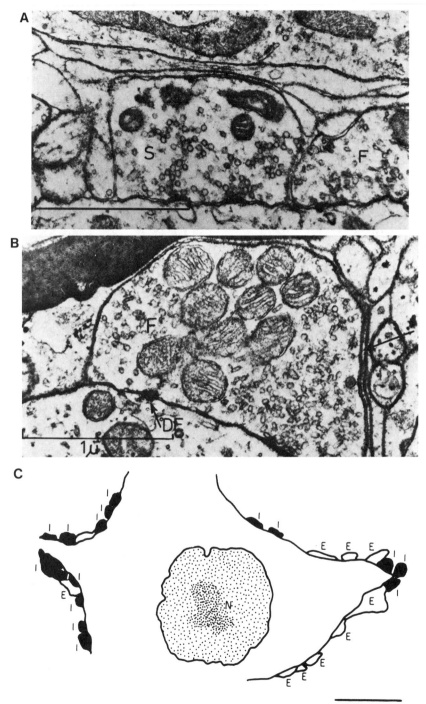

Different types of boutons are not distributed randomly on the motoneuron surface. Although intermingled with boutons of other types on all regions of the motoneuron surface (Fig. 1C), F-type synapses occur with more frequency on the cell body and axon hillock than on the dendrites. The converse is true for small distal dendrites (6,15-22). There is also some evidence that F-boutons are derived from segmental sources (i.e., interneurons and propriospinal neurons) (14,18), but further identification of the source of these boutons has not been possible.

B. "Direct" Inhibition

Almost 40 years ago Lloyd described the results of experiments in which stimulation of large muscle afferents (group Ia afferents) not only produced monosynaptic excitation of motoneurons but also inhibition of antagonstic motoneurons (34-37). Because of the short latency of the inhibition Lloyd felt that a monosynaptic arc was involved; hence he applied the term "direct inhibition" to the inhibitory process. This idea was refuted by later studies in which data obtained by means of intracellular recordings indicated that the latency of the inhibitory postsynaptic potential (IPSP) in alpha motoneurons was invariably 0.8 msec longer than the latency of the excitatory postsynaptic potential (EPSP) evoked in the same motoneurons by activation of the appropriate group Ia afferents (38). These results were correctly interpreted to indicate that interneurons (now designated as Ia inhibitory interneurons) are interposed between the afferent fibers and the motoneurons. Therefore, a more appropriate term than direct inhibition would be "disynaptic inhibition." The terms "segmental inhibition" and "reciprocal inhibition" have also been used to describe the process.

1. The Ia Inhibitory Postsynaptic Potential

Inhibitory postsynaptic potentials (Ia IPSPs) were first observed by means of intracellular recordings from cat alpha motoneurons in response to volleys in group Ia afferent fibers from spindles located in a muscle antagonistic to the one supplied by the motoneurons under study (39) (Fig. 2A). Such Ia inhibitory postsynaptic potentials have a central latency of 1.2-1.6 msec (38,40), a brief rising phase (time-to-peak, 1.0-1.5 msec), and a slower, approximately exponential decay (1/2 decay time, 1.5-3.5 msec) (41-43; cf. 44). The time constant of decay is about the same as the membrane time constant determined by passing current pulses across the motoneuron membrane (Fig. 1B). The amplitude of inhibitory postsynaptic potentials varies depending upon the Ia afferents stimulated, the target motoneuronal pool, and the particular type of motoneuron within the pool (45-48).

The inhibitory postsynaptic potential evoked by stimulation of the Ia afferents in a muscle nerve is a composite potential composed of "unit" potentials

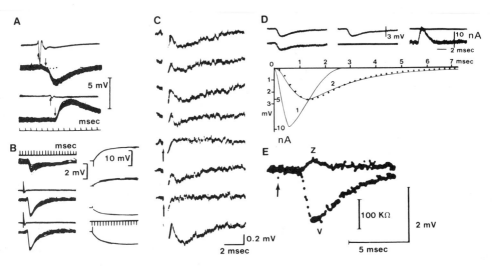

Figure 2 Spinal postsynaptic potentials. A, Intracellular responses from probable sartorius motoneuron (lower traces) and from dorsal root entry zone (upper traces). In the dorsal root traces, the upward deflection signals positivity and the first reversal point indicted by first arrow signals approximate time of entry of volley into spinal cord. IPSP evoked by stimulation of group Ia fibers in quadriceps nerve and EPSP by stimulation of hamstring nerve. Note longer latency of IPSP. Records formed by superimposition of about 40 traces. B, IPSPs produced by different strengths of stimulation of group Ia afferents in quadriceps nerve and recorded in hamstrings motoneuron (lower traces on left). Upper traces are from appropriate dorsal root. Traces on right are intracellular potentials produced by depolarizing (12 and 6 × 10^{-9} amps) and hyperpolarizing (6 and 12 × 10^{-9} amps) pulses. Records formed from superimposition of about 40 traces. C, Monosynaptic IPSPs evoked in a motoneuron by constant pulses (at a rate of 1 Hz) of current passed through pair of electrodes placed in the spinal gray matter. Some of the stimuli failed to evoke a detectable IPSP, as indicated by arrows. D, Membrane current during the IPSP. Left traces show IPSP recorded with two intracellular microelectrodes placed in a hamstring motoneuron. The potential was elicited by a Ia volley in the quadriceps nerve. Middle traces show voltage (upper) and current (lower) recordings while neuron is unclamped. Right traces show membrane voltage clamped at the resting membrane potential and the IPSP current during the IPSP. The graph is a tracing (1) of the IPSP current (tracing reversed) and the actual IPSP (2). The IPSP calculated from the IPSP current and the membrane resistance (based on the cell as a simple resistance-capacitance circuit) is graphed by the dots and agrees remarkably well with the actual IPSP. E, IPSP (V) and associated in-phase impedance change (Z) arising from superimposed baselines. Arrow indicates shock artifact from stimulation of hamstring nerve. Upward deflection of Z indivates impedance increase. Records are formed from superimposition of about 150 traces. (A from Ref. 38; B from Ref. 43; C from Ref. 50; D from Ref. 66; E from Ref. 67.)

(Fig. 1C) (44,49,50). Each unit potential is presumably produced by release of inhibitory transmitter from the terminals of one Ia interneuron. Estimations of the amplitude of unit inhibitory postsynaptic potentials are difficult to obtain, since the inhibitory pathway is disynaptic. This factor complicates the relationship between Ia fiber firing and the production of unit inhibitory synaptic potentials. The problem has been approached by stimulating single interneurons, but monosynaptic unit inhibitory postsynaptic potentials evoked in response to interneuron stimulation fluctuate considerably in size (50) and are of very small average amplitude, usually less than 0.1 mV (44,50,51). The fluctuations in amplitude suggests that the unit inhibitory postsynaptic potentials are in turn composed of "quanta" (50), but the nature of such quanta is still in doubt and the analogy to quantal transmission at other synapses is open to question.

The inhibitory postsynaptic potentials produced in motoneurons by afferent volleys in nerves containing group Ib, II, III, and IV fibers have slower time courses than the inhibitory postsynaptic potentials evoked by Ia volleys (e.g., 52,53). It is felt that the slower time course reflects temporal dispersion in the pathways leading to the inhibitory potential rather than any difference in the mechanism of the inhibitory postsynaptic potential (4).

a. Ionic mechanism. Early experimental investigations of the Ia inhibitory postsynaptic potential indicated that the hyperpolarization was accompanied by an increased membrane conductance (54,55) and could be altered by varying the membrane potential or by the injection of Cl^- ions (41) (Fig. 3C,D). These data were interpreted as indicating that the inhibitory postsynaptic potential was caused by a great increase in the flux of an ion or ions across the postsynaptic membrane of the motoneuron (56).

When the membrane potential of the motoneuron was increased past -80 mV the Ia Inhibitory postsynaptic potential was reversed to a depolarizing potential (Fig. 3A). It was therefore assumed that the reversal potential of the inhibitory postsynaptic potential was midway between a K^+ equilibrium potential of -90 mV and a presumed Cl^- equilibrium potential of -70 mV. This led to the conclusion that the inhibitory transmitter increased membrane permeability to K^+ and to Cl^- ions, allowing both these ions to move down their electrochemical gradients (41,56,57). However, the hypothesis of a dual ionic mechanism for the generation of inhibitory postsynaptic potentials has been challenged. Earlier analyses of the problem had been carried out under the assumption that Cl^- is distributed   passively across the membrane. It now appears that the internal Cl^- concentration of motoneurons is maintained at a lower level than that dictated by passive ionic distribution. Presumably, an active extrusion process (i.e., a Cl^- pump) is responsible for reducing internal Cl^-.

The evidence for this hypothesis is based on experiments that have utilized NH_4^+ ions (Fig. 3E). Administration of NH_4^+ ions reduces the hyperpolarization accompanying inhibitory postsynaptic potentials in cat motoneurons

(58,59), but it does not affect the postsynaptic membrane conductance change. There are no other alterations in electric membrane properties. There is a reversible shift of the inhibitory postsynaptic potential reversal potential in a depolarizing direction toward the resting membrane potential. In addition, the depolarizing effect of intracellularly injected Cl^- on the Ia inhibitory postsynaptic potential reversal potential is enhanced and the recovery time of the inhibitory postsynaptic potential after Cl^- injection is prolonged. The results suggest that NH_4^+ ions block the active extrusion of Cl^- ions responsible for maintaining the high Cl^- gradient necessary for hyperpolarizing synaptic inhibition.

Furthermore, little or no change was observed in the reversal potential of the inhibitory postsynaptic potential following injection of K^+ ions into motoneurons (60). In contrast, changing the intracellular Cl^- concentration by passing electric current of appropriate polarity through an intracellular microelectrode filled with a Cl^- salt results in a prompt conversion of the hyperpolarizing inhibitory postsynaptic potential to a depolarizing potential (41).

The problem has been recently studied in the isolated frog spinal cord maintained in vitro (61). In these experiments advantage was taken of the fact that in frog motoneurons the inhibitory postsynaptic potential produced by stimulating afferents is frequently a depolarizing potential. In contrast to the situation in cat motoneurons, frog motoneurons have an inwardly directed Cl^- pump. In the frog, therefore, there is a great difference between the depolarizing Cl^- equilibrium potential and the hyperpolarizing K^+ equilibrium potential. Simultaneous measurements of the internal and external Cl^- and K^+ activities by means of ion-sensitive microelectrodes indicated that the calculated Cl^- equilibrium potential deviated little from the reversal potential of the inhibitory postsynaptic potential. No changes of internal K^+ activity during the inhibitory postsynaptic potential were observed.

In sum, there seems to be little objection at the present time to the idea that an increased permeability to Cl^- is the sole basis for the Ia inhibitory postsynaptic potential in spinal motoneurons.

Attempts have been made to define the properties of the ionic permeability mechanism of the activated postsynaptic membrane of cat and toad motoneurons by substituting foreign anions for Cl^- (Fig. 2F). Various species of anions have been injected into the interior of the neuron and measurements made of the sign of the Ia inhibitory postsynaptic potential (41,62-64). Injection of Cl^- and a variety of other anions (e.g., Br^-, NO_3^-, SCN^-) with a hydrated diameter smaller than 2.9 Å changed the inhibitory postsynaptic potential to a depolarizing potential. The results were explained by assuming that the activated inhibitory subsynaptic membrane is permeable to these ions. On the other hand, injection of larger anions (e.g., HCO_3^-, SO_4^{2-}, $H_2PO_4^{2-}$) had no effect on the inhibitory postsynaptic potential. It was assumed that the

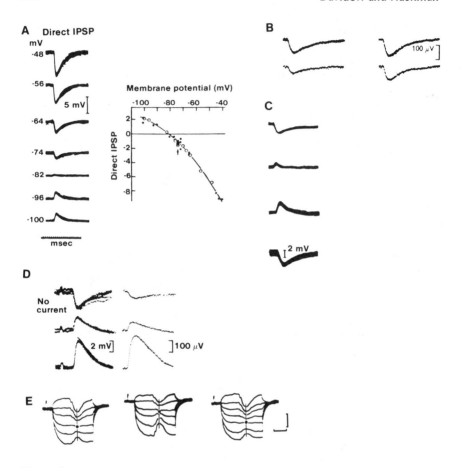

Figure 3 Mechanism of the inhibitory postsynaptic potential. A, Equilibrium potential of the IPSP. Recordings from hamstring motoneuron formed by superimposition of about 40 traces in response to quadriceps volley. The membrane potential was preset at the potentials indicated on each record by means of a steady background current passed through an intracellular double-barreled microelectrode. The resting membrane potential was –74 mV. The graph plots the results of the experiment partly illustrated by the traces. The abscissa indicates the membrane potential and the ordinate the amplitude of the IPSP. Arrow indicates resting membrane potential. By, Unitary IPSPs evoked in two different motoneurons by stimulation of a single Ia inhibitory interneuron. The left traces were taken at the resting membrane potential and the corresponding right traces after a depolarization of the motoneuron membrane. All traces are averaged records. C, Permeability of the postsynaptic inhibitory membrane to Cl⁻ ions. Records of IPSPs recorded from a hamstring motoneuron. Upper record is control recording. Next two records demonstrate reversal of the

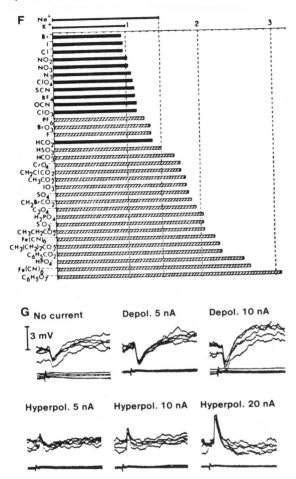

potential by diffusion of Cl⁻ ions from intracellular microelectrode. In the lowest trace the IPSP is reversed to its original hyperpolarizing direction by lowering the membrane potential by the passage of current from –59 mV to –27 mV. D, Reversal of unitary and compound IPSPs by Cl⁻ ions. Left traces are compound IPSPs evoked in a hamstring motoneuron; right traces are unitary IPSPs elicited by stimulating a single Ia interneuron. The upper traces are controls and the next two sets of traces were taken after the diffusion of ions from an intracellular microelectrode filled with a solution of KCl. All traces are averaged potentials. E, Effects of extracellularly applied NH_4^+ ions on equilibrium potential of IPSP. Series of IPSPs at different membrane potentials. Series on left before application; in center during iontophoresis of NH_4^+ ions; right 4 minutes inhibitory membrane is not permeable to these larger anions. On the basis of experiments using large numbers of anions, it was proposed that the inhibitory membrane of motoneurons behaves as a sieve with pores of a precisely standardized size that allow movement of small hydrated ions (4). Ions with a larger hydrated diameter than the pore size would not penetrate the membrane. It is believed that the ionic channels lack any chemical specificity for anions. There is merely a discrimination among anions based on size.

This hypothesis—which has great appeal because of its simplicity—does not satisfy the available data of at least one other inhibitory synapse. In crayfish muscle (65) ionic mobility across the membrane (as measured by conductance) is not directly related to the hydrated diameter of anions. In this particular inhibitory membrane, the conductance change during the inhibitory postsynaptic potential was found to be graded with respect to the anionic species studied—a finding that is inconsistent with the sieve hypothesis. It was suggested that the pores are not simple channels, but rather they interact with anions passing through the membrane. Obviously, more data is needed with regard to postsynaptic inhibition in motoneurons.

Attempts have been made to directly measure the current generating the Ia inhibitory postsynaptic potential. Since most of the inhibitory synapses are believed to be located near the somata of cat motoneurons, a reasonable voltage clamp of the potential can be obtained (66) (Fig. 2D). Peak values of the inhibitory current from such an investigation were about 10 nÅ. The current reached a peak in about 0.8 msec and had a duration of about 2.5 msec. These data agree well with the earlier calculations of Curtis and Eccles (43) based on measurements of the time constant and restivity of the motoneuron membrane.

The ionic mechanism of other inhibitory synapses on motoneurons has not

---

Figure 3 *(continued)*
after cessation of iontophoric current. Note the depolarizing shift in the IPSP equilibrium potential. Calibration: 10 mV, 20 msec. F, Diagram indicating the correlation between the ion size of various anions and their ability to reverse the IPSP after intracellular injection. The length of the bars indicates the calculated ion size in aqueous solution. The black bars are for anions effective in inverting the IPSP; hatched bands for ineffective anions. The size of the hydrated sizes of Na^+ and K^+ ions are shown above the length scale. The size of the K^+ ion was taken as one. G, Reversal of Ia IPSP by injection of current through a microelectrode filled with KCl. Intracellular recording (upper records consisting of five superimposed sweeps) from hamstring motoneuron. IPSP evoked by volley in quadriceps nerve at 1.5 × threshold for the most excitable fibers in the nerve. DC currents of indicated strength and polarity were passed through the recording microelectrode for 5-7 sec. Bottom records are from the L7 dorsal root entry zone. Note diphasic reversal of IPSP. (A and C from Ref. 55; B and D from Ref. 81; E from Ref. 58; F from Ref. 63; G from Ref. 68.)

been as extensively investigated as that of the Ia inhibitory synapse. It is thought, however, that other inhibitory synapses in the cord operate by the same Cl⁻ permeability mechanism.

b. Location of Ia inhibitory synapses. It is thought that the inhibitory synaptic terminals of Ia interneurons are predominantly located on or near the somata of cat motoneurons (44). This assumption is based on the following evidence:

(1) The majority of Ia inhibitory postsynaptic potentials are accompanied by a change in conductance that is readily detectable by a microelectrode placed in the soma (66,67).
(2) The falling phase of the Ia inhibitory postsynaptic potential closely resembles the time course of the membrane response to the injection of a current pulse into the cell soma (43).
(3) The amplitude of the Ia inhibitory postsynaptic potential is sensitive to small changes in transmembrane potential (41,66).
(4) The Ia inhibitory postsynaptic potential is readily reversed in sign by the diffusion of Cl⁻ ions from an intrasomatic microelectrode (41).

On the other hand, it is now realized that in some cases the reversal of the Ia inhibitory postsynaptic potential to both current and Cl⁻ injection is biphasic with a differential reversal of early and later parts of the potential (Fig. 3G) (41,44,66). Such a nonuniform reversal suggests that a proportion of the inhibitory synapses responsible for generating the Ia inhibitory postsynaptic potential may be located at sites electrically remote from the soma. It is thought that these sites are on proximal dendrites.

c. Mechanism of Ia inhibition. It is widely accepted that Ia inhibitory postsynaptic potentials exert their inhibitory action on the excitability of motoneurons by a combination of hyperpolarization and increased ionic conductance (43,54,55). The hyperpolarization occurring during the inhibitory postsynaptic potential shifts the cell membrane potential away from threshold for the action potential. The increased conductance of the subsynaptic membrane reduces the size of the excitatory postsynaptic potential, since any shift in charge across the motoneuron membrane (e.g., an inward flow of Na⁺ ions during the excitatory postsynaptic potential) would produce a smaller potential change at the membrane. In other words, the motoneuron membrane is "short-circuited" by the increased conductance. In addition, any depolarizing tendency exerted on the motoneuron membrane caused by increased inward current is automatically compensated for by an accompanying influx of Cl⁻ ions.

It is difficult, however, to assess the relative contribution of the hyperpolarization and the conductance change to the inhibitory action of the inhibitory postsynaptic potential. It is generally believed that the maximum depression is produced by the initial brief phase of high ionic conductance that lasts about 2 msec (55). A smaller residual depression is caused by the

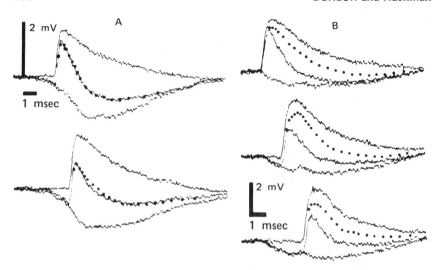

Figure 4 Interaction of IPSPs and EPSPs. Averaged PSP records. Column A demonstrates the linear summation of an EPSP produced by a lateral gastroc-nemius volley (upper traces) and an IPSP evoked by a flexor digitorum longus volley (lower traces) when the two PSPs were generated together (middle trace). The dots represent the algebraic summation of the top and bottom potentials in each case. The linear summation is taken to indicate that the two sets of PSPs were at some distance from each other sufficient to prevent mutual interaction. Nonlinear summation is seen in column B where the EPSP was produced by stimulation of the nerve from the lateral gastrocnemius and the IPSP by stimula-tion of the nerve from the extensor digitorum longus. The nonlinear summation is taken to indicate that the generators of the two types of PSPs were electro-tonically close enough to mutually interact. (From Ref. 69.)

hyperpolarization of the inhibitory postsynaptic potential. The transient altera-tion in conductance measured by voltage clamp (66) and by impedance bridge lasts up to 2 msec (Fig. 2E). Furthermore, there is often a very effective non-linear interaction between inhibitory postsynaptic potentials and excitatory postsynaptic potentials (Fig. 4) (43,68,69)—an effect expected of two potentials produced by conductance increases.

On the other hand, the inhibitory action of the inhibitory postsynaptic potential in trochlear motoneurons was considerably reduced when the hyper-polarization, but not the conductance increase, was reduced by blocking the Cl^- pump with NH_4^+ (70). It was concluded that shunting caused by an increased conductance represented only a minor part of the total inhibition and that the hyperpolarization is the major factor in producing inhibition. A compli-cating factor in interpreting these results, however, is the fact that inhibition of the Cl⁻ pump not only reduces the hyperpolarization, but also decreases the electrochemical gradient for Cl⁻ ions. This results in a decreased driving force for the anion, and thus a decreased ability to compensate for depolarizing inward currents.

It is generally recognized that the distribution of Ia inhibitory synapses on the soma between the main excitatory inputs on dendrites and the site of action of potential generation in the initial segment of the motoneuron puts this inhibitory system in a strategic position to reduce the probability of impulse initiation. Inhibitory synapses located on dendrites far from the initial segment would not have such a role. The Ia inhibitory system is thus ideally located to be a potent regulator of motoneuron activity.

2. Ia Inhibitory Interneurons

The Ia inhibitory interneuron is intercalated between group Ia fibers and the motoneurons innervating muscles with antagonistic functions. As such it should be monosynaptically excited by volleys in group Ia afferents. Early investigations indicated that a population of interneurons with monosynaptic excitatory postsynaptic potentials from that source were located in the dorsolateral gray matter of the cord in the so-called "intermediate nucleus of Cajal" (71-73). More recent investigations have shown that neurons with the requisite properties are found in the ventral horn (discussed later).

At first, the Ia inhibitory interneuron was regarded mainly as a convenient means to enable the spinal cord to use a single afferent input to produce excitation of one group of motoneurons and inhibition of another set (38). It was soon realized, however, that the interneuron might also function as a simple "integrative center" (45). This idea is now firmly established, since it is now evident that a given Ia inhibitory interneuron can receive a wide and diverse convergence of excitatory and inhibitory inputs from a variety of segmental and descending sources (74-76).

The complex pattern of convergence of segmental and suprasegmental inputs (77-83) clearly allows these particular interneurons to be distinguished from other classes of interneurons and permits an individual neuron to be identified as an Ia interneuron. It now appears that Ia inhibitory interneurons have the following properties:

1. There is convergence of a number of Ia afferents on a given interneuron (40). There is also a convergence of Ia afferents from several different synergistic muscles on Ia inhibitory interneurons (80,91,84,85). This latter finding is the basis for the observation that in most species of motoneurons Ia inhibition can be elicited by stimulation of Ia afferents from several muscles (45).

The pattern of convergence of Ia afferents resembles that found in the corresponding alpha motoneurons (80,84).

2. High-threshold primary afferent fibers from muscle, skin, and joints, usually, but not always (86), exert a facilitatory effect upon Ia inhibitory interneurons through polysynaptic pathways (87).

3. Ia inhibitory interneurons are inhibited by volleys in motor axon collaterals. In other words, antidromic volleys that inhibit a group of alpha motoneurons also inhibit the corresponding Ia inhibitory interneurons (46,79,80, 83-85). The inhibition from motor axon collaterals appears to be unique for this species of interneuron.

4. Ia inhibitory interneurons excited by volleys in one functional group of large muscle afferents are disynaptically inhibited by volleys in Ia afferents from antagonistic muscles. This inhibition is mediated by the "opposite" Ia interneurons (85). In other words, there is a mutual inhibition between different functional groups of Ia inhibitory interneurons.

5. Ia inhibitory interneurons are under the influence of a variety of descending pathways that are also known to influence alpha motoneurons. Thus, the vestibulospinal (74,88-90), the rubrospinal (74,90,91), and the corticospinal (90,92-94) tracts mono- or polysynaptically excite, and sometimes inhibit, Ia inhibitory interneurons.

6. Propriospinal systems monosynaptically excite interneurons mediating Ia inhibition (95,96).

An important conclusion can be drawn from this data—there is a striking parallelism of afferent inputs on alpha motoneurons and on Ia inhibitory interneurons with the same monosynaptic Ia input.

Ia inhibitory interneurons—identified by the findings of monosynaptic excitation from Ia afferents and inhibition from recurrent motor axon collaterals —were first located by estimating the position of the tip of intracellular electrodes (80). They appeared to be situated within an area just dorsal and dorsomedial to the motor nuclei of the ventral horn in Rexed's lamina VII. This conclusion was confirmed by intracellular injection studies (97). No somatotopic organization is evident in the population of Ia interneurons, but the interneurons innervated by a particular muscle nerve are usually found in the same spinal segment at which the afferents from that nerve entered the spinal cord (97).

Such injection studies have demonstrated that Ia inhibitory interneurons are fairly uniform in size, with an average soma diameter of about $20 \times 30 \ \mu m$ (97). They have four to five dendrites that extend considerable distances (300-600 μm). Electrophysiologic and histologic investigations have indicated that such neurons have relatively long myelinated axons that may project either rostrally or caudally in either the ventral or lateral funiculi for two or three segments (80, 81,97) before reentering the ventral gray matter to make synaptic contact with motoneurons as well as other interneurons (97,98).

The available evidence suggests that about 70 Ia inhibitory interneurons may converge to synapse on one alpha motoneuron (44). Conversely, a single Ia interneuron may synapse on about 1/5 of the motoneurons in a pool (44).

3. Function of Ia Inhibition

The concept of reciprocal innervation as conceived by Sherrington (99) indicated that one muscle of an antagonistic pair is relaxed as its mechanical opponent actively contracts. The work of Lloyd (35,36) demonstrated that the process involved the large afferent fibers arising from the primary endings of muscle spindles. He specified that these fibers not only excited the motoneurons of that particular muscle and muscles of like function, but that they also inhibited the motoneurons of antagonistic muscles acting at the same joint. The rule of reciprocity in which a strict reciprocal innervation exists at a given joint has been generally accepted (e.g., 45,100). The patterns of reciprocal inhibition have been mainly studied in the cat, but the same types of patterns have also been demonstrated in the monkey (93) and in man (101,102).

It must be realized, however, that in a number of motor nuclei the reciprocal Ia inhibitory actions are organized in a more complex manner (45) than was originally postulated. Thus, Ia afferents from muscles other than strict mechanical antagonists can inhibit a given motoneuronal pool. The complexities presumably arise from the fact that many muscles have more than one action and that some muscles act at more than one joint.

In many muscular contractions evoked by activity in descending or segmental spinal pathways there appears to be a central coactivation of alpha and gamma motoneurons. The functional significance of the alpha-gamma linkage has been extensively reviewed (103,104) and will not be discussed here at length. However, it must be emphasized that motoneuronal discharges during a variety of movements appear to depend upon spatial facilitation from inputs directly exciting alpha motoneurons and from the same inputs indirectly exciting the same motoneurons by activating gamma motoneurons.

The two principles—"alpha-gamma coactivation" and "reciprocal innervation"—have now been coupled (75,76). To produce smooth well-coordinated movements it would seem important to coordinate reciprocal inhibition of antagonist muscles with the excitation of agonists (78,91). It is hypothesized that neuronal inputs that elicit alpha-gamma linked movements excite not only alpha and gamma motoneurons, but also Ia inhibitory interneurons projecting to motoneurons of antagonistic muscles. Since the alpha motoneurons and the corresponding interneurons would both be governed by a similar convergence of direct alpha and indirect gamma inputs, the term "alpha-gamma linkage in reciprocal inhibition" has been applied to the process (91).

Major support for this hypothesis is given by the existence of parallel connections on the three types of neurons (see Sec. II.B.2; see also 75,76,83 for refs.).

C. Autogenetic Inhibition

In general, Ib afferent fibers from Golgi tendon organs (GTO) in a given muscle are considered the main source of inhibition directed back to the motoneurons supplying that muscle—so-called "autogenetic inhibition." However, the reflex actions of Ib afferents are not as well understood as those of Ia afferents. In part, this may be attributed to the difficulty in selectively stimulating Ib afferent fibers and in part to previous failures to appreciate the extensive control exerted on Ib reflex pathways by activity in supraspinal structures and in other segmental systems. For example, there are great differences in the spinal actions of Ib afferents when these are studied in intact, spinal, or decerebrate animals (e.g., cf. 37,52,105).

Major pioneer contributions to understanding the function of Ib muscle afferents were made by Laporte and Lloyd (37). These workers investigated the complex reflex effects of graded electrical stimulation of muscle nerves and hypothesized that afferents from Golgi tendon organs were responsible for disynaptic inhibition of motoneurons to homonymous and synergistic muscles (as well as for disynaptic excitation of antagonist motoneurons). These findings were in large measure confirmed by intracellular recordings from motoneurons (52,105), but both inhibitory and excitatory actions evoked by group Ib afferents from Golgi tendon organs were found more widely distributed than shown by the original observations of Laporte and Lloyd.

It appears that both excitatory and inhibitory effects from Ib afferents are relayed in pathways involving two or three interneurons (37,105). It also appears that afferent information from Golgi tendon organs from a particular muscle affects nearly all the major motoneuron groups of a limb (106). Conversely, Ib afferents from different muscles converge on the interposed interneurons (107). These effects are true of Ib afferents from both extensor and flexor muscles.

1. Ib Interneurons

Available evidence indicates that interneurons mediating Ib effects are located in the intermediate nucleus in laminae V and VI (72,82,98,108-115). Thus it has been difficult to define precisely the properties of these cells because they receive such a wealth of convergent inputs from other types of segmental afferents and such an extensive innervation from supraspinal sources. The problem is also complicated by the fact that there are many other types of interneurons in the intermediate nucleus (e.g., interneurons mediating presynaptic inhibition from group I fibers; interneurons transmitting information to long ascending tracts).

Of particular interest is the finding that many of these group Ib-activated interneurons are also monosynaptically excited by impulses in Ia fibers from the same, from synergistic, and from other muscles (72,109,112,113,115). This means that classic ideas about the inhibitory reflex functions of Ia inputs to the spinal cord—namely, that they mediate reciprocal inhibition between antagonistic muscles operating at the same joint—now have to be revised to include another function, that of autogenetic inhibition (116). It also means that autogenetic inhibition can no longer be considered the sole province of Ib fibers. It does appear, however, that the amount of autogenetic inhibition exerted by Ia afferents is less than that exerted by Ib afferents. In addition, there are interneurons in laminae V and VI that primarily appear to subserve reflexes from tendon organs and that are not influenced by Ia fibers (113).

Ib interneurons are di- or trisynaptically excited by impulses in cutaneous afferents, and oligosynaptically from joint afferents (107,109,117,118). In fact, this pattern of extensive convergence has raised the question of whether these particular cells are primarily related to the Ib afferents or are intercalated in other reflex pathways primarily activated by cutaneous or joint or other types of muscle afferents (117). It may be that such interneurons are shared by many segmental systems and their activity may only partially relate to the activation of tendon organs.

The Ib reflex pathway is extensively regulated by supraspinal structures. For example, Ib interneurons receive monosynaptic excitation from the corticospinal and rubrospinal tracts (91,94,112,114,119) and inhibition from the dorsal reticulospinal and the noradrenergic reticulospinal systems (120,121). It has been suggested that convergence of descending pathways from supraspinal structures permits the brain to set the sensitivity of segmental Ib pathways (118). The importance of such effects is shown by observations that Ib interneurons are often not very effectively excited by Ia or by Ib afferents and that their activation often requires facilitation by descending pathways (or by other segmental inputs) (91,117,118).

Intracellular staining of cells identified as Ib interneurons on the basis of excitation by Ib and cutaneous afferents and excitation by descending tracts shows that they project to the motor nuclei (98,111,113).

2. Function of Autogenetic Inhibition

In view of the findings that most, if not all, of the pathways activated by Ib afferents are also shared by inputs from other muscle, cutaneous, and joint receptors, it is difficult at this time to propose a comprehensive statement concerning the function of Ib inhibition in isolation from other afferent systems. This task is compounded by the extensive convergence from different supraspinal areas that can set the sensitivity of the Ib reflex pathways. Older ideas that Golgi tendon organs served to "protect" muscle from excessive stretch must be discarded. The concept that the sole function of these receptors is to regulate muscle tension or force (121a) has to be reevaluated.

It appears more realistic to consider that the inhibitory effects of Golgi tendon organs are part of a complex system regulating movement by inputs from a variety of different types of afferents, all capable of activating the same pathways. It may also be that only a minor part of the Ib inhibitory action is autogenetic. It must also be realized that Ib afferents are responsible for presynaptic inhibition of transmission in a variety of other afferent systems (see Sec. III.B.2c).

D. Other Spinal Inhibitions

1. Inhibition by High-Threshold Afferents

In general, electrical stimulation of high-threshold muscle, cutaneous, and joint afferents results in a flexion reflex (122,123) with the production of excitatory postsynaptic potentials in flexor motoneurons and inhibitory postsynaptic potentials in extensor motoneurons (53,123). Since under appropriate conditions electrical stimulation of these afferents could evoke a flexion reflex, they were thought to comprise a system of "flexor reflex afferents" (FRA) (123) with a more or less uniform reflex function (53). This unitary and simplistic formulation is now difficult to support.

It has been realized for many years that the reflex responses to stimulation of flexor reflex afferent depend upon the state of the preparation. For example, in the decerebrate cat, volleys in the flexor reflex afferents are almost without effect (124,125). Presumably, this phenomenon is a result of a tonic inhibition by supraspinal structures of the interposed interneurons, since section of the spinal cord releases the expected excitatory and inhibitory actions (125). In addition, different lesions in the brainstem have been shown to convert the effect of stimulating different high-threshold afferents from excitation to inhibition or vice versa (123). Supraspinal structures appear to have the ability to switch the pathways activated by flexor reflex afferents, presumably by actions on interneurons.

As recently reviewed by Baldissera et al. (76), an astonishing variety of inhibitory effects can be attributed to activation of afferents comprising the flexor reflex afferents. This complexity arises because, although the flexor reflex afferents show extensive convergence onto common interneurons, each of the specific afferents in the flexor reflex afferent system has additional and more specialized effects. In addition, the flexor reflex afferents can activate parallel, and often antagonistic, reflex effects depending upon the state of various supraspinal centers.

2. Recurrent Inhibition

This important form of inhibition is reviewed in Chapter 11 of the present volume (126).

3. Remote Inhibition

The term "remote inhibition" was introduced by Frank (127) to indicate an inhibition exerted by synapses located so far out on dendrites of motoneurons that the usual membrane changes associated with postsynaptic inhibition were not detected by a microelectrode in the motoneuron soma (see Sec. III.B.3.b). A number of workers have reported inhibitory effects that could be attributed to such synapses (e.g., 127-135), but in most of these cases changes in the potential, conductance, or excitability were detected coincident with the inhibition. It is difficult to study the properties of such synapses and most discussion of the problem has focused on distinguishing such inhibitions from presynaptic inhibition.

III. PRESYNAPTIC CONTROL MECHANISMS

A variety of control mechanisms exerted at the level of the primary afferent fiber terminal modulate the transmission of sensory impulses coming from the periphery. Investigation of presynaptic control has largely been focused upon presynaptic inhibition as described by Eccles and coworkers, but recent work indicates that control of afferent inputs may be a more complicated process than has hitherto been thought. Apparently, several different types of control can be exerted over impulses entering the spinal cord via primary afferent fibers.

A. Early Investigations

Gasser and his colleagues (136-138), who systematically examined the various components of the cord potentials produced by an afferent volley, recorded a slow positive wave (P wave) from the dorsum of the cord following peripheral nerve stimulation. They suspected a possible connection between the P wave and previously reported long-duration inhibitions of flexor reflexes (139-141), since both processes had a similar time course.

Barron and Matthews (142), who popularized the recording of potentials electrotonically propagated along primary afferent fibers, reported that afferent volleys evoked a long-duration depolarization of the intraspinal portion of afferent fibers—the dorsal root potential (DRP). They postulated that the same potential generator was responsible for both the P wave and for the dorsal root potential and, in agreement with Gasser, concluded that there was a causal relationship between the depolarizing process and the flexor reflex inhibition.

The significance of much of this work was lost sight of in the next two decades, principally because of the excitement engendered by the discovery of the inhibitory postsynaptic potential. A cogent observation, however, was made by Frank and Fuortes (5), who noted that monosynaptic excitatory postsynaptic potentials recorded in extensor motoneurons could be reduced in size by conditioning volleys in Ia afferent fibers from flexor muscles. The importance of this observation resided in the finding that such volleys could produce the inhibition without altering the membrane properties of the postsynaptic neurons.

These data were rapidly confirmed by Eccles and his colleagues (4,143) and were linked to the previous work on depolarization of afferent fibers by the demonstration of a like time course of Ia afferent fiber depolarization and the type of inhibition reported by Frank and Fuortes (5). It was concluded that the diminution of the Ia excitatory postsynaptic potentials was caused by a diminished excitatory action of the presynaptic action potentials in Ia fiber terminals and the process was designated "presynaptic inhibition" (4,143).

B. The Eccles' Hypothesis

An extensive series of investigations conducted in the early 1960s by Eccles et al. led to the formulation of a hypothesis for the mechanism of presynaptic inhibition.

The precise correlation of the time course of the presynaptic inhibition of Ia-evoked excitatory postsynaptic potentials and the depolarization of presynaptic fibers (144–147) produced the formulation that presynaptic depolarization is the *causal* factor in the inhibition responsible for the excitatory postsynaptic potential reduction.

The presynaptic depolarization was believed responsible for depressing the amplitude of the presynaptic spike potential. In turn, the reduced size of the afferent spike caused a reduction in the amount of transmitter released from the afferent terminal (148,149).

The presynaptic depolarization was named primary afferent depolarization (PAD). It was thought to be caused by the prolonged action of a inhibitory chemical transmitter acting on the presynaptic terminal to produce a high permeability to ions (144,148,150). The inhibitory transmitter was postulated to be released from axoaxonic synapses located on or close to the synaptic terminals of afferent fibers.

A polysynaptic reflex pathway that included at least two interneurons was thought responsible for activating the axoaxonic synapse (144,148).

The hypothesis has been subjected to extensive experimental testing in the past two decades. Some of its provisions have been fully accepted; some are still in dispute.

1. Axoaxonic Synapses

Soon after axoaxonic synapses were first postulated on physiologic grounds they were described in the spinal cord by Gray (151). These early observations have been repeatedly verified (Fig. 5) and axoaxonic contacts have been demonstrated in electron micrographs of mammalian dorsal horn (152–155), Clarke's column

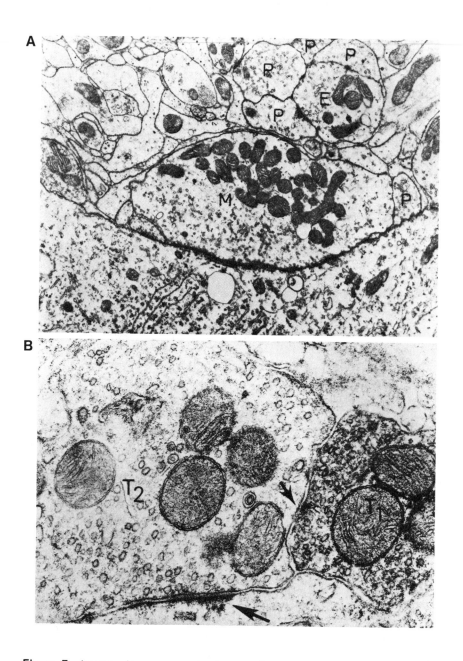

Figure 5 Axoaxonic synapses. A, Axoaxonic synapses on a motoneuron. M-bouton (M) covered by several smaller P-boutons (P). B, Axoaxonic synapse in lamina II. Immunocytochemical staining of a glutamic acid decarboxylase (GAD)-containing terminal (T_1) that is presynaptic to a second terminal (T_2) (small arrow) that in turn makes synaptic contact with a dendrite (large arrow). (A from Ref. 6; B from Ref. 159.)

(156,157), and the motor nuclei (6,158,159; cf. 15,17,160). They have also been described in the amphibian spinal cord, where they appear to be located at the base of the dorsal horn (12,161-163)—the precise location of the neuronal elements generating primary afferent depolarization.

Axoaxonic contacts in the mammalian motor nuclei consist of small (250-400 Å) boutons (P-boutons in the terminology of Conradi [6]) containing flattened or irregularly shaped vesicles that are apposed to the convex side of larger (4-7 μm) axonal terminals (M-boutons). In turn, the M-boutons, which contain spherical vesicles, synapse on the somata and proximal dendrites of motoneurons (6,12). Several P-boutons can contact one M-bouton and some P-boutons are apposed both at M-boutons and at the motoneuron membrane (6). Degeneration and injection studies have shown that dorsal root terminals are the postsynaptic elements in the axoaxonic appositions in both mammalian and frog cords (6,158,163).

2. Primary Afferent Depolarization

Afferent fiber volleys entering the spinal cord through the dorsal roots usually change the potential of presynaptic terminals and preterminal regions of neighboring afferents. Such presynaptic potential changes may be measured in several different ways (Fig. 6; see Schmidt [9] for complete discussion). The most frequently used method is the recording of dorsal root potentials from a dorsal root or rootlet. Although observations of such potentials were first reported almost 100 years ago (164), full descriptions were first given by Barron and Matthews (142,165).

Dorsal root potentials, usually recorded by means of two electrodes placed on a root—one close to the spinal cord and the other at a distance toward the cut end of the root, are most frequently negative in direction. There is general agreement that negative dorsal root potentials—DRP$_V$ in the terminology of Lloyd and McIntyre (166,167)—are produced by the electrotonic spread of a depolarozation generated in the terminal arborizations or in the terminals of afferent fibers and as such are an indication of primary afferent depolarization.

Primary afferent depolarization may be directly observed by intracellular recording from afferent fibers, but such recording is possible only in the dorsal region of the cord where the fibers are relatively corase (145,148,168-176). Alternatively, depolarization of afferent fibers may be tested indirectly by measuring their excitability by brief current pulses applied through an extracellular microelectrode (145,168,177,178). It is assumed that the excitability of afferent fibers is a function of the membrane potential.

a. Characteristics of primary afferent depolarization. Primary afferent depolarization can be evoked by electrical stimulation of large- and small-diameter myelinated and unmyelinated fibers in both cutaneous and muscle nerves (e.g., 144,145,179-185) and by stimulation of visceral nerves (186-188).

The latency of primary afferent depolarization has usually been considered to be 2-4 msec depending upon whether cutaneous or muscle afferents were stimulated (cf. 145,170,171,177). These values were obtained from measurements of the activity in populations of afferent fibers. A more recent analysis of the problem yielded minimal segmental latencies of 1.7-2.0 msec for primary afferent depolarization measured in single fibers and elicited by electrical stimuli applied to peripheral nerves (189). Furthermore, the latency was similar for primary afferent depolarization produced by stimulation of group I and of cutaneous afferents. Under most conditions, primary afferent depolarization usually slowly increases in amplitude over a period of 10-20 msec to a summit. The depolarization can persist for 200-300 msec in the cat and as long as 1000 msec in the frog when sucrose gap recordings are used (Fig. 6F). It is difficult to give exact figures for the duration, since intrafiber recordings and dorsal root potentials are distorted by electrotonic decrement of potential. In addition, most workers have used an AC-coupled recording system with a 1-second time constant to record dorsal root potentials. Such recording conditions can artifactually and substantially shorten the record by filtering out the slower components of the potential. Furthermore, the duration of primary afferent depolarization is a function of the type of fiber stimulated and whether or not repetitive stimuli have been used (e.g., 145,170,177).

b. Localization of primary afferent depolarization. The location of the site of maximum depolarization produced in primary afferent fibers has been ascertained by measurements of the intraspinal field potential occurring during primary afferent depolarization and by tests of the excitability of these fibers at various locations along their intramedullary course. The magnitude of primary afferent depolarization appears considerably greater in the preterminal and terminal regions of the afferent fibers than it is in the more proximal parts of these fibers. The evidence indicates that primary afferent depolarization is generated by a sink of membrane current in the terminal arborizations of the afferent fibers. The locus of primary afferent depolarization produced by volleys in group Ia fibers appears to be in the motor nucleus (145,168). A second site is located in the intermediate nucleus. There is some disagreement, however, with regard to cutaneous afferents. Wall and his coworkers (190-192) have indicated the major sink produced by cutaneous volleys to lie in the substantia gelatinosa, but Eccles and colleagues (144,168) have localized the site to lamina IV, at the base of the dorsal horn.

c. Mechanisms. There are three major hypotheses regarding the genesis of primary afferent depolarization. The mechanism has been attributed to: (1) current flows generated by interneurons, (2) the action of a specific chemical transmitter, and (3) a change in the ionic constitution of the extracellular space.

Current flows. It was originally proposed by Barron and Matthews (142) that the dorsal root potential was produced by electrical fields generated by the

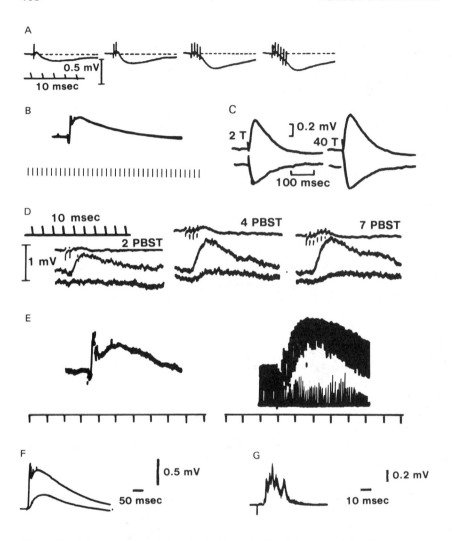

Figure 6 Primary afferent depolarization. A, Cord dorsum potentials produced by group I afferent volleys. The monopolar recording was taken from the cord surface just medial to the L7 dorsal root entry zone with an indifferent electrode on the back musculature. Potentials produced by just maximal stimuli for group I fibers contained in nerve to peroneal muscles and deep peroneal nerve. The prolonged positive wave (downward) is the P wave. B, Dorsal root potential recorded from a barbiturate-anesthetized cat in response to a cutaneous volley. Recording from lumbar dorsal root with a DC amplifier. Note dorsal root reflex. Calibration marked in 10 msec. C, Dorsal root potentials (upper traces) and cord dorsum potentials (P waves); lower traces). DRPs recorded from caudal L6 rootlet in response to afferent volleys (2 and 40 × threshold) in superficial

firing of interneurons. Although this theory was in vogue for some time (166, 193-196), it has been disproved by the recent experiments of Glusman and Rudomín (197). In these experiments performed on the frog spinal cord, primary afferent depolarization—measured by means of field potentials—disappeared following section of dorsal roots. This finding indicates that the afferent fibers contained in the dorsal roots were generating the extracellular currents associated with primary afferent depolarization rather than the interneurons that remained undisturbed by the root section.

Chemical transmission. The idea that primary afferent depolarization was caused by the action of a specific transmitter was first proposed by Fatt (198) and by Koketsu (172) who, however, differed in their ideas about the site of release of the transmitter. Fatt hypothesized that it could be liberated from activated afferent terminals and Koketsu thought that it might be released from interneuronal terminals.

Evidence compatible with the idea that at least part of primary afferent depolarization is caused by the action of a transmitter includes the following:

(1) Axoaxonic synapses are present on the terminals of afferent fibers (see Sec. III.B.1).
(2) Primary afferent depolarization has a central latency of several msec—a latency compatible with a synaptic process involving at least two synapses (see Sec. III.B.2.a).

---

peroneal nerve. D, Intracellular recording of PAD from quadriceps primary afferent fiber at the rostral L6 segmental level (middle traces). Upper traces from dorsal root entry zone; lower traces from microelectrode after withdrawal from fiber. Note depolarization of fiber produced by repetitive stimulation delivered to posterior biceps-semitendinosus nerve at strength maximum for group I fibers. E, Comparison of time course of dorsal root potential and excitability changes in terminal arborization of sural nerve fibers. In left trace, DRP is shown. In right trace, the excitability of the sural nerve endings was measured by stimulating the terminals by means of an electrode placed among them and recording the antidromic action potential in the nerve at the periphery. An increase in excitability is assumed to mean a depolarization of the membrane of the nerve endings and is reflected as an increase in the amplitude of the antidromic compound action potential. Calibration marked in 10 msec. F, Dorsal root potentials recorded from the isolated frog spinal cord. Superimposed oscilloscope sweeps of DRPs evoked by stimulation of an adjacent dorsal root (larger trace) and ventral root of same segment (smaller trace). G, Dorsal root reflex monophasically recorded from the distal end of the dorsal root of an isolated frog cord. Record obtained by superimposing 10 traces. (A and D from Ref. 145; C from Ref. 144; B and E from Ref. 177; F from Ref. 163a.)

(3) Primary afferent depolarization demonstrates spatial and temporal facilitation (145,168)—properties invariably associated with a synaptic relay in neuronal pathways.

(4) Primary afferent depolarization is evoked in different types of primary afferent fibers with remarkable specificity with respect to the types of input that produce the depolarization (9) (see Sec. III.B.2.c).

(5) In the isolated frog cord primary afferent depolarization is substantially (>90%) reduced by exposure of the cord to Ringer's solution containing concentrations of Mg^{2+}, Mn^{2+}, Co^{2+}, or La^{3+} ions sufficient to block synaptic transmission (199-203).

(6) There is a formidable body of evidence implicating gamma-aminobutyric acid (GABA) as the neurotransmitter involved in the production of primary afferent depolarization (204). In particular, a number of pharmacologic antagonists of the action of this amino acid at synaptic sites reduce primary afferent depolarization (see Sec. III.B.3.c).

It should be noted that all of this evidence is indirect, and while all of it is necessary, none of it is sufficient to confirm the idea that primary afferent depolarization is a synaptic process.

On the other hand, as indicated by Eccles, if primary afferent depolarization is synaptically generated, it should have properties similar to those of a variety of other depolarizing chemical synapses. In particular, there should be an increased ionic conductance and the depolarization should have an equilibrium potential more positive than the resting membrane potential (4,143). Precise analysis of the problem is made difficult by the complexity of the intact spinal cord. As a result, unequivocal data with regard to the ionic mechanisms of primary afferent depolarization is not available.

Primary afferent depolarization recorded intracellularly in an afferent fiber has been reported to be augmented by hyperpolarizing and decreased by depolarizing the fiber by means of current passed through the recording microelectrode (170,204a). However, the changes in amplitude produced in this way were relatively small, and in other experiments the results were indecisive (148). It must be realized, however, that the polarizing currents were applied far from the terminal region of the afferent fiber, the site of the presumed conductance change.

Primary afferent depolarization is increased in size by the hyperpolarization of afferent terminals occurring during the after-hyperpolarization and the hyperpolarization that follows tetanization (145,148,170), but the rising phase of the potential was changed very little. One would expect the rising phase to be steeper if the hyperpolarization produced its effects by increasing the driving current responsible for a synaptic potential.

Attempts to change the membrane potential of terminals by means of current passed across the cord by extrinsic electrodes has also yielded indecisive results. It is true that depolarization of intraspinal afferent fibers by this method can reduce the amplitude of the dorsal root potential (148), but reversal of the current to hyperpolarize the fibers produced similar effects—perhaps as a result of blocking transmission in the pathway responsible for producing primary afferent depolarization.

Padjen and his colleagues have been more successful in defining the mechanism of primary afferent depolarization (205). Intrafiber recordings from afferents in the isolated frog cord maintained in sucrose gap demonstrated a reduced membrane resistance during primary afferent depolarization. Furthermore, the amplitude of primary afferent depolarization was augmented by fiber hyperpolarization and reduced by fiber depolarization. These changes in fiber potential were produced by the application of current to the whole root by a bridge circuit. Padjen et al. (205) were not able to reverse primary afferent depolarization by depolarization. This latter finding was attributed to delayed rectification in afferent fibers, but as recently emphasized (206), it is impossible to establish the chemical synaptic nature of primary afferent depolarization without demonstration of a true reversal potential.

It has been hypothesized that primary afferent depolarization could be caused by an increased permeability to Na^+ and/or Cl^- ions and attempts have been made at defining the mechanism of primary afferent depolarization by means of ion substitution. In such experiments, advantage has been taken of the fact that the frog and neonatal rat spinal cords may be maintained by a superfusing salt solution, but the results have not yielded definitive answers. In large part, this is because of the effects of such ion substitution upon afferent inputs and upon the complex interneuronal population of the cord. In part, it is a result of the limitations inherent in extracellular recording.

The dorsal root potential evoked in the frog spinal cord by dorsal root stimulation has been reported to vary linearly with the logarithmic Na^+ concentration in the superfusate (207), but this effect probably results from a block of impulse activity in the afferent fibers and from reduction of excitatory synaptic activity in the interneurons producing the dorsal root potential, rather than from a direct effect on the ionic process generating the potential.

The dorsal root potential evoked by dorsal root stimulation is markedly prolonged by superfusion of the isolated frog cord with Cl^--free Ringer's solution (208,209). Again, this effect is probably not the result of a direct action on primary afferent depolarization, but is caused by a block of Cl^--dependent spinal postsynaptic inhibition, resulting in increased interneuronal activity of the cord. This idea is supported by the finding of a concomitant increase of polysynaptic reflex activity in low Cl^- solutions. On the other hand, an early component of the dorsal root potential produced in the frog cord by afferent fiber stimulation (Fig. 8B) and the dorsal root potential elicited by ventral root volleys are both reduced by exposure of the cord to low Cl^- Ringer's solution (208,209); so are the dorsal root potentials evoked in the isolated neonatal rat spinal cord (210, 211). In sum, although complicated by a variety of experimental factors, the results of these experiments are compatible with the idea that at least part of primary afferent depolarization is the result of a change in Cl^- permeability.

GABA-induced primary afferent depolarization. Many reports have shown that GABA depolarizes primary afferent fibers. This effect is thought to be caused by an action of the amino acid on specific receptors located on the afferent terminals (212). Extensive efforts have been made to determine the mechanism of this depolarization, since it should shed light on the mechanism of primary afferent depolarization. There is data indicating that the GABA response on the terminals of the isolated frog cord is abolished in Na^+-free Ringer's solution (208,213,214), but other experiments with Na^+ substitution have indicated that the GABA-evoked depolarization of primary afferent fibers is depressed only when the Na^+ concentration is substantially reduced (i.e., $<10\%$), and that at intermediate levels of the cation the response can actually be augmented (211,215). On the other hand, reduction of the Cl^- level in the Ringer's solution superfusing the frog and neonatal rat cord has been reported to depress the GABA-induced depolarization (208,211,213,215,216). Thus, the weight of evidence would seem to indicate that Cl^- ions mediate at least part of primary afferent depolarization, but the contribution of Na^+ ions to the process is still unclear.

GABA and dorsal root ganglion cells. Recent investigations have indicated that GABA depolarizes the somata of primary afferent neurons (217). Pharmacologically, the depolarization closely resembles that produced by GABA on the terminals of the same neurons (e.g., 217,218). Intracellular investigations on neurons in the intact ganglion and in culture have indicated that the depolarization is caused by an increased conductance to Cl^- ions (Fig. 7A) (215,218-223). Furthermore, while the reversal potential of the depolarization is related to the logarithmic Cl^- concentration (Fig. 7b), it is unaffected by changing the external Na^+, K^+, or Ca^{2+} concentrations (215,218-222,224).

Measurements of the reversal potential of the GABA-response have varied among different investigators, but all reported values are more positive than the resting membrane potential (Fig. 7b) (215,218,220,224). If it is assumed that the entire GABA-response on dorsal root ganglion cells is carried by Cl^- ions, then the Cl^- equilibrium potential must also be positive with respect to the resting membrane potential. Therefore, one would expect a "high" concentration of the anion in dorsal root ganglion cells and probably also in afferent terminals. Such a concentration gradient for Cl^- could only be explained if an inwardly directed pump maintained the intracellular level of Cl^- ions. However, attempts to block such a pump with agents that have been shown to affect Cl^- transport in other systems have not been successful (cf. 225-227).

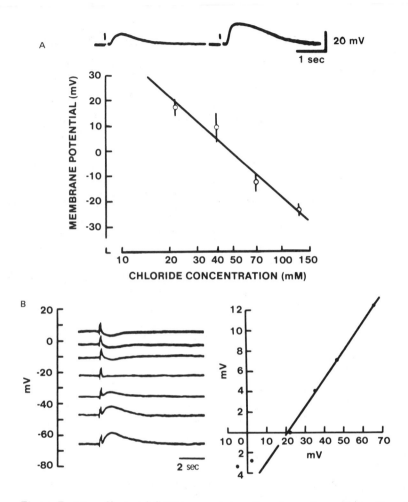

Figure 7 The effects of GABA on cat dorsal root ganglion cells in vitro. A, Cl⁻-dependency of depolarization evoked by iontophoresis of GABA. Upper left record is control response in normal Kreb's solution; upper right in medium containing 40 mM Cl⁻ demonstrating increase in rate of rise and amplitude of GABA response. The graph depicts the shifts in the GABA equilibrium potential produced by changes in the extracellular Cl⁻ concentration. B, Equilibrium potential of the GABA depolarization. The resting membrane potential was –66 mV. The graph plots the amplitudes of the GABA responses versus membrane potential. The reversal potential for the GABA response was –22 mV. (A and B from Ref. 218.)

Accumulation of Extracellular K^+. Although Barron and Matthews (142) had suggested that the dorsal root potential might be produced by alterations in extracellular ionic concentrations following neuronal impulses, the hypothesis was not explored until the development of ion-sensitive microelectrodes in the 1970s made possible precise observations of transient changes in ionic concentration.

A number of recent investigations have shown that afferent stimulation results in an increase in the concentration of K^+ ions in the extracellular space of the spinal gray matter. Furthermore, the increase is particularly high in the dorsal horn and intermediate nucleus—those loci of the cord where primary afferent depolarization is generated and where there are the largest number of axoaxonic synapses (e.g., 228-233; see review by Somjen in vol. 1 of this series for complete references [234]). Intraspinal afferent terminals are sensitive to changes in extracellular K^+ levels (213,235,236). As a result of these findings, much energy and polemic has been expended to revive the idea that K^+ is responsible for primary afferent depolarization.

Although some perspective has been achieved in defining the role of K^+, the situation is far from clear. There are a number of points that argue against the idea that increases in K^+ concentration are responsible for generating *all* of the potential change in primary afferent depolarization:

1. Although substantial quantities of the cation are released by tetanic afferent stimulation in mammalian and amphibian spinal cords (4-9.0 mM above resting levels [229-231,233,237]), only small amounts (<0.5 mM [237-240]) are accumulated following single afferent volleys.

2. The time course of the K^+ accumulation is much slower and more prolonged than the time course of primary afferent depolarization evoked by the same afferent stimuli causing the increased K^+ (237).

3. Volleys in Ia afferents produce a dorsal root potential and a concomitant increase in K^+ levels. However, primary afferent depolarization and K^+ increases can be dissociated. Conditioning volleys in flexor reflex afferents are reported to block the Ia-evoked dorsal root potential, while leaving the Ia-induced increase in K^+ levels unchanged (229).

4. Stimulation of the ventral root in the frog cord elicits a dorsal root potential (see Sec. III.B.2.c) that is not associated with any change in the extracellular K^+ concentration (233,240).

5. Some pharmacologic agents cause opposite effects on primary afferent depolarization and on K^+ accumulation (229) (see Sec. III.B.3.c). For example, barbiturates prolong, and sometimes increase, the amplitude of the dorsal root potential (241), but reduce the release of K^+ by afferent stimuli (229).

6. There is great specificity in the pathways generating primary afferent depolarization (see Sec. III.B.2.c). For example, volleys in group I afferents from

flexor muscles are reported to depress Ia excitatory postsynaptic potentials in extensor motoneurons without affecting monosynaptic excitatory postsynaptic potentials evoked from the vestibulospinal tract despite the fact that both sets of excitatory terminals are thought to be in close proximity (242). It would be expected that K^+ accumulation would affect all presynaptic terminals near to the site of K^+ release.

On the other hand, a small dorsal root potential and a small increment in the extracellular K^+ concentration can be elicited in the frog spinal cord when all synaptic transmission has been blocked by bathing the cord in high concentrations of Mg^{2+} (200,202,240). On the basis of such data it has been calculated that the increment in extracellular K^+ evoked by a single dorsal root volley in the isolated frog spinal cord could account for 10–33% of the potential change underlying the dorsal root potential (235,240).

Attention has been paid toward determining the origin of the accumulated extracellular K^+. Most of the K^+ released into the extracellular space in the spinal cord by afferent stimulation is believed to originate in synaptically activated secondary neurons; in other words, intact synaptic transmission is thought necessary for K^+ to be released—a conclusion reached because concentrations of Mg^{2+} high enough to suppress synaptic activity (10–20 mM) markedly attenuate the release of K^+ (202,240). But such high concentrations of the cation have other effects (e.g., to reduce the excitability of afferent fibers). It may well be that K^+ could be liberated by activity of the unmyelinated terminal arborization of afferent fibers (243). The problem requires further study.

Two components to primary afferent depolarization. The current picture of primary afferent depolarization generation has been further complicated by observations that suggest that more than one mechanism may be involved. Thus, although much weight with regard to the GABA hypothesis has been placed on the findings that the GABA antagonists picrotoxin and bicuculline reduce primary afferent depolarization (208,214,241,244-250), recent investigations that have utilized DC recordings from dorsal roots of the isolated frog cord have shown that these agents reduce only the early phase of the dorsal root potential; the latter portion of the potential is enlarged and prolonged even during the peak effect of the convulsants (236,251-253) (Fig. 8A). It should be realized, however, that no picrotoxin- or bicuculline-resistant dorsal root potential has been described in the mammalian spinal cord.

Since picrotoxin and bicuculline antagonize the effects of GABA in a number of synaptic sites, the most likely explanation of their ability to block the early phase of primary afferent depolarization rests with the capacity of these convulsants to exert the same antagonistic activity at GABAergic synapses located on primary afferent fibers. In other words, there is good reason to believe that the early component of primary afferent depolarization is mediated by the action of the amino acid.

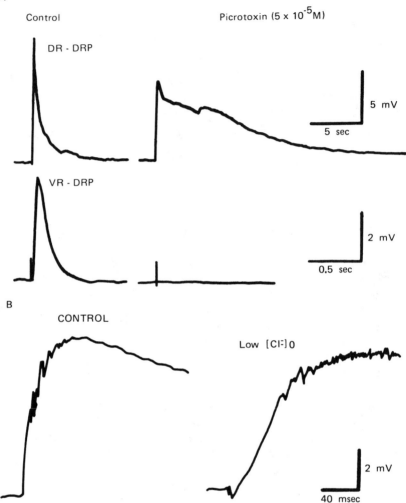

Figure 8 Effect of picrotoxin and low external chloride concentration on the dorsal root potential. A, Sucrose gap recordings from dorsal root of isolated frog spinal cord. Dorsal root potentials evoked by simulation of adjacent dorsal root (DR-DRP) and by stimulation of ventral root of same segment (VR-DRP) in normal Ringer's solution (control) and 20 min after addition of picrotoxin to superfusate. Note abolition of VR-DRP and reduction of early component of DR-DRP as well as appearance of another later depolarizing component of the DR-DRP. B, Sucrose gap recordings from frog dorsal root. DRP elicited by stimulation of adjacent dorsal root in normal Ringer's solution (left trace) and after superfusion with Ringer's solution in which 95% of the chloride was replaced with isethionate. Again, note reduction of early part of DRP and appearance of a late component. (A from Ref. 251. B from unpublished observations of J. C. Hackman and R. A. Davidoff.)

It may be that accumulation of interstitial K^+ accounts for the slow component of primary afferent depolarization (239,254). In this regard it should be noted that concentrations of picrotoxin and bicuculline that increase the amplitude of the slow phase of the dorsal root potential increase the evoked release of K^+ in the spinal cord (229,239,240,255); an augmented local level of K^+ could be the main factor in the convulsant-induced enhancement of the slow phase of primary afferent depolarization. Alternatively, a transmitter resistant to the blocking actions of picrotoxin and bicuculline may be involved in the production of primary afferent depolarization (215).

Primary afferent hyperpolarization. There are numerous reports that stimulation of afferent fibers (167,256-262) and of supraspinal structures (263-266) can hyperpolarize the terminals of inactive primary afferent fibers. This hyperpolarization—designated primary afferent hyperpolarization (PAH)—can be demonstrated by means of positive dorsal root potentials (256,258,262-264, 267-270) (Fig. 9), by intrafiber recording (260,261), and by a decreased excitability of afferent terminals (256,261,270-272).

The mechanism of primary afferent hyperpolarization is not known with certainty, but it is generally believed that it is a consequence of the suppression of tonic background activity in primary afferent depolarization-generating systems (190,256,263,273). This suppression may result from inhibition of tonically active interneurons intercalated in the pathway to afferent terminals and responsible for generating primary afferent depolarization. Active synaptic hyperpolarization of afferent terminals has also been proposed to account for some primary afferent hyperpolarization (265), but the evidence supporting this proposal is not convincing.

Controversy has arisen concerning the types of stimuli effective in evoking primary afferent hyperpolarization, but it is now generally agreed that afferent volleys in small-diameter fibers from both cutaneous and muscle nerves can hyperpolarize some large-diameter afferent fiber terminals (256-260,262). However, such hyperpolarization may only be evoked under certain conditions of stimulation (e.g., certain rates of stimulation [259]) and may be limited to a small number of recipient terminals (260). It should also be noted that some stimuli reported to elicit primary afferent hyperpolarization can also produce primary afferent depolarization.

Pathways generating primary afferent depolarization. It is unanimously agreed that volleys in cutaneous nerves are much more effective in evoking primary afferent depolarization than volleys in muscle or visceral nerves (e.g., 142,145,171,177,183,274). For example, dorsal root potentials can be obtained by activation of some single cutaneous fibers (274,275). In contrast, dorsal root potentials can be elicited only when several muscle afferent fibers are activated simultaneously. In addition, larger potential changes are produced by cutaneous than by muscle afferent volleys (e.g., 145). Dorsal root potentials can also be elicited by natural stimulation of receptors in skin and muscle (e.g., 262,271, 276-281).

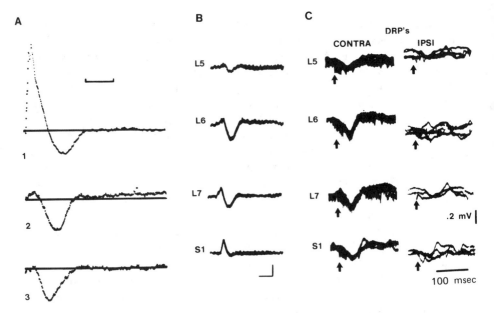

Figure 9 Primary afferent hyperpolarization. A, DRPs recorded from L7 dorsal rootlet in response to sural nerve stimulation. Top trace in response to maximal stimulation. Middle trace evoked by same stimulus but with anodal blocking of the afferent volley. A_β potentials were not seen in recordings (not illustrated) from sural nerve and it was considered that the positive DRP was mainly generated by activity in fine (i.e., A_δ and C) fibers. Bottom trace taken while anodal block was in effect and while a rostral L7 rootlet was continuously stimulated at 100 Hz. This latter stimulus generated a small steady negative DRP and eliminated the phasic negative DRP evoked by the sural nerve test shock. Each trace represents the average of eight responses. The animal was spinalized and unanesthetized. Calibration line is 100 msec. B, DRPs evoked in different dorsal root filaments in the same preparation by stimulation of the gastrocnemius-soleus nerve. Note the differing amplitudes of negative and positive DRPs in different filaments. Calibration: 100 μV, 100 msec. C, DRPs recorded from various spinal segments (L5–S1) on the same (ipsi) and on the opposite (contra) side as the site of stimulation in the nucleus reticularis gigantocellularis. The stimulus was 200 Hz, 20 msec train delivered with a monopolar electrode. (A from Ref. 258. Copyright 1970 by the American Association for the Advancement of Science. B from Ref. 261. C from Ref. 266.)

Interneurons. Although the existence of disynaptic (282) or even monosynaptic (283) pathways has been considered, it has been generally agreed that the pathway generating primary afferent depolarization is polysynaptic, involving a chain of two or possibly three serially arranged interneurons (9,143). This idea was based on early data concerning the latency of primary afferent depolarization and on the observation that the latency of synaptic action does not exceed 0.5 msec in the mammalian spinal cord. The idea of a polysynaptic pathway was supported by the slow time course of primary afferent depolarization and by the findings of spatial and temporal summation of primary afferent depolarization (143,144,284). Interneurons (so-called D-cells) with appropriate properties (e.g., excitation by suitable afferents; repetitive discharges to afferent volleys) were described by the Eccles' group in the intermediate nucleus for the case of primary afferent depolarization involving group I fibers and at the base of the dorsal horn in the case of cutaneous fibers (144).

The problem has recently been reexamined by the technique of intraspinal stimulation (189,285). Taken together with more precise data indicating a shorter latency for primary afferent depolarization than was previously thought (1.7-2.0 msec [189]) (Fig. 10A), primary afferent depolarization appears generated by a trisynaptic pathway with two interposed interneurons—the last interneuron mediating primary afferent depolarization of cutaneous fibers located in laminae III and IV (the base of the dorsal horn) and the last interneuron involved in primary afferent depolarization of group I afferents in laminae V and VI (the intermediate nucleus) (Fig. 10B). Thus, it appears that the original ideas of Eccles (143) regarding the location of the interneuronal apparatus generating primary afferent depolarization are supported. However, the data do not exclude the possibility of parallel polysynaptic pathways with interneurons located in other loci. In addition, the role of the numerous axoaxonic synapses that presumably contain GABA located in the substantia gelatinosa (158,159) and the location of their cell bodies must be ascertained.

Input-output relations. A number of relatively complex input-output patterns have been described for primary afferent depolarization that depend upon the type of afferent fibers stimulated (e.g., groups I, II, III, or IV), the origin of the fibers (e.g., phasic or tonic cutaneous receptors; receptors in extensor or flexor muscle), and the type of recipient afferent (e.g., cutaneous or muscle). In addition, descending pathways also generate primary afferent depolarization. The earlier literature has been reviewed extensively by Schmidt (9) and an update has been provided by Baldissera et al. (76).

Data concerning the input-output patterns of primary afferent depolarization have been obtained from a variety of different experimental preparations (anesthetized intact animals [e.g., 182,271]; anesthetized [e.g., 276] and unanesthetized [e.g., 180] spinal animals; decerebrate animals [e.g., 181,185]). These factors complicate analysis of published data. For example, primary afferent depolarization is increased by barbiturates and by other anesthetics (167,241,244,286). Furthermore, the excitability of primary afferent terminals is influenced by activity of supraspinal structures and there is data that a tonic control is exerted (e.g., 185,287). In addition, it appears that the excitability of

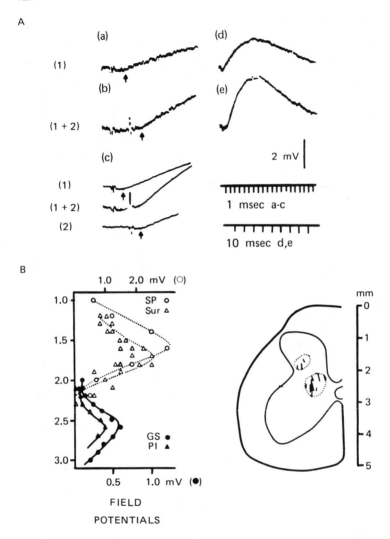

Figure 10 Latency and site of generation of primary afferent depolarization. A, Minimal latency of dorsal root potential. DRPs recorded from the most caudal filament of L6 dorsal root and evoked by single (1), two (1 + 2), and the second of two stimuli (intensity maximal for group I afferents) applied to deep peroneal nerve. Latency was measured in relation to the incoming volleys following the first and second stimulus. Records in c taken with faster sweep speed. To estimate the latency of the DRP produced by the second stimulus (presumably producing a facilitated response), the DRPs evoked by one stimulus were subtracted from the DRPs evoked by a pair. Arrows indicate the onset of the DRP. Single sweeps in a, b, d, and e; 64 averaged sweeps in c. B, Optimal

single afferent terminals fluctuates over time (288). Presumably, these fluctuations are related to alterations in the level of tonically maintained primary afferent depolarization.

Primary afferent depolarization in muscle afferents. In general, activity in muscle afferents influences other muscle afferents (Fig. 11). Thus, group Ia afferents from both extensor and flexor muscles are depolarized mainly by stimulation of group Ia and group Ib afferents from ipsilateral muscles (145,147, 168,281,289–299). Although Ia terminals were originally considered to be unaffected by activation of high-threshold muscle or cutaneous afferents (145, 269,288,293,294), such effects have now been described (262). In addition, a long-latency primary afferent depolarization can be demonstrated following the injection of DOPA (3,4-dihydroxyphenylalanine) into spinal animals (257,300). It is also now realized that cutaneous volleys can produce a mixture of primary afferent depolarization and primary afferent hyperpolarization in Ia fibers (270) and these opposite actions may cancel in measurements of population responses. Thus, subtle effects of cutaneous afferents on Ia fibers may have been overlooked.

The terminals of group Ib fibers of both extensor and flexor muscles are depolarized mainly by activity in other Ib afferents, but high-threshold muscle and cutaneous fibers are also effective (262,281,292,293). Volleys in Ia fibers do not contribute to primary afferent depolarization of Ib afferents (293).

Primary afferent depolarization in cutaneous fibers. Primary afferent depolarization is produced in cutaneous afferents by stimulation of other large and small cutaneous fibers, and by volleys in group Ib and high-threshold muscle afferents. Ia afferents do not depolarize cutaneous afferents (144,169,278,281, 290,292,301–303). Selective electrical stimulation of fine afferents in cutaneous nerves or noxious stimulation of the skin produces primary afferent depolarization in a variety of large-diameter afferent fibers (179–182,262). Conversely, the excitability of unmyelinated cutaneous afferent fibers is reported increased following electrical stimulation of large cutaneous afferents or mechanical stimulation of hair receptors served by large afferents (184,185,271,272).

---

regions for producing PAD. Graph indicates the amplitude of field potentials evoked from cutaneous (open symbols; SP, superficial peroneal nerve; Sur, sural nerve) and group I (closed symbols; GS, gastrocnemius nerve; Pl, plantaris nerve) afferents as a function of depth from the cord dorsum. Cord diagram is a reconstruction of spinal cord regions from which PAD was elicited at lowest thresholds and with shortest latency by intraspinal microstimulation. Upper and lower regions enclosed by dashed lines indicate such optimal areas for cutaneous and group I afferents, respectively. The lines within the regions indicate effective parts of individual electrode tracks. (From Ref. 189.)

FIBERS GIVING   FIBERS RECEIVING

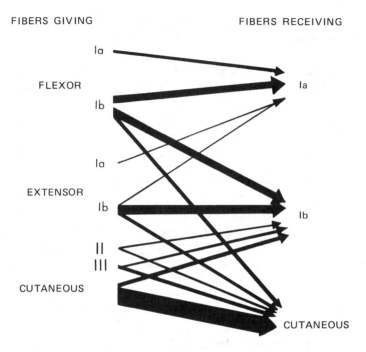

Figure 11 Diagram of afferent fibers producing depolarization of group I and large cutaneous fibers. The widths of the arrows are approximately proportional to the amounts of PAD that are produced in each case. (From Ref. 169.)

The primary afferent depolarization evoked in cutaneous afferents by stimulation of other cutaneous fibers possesses a high degree of modality and spatial specificity. For example, primary afferent depolarization can be produced by activity in large fibers from both tonic and phasic cutaneous mechanoreceptors (271,278-280,304), but primary afferent depolarization produced by activity in a particular fiber type is directed most strongly to fibers of the same type; that is, stimulation of slowly adapting mechanoreceptors produces relatively more depolarization of fiber terminals from other slowly adapting receptors than of fiber terminals from rapidly adapting receptors; conversely, primary afferent depolarization in afferents from rapidly adapting receptors is most easily elicited by stimulation of rapidly adapting receptors (271,280,304). There is also data that indicate the presence of a system in the cord that receives input mainly from myelinated nociceptor fibers and that mainly depolarizes fibers of the same type (271). Furthermore, primary afferent depolarization in cutaneous fibers appears to have a topographic organization. For example, mechanical stimulation of the skin will exert its greatest influence on cutaneous afferents coming from receptors located in contiguous skin areas (278,280).

Ventral root-evoked primary afferent depolarization. Early investigations by Barron and Matthews (142) indicated that in the frog spinal cord antidromic activation of motoneurons by ventral root volleys generate primary afferent depolarization. This observation has been confirmed on numerous occasions (e.g., 166,172,178,196,197,203,305) (Fig. 6F). Since dorsal root potentials evoked by ventral root stimulation are blocked by agents that interfere with cholinergic transmission (203,306), it is thought that the depolarization results from activation of motor axon collaterals that make cholinergic synapses on interneurons and that in turn terminate either directly on afferent fiber terminals or, more likely in view of the long latency of the depolarization (10-60 msec depending on the temperature of the preparation [cf. 196,203, 305]), do so via a chain of interneurons. Strong support for this idea is provided by the reports of Shapovalov and Shiriaev (173,174). Simultaneous intracellular recordings from frog motoneurons and from dorsal root fibers revealed long-latency (12-19 msec; temperature unspecified) depolarizations in afferent fibers after direct stimulation of single motoneurons. These depolarizations were chemically mediated, since they were blocked by substitution of Mn^{2+} for Ca^{2+} in the superfusate. Furthermore, picrotoxin antagonized the depolarizations, indicating that GABA was probably the responsible transmitter. It should be noted that the dorsal root potential elicited by ventral root stimulation is very sensitive to the actions of GABA antagonists (178,251).

In the frog, dorsal root potentials produced by antidromic stimulation of extensor motor nerves are usually larger than the dorsal root potentials produced by antidromic stimulation of flexor motor nerves (305,307). This suggests that during the powerful extensor muscle contractions that are characteristic of amphibians, there is a widespread depolarization of afferent fibers. The primary afferent depolarization appears mostly in cutaneous and extensor muscle afferent fibers (305).

It has been generally agreed that antidromic ventral root volleys fail to produce primary afferent depolarization in the mammalian spinal cord; but recently, stimulation of the third sacral ventral root in the cat has been reported to evoke bilateral dorsal root potentials in the corresponding dorsal roots (308). It may be that primary afferent depolarization elicited in this way in the cat is caused by activation of sensory afferents, which are now known to enter the cord in the ventral roots (309-311).

Dorsal root reflexes. During primary afferent depolarization antidromic discharges can sometimes be recorded from peripheral cutaneous or muscle nerves or from dorsal roots (142,165,196,282,294,312-315) (Fig. 6G). The antidromic impulses coincide with the ascending phase of primary afferent depolarization, (196) and it is believed that they arise when primary afferent depolarization is elicited by a highly synchronized afferent input producing primary afferent depolarization with a steeply rising ascending phase sufficient to reach the threshold of afferent fibers (142,294,316). Such synchronized inputs occur when a whole cutaneous nerve is stimulated electrically. There is little information concerning the elicitation of dorsal root reflexes by physiologic stimuli.

As expected from a process related to primary afferent depolarization, dorsal root reflexes are most readily observed in cutaneous nerves, but they can also be recorded in muscle nerves, particularly in cooled animals (312–314). There is general agreement that full dorsal root discharges can be elicited by stimulation of large myelinated fibers and that most of the antidromic action potentials are produced in myelinated afferents (282,313,317).

Descending pathways. Dorsal root potentials are evoked in the afferent fibers of the lumbosacral cord by activation of many supraspinal structures. These structures include the sensorimotor cortex, the brainstem, the vestibular nuclei, and the cerebellum.

Group Ia afferents appear most influenced by subcortical structures. For example, they are depolarized by stimulation of the reticular formation (318), including a dorsal midline region of the medulla that projects to the spinal cord by means of the ipsilateral medial longitudinal fasciculus (319,320). Primary afferent depolarization in Ia fibers is also produced by activation of the VIIIth cranial nerve, presumably via the vestibular nuclei and the vestibulospinal tract (321,322), and by stimulation of cerebellar structures (323).

The sensorimotor cortex is reported not to influence Ia terminals, but stimulation of the cortex does inhibit transmission in the pathway from Ia fibers that generates primary afferent depolarization in Ia fibers (324–327). Rubrospinal fibers also inhibit transmission in the same segmental pathway (328).

The cortex produces primary afferent depolarization in Ib and cutaneous fibers (324–327,329,330). The effect appears mediated by both pyramidal and extrapyramidal pathways. Since spatial facilitation has been observed between segmental and cortical inputs producing primary afferent depolarization (327, 331), it is probable that a common interneuronal pathway is activated by pathways from the cortex and from the periphery. Primary afferent depolarization in Ib and cutaneous fibers is also produced by stimulation of wide areas of the reticular formation of the brainstem (319,320,332), the vestibular nuclei, and the cerebellum (264,320-323,333).

Rudomín and his colleagues (284a,285) have recently obtained data by means of excitability measurements of single fibers that indicate that depolarization of terminals is not restricted to primary afferent fibers, but that it may also be produced in the descending terminals of the corticospinal and rubrospinal systems. Thus, these terminals—but not those of the vestibulospinal tract—are depolarized by group I and by cutaneous volleys. There appears to be some specificity in the process, since volleys in certain specific afferent nerves more effectively depolarize the rubrospinal terminals than volleys in other sensory nerves. It should be noted that the changes of excitability generated in descending terminals are small compared to those produced in primary afferent terminals by the same conditioning stimuli.

The mechanism of the depolarization of descending fiber terminals is not known, but a process involving GABA appears unlikely, since iontophoretic injections of the amino acid either do not affect the descending terminals or hyperpolarize them (285).

3. Presynaptic Inhibition

To reiterate (see Sec. III.B), Eccles and his colleagues (4,9,143) defined presynaptic inhibition as the depression of excitatory postsynaptic potentials unaccompanied by concomitant change in postsynaptic excitability. Primary afferent depolarization was implicated as the causal step in the presynaptic inhibitory process because of the close correspondence between the time course of primary afferent depolarization and presynaptic inhibition and because of the similar pharmacologic responsiveness of the two phenomena to picrotoxin (4,143).

Alternatively, as first proposed by Frank (127), the depression of excitatory postsynaptic potentials could be caused by postsynaptic inhibition exerted on the dendrites electrotonically distant from the soma—so-called "remote inhibition" (see Sec. II.D.3). A microelectrode located in the soma would be unable to detect any voltage or conductance changes produced by such remote postsynaptic inhibition.

The only spinal pathway in which these hypotheses have been investigated in depth is the Ia afferent fiber system that makes monosynaptic contact with alpha motoneurons.

a. Time course. There is little disagreement that the time course of the depression of the Ia excitatory postsynaptic potential produced by Ia conditioning volleys is qualitatively similar to the time course of the primary afferent depolarization in Ia afferents evoked by the same types of conditioning stimuli (cf. latency and duration of Ia excitatory postsynaptic potential depression and primary afferent depolarization [e.g., 145,147,148,168,171,172,177,241,334, 335]) (Fig. 12A). In addition, inferences about changes in Ia excitatory postsynaptic potentials have been made from measurements of changes in monosynaptic reflex transmission following stimuli that produce primary afferent depolarization in Ia fibers (241,336). Again, the time courses of the two phenomena—reflex depression and primary afferent depolarization—are very similar.

Interpretation of the correlation is complicated by reports that stimuli used to evoke primary afferent depolarization can also produce concomitant postsynaptic inhibitions (see Sec. II.D.3). Such postsynaptic processes may contaminate measurements of excitatory postsynaptic potential amplitude.

b. Measurement of postsynaptic conductance. Measurements of postsynaptic conductance changes in alpha motoneurons following stimuli that evoke primary afferent depolarization have been the focus of major efforts both to support and to discredit the Eccles' hypothesis of presynaptic inhibition. It is felt that the hypothesis is supported by evidence that indicates a lack of

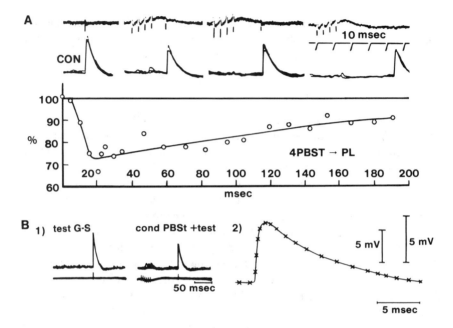

Figure 12 Presynaptic inhibition. A, Depression of a monosynaptic EPSP by afferent volleys. The amplitude of the monosynaptic EPSP (CON) recorded in a plantaris motoneuron is depressed by four group I conditioning volleys in the nerve to the hamstrings. The intervals between the conditioning and test volleys are seen in the upper traces recorded from the dorsal root entry zone. The graph illustrates the time course of the depression of the EPSP (as a percentage of control) for the experiment partially illustrated in the traces. B, Depression of homonymous EPSP in gastrocnemius motoneuron by conditioning volleys in hamstring nerve. Upper traces are intracellular records and lower traces are from dorsal root entry zone. B_1, Left trace—unconditioned control; right trace—conditioning volleys evoked at a stimulus of 1.6× threshold, which was submaximal for group I afferents. B_2, The graph represents the time course of the unconditioned (crosses) and conditioned (continuous line) EPSP as plotted from traces in B_1. Note two different voltage calibrations. (A from Ref. 147; B from Ref. 334.)

postsynaptic effects and is disproved by data that demonstrate such effects. However, since the two processes of inhibition are not mutually exclusive, this reasoning is probably fallacious (discussed later).

   There are many examples of Ia excitatory postsynaptic potential depression without concomitant postsynaptic conductance or potential changes (e.g., 5,127,130,135,147,242,334,335,337). In particular, a number of investigations have indicated that the falling phase of the composite Ia excitatory postsynaptic potential is unchanged during primary afferent depolarization (130,132,147, 242,334,335,337; cf. 135) (Fig. 12B). Since available data indicate that the Ia excitatory postsynaptic potential is a composite potential produced by the activation of both somatic and dendritic synapses (338), the decay of the falling phase should be very sensitive to inhibitory postsynaptic potentials generated far out on motoneuron dendrites.

Other investigations have shown that conditioning volleys that evoke primary afferent depolarization produce no change in the threshold current required for generation of an impulse (127,132), do not alter the membrane potential changes caused by a depolarizing or hyperpolarizing pulse of current (334), and do not affect monosynaptic excitatory postsynaptic potentials evoked by volleys in descending tracts (242,334) even when such excitatory postsynaptic potentials are in electrotonic proximity to Ia excitatory postsynaptic potentials.

On the other hand, there is data that show postsynaptic changes. For example, afferent volleys that produce primary afferent depolarization in Ia terminals have been reported to cause long-lasting inhibitory postsynaptic potentials (130,134,135) (Fig. 13A). A remote dendritic location for the synapses generating the long-lasting inhibitory postsynaptic potentials was demonstrated by the findings that the inhibitory postsynaptic potentials were relatively insensitive to intracellular injection of Cl^- ions or current (130). But, the problem is complicated. For example, inhibitory postsynaptic potentials can be evoked in some cases by volleys that do not influence the Ia excitatory postsynaptic potential, and conversely Ia excitatory postsynaptic potentials can sometimes be depressed by stimuli that do not produce detectable postsynaptic hyperpolarization (130). On the other hand, maximum excitatory postsynaptic potential depression was obtained with group I afferent conditioning volleys, whereas the inhibitory postsynaptic potential continued to grow with the recruitment of group II and III fibers.

The repetitive discharge of alpha motoneurons caused by injected depolarizing current is reduced by conditioning stimuli that are believed to produce presynaptic inhibition (130,132,339). Reduction of such repetitive firing is clearly the result of a postsynaptic change. Other studies, however, have shown that inhibition of repetitive discharge appeared only when stimuli at, or above, the threshold for eliciting long-lasting inhibitory postsynaptic potentials were used (130) (Fig. 13B). In addition, Carlen et al. (135) were able to demonstrate a postsynaptic conductance in almost all alpha motoneurons following minimal conditioning stimuli normally associated with the production of primary afferent depolarization. In this investigation, the decay of injected short current pulses was analyzed before and after conditioning volleys. The voltage changes produced by such pulses should be sensitive to alterations in distal as well as in proximal dendritic conductance (340).

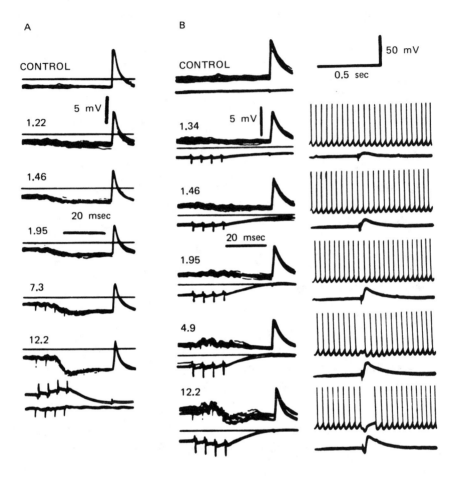

Figure 13 Postsynaptic changes produced by afferent inputs. A, Intracellular recording (K citrate electrode) from gastrocnemius-soleus motoneuron showing effects of four hamstring afferent volleys on resting membrane potential and monosynaptic EPSP. Strength of afferent stimuli expressed as multiples of threshold voltage for group I fibers. First trace (control) is unconditioned record. The bottom two traces are the cord dorsum response and the extracellular field potential. Each record consists of about 10 superimposed traces. B, Intracellular recordings (K citrate electrode) from gastrocnemius-soleus motoneuron demonstrating the effect of four hamstring volleys on the monosynaptic EPSP (left column) and on the repetitive discharge evoked by injection of current (right column). Hyperpolarizing potential (IPSP) partially masked by admixed EPSP. Note inhibition of cell firing at 1.95× threshold. In both columns the cord dorsum potentials are shown beneath the intracellular records. (A from Ref. 130; B from Ref. 129.)

In sum, it appears that postsynaptic changes can be generated by some afferent volleys that have previously been considered to produce only presynaptic inhibition. In many cases, small changes in the strength of the current used to stimulate afferent nerves is the determining factor in deciding whether presynaptic or postsynaptic changes are evoked. But there is no reason why primary afferent depolarization and presynaptic inhibition cannot be coincident with postsynaptic inhibition. Postsynaptic inhibition and presynaptic inhibition may very well be caused by activation of the same interneurons—such interneurons making axoaxonic contacts with afferent terminals and axodendritic synapses with neurons (e.g., 154,158,197). In such a situation primary afferent depolarization and postsynaptic inhibition would be inseparable.

c. *Pharmacologic observations.* Eccles and his colleages (241) reported that picrotoxin reduced the dorsal root potential and the concomitant inhibition of monosynaptic reflexes produced by afferent volleys that, in other studies, evoked a reduction in the Ia excitatory postsynaptic potential. On the other hand, they observed that strychnine increased primary afferent depolarization and inhibition of monosynaptic reflexes. These observations have been amply confirmed (see 10 for refs). At the time these experiments were performed the identity of the transmitters responsible for spinal inhibition were unknown. As a result it was felt that the data permitted a sharp distinction to be made between presynaptic and postsynaptic inhibition. However, it is now known that GABA hyperpolarizes motoneurons in a manner similar to that of glycine (341, 342). There are also examples of postsynaptic inhibition in the spinal cord sensitive to picrotoxin (133,134) or to bicuculline (343,344) and that are therefore presumably generated by the action of GABA. There is also histologic evidence that GABAergic terminals make synaptic contact with motoneurons (159). Thus, the sharp pharmacologic distinction between presynaptic and postsynaptic inhibition can no longer be made and such data cannot be used to support the Eccles' hypothesis.

d. *Possible mechanisms.* There are a number of possible ways by which presynaptic mechanisms can modulate the release of transmitter from primary afferent terminals. Eccles (147,148) first postulated that depolarization of afferent terminals diminished the amplitude of the action potential in the terminals and that this change in the action potential in turn reduced the output of transmitter. It was assumed that the size of the excitatory postsynaptic potential is related to the size of the presynaptic action potential and that the action potential amplitude is a function of the membrane potential. It was also assumed that, as at other synapses (e.g., 345,346), there is a very steep relationship between the size of the action potential in afferent terminals and the release of transmitter such that small changes in spike size can greatly affect postsynaptic potentials. No mention was made of possible mechanisms by which a smaller action potential would release less transmitter.

None of the above assumptions can be directly tested, since the small size of afferent terminals precludes intracellular recording. There are, however, some pertinent data. The size of the action potential recorded in the proximal portions of afferent fibers is diminished during primary afferent depolarization, but only by a few percent (148). However, such recordings may only approximate conditions at afferent terminals where primary afferent depolarization is much larger than in the more proximal portions of the fibers. The amplitude of the spike is also reduced by the passage of depolarizing currents through electrodes placed on the dorsal root or on the spinal cord (149,150). In addition, passive depolarization of afferent fibers decreases the size of the Ia excitatory postsynaptic potential evoked by volleys in the depolarized fibers (149). On the other hand, such a decrease in the excitatory postsynaptic potential might have resulted from a depolarization-induced conduction block in some of the fibers or preterminal arborizations conveying the afferent volley. Excitatory postsynaptic potentials were not reduced by the application of polarizing currents directly to dorsal roots (347), but presumably such currents significantly decremented along the afferent fibers and may not have reached the terminals.

Realization that the changes in the resting membrane and spike potentials of afferent fibers by passive depolarization were insufficient to explain the large reductions in excitatory postsynaptic potentials seen during primary afferent depolarization prompted consideration of the role that a conductance change in presynaptic terminals might play in presynaptic inhibition (4,148). An increase in conductance would shunt the currents generating the action potential in afferent terminals and result in a decrease in its size or alternatively cause a block of impulse invasion into terminals (see Sec. III.B.2.c). There is evidence that conductance changes in terminals may play an important role in presynaptic inhibition in invertebrates. (See references in Ref. 8.) At the present time, the relative importance of depolarization and conductance changes in reducing transmitter release from spinal afferent terminals is not known.

It is now thought that depolarization of a nerve terminal following an action potential leads to an increased Ca^{2+} conductance and an influx of the cation into the terminal. There is evidence that this same process may take place at the terminals of spinal afferent fibers (348). The entry of Ca^{2+} increases the internal Ca^{2+} concentration and causes the release of transmitter. The proposal of Eccles of a very steep relationship between the amount of transmitter released by afferent terminals and the amplitude of the presynaptic spike must now be updated in terms of the Ca^{2+} hypothesis. In other words, it is now required that the influx of Ca^{2+} be a very steep function of the action potential size. Unfortunately, there is no available data for spinal afferents.

There are several ways in which primary afferent depolarization could reduce the Ca^{2+} currents involved in transmitter release. It is possible that such currents are voltage sensitive and decreased by the change in membrane potential produced by primary afferent depolarization. It is also possible that such Ca^{2+} currents are reduced by the direct action of GABA. Recently, Dunlap and Fischbach (349,350) reported that application of GABA decreased the Ca^{2+} component of the action potential in the somata of cultured embryonic sensory neurons (Fig. 14). The reduction in the inward Ca^{2+} current appeared to result from a selective suppression of the voltage-sensitive Ca^{2+} conductance in these cells. It was produced by concentrations of GABA that did not cause a change in resting membrane conductance. However, caution must be exercised in evaluating the significance of these data with regard to the mechanism of presynaptic inhibition, since this effect of GABA is insensitive to conventional GABA antagonists. In addition, it appears that cultured sensory neurons may have two GABA receptors—one, an unconventional type responsible for reduction of the Ca^{2+} current, unaffected by GABA antagonists, and activated by baclofen, a GABA analogue; and a second type, a more conventional GABA receptor that causes an increased permeability to Cl^- and that is blocked by GABA antagonists (223). It is of interest that baclofen reduces monosynaptic reflexes and is thought to do so by reducing the output of excitatory transmitter from afferent terminals. (See references in Ref. 351.)

There are many suggestions in the literature that block of conduction of action potentials through the branching arborizations of afferent fibers is responsible for inhibition in the spinal cord (e.g., 142,165,191,352). Evidence relating to this mechanism is available in the work of Kuno (353). Kuno showed that the probability of occurrence of unit Ia excitatory postsynaptic potentials—presumably resulting from the release of transmitter from one synaptic bouton—is reduced by afferent volleys that are known to elicit primary afferent depolarization. If it is presumed that adequate terminal invasion by action potentials always leads to transmitter release, these data are most easily explained by implicating a failure of conduction in part of the Ia fibers. It is thought that such conduction block takes place at axonal bifurcations that are regions of low safety factor for the conduction of action potentials (354,355). A conductance increase such as that presumably occurring at the terminals of afferent fibers during primary afferent depolarization will produce shunting of current and lower the safety factor further. If shunting is substantial, conduction will be blocked. Block of conduction by a synaptic input has been demonstrated in invertebrate axons (356).

4. Functional Implications

Most investigations of the organization and function of presynaptic inhibition in the spinal cord have involved the measurement of primary afferent depolarization. The inhibition itself has only rarely been measured. It has been tacitly assumed that primary afferent depolarization causes presynaptic inhibition and that primary afferent depolarization is a sufficient indicator of the presynaptic

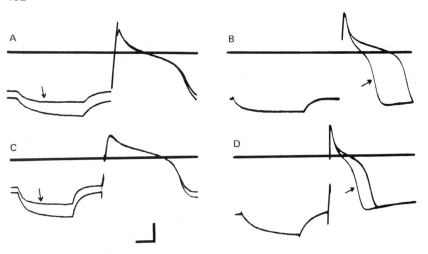

Figure 14 Effects of GABA, muscimol, and baclofen on chick dorsal root ganglion cells in culture. Each record consists of two superimposed traces of membrane hyperpolarizations followed by action potentials evoked by current pulses passed through recording electrode. Arrows indicate control traces. A and B, After application of GABA to two different cells. Cell in A showed a reduction in input resistance. Cell in B demonstrated a reduction in the duration of the action potential without detectable change in input resistance. C, After muscimol. D, After baclofen. All applied in a concentration of 10^{-4} M. Horizontal lines indicate 0 mV. Calibration: 20 mV, 2 msec. (From Ref. 223.)

inhibitory process. This is a gross simplification, but inferences about inhibition from measurements of primary afferent depolarization are still to be made because of the lack of direct data concerning the organization of the inhibition itself.

Much has been made of the negative feedback character of segmental primary afferent depolarization (e.g., 9,143). It appears that this feedback is not indiscriminate. For example, as indicated in Sec. III.B.2.c, volleys in one type of afferent tend to result in primary afferent depolarization in the same type of afferent (e.g., muscle afferents tend to influence other muscle afferents; cutaneous fibers affect cutaneous fibers). In addition, some specific afferents tend to preferentially generate primary afferent depolarization in fibers of the same sensory type (e.g., Ib afferents tend to produce primary afferent depolarization in Ib afferents). It has been suggested that negative feedback among segmental afferents allows an automatic suppression of inconsequential information so that the central sensory apparatus is free to process significant sensory inputs (303). In addition, although some specific sensory signals may be suppressed by presynaptic mechanisms, the second-order neurons are unaffected by the inhibition (303) and are still free to receive unsuppressed information.

Speculation has arisen that descending pathways exert presynaptic inhibitory controls on specific types of afferents to selectively increase or decrease particular sensory inputs (9). The mechanism has been viewed as a means of providing the central nervous system with a mechanism to determine which kinds of afferent information it "needs" or "wants" at a given time. It provides a means for supraspinal structures to selectively reduce or eliminate some inputs without affecting others. It may provide a means to regulate the transmission of information to ascending spinal pathways. It may also serve to reduce reflex control to allow supraspinal structures sole control of the motor apparatus of the spinal cord.

The idea has been proposed that presynaptic inhibition could function to increase the spatial aspects of sensory discrimination (9,280). This idea arose from considerations of the organization of afferents arising in cutaneous mechanoreceptors. The primary afferent depolarization resulting from activation of such receptors is organized in a "surround" fashion (i.e., an excited afferent exerts an effect upon the terminals of afferents innervating adjacent or surrounding areas of skin). Such an organizational pattern is thought to reduce the spatial spread of excitation by producing so-called lateral, or surround, inhibition.

Rudomín and Dutton (357,358) have provided data that indicate that primary afferent depolarization may be concerned with certain aspects of synaptic transmission other than inhibition. During primary afferent depolarization elicited by stimulation of muscle or cutaneous afferents there is a significant decrease in the variability of monosynaptic reflexes produced by constant Ia volleys, that is, there was an increased probability that a particular input would result in an expected output.

B. Other Presynaptic Mechanisms

The classic picture of presynaptic events at primary afferent terminals has been modified over the past few years by accumulating evidence that transmitters other than GABA influence the membrane potential of these terminals and by data demonstrating that the quantity of transmitter released from a terminal by an impulse depends upon the prior activity occurring at that terminal, particularly repetitive firing.

1. Presynaptic Effects of Other Transmitters

It may be postulated that several different transmitters have presynaptic effects that result in reduction of transmitter release, that is, result in presynaptic inhibition. In this regard, it should be noted that axoaxonic contacts on primary afferent terminals are numerous (6) and up to 13 synapses on a single fiber have been described. In the case of the frog cord, at least three different specific types of presynaptic profiles have been reported (163), suggesting that more than one type of transmitter may be released onto an afferent terminal.

In addition to GABA receptors, there is considerable evidence that primary afferent fibers have significant numbers of opioid receptors on their central processes (359-362). Activation of these sites by enkephalin results in inhibition of the evoked release of substance P from afferent terminals (363,364) and in hyperpolarization of the afferent terminals of fine cutaneous fibers (365-367). Both of these effects are antagonized by naloxone, indicating a specific interaction of enkephalin with opioid receptors. Thus, in this case there is presynaptic inhibition, but primary afferent terminals are hyperpolarized. The mechanisms of the hyperpolarization and of the inhibition of transmitter release are not known, but enkephalin—like GABA—is reported to block Ca^{2+} influx in cultured dorsal root ganglion cells (350).

In addition to enkephalin there are several other peptidergic systems represented in the dorsal horn that may play roles in the modulation of afferent inputs (e.g., substance P, neurotensin, somatostatin, thyrotrophin-releasing hormone, angiotensin [368-375]). Although little pharmacologic data is available concerning their roles in the spinal cord, these compounds all reportedly have potent effects on the membrane potential of afferent terminals (376-378). There is also strong evidence that norepinephrine and serotonin modulate sensory transmission at the segmental level (see 379 and 380 for refs.). These compounds can alter the membrane potential of afferent fibers (381-384), although some of the data is conflicting. Obviously, more detailed information concerning the mode of action of peptides and amines on spinal afferents is needed.

2. Presynaptic Terminal Invasion

As indicated in Sec. III.B.3.d, block of conduction of action potentials in the intraspinal arborizations of afferent fibers may be another means by which transmitter output from afferent terminals may be limited. Intraspinal failure of transmission in afferent fibers was first described by Barron and Matthews (165), who showed that impulses entering the spinal cord sometimes failed to continue into collateral branches attached to the peripheral axons if the peripheral axons were repetitively stimulated. These observations have been confirmed (385-388), but beyond this, only a few fragmentary observations on the mechanism of conduction block have been made in the spinal cord. It is postulated to occur at axonal branch points (165,387) and the effects of temperature (165), primary afferent depolarization (385), and anoxia (387) have been studied. This dearth of knowledge of the mechanism in vertebrates is in sharp contrast to the situation in invertebrates where disruption of impulse transmission has been extensively investigated and where synaptic activity (356), accumulation of K^+ ions (389,390), and hyperpolarization of axons by the action of an electrogenic Na^+ pump (391) have all been implicated as causative factors.

IV. COMMENTS

The spinal cord is constantly exposed to enormous amounts of afferent information entering the roots and messages from a variety of supraspinal structures. The information-handling capabilities of the cord are not known, but it is obvious that the neuronal apparatus of the spinal cord must have ways to process this enormous input and mechanisms to limit the input and spread of activity. This chapter has focused on some of the means that the spinal cord has available to control the transmission of information.

The transmission of information in the spinal cord is determined by the properties of the individual neurons in the cord and in particular the ways in which their excitability is determined and by the circuitry by which these neurons are connected with each other. We have attempted to show how the passage of impulses and synaptic activity may be impeded or suppressed at the level of the primary afferent fiber and its terminals and at second order neurons postsynaptic to the terminals. To do this we have described much of what is known about the structure of the pertinent synapses, the ionic mechanisms of inhibition, the properties of the interneurons involved in inhibition, the connections of the appropriate elements, and some of the functional implications of the involved circuits.

There are many unanswered questions. For example, the relative importance of pre- and postsynaptic inhibition is not known. Many statements about the function of various interneurons and circuits are only first approximations based on inferences rather than on experimentally derived data. The mechanisms involved in presynaptic inhibition are poorly understood. Particularly confusing are the ways in which synaptic transmission through one pathway affects transmission through the many interconnected and parallel pathways in the spinal cord. However, considering the progress that has been made in the understanding of the processes of inhibition in the past few decades since the application of the microelectrode, we remain optimistic that new research tools and strategies can be applied to the problems discussed here and that these, and other unanswered questions, will be explained.

ACKNOWLEDGMENTS

This work was supported in part by the Veterans Administration Medical Center Funds (MRIS 1769) and U.S. Public Health Service Grant (NS 17577).

REFERENCES

1. Weber, E. F. W., and Weber, E. H. (1845). Experimenta, quibus probatur nervos vagos votatione machinae galvanomagenticae irritatos, motem cord, retardare et adeointercipare. *Ann. Univ. Med. Milano 20*:227.

2. Sechenov, I. M. (1863). *Physiologische Studien über die Hemmungsmechanismus für die Reflexthätigkeit des Ruckenmarks im Olhirne des Frosches.* Hirschwald, Berlin.

3. Sherrington, C. S. (1906). *Integrative Action of the Nervous System.* Yale University Press, New Haven, Connecticut.

4. Eccles, J. C. (1964). *The Physiology of Synapses.* Academic Press, New York.

5. Frank, K., and Fuortes, M. G. F. (1957). Presynaptic and postsynaptic inhibition of monosynaptic reflexes. *Fed. Proc. 16*:39–40.

6. Conradi, S. (1969). On motoneuron synaptology in adult cats. *Acta Physiol. Scand. (Suppl.) 332*:5–115.

7. Burke, R. E., and Rudomín, P. (1977). Spinal neurons and synapses. In *The Handbook of Physiology, Section I: The Nervous System,* vol. 1, no. 2, E. R. Kandel (Ed.), American Physiological Society, Bethesda, Maryland, pp. 877–944.

8. Nicoll, R. A., and Alger, B. E. (1979). Presynaptic inhibition: Transmitter and ionic mechanisms. *Int. Rev. Neurobiol. 21*:217–258.

9. Schmidt, R. F. (1971). Presynaptic inhibition in the vertebrate nervous system. *Ergebn. Physiol. 63*:20–101.

10. Levy, R. A. (1977). The role of GABA in primary afferent depolarization. *Prog. Neurobiol. 9*:211–267.

11. Schmidt, R. F. (1973). Control of the access of afferent activity to somatosensory pathways. In *Handbook of Sensory Physiology,* vol. II, A. Iggo (Ed.), Springer-Verlag, Berlin, pp. 151–206.

12. Charlton, B. T., and Gray, E. G. (1966). Comparative electron microscopy of synapses in the vertebrate spinal cord. *J. Cell Sci. 1*:67–80.

13. Uchizono, K. (1966). Excitatory and inhibitory synapses in the cat spinal cord. *Jpn. J. Physiol. 16*:570–575.

14. Bodian, D. (1975). Origin of specific synaptic types in the motoneuron neuropil of the monkey. *J. Comp. Neurol. 159*:225–244.

15. McLaughlin, B. J. (1972). Dorsal root projections to the motor nuclei in the cat spinal cord. *J. Comp. Neurol. 144*:461–474.

16. Bernstein, J. J., and Bernstein, M. E. (1976). Ventral horn synaptology in the rat. *J. Neurocytol. 5*:109–123.

17. McLaughlin, B. J. (1972). The fine structure of neurons and synapses in the motor nuclei of the cat spinal cord. *J. Comp. Neurol. 144*:429–460.

18. McLaughlin, B. J. (1972). Propriospinal and supraspinal projections to the motor nuclei in the cat spinal cord. *J. Comp. Neurol. 144*:475–500.

19. Bodian, D. (1964). An electron-microscopic study of the monkey spinal cord. *Bull. Johns Hopkins Hosp. 114*:13–119.

20. Bodian, D. (1966). Synaptic types on spinal motoneurons. An electron microscopic study. *Bull. Johns Hopkins Hosp. 119*:16–45.

21. Bodian, D. (1966). Electron microscopy: Two major synaptic types on spinal motoneurons. *Science 151*:1093–1094.

22. Bodian, D. (1970). An electron microscopic characterization of classes of synaptic vesicles by means of controlled aldehyde fixation. *J. Cell. Biol. 44*:115–124.

23. Rosenbluth, J. (1962). Subsurface cisterns and their relationship to the neuronal plasma membrane. *J. Cell. Biol. 13*:405–421.

24. Gray, E. G. (1963). Electron microscopy of presynaptic organelles of the spinal cord. *J. Anat. 97*:101–106.

25. Ralston, H. J., III (1967). Synaptic morphology in ventral horn of cat spinal cord. *Anat. Rec. 157*:305–306.

26. Kawana, E., Akert, K., and Sandri, C. (1969). Zinc iodide-osmium tetroxide impregnation of nerve terminals in the spinal cord. *Brain Res. 16*: 325–331.

27. Streit, P., Akert, K., Sandri, C., Livingston, R. B., and Moor, H. (1972). Dynamic ultrastructure of presynaptic membranes at nerve terminals in the spinal cord of rats. Anesthetized and unanesthetized preparations compared. *Brain Res. 48*:11–26.

28. Akert, K., Pfenninger, K., Sandri, C., and Moor, H. (1972). Freeze-etching and cytochemistry of vesicles and membrane complexes in synapses of the C.N.S. In *Structure and Function of Synapses*, G. D. Pappas and D. P. Purpura (Eds.), Raven Press, New York, pp. 67–86.

29. Gray, E. G. (1969). Electron microscopy of excitatory and inhibitory synapses: A brief review. *Prog. Brain Res. 31*:141–155.

30. Conradi, S. (1976). Functional anatomy of the anterior horn neuron. In *The Peripheral Nerve*, D. N. Landon (Ed.), Chapman and Hall, London, pp. 279–329.

31. Uchizono, K. (1967). Inhibitory synapses on the stretch receptor neurone of the crayfish. *Nature 214*:833–834.

32. Matus, A. I., and Dennison, M. E. (1971). Autoradiographic localization, of tritiated glycine at flat-vesicle synapses in spinal cord. *Brain Res. 32*: 195–197.

33. Conradi, S., Kellerth, J.-O., and Berthold, C.-H. (1979). Electron microscopic studies of serially sectioned cat spinal α-motoneurons. II. A method for the description of architecture and synaptology of the cell body and proximal dendritic segments. *J. Comp. Neurol. 184*:741–754.

34. Lloyd, D. P. C. (1941). A direct central inhibitory action of dromically conducted impulses. *J. Neurophysiol. 4*:184–190.

35. Lloyd, D. P. C. (1946). Facilitation and inhibition of spinal motoneurones. *J. Neurophysiol. 9*:421–438.

36. Lloyd, D. P. C. (1946). Integrative pattern of excitation and inhibition in two-neuron reflex arc. *J. Neurophysiol. 9*:439–444.

37. Laporte, Y., and Lloyd, D. P. C. (1952). Nature and significance of the reflex connections established by large afferent fibres of muscular origin. *Am. J. Physiol. 169*:609–621.

38. Eccles, J. C., Fatt, P., and Landgren, S. (1956). Central pathway for direct inhibitory action of impulses in largest afferent nerve fibers to muscle. *J. Neurophysiol. 19*:75–98.

39. Brock, L. G., Coombs, J. S., and Eccles, J. C. (1952). Synaptic excitation and inhibition. *J. Physiol. (Lond.) 117*:8P.

40. Eccles, R. M., and Lundberg, A. (1958). The synaptic linkage of "direct" inhibition. *Acta Physiol. Scand. 43*:204–214.

41. Coombs, J. S., Curtis, D. R., and Eccles, J. C. (1955). The specific ionic conductances and the ionic movement across the motoneuronal membrane that produce the inhibitory postsynaptic potential. *J. Physiol. (Lond.)* *130*:326-373.

42. Coombs, J. S., Eccles, J. C., and Fatt, P. (1955). The ionic permeability of the motoneurone membrane. *J. Cell. Comp. Physiol. 46*:362-363.

43. Curtis, D. R., and Eccles, J. C. (1959). The time courses of excitatory and inhibitory synaptic actions. *J. Physiol. (Lond.) 145*:529-546.

44. Jankowska, E., and Roberts, W. J. (1972). Synaptic actions of single interneurones mediating reciprocal Ia inhibition of motoneurones. *J. Physiol. (Lond.) 222*:623-642.

45. Eccles, R. M., and Lundberg, A. (1958). Integrative pattern of Ia synaptic actions of motoneurons of hip and knee muscles. *J. Physiol. (Lond.) 144*: 271-298.

46. Hultborn, H., Jankowska, E., and Lindström, S. (1971). Relative contribution from different nerves to recurrent depression of Ia IPSP's in motoneurones. *J. Physiol. (Lond.) 215*:637-664.

47. Burke, R. E., Jankowska, E., and ten Bruggencate, G. (1970). A comparison of peripheral and rubrospinal synaptic input to slow and fast twitch motor units of triceps surae. *J. Physiol. (Lond.) 207*:709-732.

48. Burke, R. E., Rymer, W. Z., and Walsh, J. V. (1973). Functional specialization in the motor unit population of cat medial gastrocnemius muscle. In *Control of Posture and Locomotion*, R. B. Stein, K. G. Pearson, R. S. Smith, and J. B. Redford (Eds.), Plenum Press, New York, pp. 29-44.

49. Blankenship, J. E., and Kuno, M. (1968). Analysis of spontaneous subthreshold activity in spinal motoneurons of the cat. *J. Neurophysiol. 31*: 195-209.

50. Kuno, M., and Weakley, J. N. (1972). Quantal components of the inhibitory synaptic potential in spinal motoneurones of the cat. *J. Physiol. (Lond.) 224*:287-303.

51. Eide, E., Lundberg, A., and Voorhoeve, P. (1981). Monosynaptically evoked inhibitory post-synaptic potentials in motoneurones. *Acta Physiol. Scand. 53*:185-195.

52. Eccles, J. C., Eccles, R. M., and Lundberg, A. (1957). Synaptic actions on motoneurones caused by impulses in Golgi tendon organ afferents. *J. Physiol. (Lond.) 138*:227-252.

53. Eccles, R. M., and Lundberg, A. (1959). Synaptic actions in motoneurones by afferents which may evoke the flexion reflex. *Arch. Ital. Biol. 97*:199-221.

54. Araki, T., Eccles, J. C., and Ito, M. (1960). Correlation of the inhibitory postsynaptic potential of motoneurones with the latency and time course of inhibition of monosynaptic reflexes. *J. Physiol. (Lond.) 154*:354-377.

55. Coombs, J. S., Eccles, J. C., and Fatt, P. (1955). The inhibitory suppression of reflex discharges from motoneurones. *J. Physiol. (Lond.) 130*: 396-413.

56. Eccles, J. C. (1957). *The Physiology of Nerve Cells.* Johns Hopkins Press, Baltimore.
57. Coombs, J. S., Curtis, D. R., and Eccles, J. C. (1953). The action of the inhibitory synaptic transmitter. *Aust. J. Sci. 16*:1–5.
58. Lux, H.-D., Loracher, C., and Neher, E. (1970). The actions of ammonium on postsynaptic inhibition of cat spinal motoneurons. *Exp. Brain Res. 11*: 431–447.
59. Lux, H.-D. (1971). Ammonium and chloride extrusion: Hyperpolarizing synaptic inhibition in spinal motoneurons. *Science 173*:555–557.
60. Eccles, J. C., Eccles, R. M., and Ito, M. (1964). Effects of intracellular potassium and sodium injections on the inhibitory postsynaptic potential. *Proc. R. Soc. Lond. (Biol.) 160*:181–196.
61. Sonnhof, U., and Bührle, C. P. (1981). The ionic basis of the IPSP in spinal motoneurons of the frog. In *Ion-selective Microelectrodes and Their Use in Excitable Tissue*, E. Syková, P. Hnik, and L. Vyklický (Eds.), Plenum Press, New York, pp. 191–194.
62. Araki, T., Ito, M., and Oscarsson, O. (1961). Anion permeability of the synaptic and non-synaptic motoneurone membrane. *J. Physiol. (Lond.) 159*:410–435.
63. Ito, M., Kostyuk, P. G., and Oshima, T. (1962). Further study on anion permeability in cat spinal motoneurones. *J. Physiol. (Lond.) 164*:150–156.
64. Matsuura, S., and Endo, K. (1971). Anion permeability of the inhibitory subsynaptic membrane of the spinal motoneuron of the toad. *Jpn. J. Physiol. 21*:265–276.
65. Takeuchi, A., and Takeuchi, N. (1967). Anion permeability of the inhibitory post-synaptic membrane of the crayfish neuronmuscular junction. *J. Physiol. (Lond.) 191*:575–590.
66. Araki, T., and Terzuolo, C. A. (1962). Membrane currents in spinal motoneurons associated with the action potential and synaptic activity. *J. Neurophysiol. 25*:772–789.
67. Smith, T. G., Wuerker, R. B., and Frank, K. (1967). Membrane impedance changes during synaptic transmission in rat spinal motoneurons. *J. Neurophysiol. 30*:1072–1096.
68. Burke, R. E., Fedina, L., and Lundberg, A. (1971). Spatial synaptic distribution of recurrent and group Ia inhibitory systems in cat spinal motoneurones. *J. Physiol. (Lond.) 214*:304–326.
69. Rall, W., Burke, R. E., Smith, T. G., Nelson, P. G., and Frank, K. (1967). Dendritic location of synapses and possible mechanisms for the monosynaptic EPSP in motoneuron. *J. Neurophysiol. 30*:1169–1193.
70. Llinás, R., Baker, R., and Precht, W. (1974). Blockage of inhibition by ammonium acetate action on chloride pump in cat trochlear motoneurons. *J. Neurophysiol. 37*:522–532.
71. Eccles, J. C. (1969). *The Inhibitory Pathways of the Central Nervous System*. Liverpool University Press, Liverpool.

72. Eccles, J. C., Eccles, R. M., and Lundberg, A. (1960). Types of neurone in and around the intermediate nucleus of the lumbo-sacral cord. *J. Physiol. (Lond.) 154*:89–114.

73. Eccles, J. C., Fatt, P., Landgren, S., and Winsbury, G. J. (1954). Spinal cord potentials generated by volleys in the large muscle afferents. *J. Physiol. (Lond.) 125*:590–606.

74. Hultborn, H., and Udo, M. (1972). Convergence in the reciprocal Ia inhibitory pathway of excitation from descending pathways and inhibition from motor axon collaterals. *Acta Physiol. Scand. 84*:95–108.

75. Hultborn, H. (1976). Transmission in the pathway of reciprocal Ia inhibition to motoneurones and its control during the tonic stretch reflex. *Prog. Brain Res. 44*:235–255.

76. Baldissera, F., Hultborn, H., and Illert, M. (1981). Integration in spinal neuronal systems. In *Handbook of Physiology, Sect. 1, The Nervous System*, Vol. 2, *Motor Control*, V. B. Brooks (Ed.), American Physiological Society, Bethesda, Maryland, pp. 509–596.

77. Lindström, S. (1973). Recurrent control from motor axon collaterals of Ia inhibitory pathways in the spinal cord of the cat. *Acta Physiol. Scand.* (Suppl.) *392*:1–43.

78. Lundberg, A. (1970). The excitatory control of the Ia inhibitory pathway. In *Excitatory Synaptic Mechanisms*, P. Andersen and J. K. S. Jansen (Eds.), Universitetsforlaget, Oslo, pp. 333–340.

79. Hultborn, H., Jankowska, E., and Lindström, S. (1971). Recurrent inhibition from motor axon collaterals of transmission in the Ia inhibitory pathway to motoneurones. *J. Physiol. (Lond.) 215*:591–612.

80. Hultborn, H., Jankowska, E., and Lindström, S. (1971). Recurrent inhibition of interneurones monosynaptically activated from group Ia afferents. *J. Physiol. (Lond.) 215*:613–636.

81. Jankowska, E., and Roberts, W. J. (1972). An electrophysiological demonstration of the axonal projections of single spinal interneurones in the cat. *J. Physiol. (Lond.) 222*:597–622.

82. Lundberg, A. (1969). Convergence of excitatory and inhibitory action on interneurons in the spinal cord. In *The Interneuron*, M. A. B. Brazier (Ed.), University of California Press, Los Angeles, pp. 231–265.

83. Hultborn, H. (1972). Convergence on interneurones in the reciprocal Ia inhibitory pathway to motoneurones. *Acta Physiol. Scand. 85* (Suppl.) *375*:1–42.

84. Hultborn, H., and Udo, M. (1972). Convergence of large muscle spindle (Ia) afferents at interneuronal level in the reciprocal Ia inhibitory pathway to motoneurones. *Acta Physiol. Scand. 84*:493–499.

85. Hultborn, H., Illert, M., and Santini, M. (1976). Convergence on interneurones mediating the reciprocal inhibition of motoneurones. I. Disynaptic Ia inhibition of Ia inhibitory interneurones. *Acta Physiol. Scand. 96*: 193–201.

86. Hultborn, H., Illert, M., and Santini, M. (1976). Convergence on interneurones mediating the reciprocal Ia inhibition of motorneurones. II. Effects from segmental flexor reflex pathways. *Acta Physiol. Scand. 96*:351–367.

87. Fedina, L., and Hultborn, H. (1972). Facilitation from ipsilateral primary afferents of interneuronal transmission in the Ia inhibitory pathway to motoneurones. *Acta Physiol. Scand. 86*:59–81.

88. Grillner, S., and Hongo, T. (1972). Vestibulospinal effects on motoneurones and interneurones in lumbosacral cord. *Prog. Brain Res. 37*:243–262.

89. Grillner, S., Hongo, T., and Lund, S. (1966). Interaction between the inhibitory pathways from the Deiters' nucleus and Ia afferents to flexor motoneurones. *Acta Physiol. Scand. 68*(Suppl. 277):61.

90. Hultborn, H., Illert, M., and Santini, M. (1976). Convergence on interneurones mediating the reciprocal Ia inhibition of motoneurones. III. Effects from supraspinal pathways. *Acta Physiol. Scand. 96*:368–391.

91. Hongo, T., Jankowska, E., and Lundberg, A. (1969). The rubrospinal tract. II. Facilitation of interneuronal transmission in reflex paths to motoneurons. *Exp. Brain Res. 7*:365–391.

92. Illert, M., and Tanaka, R. (1978). Integration in descending motor pathways controlling the forelimb in the cat. 4. Corticospinal inhibition of forelimb motoneurones mediated by short propriospinal neurones. *Exp. Brain Res. 31*:131–141.

93. Jankowska, E., Padel, Y., and Tanaka, R. (1976). Disynaptic inhibition of spinal motoneurones from the motor cortex in the monkey. *J. Physiol. (Lond.) 258*:467–487.

94. Lundberg, A., and Voorhoeve, P. (1962). Effects from the pyramidal tract on spinal reflex arcs. *Acta Physiol. Scand. 56*:201–219.

95. Jankowska, E., Lundberg, A., and Stuart, D. (1973). Propriospinal control of last order interneurones of spinal reflex pathways in the cat. *Brain Res. 53*:227–231.

96. Illert, M., and Tanaka, R. (1976). Transmission of corticospinal IPSP's to cat forelimb motoneurones via high cervical propriospinal neurones and Ia inhibitory interneurones. *Brain Res. 103*:143–146.

97. Jankowska, E., and Lindström, S. (1972). Morphology of interneurones mediating Ia reciprocal inhibition of motoneurones in the spinal cord of the cat. *J. Physiol. (Lond.) 226*:805–823.

98. Czarkowska, J., Jankowska, E., and Sybirska, E. (1976). Axonal projections of spinal interneurones excited by group I afferents in the cat, revealed by intracellular staining with horseradish peroxidase. *Brain Res. 118*:115–118.

99. Sherrington, C. S. (1897). On reciprocal inversion of antagonistic muscles. Third Note. *Proc. R. Soc. Lond. (Biol.) 60*:414–417.

100. Eccles, J. C., Eccles, R. M., and Lundberg, A. (1957). The convergence of monosynaptic excitatory afferents onto many different species of alpha motoneurones. *J. Physiol. (Lond.) 137*:22–50.

101. Tanaka, R. (1976). Reciprocal Ia inhibition and voluntary movements in man. *Prog. Brain Res. 44*:291-302.

102. Mizuno, Y., Tanaka, R., and Yanagisawa, N. (1971). Reciprocal group I inhibition on triceps surae motoneurons in man. *J. Neurophysiol. 34*: 1010-1017.

103. Granit, R. (1970). *The Basis of Motor Control*, Academic Press, New York.

104. Matthews, P. B. C. (1972). *Mammalian Muscle Receptors and Their Central Actions*, Edward Arnold, London.

105. Eccles, J. C., Eccles, R. M., and Lundberg, A. (1957). Synaptic actions on motoneurones in relation to the two components of the group I muscle afferent volley. *J. Physiol. (Lond.) 136*:527-546.

106. Baxendale, R. H., and Rosenberg, J. R. (1977). Crossed reflexes evoked by selective activation of tendon organ afferent axons in the decerebrate cat. *Brain Res. 127*:323-326.

107. Lundberg, A., Malmgren, K., and Schomberg, E. D. (1975). Convergence from Ib, cutaneous and joint afferents in reflex pathways to motoneurones. *Brain Res. 87*:81-84.

108. Eccles, R. M. (1965). Interneurones activated by higher threshold group I muscle afferents. In *Studies in Physiology*, D. R. Curtis and A. K. McIntyre (Eds.), Springer-Verlag, New York, pp. 59-64.

109. Hongo, T., Jankowska, E., and Lundberg, A. (1966). Convergence of excitatory and inhibitory action on interneurones in the lumbosacral cord. *Exp. Brain Res. 1*:338-358.

110. Lucas, M. E., and Willis, W. D. (1974). Identification of muscle afferents which activate interneurons in the intermediate nucleus. *J. Neurophysiol. 37*:282-293.

111. Czarkowska, J., Jankowska, E., and Sybirska, E. (1976). Diameter and intranodal length of axons of spinal interneurones excited by group I afferents in the cat. *Brain Res. 118*:119-122.

112. Hongo, T., Jankowska, E., and Lundberg, A. (1972). The rubro-spinal tract. IV. Effects on interneurones. *Exp. Brain Res. 15*:54-78.

113. Jankowska, E., Johanisson, T., and Lipski, J. (1981). Common interneurones in reflex pathways from group Ia and Ib afferents in ankle extensors in the cat. *J. Physiol. (Lond.) 310*:381-402.

114. Lundberg, A., Norrsell, U., and Voorhoeve, P. (1962). Pyramidal effects on lumbosacral interneurones activated by somatic afferents. *Acta Physiol. Scand. 56*:220-229.

115. Czarkowska, J., Jankowska, E., and Sybirska, E. (1981). Common interneurones in reflex pathways from group 1a and 1b afferents of knee flexors and extensors in the cat. *J. Physiol. (Lond.) 310*:367-380.

116. Fetz, E. E., Jankowska, E., Johanssison, T., and Lipski, J. (1979). Autogenetic inhibition of motoneurones by impulses in group Ia muscle spindle afferents. *J. Physiol. (Lond.) 293*:173-195.

117. Lundberg, A., Malmgren, K., and Schomburg, E. D. (1978). Role of joint afferents in motor control exemplified by effects on reflex pathways from Ib afferents. *J. Physiol. (Lond.) 284*:327-343.

118. Lundberg, A., Malmgren, K., and Schomburg, E. D. (1977). Cutaneous facilitation of transmission in reflex pathways from Ib afferents to motoneurones. *J. Physiol. (Lond.) 265*:763-780.

119. Illert, M., Lundberg, A., and Tanaka, R. (1976). Integration in descending motor pathways controlling the forelimb in the cat. 2. Convergence on neurons mediating disynaptic cortico-motoneuronal excitation. *Exp. Brain Res. 26*:521-540.

120. Engberg, I., Lundberg, A., and Ryall, R. W. (1968). Reticulospinal inhibition of interneurones. *J. Physiol. (Lond.) 194*:225-236.

121. Anden, N. E., Jukes, M. G., and Lundberg, A. (1966). The effect of DOPA on the spinal cord. 1. Influences on transmission from primary afferents. *Acta Physiol. Scand. 67*:373-386.

121a. Houk, J. C., Singer, J. J., and Goldman, M. R. (1970). An evaluation of length and force feedback to soleus muscles of decerebrate cats. *J. Neurophysiol. 33*:784-811.

122. Sherrington, C. S. (1910). Flexion-reflex of the limb, crossed extension reflex and standing. *J. Physiol. (Lond.) 40*:28-121.

123. Holmqvist, B., and Lundberg, A. (1962). Differential supraspinal control of synaptic actions evoked by volleys in the flexion reflex afferents in alpha motoneurones. *Acta Physiol. Scand. 54*(Suppl. 186):53-64.

124. Job, C. (1953). Über autogene Inhibition und Reflexumkehr bei spinalisierten und decebrierten Katzen. *Pflugers Arch. ges. Physiol. 256*:406-418.

125. Eccles, R. M., and Lundberg, A. (1959). Supraspinal control of interneurons mediating spinal reflexes. *J. Physiol. (Lond.) 147*:565-584.

126. Pompeiano, O. (1984). Recurrent inhibition. In *Handbook of the Spinal Cord*, vols. 2 and 3, *Anatomy and Physiology*, R. A. Davidoff (Ed.), Marcel Dekker, New York, pp. 461-557.

127. Frank, K. (1959). Basic mechanisms of synaptic transmission in the central nervous system. *IRE Trans. Med. Electron. ME-6*:85-88.

128. Llinás, R., and Terzuolo, C. A. (1965). Mechanisms of supraspinal actions upon spinal cord activities. Reticular inhibitory mechanisms upon flexor motoneurons. *J. Neurophysiol. 28*:413-422.

129. Cook, W. A., Jr., and Cangiano, A. (1970). Presynaptic inhibition of spinal motoneurons. *Brain Res. 24*:521-524.

130. Cook, W. A., Jr., and Cangiano, A. (1972). Presynaptic inhibition of spinal motoneurons. *J. Neurophysiol. 35*:389-403.

131. Kellerth, J.-O. (1965). A strychnine resistant postsynaptic inhibition in the spinal cord. *Acta Physiol. Scand. 63*:469-471.

132. Kellerth, J.-O. (1968). Aspects on the relative significance of pre- and postsynaptic inhibition in the spinal cord. In *Structure and Function of Inhibitory Neuronal Mechanisms*, C. von Euler, S. Skoglund and U. Söderberg (Eds.), Pergamon Press, Oxford, pp. 197-212.

133. Kellerth, J.-O., and Szumski, A. J. (1966). Two types of stretch activated postsynaptic inhibitions in spinal motoneurones as differentiated by strychnine. *Acta Physiol. Scand. 66*:133–145.

134. Kellerth, J.-O., and Szumski, A. J. (1966). Effects of picrotoxin on stretch activated postsynaptic inhibitions in spinal motoneurones. *Acta Physiol. Scand. 66*:146–156.

135. Carlen, P. L., Werman, R., and Yaari, Y. (1980). Post-synaptic conductance increase associated with presynaptic inhibition in cat lumbar motoneurones. *J. Physiol. (Lond.) 298*:539–556.

136. Gasser, H. S., and Graham, H. T. (1933). Potentials produced in the spinal cord by stimulations of the dorsal roots. *Am. J. Physiol. 103*:303–320.

137. Hughes, J., and Gasser, H. S. (1934). The response of the spinal cord of two afferent volleys. *Am. J. Physiol. 108*:307–321.

138. Hughes, J., and Gasser, H. S. (1934). Some properties of the cord potentials evoked by a single afferent volley. *Am. J. Physiol. 108*:295–306.

139. Gerard, R. W., and Forbes, A. (1928). "Fatigue" of the flexion reflex. *Am. J. Physiol. 86*:186–205.

140. Eccles, J. C., and Sherrington, C. (1931). Studies on the flexor reflex. VI. Inhibition. *Proc. R. Soc. Lond. (Biol.) 109*:91–113.

141. Forbes, A., Querido, A., Whitaker, L. R., and Hurxtal, L. M. (1928). Electrical studies in mammalian reflexes. V. The flexion reflex in response to two stimuli as recorded from the motor nerve. *Am. J. Physiol. 85*:432–457.

142. Barron, D. H., and Matthews, B. H. C. (1938). The interpretation of potential changes in the spinal cord. *J. Physiol. (Lond.) 92*:276–321.

143. Eccles, J. C. (1964). Presynaptic inhibition in the spinal cord. *Prog. Brain Res. 12*:65–91.

144. Eccles, J. C., Kostyuk, P. G., and Schmidt, R. F. (1962). Central pathways responsible for depolarization of primary afferent fibres. *J. Physiol. (Lond.) 161*:237–257.

145. Eccles, J. C., Magni, F., and Willis, W. D. (1962). Depolarization of central terminals of group I afferent fibres from muscle. *J. Physiol. (Lond.) 160*:62–93.

146. Schmidt, R. F., and Willis, W. D. (1963). Intracellular recording from motoneurons of the cervical spinal cord of the cat. *J. Neurophysiol. 26*:28–43.

147. Eccles, J. C., Eccles, R. M., and Magni, F. (1961). Central inhibitory action attributable to presynaptic depolarization produced by muscle afferent volleys. *J. Physiol. (Lond.) 159*:147–166.

148. Eccles, J. C., Schmidt, R. F., and Willis, W. D. (1963). The mode of operation of the synaptic mechanism producing presynaptic inhibition. *J. Neurophysiol. 26*:523–536.

149. Eccles, J. C. (1961). The mechanism of synaptic transmission. *Ergebn. Physiol. 51*:299–430.

150. Eccles, J. C., Kostyuk, P. G., and Schmidt, R. F. (1962). The effect of electric polarization of the spinal cord on central afferent fibres and on their excitatory synaptic action. *J. Physiol. (Lond.) 162*:138–150.

151. Gray, E. G. (1962). A morphological basis for presynaptic inhibition. *Nature 193*:82–83.

152. Kerr, F. W. L. (1966). The ultrastructure of the spinal tract of the trigeminal nerve and the substantia gelatinosa. *Exp. Neurol. 16*:359–376.

153. Ralston, H. G., III (1965). The organization of substantia gelatinosa Rolandi in the cat lumbosacral spinal cord. *Z. Zellforsch. 67*:1–23.

154. Réthelyi, M., and Szentogothai, J. (1969). The large synaptic complexes of the substantia gelatinosa. *Exp. Brain Res. 7*:258–274.

155. Ralston, H. J., and Ralston, D. D. (1979). Identification of dorsal root synaptic terminals on monkey ventral horn cells by electron microscopic autoradiography. *J. Neurocytol. 8*:151–166.

156. Réthelyi, M. (1970). Ultrastructural synaptology of Clarke's column. *Exp. Brain Res. 11*:159–174.

157. Saito, K. (1974). The synaptology and cytology of the Clarke cell in nucleus dorsalis of the cat: An electron microscopic study. *J. Neurocytol. 3*:179–197.

158. Barber, R. P., Vaughn, J. E., Saito, K., McLaughlin, B. J., and Roberts, E. (1978). GABAergic terminals are presynaptic to primary afferent terminals in the substantia gelatinosa of the rat spinal cord. *Brain Res. 141*:35–55.

159. McLaughlin, B. J., Barber, R., Saito, L., Roberts, E., and Wu, J.-Y. (1975). Immunocytochemical localization of glutamate decarboxylase in rat spinal cord. *J. Comp. Neurol. 164*:305–322.

160. Szentagothai, J. (1968). Synaptic structure and the concept of presynaptic inhibition. In *Structure and Function of Inhibitory Neuronal Mechanisms*, C. von Euler, S. Skoglund, and U. Söderberg (Eds.), Pergamon Press, New York, pp. 15–32.

161. Uchizono, K. (1973). Structural and chemical considerations on the presynaptic inhibitory synapses. *Proc. Jpn. Acad. 49*:569–574.

162. Glusman, S., Vázquez, G., and Rudomín, P. (1976). Ultrastructural observations in the frog spinal cord in relation to the generation of primary afferent depolarization. *Neurosci. Lett. 2*:137–145.

163. Székely, G., and Kosaras, B. (1977). Electron microscopic identification of postsynaptic dorsal root terminals: A possible substrate of dorsal root potentials in the frog spinal cord. *Exp. Brain Res. 29*:531–539.

163a. Davidoff, R. A., and Hackman, J. C. (1978). Pentylenetetrazol and reflex activity of isolated frog spinal cord. *Neurology 28*:488–494.

164. Gotch, F., and Horsley, V. (1891). On the mammalian nervous system, its functions, and their localization determined by an electrical method. *Philos. Trans. R. Soc. Lond. 182*:267–526.

165. Barron, D. H., and Matthews, B. H. C. (1935). Intermittent conduction in the spinal cord. *J. Physiol. (Lond.) 85*:73–103.

166. Lloyd, D. P. C., and McIntyre, A. K. (1949). On the origin of dorsal root potentials. *J. Gen. Physiol. 32*:409–443.

167. Lloyd, D. P. C. (1952). Electrotonus in dorsal nerve roots. *Cold Spring Harbor Symp. Quant. Biol. 17*:203–219.

168. Eccles, J. C., Schmidt, R. F., and Willis, W. D. (1963). The location and the mode of action of the presynaptic inhibitory pathways on the group I afferent fibers from muscle. *J. Neurophysiol. 26*:506–522.

169. Eccles, J. C., Schmidt, R. F., and Willis, W. D. (1963). Depolarization of the central terminals of cutaneous afferent fibers. *J. Neurophysiol. 26*: 646–661.

170. Eccles, J. C., and Krnjević, K. (1959). Potential changes recorded inside primary afferent fibres within the spinal cord. *J. Physiol. (Lond.) 149*: 250–273.

171. Koketsu, K. (1956). Intracellular potential changes of primary afferent nerve fibers in spinal cords of cats. *J. Neurophysiol. 19*:375–392.

172. Koketsu, K. (1956). Intracellular slow potential of dorsal root fibers. *Am. J. Physiol. 184*:338–344.

173. Shapovalov, A. I., and Shiriaev, B. I. (1979). Unexpected features of the interaction between individual primary afferents and spinal motoneurones. *Experientia 35*:347–348.

174. Shapovalov, A. I., and Shiriaev, B. I. (1980). Recurrent interactions between individual motoneurones and dorsal root fibres in the frog. *Exp. Brain Res. 38*:115–116.

175. Shapovalov, A. I., and Shiriaev, B. I. (1979). Spontaneous miniature potentials in primary afferent fibres. *Experientia 35*:348–349.

176. Hayashida, Y. (1975). Physiological and morphological studies on the primary afferent fiber of the spinal cord. *Osaka City Med. J. 21*:35–53.

177. Wall, P. D. (1958). Excitability changes in afferent fibre terminations and their relation to slow potentials. *J. Physiol. (Lond.) 142*:1–21.

178. Davidoff, R. A. (1972). The effects of bicuculline on the isolated spinal cord of the frog. *Exp. Neurol. 35*:179–193.

179. Franz, D. N., and Iggo, A. (1968). Dorsal root potentials and ventral root reflexes evoked by non-myelinated fibers. *Science 162*:1140–1142.

180. Zimmermann, K. (1968). Dorsal root potentials after C-fiber stimulation. *Science 160*:896–898.

181. Gregor, M., and Zimmermann, M. (1973). Dorsal root potentials produced by afferent volleys in cutaneous group III fibres. *J. Physiol. (Lond.) 232*: 413–425.

182. Jänig, W., and Zimmermann, M. (1971). Presynaptic depolarization of myelinated afferent fibres evoked by stimulation of cutaneous C-fibres. *J. Physiol. (Lond.) 214*:29–50.

183. Brooks, C., McC, and Fuortes, M. G. F. (1952). The relation of dorsal and ventral root potentials to reflex activity in mammals. *J. Physiol. (Lond.) 116*:380–394.

184. Fitzgerald, M., and Woolf, C. J. (1981). Effects of cutaneous nerve and intraspinal conditioning on C-fiber afferent terminal excitability in decerebrate spinal rats. *J. Physiol. (Lond.) 318*:25–39.

185. Calvillo, O. (1978). Primary afferent depolarization of C fibres in the spinal cord of the cat. *Can. J. Physiol. Pharmacol. 56*:154–157.

186. Selzer, M., and Spencer, W. A. (1969). Interactions between visceral and cutaneous afferents in the spinal cord: Reciprocal primary afferent fiber depolarization. *Brain Res. 14*:349–366.

187. Hancock, M. B., Willis, W. D., and Harrison, F. (1970). Viscerosomatic interactions in lumbar spinal cord of the cat. *J. Neurophysiol. 33*:46–58.
188. Duda, P., Kostyuk, P. G., and Preobrazhenskii, N. N. (1966). Inhibition of synaptic potentials in motoneurons during repetitive visceromotor stimulation. *Bull. Exp. Biol. Med. USSR 62*:3–7.
189. Jankowska, E., McCrea, D., Rudomín, P., and Syková, E. (1981). Observations on neuronal pathways subserving primary afferent depolarization. *J. Neurophysiol. 46*:506–516.
190. Wall, P. D. (1964). Presynaptic control of impulses at the first central synapse in the cutaneous pathway. In *Progress in Brain Research. Physiology of Spinal Neurons*, vol. 12, J. C. Eccles and J. P. Schade (Eds.), Elsevier, Amsterdam, pp. 92–115.
191. Howland, B., Lettvin, J. Y., McCulloch, W. S., Pitts, W., and Wall, P. D. (1955). Reflex inhibition by dorsal root interaction. *J. Neurophysiol. 18*:1–17.
192. Wall, P. D. (1962). The origin of a spinal cord slow potential. *J. Physiol. (Lond.) 164*:508–526.
193. Bonnet, V., and Bremer, F. (1952). Les potentials synaptiques et la transmission nerveuse centrale. *Arch. Int. Physiol. Biochim. 60*:33–93.
194. Eccles, J. C. (1939). The spinal cord and reflex action. *Ann. Rev. Physiol. 1*:363–384.
195. Bremer, F., and Bonnet, V. (1949). Les potentials synaptiques et leur interprétation. *Arch Sci. Physiol. 3*:489–520.
196. Eccles, J. C., and Malcolm, J. L. (1946). Dorsal root potentials of the spinal cord. *J. Neurophysiol. 9*:139–160.
197. Glusman, S., and Rudomín, P. (1974). Presynaptic modulation of synaptic effectiveness of afferent and ventrolateral tract fibers in the frog spinal cord. *Exp. Neurol. 45*:474–490.
198. Fatt, P. (1954). Biophysics of junctional transmission. *Physiol. Rev. 34*: 674–710.
199. Adair, R., and Davidoff, R. A. (1977). Studies on the uptake and release of [^{3}H]β-alanine by frog spinal cord slices. *J. Neurochem. 29*:213–220.
200. Vyklický, L., Syková, E., and Mellerova, B. (1976). Depolarization of primary afferents in the frog spinal cord under high Mg^{2+} concentrations. *Brain Res. 117*:153–156.
201. Smith, D., and Dambach, G. (1979). Extracellular K^+, Ca^{++} and Mg^{++} effects on the dorsal root potential of isolated frog spinal cord. *The Pharmacologist 21*:244.
202. Syková, E., and Vyklický, L. (1977). Changes of extracellular potassium activity in isolated spinal cord of frog under high Mg^{++} concentration. *Neurosci. Lett. 4*:161–165.
203. Grinnell, A. D. (1966). A study of the interaction between motoneurones in the frog spinal cord. *J. Physiol. (Lond.) 182*:612–648.
204. Nistri, A. (1983). Spinal cord pharmacology of GABA and chemically related amino acids. In *Handbook of the Spinal Cord*, vol. 1, *Pharmacology*, R. A. Davidoff (Ed.), Marcel Dekker, New York, pp. 45–102.

205. Padjen, A., Nicoll, R. A., and Barker, J. L. (1973). Synaptic potentials in the isolated frog spinal cord using sucrose gap techniques. *J. Gen. Physiol.* 61:270-271.

206. Rudomín, P., Stefani, E., and Werman, R. (1979). Voltage sensitivity of small focal transient potassium depolarizations in snail neurons: Relevance for diagnosis of chemical synaptic activity. *J. Neurophysiol.* 42: 912-924.

207. Carlson, C. B. (1964). Sodium and the dorsal root potential. *J. Physiol. (Lond.)* 172:295-304.

208. Barker, J. L., and Nicoll, R. A. (1973). The pharmacology and ionic dependency of amino acid responses in the frog spinal cord. *J. Physiol. (Lond.)* 228:259-277.

209. Katz, B., and Miledi, R. (1963). A study of spontaneous miniature potentials in spinal motoneurones. *J. Physiol. (Lond.)* 168:389-422.

210. Preston, P. R., and Wallis, D. I. (1980). The pharmacology of dorsal root potentials recorded from the isolated spinal cord of the neonate rat. *Gen. Pharmacol.* 11:527-534.

211. Otsuka, M., and Konishi, S. (1976). GABA in the spinal cord. In *GABA in Nervous System Function*, E. Roberts, T. N. Chase, and D. B. Tower (Eds.), Raven Press, New York, pp. 197-202.

212. Nistri, A., and Constanti, A. (1979). Pharmacological characterization of different types of GABA and glutamate receptors in vertebrate and invertebrates. *Prog. Neurobiol.* 13:117-235.

213. Barker, J. L., and Nicoll, R. A. (1972). Gamma-aminobutyric acid: Role in primary afferent depolarization. *Science* 176:1043-1045.

214. Constanti, A., and Nistri, A. (1976). A comparative study of the action of γ-aminobutyric acid and piperazine on the lobster muscle fibre and the frog spinal cord. *Br. J. Pharmacol.* 57:347-358.

215. Nishi, S., Minota, S., and Karczmar, A. G. (1974). Primary afferent neurones: The ionic mechanism of GABA-mediated depolarization. *Neuropharmacology* 13:215-219.

216. Kudo, Y., Ake, N., Goto, S., and Fukuda, H. (1975). The chloride-dependent depression by GABA in the frog spinal cord. *Eur. J. Pharmacol.* 32: 251-259.

217. DeGroat, W. C. (1972). GABA-depolarization of a sensory ganglion: Antagonism by picrotoxin and bicuculline. *Brain Res.* 38:429-432.

218. Gallagher, J. P., Higashi, H., and Nishi, S. (1979). Characterization and ionic basis of GABA-induced depolarizations recorded *in vitro* from cat primary afferent neurones. *J. Physiol. (Lond.)* 275:263-282.

219. Feltz, P., and Rasminsky, M. (1974). A model for the mode of action of GABA on primary afferent terminals: Depolarizing effects of GABA applied iontophoretically to neurones of mammalian dorsal root ganglia. *Neuropharmacology* 13:553-563.

220. Obata, K. (1974). Transmitter sensitivities of some nerve and muscle cells in culture. *Brain Res.* 73:71-88.

221. Hösli, L., Andres, P. F., and Hösli, E. (1977). Action of GABA on neurones and satellite glial cells of cultured rat dorsal root ganglia. *Neurosci. Lett. 6*:79–83.

222. Deschenes, M., Feltz, P., and Lamour, Y. (1976). A model for an estimate *in vivo* of the ionic basis of presynaptic inhibition: An intracellular analysis of the GABA-induced depolarization in rat dorsal root ganglia. *Brain Res. 118*:486–493.

223. Dunlap, K. (1981). Two types of γ-aminobutyric acid receptors on embryonic sensory neurones. *Br. J. Pharmacol. 74*:579–585.

224. Choi, D. W., and Fischbach, G. D. (1981). GABA conductance of chick spinal cord and dorsal root ganglion neurons in cell culture. *J. Neurophysiol. 45*:605–620.

225. Iles, J. F., Jack, J. J. B., and Lewis, G. H. (1979). Dorsal root potentials and presynaptic depolarization: Actions of ammonia. *J. Physiol (Lond.) 296*:98P.

226. Nicoll, R. A. (1978). The blockade of GABA mediated responses in the frog spinal cord by ammonium ions and furosemide. *J. Physiol. (Lond.) 283*:121–132.

227. Wojtowicz, J. M., and Nicoll, R. A. (1982). Selective action of piretanide on primary afferent GABA responses in the frog spinal cord. *Brain Res. 236*:173–181.

228. Kříž, N., Syková, E., Ujec, E., and Vyklický, L. (1974). Changes of extracellular potassium concentrations induced by neuronal activity in the spinal cord of the cat. *J. Physiol. (Lond.) 238*:1–15.

229. Bruggencate, G. ten, Lux, H. D., and Liebl, L. (1974). Possible relationship between the extracellular potassium activity and presynaptic inhibition in the spinal cord of the cat. *Pflugers Arch. ges. Physiol. 349*:301–307.

230. Lothman, E. W., and Somjen, G. G. (1975). Extracellular potassium activity, intracellular and extracellular potential responses in the spinal cord. *J. Physiol. (Lond.) 252*:115–136.

231. Krnjević, K., and Morris, M. E. (1974). Extracellular accumulation of K^+ evoked by activity of primary afferent fibers in the cuneate nucleus and dorsal horn of cats. *Can. J. Physiol. Pharmacol. 52*:852–871.

232. Sonnhof, U., Richter, D. W., Parekh, N., and Grafe, P. (1977). Changes in extracellular potassium concentration, pO_2 and intracellular potential in frog spinal motoneurons. *Pflugers Arch. 368*:R30.

233. Syková, E., Shirayev, N., Kříž, N., and Vyklický, L. (1976). Accumulation of extracellular potassium in the spinal cord of frog. *Brain Res. 106*:413–417.

234. Somjen, G. G. (1983). Spinal fluids and ions. In *Handbook of the Spinal Cord*, vol. 1, *Pharmacology*, R. A. Davidoff (Ed.), Marcel Dekker, New York, pp. 329–380.

235. Shefner, S. A., and Levy, R. A. (1981). The contribution of increases in extracellular potassium to primary afferent depolarization in the bullfrog spinal cord. *Brain Res. 205*:321–335.

236. Davidoff, R. A., Hackman, J. C., and Osorio, I. (1980). Amino acid antagonists do not block the depolarizing effects of potassium ions on frog primary afferents. *Neuroscience 5*:117–126.

237. Kříž, N., Syková, E., and Vyklický, L. (1975). Extracellular potassium changes in the spinal cord of the cat and their relation to slow potentials, active transport and impulse transmission. *J. Physiol. (Lond.) 249*:167–182.

238. Vyklický, L., Syková, E., and Kříž, N. (1975). Slow potentials induced by changes of extracellular potassium in the spinal cord of the cat. *Brain Res. 87*:77–80.

239. Syková, E., and Vyklický, L. (1978). Effects of picrotoxin on potassium accumulation and dorsal root potentials in frog spinal cord. *Neuroscience 3*:1061–1067.

240. Nicoll, R. A. (1979). Dorsal root potentials and changes in extracellular potassium in the spinal cord of the frog. *J. Physiol. (Lond.) 290*:113–127.

241. Eccles, J. C., Schmidt, R. F., and Willis, W. D. (1963). Pharmacological studies on presynaptic inhibition. *J. Physiol. (Lond.) 168*:500–530.

242. Rudomín, P., Nuñez, R., and Madrid, J. (1975). Modulation of synaptic effectiveness of Ia and descending fibers in cat spinal cord. *J. Neurophysiol. 38*:1181–1195.

243. Krnjević, K., and Morris, M. E. (1972). Extracellular K^+ activity and slow potential changes in spinal cord and medulla. *Can. J. Physiol. Pharmacol. 50*:1214–1217.

244. Schmidt, R. F. (1963). Pharmacological studies on the primary afferent depolarization of the toad spinal cord. *Pflugers Arch. ges. Physiol. 277*:325–346.

245. Tebēcis, A. K., and Phillis, J. W. (1969). The use of convulsants in studying possible functions of amino acids in the toad spinal cord. *Comp. Biochem. Physiol. 28*:1303–1315.

246. Levy, R. A., Repkin, A. H., and Anderson, E. G. (1971). The effect of bicuculline on primary afferent terminal excitability. *Brain Res. 32*:261–265.

247. Davidoff, R. A. (1972). Gamma-aminobutyric acid antagonism and presynaptic inhibition in the frog spinal cord. *Science 175*:331–333.

248. Levy, R. A. (1975). The effect of intravenously administered γ-aminobutyric acid in afferent fiber depolarization. *Brain Res. 92*:21–34.

249. Gmelin, G., and Cerletti, A. (1976). Electrophoretic studies on presynaptic inhibition in the mammalian spinal cord. *Experientia 32*:756.

250. Curtis, D. R., Lodge, D., and Brand, S. S. (1977). GABA and spinal afferent terminal excitability in the cat. *Brain Res. 130*:360–363.

251. Barker, J. L., Nicoll, R. A., and Padjen, A. (1975). Studies on convulsants in the isolated frog spinal cord. II. Effects on root potentials. *J. Physiol. (Lond.) 245*:537–548.

252. Osorio, I., Hackman, J. C., and Davidoff, R. A. (1979). GABA or potassium: Which mediates primary afferent depolarization? *Brain Res. 161*:183–186.

253. Shirasawa, Y., and Koketsu, K. (1975). The effect of picrotoxin on the dorsal root potential of bullfrog spinal cords. *Kurume Med. J. 22*:1-4.

254. Krnjević, K., and Morris, M. E. (1975). Correlation between extracellular focal potentials and K⁺ potentials evoked by primary afferent activity. *Can. J. Physiol. Pharmacol. 53*:912-922.

255. Somjen, G. G. (1970). Evoked sustained focal potentials and membrane potential of neurons and of unresponsive cells of the spinal cord. *J. Neurophysiol. 33*:562-582.

256. Mendell, L. M., and Wall, P. D. (1964). Presynaptic hyperpolarization: A role for fine afferent fibres. *J. Physiol. (Lond.) 172*:274-294.

257. Anden, N. E., Jukes, M. G. M., Lundberg, A., and Vyklický, L. (1966). The affect of DOPA on the spinal cord. 3. Depolarization evoked in the central terminals of ipsilateral Ia afferents by volleys in the flexor reflex afferents. *Acta Physiol. Scand. 68*:322-336.

258. Dawson, G. D., Merrill, E. G., and Wall, P. D. (1970). Dorsal root potentials produced by stimulation of fine afferents. *Science 167*:1385-1387.

259. Mendell, L. (1970). Positive dorsal root potentials produced by stimulation of small diameter muscle afferents. *Brain Res. 18*:375-379.

260. Hodge, C. J., Jr. (1972). Potential changes inside central afferent terminals secondary to stimulation of large and small diameter peripheral nerve fibers. *J. Neurophysiol. 35*:30-43.

261. Mendell, L. (1972). Properties and distribution of peripherally evoked presynaptic hyperpolarization in cat lumbar spinal cord. *J. Physiol. (Lond.) 226*:769-792.

262. Burke, R. E., Rudomín, P., Vyklický, L., and Zajac, F. E. (1971). Primary afferent depolarizaion and flexion reflexes produced by radiant heat stimulation of the skin. *J. Physiol. (Lond.) 213*:185-214.

263. Lundberg, A., and Vylický, L. (1966). Inhibition of transmission to primary afferents by electrical stimulation of the brain stem. *Arch. Ital. Biol. 104*:86-97.

264. Cangiano, A., Cook, W. A. Jr., and Pompeiano, O. (1969). Cerebellar inhibitory control of the vestibular reflex pathways to primary afferents. *Arch. Ital. Biol. 107*:341-364.

265. Chan, S. H. H., and Barnes, C. D. (1971). Presynaptic facilitation: Positive dorsal root potentials evoked from brain stem reticular formation in lumbar cord. *Brain Res. 28*:176-179.

266. Owen, M. P., and Hodge, C. J., Jr. (1973). Positive dorsal root potentials evoked by stimulation of the brain stem reticular formation. *Brain Res. 54*:305-308.

267. Levy, R. A., and Anderson, E. G. (1974). The role of γ-aminobutyric acid as a mediator of positive dorsal root potentials. *Brain Res. 76*:71-82.

268. Hongo, T., Jankowska, E., and Lundberg, A. (1972). The rubrospinal tract. III. Effects on primary afferent terminals. *Exp. Brain Res. 15*:39-53.

269. Lund, S., Lundberg, A., and Vyklický, L. (1965). Inhibitory action from the flexor reflex afferents on transmission to Ia afferents. *Acta Physiol. Scand. 64*:345-355.

270. Rudomín, P., Nuñez, R., Madrid, J., and Burke, R. E. (1974). Primary afferent hyperpolarization and presynaptic facilitation of Ia afferent terminals induced by large cutaneous fibers. *J. Neurophysiol. 37*:413-429.

271. Whitehorn, D., and Burgess, P. R. (1973). Changes in polarization of central branches of myelinated mechanoreceptor and nociceptor fibers during noxious and innocuous stimulation of the skin. *J. Neurophysiol. 36*:226-237.

272. Hentall, I. D., and Fields, H. L. (1979). Segmental and descending influences on intraspinal thresholds of single C-fibers. *J. Neurophysiol. 42*: 1527-1537.

273. Lundberg, A. (1964). Supraspinal control of transmission in reflex paths to motoneurones and primary afferents. In *Progress in Brain Research. Physiology of Spinal Neurons*, vol. 12, J. C. Eccles and J. P. Schade (Eds.), Elsevier, Amsterdam, pp. 196-221.

274. Fessard, A., and Matthews, B. H. C. (1939). Unitary synaptic potentials. *J. Physiol. (Lond.) 95*:398-418.

275. Matthews, B. H. C. (1966). Single fibre activation of central nervous activity. In *Muscular Afferents and Motor Control*, R. Granit (Ed.), Almqvist and Wiksell, Stockholm, pp. 227-233.

276. Schmidt, R. F., Trautwein, W., and Zimmermann, M. (1966). Dorsal root potentials evoked by natural stimulation of cutaneous afferents. *Nature 212*:522-523.

277. Sontag, K. H. (1974). Dorsal root potential and inhibition of monosynaptic extensor reflex induced by natural stretch of pretibial muscles in cats. *Arch. Ital. Biol. 112*:48-59.

278. Schmidt, R. F., Senges, J., and Zimmermann, M. (1967). Presynaptic depolarization of cutaneous mechanoreceptor afferents after mechanical skin stimulation. *Exp. Brain Res. 3*:234-247.

279. Jänig, W., Schmidt, R. F., and Zimmermann, M. (1967). Presynaptic depolarization during activation of tonic mechanoreceptors. *Brain Res. 5*: 514-516.

280. Jänig, W., Schmidt, R. F., and Zimmermann, M. (1968). Two specific feedback pathways to the central afferent terminals of phasic and tonic mechanoreceptors. *Exp. Brain Res. 6*:116-129.

281. Devanandan, M. S., Eccles, R. M., and Yokota, T. (1965). Depolarization of afferent terminals evoked by muscle stretch. *J. Physiol. (Lond.) 179*: 417-429.

282. Casey, K. L., and Oakley, B. (1972). Intraspinal latency, cutaneous fiber composition, and afferent control of the dorsal root reflex in cat. *Brain Res. 47*:353-369.

283. Van Harreveld, A., and Niechaj, A. (1970). A possibly monosynaptic component of the dorsal root potential. *Brain Res. 19*:105-116.

284. Rudomín, P. (1966). Pharmacological evidence for the existence of interneurons mediating primary afferent depolarization in the solitary tract nucleus of the cat. *Brain Res. 2*:181-183.

284a. Rudomín, P., Jankowska, E., and Madrid, J. (1978). Presynaptic depolarization of cortico-spinal and rubro-spinal terminal arborizations produced by conditioning volleys to sensory nerves. *Soc. Neurosci. Abst. 4*:571.

285. Rudomín, P., Engberg, I., and Jiménez, I. (1981). Mechanisms involved in presynaptic depolarization of group I and rubrospinal fibers in cat spinal cord. *J. Neurophysiol. 46*:532–548.

286. Nicoll, R. A. (1975). Presynaptic action of barbiturates in the frog spinal cord. *Proc. Natl. Acad. Sci. USA 72*:1460–1463.

287. Carpenter, D., Engberg, I., Funkenstein, H., and Lundberg, A. (1963). Decerebrate control of reflexes to primary afferents. *Acta Physiol. Scand. 59*:424–437.

288. Rudomín, P., and Dutton, H. (1969). Effects of muscle and cutaneous afferent nerve volleys on excitability fluctuations of Ia terminals. *J. Neurophysiol. 32*:158–169.

289. Barnes, C. D., and Pompeiano, O. (1970). Presynaptic and postsynaptic effects in the monosynaptic reflex pathway to extensor motoneurons following vibration of synergic muscles. *Arch. Ital. Biol. 108*:259–294.

290. Cook, W. A., Jr., Neilson, D. R., Jr., and Brookhart, J. M. (1965). Primary afferent depolarization and monosynaptic reflex depression following succinylcholine administration. *J. Neurophysiol. 28*:290–311.

291. Decandia, M., Provini, L., and Táborříková, H. (1967). Presynaptic inhibition of monosynaptic reflex following the stimulation of nerves to extensor muscles of the ankle. *Exp. Brain Res. 4*:34–42.

292. Devanandan, M. S., Eccles, R. M., and Stenhouse, D. (1966). Presynaptic inhibition evoked by muscle contraction. *J. Physiol. 185*:471–485.

293. Eccles, J. C., Schmidt, R. F., and Willis, W. D. (1963). Depolarization of central terminals of group Ib afferent fibers of muscle. *J. Neurophysiol. 26*:1–27.

294. Eccles, J. C., Kozak, W., and Magni, F. (1961). Dorsal root reflexes of muscle group I afferent fibers. *J. Physiol. (Lond.) 159*:128–146.

295. Schmidt, R. F., and Willis, W. D. (1963). Depolarization of central terminals of afferent fibers in cervical spinal cord of the cat. *J. Neurophysiol. 26*:44–59.

296. Decandia, M., Gasteiger, E. L., and Mann, M. D. (1968). Escape of the extensor monosynaptic reflex from presynaptic inhibition. *Brain Res. 7*:317–319.

297. Decandia, M., Gasteiger, E. L., and Mann, M. D. (1971). Excitability changes of extensor motoneurons and primary afferent endings during prolonged stimulation of flexor afferents. *Exp. Brain Res. 12*:150–160.

298. Barnes, C. D., and Pompeiano, O. (1970). Presynaptic inhibition of extensor monosynaptic reflex by Ia afferents from flexors. *Brain Res. 18*:380–383.

299. Barnes, C. D., and Pompeiano, O. (1970). Inhibition of monosynaptic extensor reflex attributable to presynaptic depolarization of the group Ia afferent fibers produced by vibration of flexor muscle. *Arch. Ital. Biol. 108*:233–258.

300. Bergman, J., Burke, R., Fedina, L., and Lündberg, A. (1974). The effect of DOPA on the spinal cord. 8. Presynaptic and "remote" inhibition of transmission from Ia afferents to alpha motoneurones. *Acta Physiol. Scand. 90*:618–639.

301. Schmidt, R. F., Senges, J., and Zimmermann, M. (1967). Excitability measurements at the central terminals of single mechano-receptor afferents during slow potential changes. *Exp. Brain Res. 3*:220–233.

302. Vyklický, L., and Tabin, V. (1966). Primary afferent depolarization evoked by adequate stimulation of skin receptors. *Physiol. Bohemoslov. 15*:89–97.

303. Eccles, J. C., Kostyuk, P. G., and Schmidt, R. F. (1962). Presynaptic inhibition of the central actions of flexor reflex afferents. *J. Physiol. (Lond.) 161*:258–281.

304. Brown, A. G., and Hayden, R. E. (1972). Presynaptic depolarization produced by and in identified cutaneous afferent fibres in the rabbit. *Brain Res. 38*:187–192.

305. Carpenter, D. O., and Rudomín, P. (1973). The organization of primary afferent depolarization in isolated spinal cord of the frog. *J. Physiol. (Lond.) 229*:471–493.

306. Kiraly, J. K., and Phillis, J. W. (1961). Action of some drugs on the dorsal root potentials of the isolated toad spinal cord. *Br. J. Pharmacol. 17*:224–231.

307. Richens, A. (1969). The action of general anesthetic agents on root responses of the frog isolated spinal cord. *Br. J. Pharmacol. 36*:294–311.

308. Niechaj, A., Lupa, K., and Ozóg, M. (1977). Dorsal root potentials evoked by stimulation of ventral roots in the lower sacral cord of the cat. *Brain Res. 137*:356–360.

309. Clifton, G. L., Coggeshall, R. E., Vance, W. H., and Willis, W. D. (1976). Receptive fields of unmyelinated ventral root afferent fibres in the cat. *J. Physiol. (Lond.) 256*:573–600.

310. Coggeshall, R. E., Coulter, J. D., and Willis, W. D. (1974). Unmyelinated axons in the ventral roots of the cat lumbosacral enlargement. *J. Comp. Neurol. 153*:39–58.

311. Applebaum, M. L., Clifton, G. L., Coggeshall, R. E., Coulter, J. D., Vance, W. H., and Willis, W. D. (1976). Unmyelinated fibres in the sacral 3 and caudal 1 ventral roots of the cat. *J. Physiol. (Lond.) 256*:557–572.

312. Toennies, J. F. (1938). Reflex discharge from the spinal cord over the dorsal roots. *J. Neurophysiol. 1*:378–390.

313. Brooks, C. McC., and Koizumi, K. (1956). Origin of the dorsal root reflex. *J. Neurophysiol. 19*:61–74.

314. Brooks, C. McC., Koizumi, K., and Malcolm, J. L. (1955). Effects of changes in temperature on reactions of spinal cord. *J. Neurophysiol. 18*:205–216.

315. Toennies, J. F. (1939). Conditioning of afferent impulses by reflex discharges over the dorsal roots. *J. Neurophysiol. 2*:515–525.

316. Tregear, R. T. (1958). The relation of antidromic impulses in the dorsal root fibres to the dorsal root potential in the frog. *J. Physiol. (Lond.) 142*: 343-359.

317. Megirian, D. (1968). Centrifugal discharges in cutaneous afferent volleys in the acutely spinal phalanger, *Trichosurus vulpecula. Arch. Ital. Biol. 106*: 343-352.

318. Chan, S. H. H., and Barnes, C. G. (1972). A presynaptic mechanism evoked from brain stem reticular formation in the lumbar cord and its temporal significance. *Brain Res. 45*:101-114.

319. Carpenter, D., Engberg, I., and Lundberg, A. (1962). Presynaptic inhibition in the lumbar cord evoked from the brain stem. *Experientia 18*:450-451.

320. Carpenter, D., Engberg, I., and Lundberg, A. (1966). Primary afferent depolarization evoked from the brain stem and the cerebellum. *Arch. Ital. Biol. 104*:73-85.

321. Cook, W. A., Jr., Cangiano, A., and Pompeiano, O. (1969). Dorsal root potentials in the lumbar cord evoked from the vestibular system. *Arch. Ital. Biol. 107*:275-295.

322. Cook, W. A., Jr., Cangiano, A., and Pompeiano, O. (1969). Vestibular control of transmission in primary afferents to the lumbar spinal cord. *Arch. Ital. Biol. 107*:296-320.

323. Cangiano, A., Cook, W. A., Jr., and Pompeiano, O. (1969). Primary afferent depolarization in the lumbar cord evoked from the fastigial nucleus. *Arch. Ital. Biol. 107*:321-340.

324. Anderson, P., and Sears, T. A. (1962). Presynaptic inhibitory action of cerebral cortex on the spinal cord. *Nature 194*:740-741.

325. Andersen, P., Eccles, J. C., and Sears, T. A. (1964). Cortically evoked depolarization of primary afferent fibers in the spinal cord. *J. Neurophysiol. 27*:63-77.

326. Carpenter, D., Lundberg, A., and Norrsell, U. (1962). Effects from the pyramidal tract on primary afferents and on spinal reflex actions to primary afferents. *Experientia 18*:337-338.

327. Carpenter, D., Lundberg, A., and Norrsell, U. (1963). Primary afferent depolarization evoked from sensorimotor cortex. *Acta Physiol. Scand. 59*: 126-142.

328. Rudomín, P., and Jankowska, E. (1981). Presynaptic depolarization of terminals of rubrospinal tract fibers in intermediate nucleus of cat spinal cord. *J. Neurophysiol. 46*:517-531.

329. Abdelmoumene, M., Besson, J.-M., and Aléonard, P. (1970). Cortical areas exerting presynaptic inhibitory action on the spinal cord in cat and monkey. *Brain Res. 20*:327-329.

330. Calma, I., and Quayle, A. A. (1971). Supraspinal control of the presynaptic effects of forepaw and hindpaw skin stimulation in the cat under chloralose anaesthesia. *Brain Res. 33*:101-114.

331. Hongo, T., and Jankowska, E. (1967). Effects from the sensorimotor cortex on the spinal cord in cats with transected pyramids. *Exp. Brain Res. 3*:117–134.
332. Martin, R. F., Haber, L. H., and Willis, W. D. (1979). Primary afferent depolarization of identified cutaneous fibers following stimulation in medial brain stem. *J. Neurophysiol. 42*:779–790.
333. Cook, W. A., Jr., Cangiano, A., and Pompeiano, O. (1968). Vestibular influences on primary afferents in the spinal cord. *Pflugers Arch. ges. Physiol. 299*:334–338.
334. Eide, E., Jurna, I., and Lundberg, A. (1968). Conductance measurements from motoneurons during presynaptic inhibition. In *Structure and Function of Inhibitory Neuronal Mechanisms*, C. von Euler, S. Skoglund and U. Söderberg (Eds.), Pergamon Press, Oxford, pp. 215–219.
335. Sypert, G. W., Munson, J. B., and Fleshman, J. W. (1980). Effect of presynaptic inhibition on axonal potentials, terminal potentials, focal synaptic potentials, and EPSP's in cat spinal cord. *J. Neurophysiol. 44*:792–803.
336. Eccles, J. C., Schmidt, R. F., and Willis, W. D. (1962). Presynaptic inhibition of the spinal monosynaptic reflex pathway. *J. Physiol. (Lond.) 161*: 282–297.
337. Rudomín, P., Burke, R. E., Nuñez, R., Madrid, J., and Dutton, H. (1975). Control by presynaptic correlation: A mechanism affecting information transmission from Ia fibers to motoneurons. *J. Neurophysiol. 38*:267–284.
338. Sypert, G. W., and Munson, J. B. (1984). Excitatory synapses. In *Handbook of the Spinal Cord*, vols. 2 and 3, *Anatomy and Physiology*. R. A. Davidoff (Ed.), Marcel Dekker, New York, pp. 315–384.
339. Granit, R. (1968). The case for presynaptic inhibition by synapses on the terminals of motoneurons. In *Structure and Function of Inhibitory Neuronal mechanisms*, C. von Euler, S. Skogland and U. Söderberg (Eds.), Pergamon Press, Oxford, pp. 183–195.
340. Jack, J. J. B., Noble, D., and Tsien, R. W. (1975). *Electric Current Flow in Excitable Cells*. Clarendon Press, Oxford.
341. Krnjević, K., Puil, E., and Werman, R. (1977). GABA and glycine actions on spinal motoneurons. *Can. J. Physiol. Pharmacol. 55*:658–669.
342. Curtis, D. R., Hösli, L., Johnston, G. A. R., and Johnston, I. H. (1968). The hyperpolarization of spinal motoneurones by glycine and related amino acids. *Exp. Brain Res. 5*:235–258.
343. Lodge, D., Curtis, D. R., and Brand, S. J. (1977). A pharmacological study of the inhibition of ventral group Ia-excited spinal interneurones. *Exp. Brain Res. 29*:97–105.
344. Game, C. J. A., and Lodge, D. (1975). The pharmacology of the inhibition of dorsal horn neurones by impulses in myelinated cutaneous afferents in the cat. *Exp. Brain Res. 23*:75–84.
345. Takeuchi, A., and Takeuchi, N. (1962). Electrical changes in pre- and postsynaptic axons of the giant synapse of *Loligo. J. Gen. Physiol. 45*:1181–1193.

346. Katz, B., and Miledi, R. (1967). A study of synaptic transmission in the absence of nerve impulses. *J. Physiol. (Lond.) 192*:407–436.

347. Eccles, J. C., and Krnjević, K. (1959). Presynaptic changes associated with post-tetanic potentiation in the spinal cord. *J. Physiol. (Lond.) 149*:274–287.

348. Sastry, B. R. (1979). Calcium and action potentials in primary afferent terminals. *Life Sci. 24*:2193–2200.

349. Dunlap, K., and Fischbach, G. D. (1978). Neurotransmitters decrease the calcium component of sensory neurone action potentials. *Nature 276*: 837–839.

350. Dunlap, K., and Fischbach, G. D. (1981). Neurotransmitters decrease the calcium conductance activated by depolarizing embryonic chick sensory neurones. *J. Physiol. (Lond.) 317*:519–535.

351. Davidoff, R. A., and Hackman, J. C. (1983). Drugs, chemicals and toxins: Their effects on the spinal cord. In *Handbook of the Spinal Cord*, vol. 1, *Pharmacology*, R. A. Davidoff (Ed.), Marcel Dekker, New York, pp. 409–476.

352. Renshaw, B. (1946). Observations on interaction of nerve impulses in the gray matter and on the nature of central inhibition. *Am. J. Physiol. 146*: 443–448.

353. Kuno, M. (1964). Mechanism of facilitation and depression of the excitatory synaptic potential in spinal motoneurones. *J. Physiol. (Lond.) 175*: 100–112.

354. Waxman, S. G. (1972). Regional differentiation of the axon: A review with special reference to the concept of the multiplex neuron. *Brain Res. 47*:269–288.

355. Waxman, S. G. (1975). Integrative properties and design principles of axons. *Int. Rev. Neurobiol. 18*:1–40.

356. Spira, M. E., Yarom, Y., and Parnas, I. (1976). Modulation of spike frequency by regions of special axonal geometry and by synaptic inputs. *J. Neurophysiol. 39*:882–899.

357. Rudomín, P., and Dutton, H. (1967). Effects of presynaptic and postsynaptic inhibition on the variability of the monosynaptic reflex. *Nature 216*: 292–293.

358. Rudomín, P., and Dutton, H. (1969). Effects conditioning of afferent volleys on variability of monosynaptic responses of extensor motoneurons. *J. Neurophysiol. 32*:130–157.

359. LaMotte, C., Pert, C. B., and Snyder, S. H. (1976). Opiate receptor binding in primate spinal cord: Distribution and changes after dorsal root section. *Brain Res. 112*:407–412.

360. Jessell, T., Tsunoo, A., Kanazawa, I., and Otsuka, M. (1979). Substance P: Depletion in the dorsal horn of rat spinal cord after section of the peripheral processes of primary sensory neurons. *Brain Res. 168*:247–260.

361. Gamse, R., Holzer, P., and Lembeck, F. (1979). Indirect evidence for presynaptic location of opiate receptors on chemosensitive primary sensory neurones. *Naunyn Schmiedebergs Arch. Pharmacol. 308*:281–285.

362. Fields, H. L., Emson, P. C., Leigh, B. K., Gilbert, R. F. T., and Iversen, L. L. (1980). Multiple opiate receptor sites on primary afferent fibres. *Nature 284*:351–353.

363. Jessell, T. M., and Iversen, L. L. (1977). Opiate analgesics inhibit substance P release from rat trigeminal nucleus. *Nature 268*:549–551.

364. Mudge, A. W., Leeman, S. E., and Fischbach, G. D. (1979). Enkephalin inhibits release of substance P from sensory neurons in culture and decreases action potential duration. *Proc. Natl. Acad. Sci. USA 76*:526–530.

365. Sastry, B. R. (1978). Morphine and met-enkephalin effects on sural A afferent terminal excitability. *Eur. J. Pharmacol. 50*:269–273.

366. Sastry, B. R. (1979). Presynaptic effects of morphine and methionine-enkephalin in feline spinal cord. *Neuropharmacology 18*:367–375.

367. Evans, R. H., and Hill, R. G. (1978). Effects of excitatory and inhibitory peptides on isolated spinal cord preparations. In *Iontophoresis and Transmitter Mechanisms in the Mammalian Central Nervous System*, R. W. Ryall and J. S. Kelly (Eds.), Elsevier-North Holland, Amsterdam, pp. 101–103.

368. Ljungdahl, A., Hökfelt, T., and Nilsson, G. (1978). Distribution of substance P-like immunoreactivity in the central nervous system of the rat. I. Cell bodies and nerve terminals. *Neuroscience 3*:861–943.

369. Barber, R. P., Vaughn, J. E., Selmmon, J. R., Salvaterra, P. M., Roberts, E., and Leeman, S. E. (1979). The origin, distribution and synaptic relationships of substance P axons in rat spinal cord. *J. Comp. Neurol. 184*: 331–352.

370. Uhl, G. R., Kuhar, M. J., and Snyder, S. H. (1978). Neurotensin: Immunohistochemical localization in rat central nervous system. *Proc. Natl. Acad. Sci. USA 74*:4059–4063.

371. Uhl, G. R., Goodman, R. R., and Snyder, S. H. (1979). Neurotensin-containing cell bodies, fibers and nerve terminals in the brain-stem of the rat: Immunohistochemical mapping. *Brain Res. 167*:77–91.

372. Innis, R. B., Corréa, F. M., Uhl, G. R., Schneider, B., and Snyder, S. H. (1979). Cholecystokinin octapeptide-like immunoreactivity: Histochemical localization in rat brain. *Proc. Natl. Acad. Sci. USA 76*:521–525.

373. Forssmann, W. G. (1978). A new somatostatinergic system in the mammalian spinal cord. *Neurosci. Lett. 10*:293–297.

374. Kardon, F. C., Winokur, A., and Utiger, R. D. (1977). Thyrotropin-releasing hormone (TRH) in rat spinal cord. *Brain Res. 122*:578–581.

375. Fuxe, K., Ganten, D., Hökfelt, T., and Bolme, P. (1976). Immunohistochemical evidence for the existence of angiotension II–containing nerve terminals in the brain and spinal cord of the rat. *Neurosci. Lett. 2*:229–234.

376. Konishi, S., and Otsuka, M. (1974). The effects of substance P and other peptides on spinal neurons of the frog. *Brain Res. 65*:397–410.

377. Phillis, J. W., and Kirkpatrick, J. R. (1979). Actions of various gastrointestinal peptides on the isolated amphibian spinal cord. *Can. J. Physiol. Pharmacol. 8*:887–899.

378. Padjen, A. L. (1977). Effects of somatostatin on frog spinal cord. *Soc. Neurosci. Abst. 3*:411.

379. Fields, H. L., and Basbaum, A. I. (1978). Brainstem control of spinal pain-transmission neurons. *Ann. Rev. Physiol. 40*:217–248.

380. Hodge, C. J., Woods, C. I., and Delatizky, J. (1980). Noradrenalin, serotonin, and the dorsal horn. *J. Neurosurg. 52*:674–685.

381. Hackman, J. C., Wohlberg, C. J., and Davidoff, R. A. (1982). The effects of epinephrine and norepinephrine on frog primary afferent fibers. *Soc. Neurosci. Abst. 8*:483.

382. Tebēcis, A. K., and Phillis, J. W. (1967). The effects of topically applied biogenic monoamines on the isolated toad spinal cord. *Comp. Biochem. Physiol. 23*:553–563.

383. Jeftinija, S., Semba, K., and Randíc, M. (1981). Norepinephrine reduces excitability of single cutaneous primary afferent C-fibers in the cat spinal cord. *Brain Res. 219*:456–463.

384. Shirasawa, Y., and Koketsu, K. (1977). Action of 5-hydroxytryptamine on isolated spinal cord of bullfrogs. *Jpn. J. Pharmacol. 27*:23–29.

385. Chung, S.-H., Raymond, S. A., and Lettvin, J. Y. (1970). Multiple meaning in single visual units. *Brain Behav. Evol. 3*:72–101.

386. Fuortes, M. G. F. (1951). Action of strychnine on the 'intermittent conduction' of impulses along the dorsal columns of the spinal cord of frogs. *J. Physiol. (Lond.) 112*:42P.

387. Wall, P. D., Lettvin, J. Y., McCulloch, W. S., and Pitts, W. H. (1955). Factors limiting the maximum impulse transmitting ability of an afferent system of nerve fibres. In *3rd London Symposium on Information Theory*. Butterworth, London, pp. 329–344.

388. Raymond, S. A., and Lettvin, J. Y. (1969). Influences on axonal conduction. *Quart. Prog. Report No. 92, Research Lab. of Electronics*, Massachusetts Institute of Technology, pp. 431–435.

389. Grossman, Y., Parnas, I., and Spira, M. E. (1979). Ionic mechanisms involved in differential conduction of action potentials at high frequency in a branching axon. *J. Physiol. (Lond.) 295*:307–322.

390. Smith, D. O. (1980). Mechanisms of action potential propagation failure at sites of axon branching in the crayfish. *J. Physiol. (Lond.) 301*:243–259.

391. Van Essen, D. C. (1973). The contribution of membrane hyperpolarization to adaptation and conduction block in sensory neurones of the leech. *J. Physiol. (Lond.) 230*:509–534.

11
RECURRENT INHIBITION

Ottavio Pompeiano   *Institute of Human Physiology, University of Pisa,*
Pisa, Italy

I. INTRODUCTION

In 1941, Renshaw (1) demonstrated that antidromic impulses traveling in motor axons could inhibit the reflex response of alpha motoneurons innervating the same or synergistic muscles. He identified (2) a population of spinal cord interneurons that responded to stimulation of motor axons and suggested that this effect was mediated by the recurrent axon collaterals described in anatomic studies by Golgi (3,4) and Cajal (5). Later, Eccles et al. (6) showed that these interneurons, termed Renshaw (R) cells, in turn inhibit alpha motoneurons. The recurrent inhibitory pathway has been subjected to extensive physiologic studies (see 7-23 for reviews).

. Renshaw cells are small neurons located in the ventral horn, medial to the motoneuronal columns. They have long axonal branches that course within the ventromedial funiculus before spreading into the gray matter to innervate their target neurons (Fig. 1; see Sec. II). It is well established that R-cells inhibit not only some groups of alpha motoneurons but also gamma motoneurons, interneurons mediating reciprocal Ia inhibition of motoneurons (i.e., Ia inhibitory interneurons), other R-cells, ascending tract cells (in particular cells of origin of the ventral spinocerebellar tract, VSCT neurons), and finally sympathetic and parasympathetic preganglionic neurons (see Sec. IV). Not all motoneurons give

461

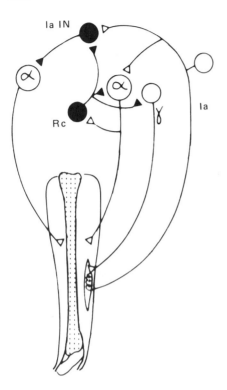

Figure 1 Schematic illustration of collateral connections from the same Renshaw cell (Rc) to synergistic alpha motoneurons, gamma motoneurons, and the Ia inhibitory interneurons (IaIN) supplied with monosynaptic excitation by the Ia afferents originating from the synergistic muscles. These Ia interneurons impinge on antagonistic alpha motoneurons. Black cells represent inhibitory interneurons.

rise to recurrent collaterals (see Sec. III.A). Moreover, not all motoneurons that contribute recurrent collaterals are equally effective in driving the R-cells, nor are all motoneurons equally sensitive to recurrent inhibition. In addition, recurrent collaterals of alpha motor axons can establish synaptic contacts not only with R-cells but also directly with homonymous alpha motoneurons without interposed interneurons. This connection may lead to activation of neighbouring motoneurons when some units are excited within a given motor nucleus.

R-cells are influenced not only from motor axon collaterals but also from segmental (see Sec. III.B) and supraspinal descending systems of different origin (see Sec. III.C). Although some data is available concerning these systems, further experiments are required to define the physiologic conditions under which the different segmental and supraspinal descending pathways act on the recurrent inhibitory circuit, either indirectly (i.e., by exciting or inhibiting the alpha motoneurons) or directly, by exciting or inhibiting the R-cells. While in the former condition the R-cell discharge would reflect changes in the motoneuronal output, in the latter condition the R-cell discharge would determine changes in the activity of alpha motoneurons and other target neurons. These and other findings indicate the important role that R-cells may exert in the control of posture and movement (see Sec. V).

This review is concerned with the neurophysiologic basis of recurrent inhibition. Mention will be made of acetylcholine, the transmitter substance involved in the excitatory contacts between recurrent collaterals of alpha motoneurons and R-cells and the postsynaptic membrane involving both muscarinic and nicotinic receptors (6,24–32; cf. 33). There is also evidence that there are two types of R-cells, one type releasing gamma-aminobutyric acid (GABA) and the other glycine as transmitter substances (34). However, the functional organization of these two populations of R-cells is not fully understood.

II. LOCATION AND MORPHOLOGY OF RENSHAW CELLS

Attempts to identify R-cells by purely anatomic procedures (cf. 19) did not lead to unequivocal results. Reliable information concerning the location of R-cells was, however, obtained by physiologists. R-cells are activated orthodromically when motor axons are stimulated (2,6,35); in particular, at a given segmental level the population of R-cells tends to discharge synchronously during the initial part of their burst responses. This synchronous discharge results in a characteristic oscillatory field potential (6,36,37). In the lumbar segments of the cat spinal cord, the region of maximum negativity of the R-cell field potential lies in the ventral horn region where the motor axons leave the gray matter (6). The antidromic field potentials evoked in the ventral horn of the deafferented cat spinal cord by stimulation of motor axons in peripheral nerve have been investigated by Willis et al. (38), who found that the R-cell potentials showed a maximum sink in the ventral part of Rexed's lamina VII (39–41), ventromedial to the main motor nuclei. This is the same region in which records from individual R-cells antidromically activated by ventral root stimulation have been obtained (Fig. 2C) (2,42–45; cf. 46,47). Such a location was verified by intracellular Procion Yellow (48–51) and horseradish peroxidase (HRP) (52) staining of physiologically identified R-cells.

Axon collaterals of triceps surae alpha motoneurons intracellularly injected with HRP make synaptic contact with neurons located ventrally in lamina VII (53; see Sec. III.A). These neurons, thought to be R-cells, showed elongated contours of cell bodies as observed in the mid-nucleolus plane (54). In terms of size, the neurons studied ultrastructurally fell within the upper part of the range given by those studied light microscopically by the same authors (mean diameters 21-33 and 11-36 μm, respectively). The lower values (10-26 μm) reported by previous investigators in light microscopic observations after intracellular injection with Procion Yellow (48-51) or HRP (52) were probably caused by some cytotoxicity of Procion Yellow with ensuing shrinkage of the injected neuron and to differences in fixation and measuring procedures. The number of dendrites of each neuron varied between three and eight (52,54) and the corresponding axon originated from cell bodies or dendrites (54).

In the limb segments of the spinal cord R-cells have ipsilateral, not contralateral projections (6,44,55). The length and spatial distribution of these ipsilaterally projecting axons have been discussed extensively in the past (cf. 17, 56-61). The observation that R-cells inhibited primarily motoneurons in close proximity (6) led to the conclusion that R-cells are probably Golgi type II neurons (62; cf. 56,57,60). Attempts to identify them morphologically were therefore aimed primarily at finding cells with short axons that do not leave the gray matter. The inability to find such neurons in anatomic studies (5,56, 57,60,63) caused some authors to deny the existence of R-cells (56; cf. 64,65). Actually, the presence of "R-elements" within the motor nucleus led Erulkar et al. (64) to suggest that these elements are synaptic endings of motoneuron recurrent collaterals. This hypothesis is no longer tenable because of all the electrophysiologic and the direct morphologic evidence discussed previously. The alternative possibility is that these neurons are funicular cells (17,48,51, 52,57-60,66). It is known, in fact, that motoneurons may be inhibited or facilitated by antidromic volleys in several (three) ventral roots (2,67-69). Since the motor axon collaterals terminate within one half segment of the parent soma (57; see Sec. III.A), R-cells must have long axons projecting more than one segment. Indeed, in the ventral part of lamina VII there are interneurons that project ipsilaterally and terminate within a few segments (59). It remained, however, for Jankowska and Smith (70; cf. 47) to explore the spinal cord in a search for sites from which single R-cells could be activated antidromically and to find that in the lower lumbar segments R-cell axons: (1) can project over distances of more than 12 mm rostrally or caudally; (2) run in the ipsilateral ventromedial funiculus before spreading into the gray matter to innervate their target neurons; (3) are likely to terminate both within motor nuclei (mainly at short distances, corresponding to about 4 mm from their somata; cf. 6) and in an area dorsomedial and medial to them;* and (4) have a maximal conduction velocity of about 30 m/sec. It is known that the target

*The finding that a single R-cell gives off terminals to motoneurons only within 4 mm of its cell body suggests that divergence of single cells cannot include an entire motoneuron pool, whose cells can extend over as much as 10 mm in the cat spinal cord (71).

cells of R-cells are located in well-defined parts of the ventral horn motor nuclei (alpha and gamma motoneurons: Sec. IV.A.1 and 2) and the areas just dorsal and medial to them (Ia inhibitory interneurons: Sec. IV.A.3 and 4) or medial (Renshaw cells: Sec. IV.A.5). In contrast to the lower lumbar segments, where R-cells are located in the medial part of the ventral horn, in lower sacral segments R-cells were found in the lateral part of the ventral horn. Their projections were likewise over long distances and were crossed as well as uncrossed (47,72). Correspondingly, both crossed and uncrossed recurrent inhibition could be elicited in motoneurons of tail muscles in lower sacral segments (72).

III. AFFERENT ACTIONS ON RENSHAW CELLS

A. Recurrent Collaterals

The recurrent axon collaterals of alpha motoneurons have been anatomically investigated with the Golgi technique by several investigators (3–5,57,60,66,73). Recent studies of recurrent axon collaterals of triceps surae alpha motoneurons identified by means of intracellular staining with HRP have verified (53,74–77; cf. 78) that axon collaterals terminate ipsilaterally in the ventral part of lamina VII, where R-cells are located (Fig. 2A,B). However, in addition, a termination on homonymous alpha motoneurons has been demonstrated (79). These collaterals are probably excitatory in function.*

The qualitative and quantitative features of intracellularly HRP-stained triceps surae alpha motoneuron axon collateral arborizations in lamina VII, including synaptic contacts with neurons suggested to represent R-cells, have been studied by means of light and electron microscopy (53,81). The same authors have also described the ultrastructural features of the axon collateral terminals on alpha motoneurons (82). Synaptic boutons of collaterals in the ventral part of Rexed's lamina VII exhibited spherical synaptic vesicles and made synaptic contacts with cell bodies and proximal dendrites of neurons assumed to be R-cells and with dendrites of unknown origin, some of them attributed to alpha motoneurons. The majority of the collateral boutons contacting alpha motoneurons were structurally indistinguishable from those contacting presumed R-cells. However, only 2–3% of the axon collateral boutons in lamina VII made direct contact with alpha motoneurons.

Not all motor axons give off recurrent collaterals (5,57,60,73,82a). For instance, it appears from anatomic studies that 20–30% of ankle extensor motoneurons (57) and also motoneurons of extrinsic eye muscles (5) lack recurrent

---

*There is at least one situation in mammals in which axon collaterals of motoneurons have been found in the absence of significant recurrent inhibition (medial rectus motoneurons [80]).

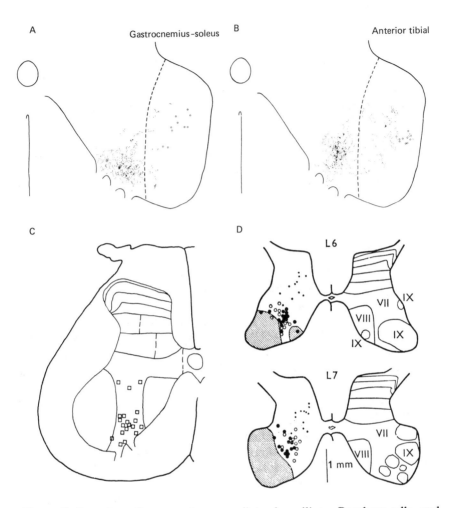

Figure 2 Location of recurrent axon collateral swellings, Renshaw cells, and interneurons of the group Ia pathway. A,B, Transverse distribution in the L7 ventral horn of 644 axon collateral swellings originating from 10 GS alpha motoneurons (A) and 818 axon collateral swellings from 10 tibial alpha motoneurons (B). The circles indicate the position of the parent cell bodies. The dashed lines show the medial border of the motor nuclei. C, Position of 19 Renshaw cells reconstructed after recordings. Most of the Renshaw cells were located in the ventral part of Rexed's lamina VII, although a few were found more dorsally in lamina VII. D, Location of interneurons monosynaptically excited by Ia afferents. Filled (●) and open (○) circles denote group A and group B interneurons inhibited from motor axon collaterals. Both groups of cells were not invaded antidromically, but only group A cells can be classified as interneurons with confidence. Points (·) denote interneurons not inhibited. The hatched areas indicate the extent of motor nuclei. The right side of the diagrams show Rexed's laminae. (A and B from Ref. 76; C from Ref. 17; D from Ref. 58.)

collaterals and recurrent effects are apparently absent in about 20% of alpha motoneurons innervating the hindlimb musculature (6), in motoneurons innervating the eye muscles of the cat (80,83), and in the motoneurons innervating the diaphragm (84,85); see Sec. IV.B). The existence of recurrent axon collaterals has been correlated with the motoneuron species (76); in particular, collaterals were always given off by motoneurons innervating long muscles at the ankle or knee, but they were absent in the case of motoneurons of short plantar muscles of the foot. This finding indicates that recurrent inhibition is primarily concerned with the control of proximal muscles (limb position) rather than of the distal ones (movement of the digits). Motor axon collaterals are distributed over only a distance of less than 1 mm from their parent cell bodies (76,77; see, however, 57,60 for immature kittens); consequently, excitation can be obtained only from motoneurons located in the immediate neighborhood of a given R-cell (35,59,86–88). Since some motoneuronal nuclei can be as long as 10 mm in the cat cord, only part of a motor nucleus may project to a given R-cell (71,89).

When R-cells receive axon collaterals of motoneurons belonging to a given pool, the problem arises as to whether all the alpha motoneurons that belong to this motor nucleus contribute the same number of axon collateral branches and boutons on R-cells. It is known that the physiologic properties of the motoneurons and the corresponding motor units are in part related to cell size (90). Moreover, there are differences depending on the properties of the neurons themselves and the muscle fiber they innervate (21).

Attempts have been made to study differences in the relative effectiveness of different sizes of motor axons to excite R-cells by graded differential blocking of larger fibers of the gastrocnemius nerve (91). It appeared from this study that most of the R-cells received a more or less homogeneous input from motor axons of different diameters. However, since branching normally occurs in the motor axons to the gastrocnemius muscle (92–95), the larger motor axons at the ventral root level may not necessarily contribute to the larger motor axons at various distances from the muscle.

Experiments in which the gain of responses of different sizes of gastrocnemius-soleus (GS) motoneurons to increasing frequency of discharge of the proprioceptive Ia input elicited by static or dynamic stretch of the homonymous muscle was evaluated led to the conclusion that large motoneurons were more effective than small motoneurons in driving the related R-cells for comparable frequencies of discharge of the Ia input (96–98; see Sec. III.B.1). Actually, other parameters, in addition to cell size, contribute to the determination of the efficacy of motoneurons of different sizes in driving R-cells. Anatomic investigations by Cullheim and Kellerth (77) have, in fact, shown that the number of synaptic contacts of recurrent collaterals of a motoneuron is correlated with the motor unit type. In the case of motoneurons of triceps surae, collaterals were much more numerous for fast-twitch, fast-fatiguing (FF) units (which are usually of larger size) than for tast-twitch, fatigue-resistant (FR) or slow-twitch, fatigue-resistant (S) units and were particularly sparse for S-units of the soleus, which are usually of small size. Although the degree of collateralization per se does not allow final predictions about the synaptic linkage and potency, these findings are compatible with the view that the R-cells are activated more effectively by large phasic alpha motoneurons than small tonic ones (see 20,22).

In the lumbar cord each R-cell can be excited not only by motor axons in an individual nerve, but also by stimulation of motor axons in different peripheral nerves (2,6,35,62,68,86,99–102). The convergence of these recurrent collaterals is not randomly organized, but follows rather specific patterns. In particular, the greatest excitatory convergence was seen with axons supplying functionally synergistic muscles, but not with axons supplying strict antagonists. In fact, in a recent study (102) it was shown that some R-cells received convergence of excitation from posterior biceps, semitendinosus, and peroneal nerves whose muscles are flexors of the knee or ankle, while other R-cells received convergent excitation from gastrocnemius-soleus, plantaris, and flexor digitorum longus muscles, which are extensors at the ankle and of some digits but flexors of other digits. Moreover, negative correlations were found between the knee flexors (posterior biceps, semitendinosus) and the ankle and digit extensors (gastrocnemius-soleus, plantaris, and flexor digitorum longus nerves), but this was mainly owing to the semitendinosus than to the posterior biceps component of the combined nerve.*

Eccles et al. (35) proposed that R-cells tend to be excited from axons of adjacent motor nuclei, although they noted exceptions. However, according to Ryall (102), there were some correlations that did not fit the proximity theory. Examples include the positive correlations between posterior biceps-semitendinosus and peroneal nerves and between gastrocnemius-soleus and flexor digitorum longus nerves. Although somewhat oversimplified, in general, it may be concluded that the pattern of excitation of R-cells follows flexor, extensor patterns of innervation and is similar to the pattern of recurrent inhibition of motoneurons (68). Thus, the pattern of recurrent inhibition of motoneurons is established to a large degree by the pattern of axon collateral convergence on different populations of R-cells, rather than by the pattern of convergence of R-cell axons on motoneurons. The excitatory convergence on R-R-cells is evidently complex and the patterns of recurrent inhibition of motoneurons will represent a second order of complexity that could well account for the differences in patterns observed. It is of interest that the distribution of

---

*A more selective excitatory convergence from functional synergists was actually found in a study of the less intense disynaptic excitation of R-cells via the motoneurons after afferent volleys in group Ia fibers (103).

recurrent inhibition in the cervical cord closely resembled that described in the lumbosacral cord (104). Even in this instance, the dependence of the location of a motoneuron on its function was regarded as a factor explaining deviations of the distribution of recurrent inhibition from the rule of proximity (see also 100).

In contrast to alpha motoneurons, gamma motoneurons only occasionally give rise to recurrent collaterals. In fact, only one out of 13 gamma motoneurons so far investigated following intracellular injection of HRP showed axon collaterals (78,105,106). This finding correlates well with the results of electrophysiologic experiments showing that activation of both gamma and alpha motor axons has no greater influence on R-cells than activation of alpha motor axons alone (6,107), and that antidromic volleys in gamma motor axons after a selective blockage of alpha motor axons may cause a liminal excitation only of a few R-cells (91). The conclusion of these experiments, that is, that gamma motoneurons do not significantly contribute recurrent collaterals to R-cells, is supported by the fact that maximal alpha efferent antidromic volleys elicited the maximum degree of recurrent inhibition (107) or the largest inhibitory postsynaptic potentials (IPSPs) in alpha motoneurons (6). Indeed, raising the strength of electrical stimulation to elicit an antidromic volley in gamma as well as in alpha motor axons never produced or increased recurrent inhibition in either type of motoneuron (108-110). The lack of participation of gamma axons in the recurrent inhibition of both alpha and gamma motoneurons suggests that the control of R-cells comes exclusively from alpha motoneurons. Future experiments, however, are required to find out whether beta motoneurons, which innervate both skeletomotor and fusimotor fibers (110a), contribute recurrent collaterals to R-cells. It has already been reported that the number of collateral terminations of alpha motoneuron axons decreases with axon diameter (76), so that the almost complete lack of gamma collaterals could be regarded as an extension of that relationship.

Much of our knowledge on the physiologic characteristics of the response of R-cells to antidromic stimulation of ventral roots or of peripheral nerves in the deafferented preparation has come from extracellular recording experiments. Preliminary experiments have excluded the idea that afferents in ventral roots are responsible for excitation of R-cells (111). The recurrent axon collaterals have strong synaptic linkage with R-cells, as shown by the fact that single antidromic motor axon volleys produce a characteristic burst of firing in R-cells, with an initial frequency of up to 1500/Hz (Fig. 3A, upper record) (cf. 2,6,44, 68). The shortest central latency of the first spike is 0.5-0.7 msec (2,6,36)— a latency that allows sufficient time for a synaptic delay following the entry of the antidromic volley into the spinal cord. This initial response is often followed, 50 msec after activation, by a pause in firing and then by a late response (31,86). Surprisingly, dihydro-β-erytroidine depresses the initial

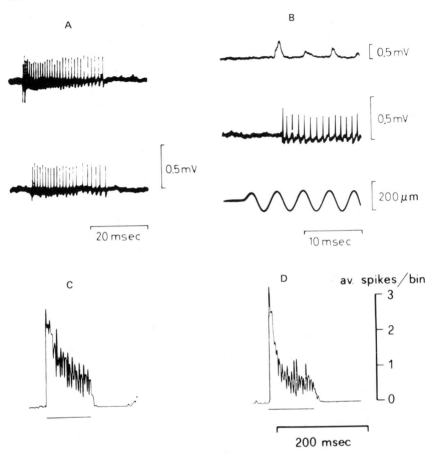

Figure 3 Responses of Renshaw cells to electrically and mechanically induced GS nerve volleys. Experiments were performed on decerebrate cats. The L6–S1 ventral roots were cut and the animal paralyzed with gallamine triethiodide (Flaxedil). The GS muscle was set at 8 mm of initial extension. A, The upper record represents the response of a Renshaw cell to single shock stimulation of the central end of the L7 ventral root [0.2 msec pulse, 1.6 times the alpha threshold (T)]; the lower record shows the effect of stimulation of the ipsilateral GS nerve with a 0.2-msec pulse, 2 times the T for group I afferents; the unit was disynaptically excited by the electrically induced group I volley. B, Response of the same Renshaw cell to longitudinal vibration of the ipsilateral GS muscle at 220 Hz, 140 μm peak-to-peak amplitude (middle record). The latency of this discharge is 0.84 msec if compared with that of the segmental monosynaptic reflex induced by the first stroke of the vibrator (upper record). The lower record represents the output of the photoelectric length meter. A lengthening movement is indicated by a downward deflection in the record of

discharge of the R-cell response to stimulation of motor axons (6,24,26,27,31, 37,112,113), but it does not affect the late discharge. On the other hand, atropine has only a slight effect on the initial burst (6,31), but it is able to block the late discharge (31,86). These findings have led to the suggestion that the early discharge depends upon the activation of nicotinic receptors by acetylcholine, whereas the late discharge is the result of the interaction of acetylcholine with muscarinic receptors.

With intracellular recordings from the cell body of R-cells, the excitatory postsynaptic potential (EPSP) that underlies the initial response has a brief intense phase, often with a spikelike peak, and a prolonged falling phase that may last over 50 msec (6,35; cf. 17). These observations have been thought to indicate that transmitter action has an intense initial phase and a later prolonged phase. Further experiments (114) revealed that by grading the stimulus intensity the recurrent excitatory postsynaptic potential of R-cells had a monophasic time course, longer than 50 msec, rather than the complex pattern previously described. The spikelike peak that was frequently seen superimposed on the excitatory postsynaptic potential is actually an action potential (6,21; cf. 51); this gave the appearance of an excitatory postsynaptic potential with an initial fast and a later slow component, as revealed by previous authors (6,17,35). Moreover, the recurrent excitatory postsynaptic potential was not followed by a hyperpolarization phase (114). This finding excludes the hypothesis (31) that the pause might be due to a hyperpolarization following the excitatory postsynaptic potential. However, after bursts of impulses there was a distinct afterhyperpolarization, which reached a peak about 100 msec after the onset of the burst (114). The fact that the length of the pause in the discharge of a R-cell depends on the duration of the initial response in that particular cell (115) suggests that an after-hyperpolarization, generated by action potentials in R-cells, is an important factor in producing the pause. Mutual inhibition of R-cells may

---

the sine wave. C,D, Sequential pulse density histograms (SPDHs) showing the response of another Renshaw cell to both mechanically and electrically induced GS volleys. As shown for the previous unit this Renshaw cell was also disynaptically excited by electrical stimulation of the group Ia afferents in the GS nerve. For each record 50 sweeps taken at a repetition rate of 0.25 Hz were accumulated, using 128 bins with a dwell time/bin of 2 msec. C, Effects of vibration of the GS muscle for 100 msec at 200 Hz, 180 μm, D, Effects of repetitive electrical stimulation of the GS nerve for 100 msec at 200 Hz, 0.2 msec pulses, 2T. The threshold for the response of this Renshaw cell to electrically induced GS volleys corresponded to 1.1T. In this and next figures, the scale near the computer record represents the average number of spikes per bin. (From Refs. 163 and 164.)

also contribute to this depression (see Sec. IV.A.5). All the effects described previously were elicited by stimulation of ipsilateral motor axons; stimulation of contralateral motor axons had no effect on R-cells (2,44).

The activity of a R-cell results from a combination of two variable inputs: (1) the number of active alpha motoneurons converging on the R-cell (spatial summation), and (2) their discharge frequency (temporal summation). This has been studied either with antidromic stimulation (this Sec.) or with orthodromic stimulation (see Sec. III.B.1). With regard to the effect of the first input variable, antidromic activation of R-cells secondary to graded stimulation of ventral roots or nerves from deafferented muscles has revealed that the number of discharges of these interneurons increases with the amount of synchronous motor output over a wide range (2,6,112; cf. 91). As to the effect of frequency variation, quantitative aspects of spinal motor activity and recurrent inhibition have been dealt with by Granit et al. (116), and Granit and Renkin (117, cf. 118). In particular, Granit and Renkin (117) have demonstrated that the antidromic inhibition of single alpha motoneurons did not increase indefinitely with increasing frequency of conditioning stimulation, but rather had a saturating characteristic.

It was originally reported by Renshaw (2) that successive stimuli to motor axons interact at the level of R-cells, as shown by the shortening of the burst response of a second stimulus following a first one. Following this observation, Haase (119) showed that the discharge rate of R-cells increased with increasing frequency of antidromic stimulation, whereas the number of spikes per stimulus decreased. This "transformation" of the interneuronal discharge pattern with stimulus frequency leads to a nonlinear, saturating static characteristic, which is also found under condition in which only one or at most a few motor axons activate a R-cell (120-122). These results could explain the inhibitory curves of Granit and Renkin (117). More detailed investigations by Cleveland et al. (123) indicated that the static response characteristic of R-cells follows the functional form of a rectangular hyperbola that approaches saturation with increasing stimulus frequency (cf. 97). On the average, the stimulus frequency at which the discharge rate reaches half its saturation value lies between 10 and 15 Hz. Saturation of this response may depend upon different mechanisms, including depletion of transmitter from motor axon collaterals (cf. 124).

The findings reported previously have received further support from the results of experiments with intracellular recordings from individual motoneurons and simultaneously recorded R-cells (122,125-127). When the motoneuron was silent, the R-cell exhibited virtually no spontaneous activity. Injection of current induced a correlated pattern of discharge from both cells. Each motoneuron spike was followed by two to three spikes from the R-cell. Moreover, in some cases a repetitive discharge of a single motoneuron produced firing of the R-cell at a much higher frequency. The relation between input frequency and output frequency was roughly linear up to a motoneuron frequency of 20 Hz and appeared to flatten out thereafter (122).

Since the recurrent inhibition stemming from one motoneuron may exert considerable influence on its neighbors and perhaps even on itself, then one would expect some change in discharge characteristics of the motoneuron for frequencies > 20-30 Hz, when recurrent inhibition would no longer increase in proportion to motoneuron frequency. Indeed, this coincides with the frequency range in which the transition from primary to secondary range occurs in the current-frequency relation of many motoneurons (16,18). Failure of the R-cell to follow the motoneuron above the transition point would result in inhibition becoming less in relation to excitatory drive, thus causing motoneuron frequency to climb at a greater rate (secondary range) than before (primary range).

B. Segmental Afferents

Much of the work performed to evaluate the physiologic properties of the R-cells studied the activity of these interneurons induced by antidromic volleys following stimulation, either of ventral roots or of peripheral muscle nerves in deafferented animals. While this is a useful method to identify R-cells and to distinguish them from other interneurons in the spinal cord, they undoubtedly represent unphysiologic conditions to induce firings of R-cells. In fact, the temporal pattern of discharge of motoneurons activated orthodromically is different from that induced by electrical stimulation of the alpha efferent fibers. Moreover, while small tonic motoneurons with small axons are usually excited by reflex action at lower threshold than are the larger phasic motoneurons with larger axons (107,128-136; cf. 10,11,16,18,90,137), weak electrical stimuli to the motor axons will excite the larger ones first. R-cells can be influenced synaptically by volleys entering the spinal cord via dorsal roots (2,6,27,31,36, 88,138). The effects of selective stimulation of different populations of primary afferents on the discharge of R-cells will be discussed subsequently.

1. Group Ia Muscle Afferents

Group Ia afferent volleys originating from the primary endings of muscle spindles monosynaptically excite the motoneurons innervating homonymous and synergistic muscles (139,140; cf. 90). Activation of the same pathway also evokes a polysynaptic (128,141-149; cf. 18,150 for refs.), usually oligosynaptic (di- and trisynaptic) excitation of these hindlimb motoneurons (139,141,142, 151-158).* The related interneurons excited by group Ia volleys are probably located in laminae V-VI (159,160).

*Oligosynaptic excitation of homonymous motoneurons may also be evoked by impulses in Golgi tendon organs (158).

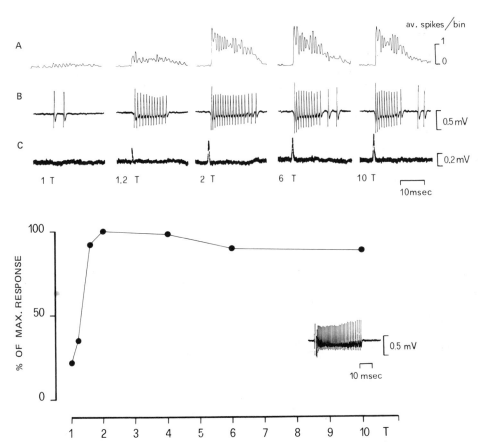

Figure 4 Response of a Renshaw cell to orthodromic volleys elicited by single shock stimulation of the GS nerve with increasing stimulus intensities. Experiments were performed on a precollicular decerebrated cat. The L6–S1 ventral roots were cut and the animal paralyzed with gallamine triethiodide (Flaxedil). GS muscle was slack. A, SPDHs showing the responses of a Renshaw cell to orthodromic volleys elicited by single shock stimulation of the GS nerve with 0.2-msec pulses of progressively increasing intensities expressed in multiples of the threshold (T) for the group I volley, as indicated below the corresponding records (C). On the whole, 50 sweeps taken at a repetition rate of 0.2 Hz were accumulated for each of the computer records, using 128 bins with a dwell time/bin of 0.5 msec. Note the progressive increase in amplitude of the Renshaw cell discharge for stimulus intensities up to 2T, and the reduced duration of the response for stimulus intensities higher than 2T. B, Single specimens of the averaged records are shown for each of the stimulus intensities used in A. In this and all subsequent records negativity is shown upward. C, Monosynaptic reflexes recorded from the ipsilateral L7 ventral root following single shock

There have been great difficulties in the past in observing R-cell excitation following electrical stimulation of the low-threshold group Ia muscle fibers (88). Electrically induced group Ia volleys are unable to monosynaptically excite R-cells; however, by producing a prominent monosynaptic excitation of motoneurons they can disynaptically excite R-cells via motor axon collaterals (Fig. 3A, lower record) (31,61,161–164; cf. 13). According to some authors, this phenomenon occurred particularly when a large monosynaptic discharge was elicited by the orthodromic volley (2,6,61); moreover, it appeared that small reflex ventral root volleys (in small fibers) elicited much smaller R-effects than similarly sized antidromic volleys (in large fibers) (61). These findings support the hypothesis originally put forward by Granit et al. (107) and Eccles et al. (68) that activation of large motor axons produces a much larger excitatory effect on R-cells firing than activation of small motor axons.

The relation between size of the monosynaptic reflex and the R-cell discharge has also been investigated. Although this relation varies from one R-cell to another (165; see also 91), the input–output relation is linear when the summed activity in a pool of R-cells is considered (61,91,161,162,164–167; cf. 16). Figure 4 illustrates the typical development of response of one R-cell to orthodromic volleys elicited by single shock stimulation of the gastrocnemius-soleus nerve with increasing stimulus intensities expressed in multiples of the threshold (T) for the group Ia fibers. Simultaneous recording in the same preparation of the ventral root discharge indicated that the induced discharge of the R-cell appeared with a latency of 0.86 msec after the beginning of the segmental monosynaptic reflex, and suggests that the R-cell was excited via the monosynaptic discharge of motoneurons. Moreover, the magnitude of the unit discharge (Fig. 4A,B) increased in parallel with the average amplitude of the monosynaptic reflex induced by single shock stimulus applied to the gastrocnemius-soleus nerve (Fig. 4C), to reach a maximum value at about 1.6–2.0T, that is, when all the group Ia afferents had been recruited by the stimulus.

---

stimulation of the GS nerve at increasing stimulus intensities. Time calibration in C applies also to A and B. The latency of the Renshaw cell discharge with respect to the foot of the segmental monosynaptic reflex, evaluated on higher sweep speed, was 0.86 msec, and indicates that the reflex discharge of the motoneurons monosynaptically excited the Renshaw cell. The diagram illustrates the development of the response of this Renshaw cell as a function of the intensity of stimulation (T) applied to the ipsilateral GS nerve. The magnitude of the response is expressed in % of the maximum number of spikes elicited by the orthodromic GS volley within the first 40 msec after the stimulus. Each dot represents the mean of 50 trials. The inset record represents the response of the Renshaw cell to single shock stimulation of the ipsilateral L7 ventral root with a 0.2-msec pulse, 3 times the alpha threshold. (From Ref. 164.)

The observation that a linear relation between reflex size and early unit discharge emerges when the responses of all the R-cells are averaged, or when the summed activity of a pool of R-cells is estimated by recording the recurrent inhibition in their target motoneurons, cannot be taken as an evidence that small tonic motoneurons recruited by the smallest monosynaptic discharges are as efficient in producing recurrent inhibition as are large phasic motoneurons (165). In fact, the size of the monosynaptic reflex recorded in ventral roots is not linearly related to the number of recruited motor units, since larger motor axons will contribute more to the size of the monosynaptic reflex than smaller ones. Moreover, the number of spikes in a R-cell burst is not linearly related to the excitatory input because the R-cell firing saturates with large responses. Therefore, in most cases the contribution of small motoneurons to R-cell excitation will be overestimated. The observed linear relation might actually be taken to indicate that large motoneurons contribute more than do small ones.

The hypothesis that large phasic motoneurons are more effective in exciting R-cells than small motoneurons is supported by the results of experiments in which the activity of R-cells was recorded during static and dynamic muscle stretches. R-cells coupled to gastrocnemius-soleus motoneurons were tonically active during maintained stretch of the de-efferented gastrocnemius-soleus muscle and this tonic discharge increased by increasing stretch lengths (96,97, 167,168; cf. 20,118). However, a burst of high-frequency discharge occurred during the phasic part of ramp stretch of the gastrocnemius-soleus muscle at rates exceeding 20-30 mm/sec (168). In these experiments the possible contribution of primary and secondary endings of muscle spindles to the R-cell responses was not evaluated.

Pompeiano et al. (169) utilized individual sinusoidal stretches of the de-efferented gastrocnemius-soleus muscle of short and constant duration, but of variable amplitude, and found that in decerebrate cats the responses of R-cells disynaptically excited by electrical stimulation of the group Ia afferents from the gastrocnemius-soleus nerve were length dependent. These responses were attributed to stimulation of the primary endings of muscle spindles, since: (1) they occurred at a threshold amplitude of 5-20 μm and reached maximum development with an amplitude of vibration of about 70-80 μm or less, which selectively stimulated all the primary endings of the muscle spindles (170-172); (2) there was a close parallel between the development of the R-cell response and that of the segmental monosynaptic reflex; (3) the central latency between the onset of the monosynaptic reflex produced by the sinusoidal stretch and the first spike of the R-cell discharge was compatible with the conclusion that a disynaptic excitation of the R-cells occurred, which depended upon monosynaptic reflex discharges of the gastrocnemius-soleus motoneurons following mechanical stimulation of the Ia afferents (see also Fig. 3B). The same population of R-cells was also submitted to a family of individual stretches of the de-efferented gastrocnemius-soleus muscle of the same amplitude (130–180 μm), but of different durations. Large-amplitude sinusoidal stretches, supramaximal for producing excitation of all the primary endings of muscle spindles, produced a smooth sinusoidal modulation of R-cell discharges for velocities of stretch ranging from 0.05 to 0.1 mm/sec. When the velocity of stretch increased from 0.1 to about 0.3 mm/sec there were some departures from the smooth change in discharge rate induced by the sinusoidal stretch. These departures were caused by the appearance of burstlike activity of the R-cell. However, for velocities of stretch at or >0.5 mm/sec a sudden and short-lasting burst of high-frequency discharge of the R-cell appeared at shorter latency with respect to the beginning of the sinusoidal stretch; this response reached the maximum amplitude for a velocity of stretch of about 10–20 mm/sec. Higher values did not modify the response (Fig. 5). There is, therefore, a critical velocity of stretch at which the pattern of response of R-cells changes from the sinusoidally modulated type, to the burstlike type.

The increased discharge of R-cells with increasing velocity of muscle stretch did not depend upon recruitment of spindle receptors, since the amplitudes of sinusoidal stretches used excited all the primary endings of muscle spindles, but actually depended upon recruitment of motoneurons. This recruitment varied according to the different spatiotemporal patterns of discharge of the spindle receptors, which was obviously asynchronous during the slow sinusoidal stretch, but became more and more synchronized with increasing velocity of stretches. Saturation of the response occurred at velocities of stretch that produced a synchronous driving of the spindle receptors, during which the induced action potentials appeared at a constant position with regard to the vibration cycle (170,173). Since the small tonic motoneurons are more readily excited than the large phasic motoneurons (130,131; cf. 16,90), it was postulated that the smooth changes in the discharge rate of the R-cells to sinusoidal stretches of low velocity (up to 0.1–0.3 mm/sec) depend exclusively upon activation of small tonic motoneurons. On the other hand, the quick large amplitude response of the R-cells to high-velocity sinusoidal stretches (at or >0.5 mm/sec) may depend upon recruitment of large phasic motoneurons. Therefore, it seems that the same R-cell may receive recurrent collaterals of both tonic and phasic motoneurons and that the postsynaptic efficacy of the phasic motoneurons on the R-cells is greater than that of the tonic ones.

A quantitative evaluation of the sensitivity of R-cells to static and dynamic stretch of the gastrocnemius-soleus muscle was obtained in decerebrate cats. The discharge rate of R-cells, disynaptically excited by group Ia volleys in the gastro-cnemius-soleus nerve, to increasing frequency of discharge of the Ia input elicited either by static stretch or by longitudinal vibration of the de-efferented homonymous muscle was recorded (96,97). In one group of experiments the discharge rate of such R-cells in response to increasing levels of static stretch was

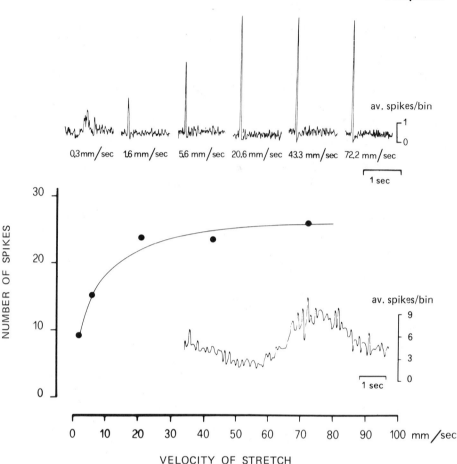

Figure 5 Effect of changing velocity of a sinusoidal stretch on the discharge activity of a Renshaw cell. Experiment performed in a decerebrate cat with GS muscle de-efferented and set at 8 mm of initial extension. Responses of a Renshaw cell, disynaptically excited by electrical stimulation of the group Ia afferents in the GS nerve, following single sinusoidal stretches of similar amplitude (130 μm), but with different velocities indicated at the bottom of each record. These values correspond to frequencies of sinusoidal stretch of 1.2 Hz, 6.1 Hz, 21.5 Hz, 79.3 Hz, 166.7 Hz, and 277.8 Hz, respectively. Thirty sweeps were accumulated for each of the computer records using 128 bins with a dwell time of 10 msec per bin. The graph illustrates the net number of spikes elicited by individual sinusoidal stretches at the amplitude indicated previously and for increasing velocities of stretch. The inset shows the response of the same Renshaw cell to a very slow sinusoidal stretch of 180 μm amplitude, at a frequency of 0.154 Hz (velocity of stretch, 0.055 mm/sec). (From Ref. 169.)

calculated. The discharge rate of the R-cells corresponded on the average to 31.5 ± 23.2, S.D. imp./sec when the gastrocnemius-soleus muscle was slack or at 0 mm extension (i.e., producing a muscle tension of about 20 gr); on the other hand, the discharge frequency of R-cells linearly increased in most instances with increasing levels of muscle extension ranging from 0 to 8 mm. A slight depression of the response, however, occurred during higher levels of static stretch—a phenomenon probably caused by stimulation of Golgi tendon organs and/or secondary endings of muscle spindles. The slope of the linear part of the curve corresponded on the average to 0.89 imp./sec/mm (n = 22 R-cells). Since the average discharge rate of primary spindle receptors recorded from the de-efferented gastrocnemius-soleus muscle corresponded to 2.62 imp./sec/mm (cf. 174,175), it appears that on the average the same R-cells increased their firing rate by 0.34 imp./sec per each imp./sec in the Ia afferents (Fig. 6A, line 1). It should be mentioned that the output frequency of individual alpha motoneurons is relatively independent of muscle length, so that the enhanced activity of R-cells with greater stretches may depend upon recruitment of more motor units (see later on).

In a second group of experiments the discharge rate of R-cells coupled to gastrocnemius-soleus motoneurons was evaluated in response to increasing parameters of longitudinal vibration applied to the de-efferented gastrocnemius-soleus muscle. It is known that small-amplitude, high-frequency longitudinal vibration of the gastrocnemius-soleus muscle induces a repetitive discharge of the Ia afferents (170-172) that is transmitted monosynaptically and probably also polysynaptically to both the homonymous and the heteronymous motoneurons. The induced discharge of the corresponding motoneurons (see 176 for ref.) then leads to a reflex contraction of the vibrated muscle in an animal with intact dorsal roots (177–180). Vibration of the de-efferented gastrocnemius-soleus muscle at a frequency of 200 Hz, 180 μm peak-to-peak amplitude for 1 sec produced a sudden increase in the discharge frequency of R-cells during the first 100 msec, which gradually decreased to a steady lower level.* The mean discharge rate of 24 R-cells calculated during both the first 100 msec (phasic response) and the last 500 msec of the 1-sec vibration period (tonic response) was linearly related to the frequency of vibration, at least up to the frequencies of vibration of 150-200 Hz for the phasic response and 100–150 Hz for the tonic response (Fig. 7). This finding can be compared to the observation that the responses of R-cells are directly proportional to antidromic tetanization of the ventral roots from 5 to 10 Hz up to a maximum of about 30–40 Hz (97,116, 117,119–123,182,184; cf. 10,11,16,18,137).

---

*Adaptation of the responses of R-cells to vibration resembled that occurring with both orthodromic (97,181) and antidromic tetanization (6,124,182-185).

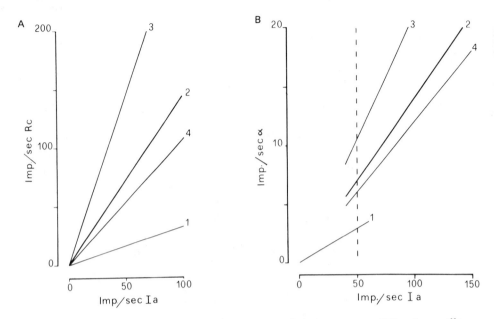

Figure 6 Comparison of the gain constants of the responses of Renshaw cells and GS alpha motoneurons to static stretch and vibration of the homonymous muscle. Experiments were performed in precollicular decerebrate cats with de-efferented GS muscle and paralysis induced with gallamine triethiodide (Flaxedil). A, Relation between the discharge rate of Renshaw cells, disynaptically excited by electrical stimulation of group Ia afferents in GS nerve, and the discharge rate in the Ia afferents from the GS muscle during: (1) static stretch (n = 22; slope = 0.34 imp./sec in Renshaw cells per imp./sec in the Ia afferents); (2) vibration for 1 sec at the amplitude of 180 μm (n = 24; slope = 1.45 imp./sec in Renshaw cells per imp./sec in the Ia afferents; linear correlation coefficient >0.97). Lines 3 and 4 refer to the phasic and the tonic component of the Renshaw cell responses to muscle vibration (n = 24; slope = 2.90 and 1.08 imp./sec in Renshaw cells per imp./sec in the Ia afferents; linear correlation coefficients >0.97 and >0.96, respectively). B, Relation between the discharge rate of GS motoneurons and the discharge rate in the Ia afferents from the homonymous muscle during: (1) static stretch (n = 21; slope = 0.059 imp./sec in motoneurons per imp./sec in the Ia afferents, corresponding to a decoding ratio, DR = 17.0); (2) vibration for 1-sec periods at the amplitude of 156–209 μm (n = 94; slope = 0.14 imp./sec in motoneurons per imp./sec in the Ia afferents; DR = 7.14; linear correlation coefficient >0.90). Lines 3 and 4 refer to the phasic and the tonic component of the motoneuronal responses to muscle vibration (n = 77; slope = 0.21 and 0.12 imp./sec in motoneurons per imp./sec in the Ia afferents; DR = 4.76 and 8.33, respectively; linear correlation coefficients >0.85 for both values). Note the low gain of the slopes relating firing rate of Renshaw cells—or motoneurons—to firing rate of the Ia afferents during static stretch with respect to vibration. (A from Ref. 97; B from Ref. 98.)

Since the vibration was of sufficient amplitude to produce driving of nearly all primary endings of the muscle spindles, if applied to the appropriately extended de-efferented muscle (170-172), the slope of the stimulus-response curve could be expressed as an increase in the discharge rate of R-cells per imp./sec in the Ia afferents. It appears that the discharge rate of the 24 R-cells increased on the average by 1.45 imp./sec per each imp./sec in the Ia afferents (Fig. 6A, line 2). This mean value is 4.3 times higher than that obtained during static stretch. On the other hand, the discharge of the same R-cells increased on average by 2.90 and 1.08 imp./sec per imp./sec in the Ia afferents during the phasic and the tonic component of the response (Fig. 6A, lines 3 and 4, respectively).

The discrepancies in the gain factors, relating the changes in the firing rate of the same R-cell to the frequencies of discharge of the Ia afferents induced during static stretch and vibration have been explained by assuming that the spatiotemporal pattern of the stretch receptors' input produced asynchronously during static stretch is mainly effective on small, tonic motoneurons (107,128, 130,131,186-190; cf. 16,90), while that produced synchronously during muscle vibration is effective not only on small tonic but also on large phasic moto-neurons (132,133,191-193). Moreover, during static stretch the fraction of active motoneurons (of small size) would fire in a narrow range at low frequency, whereas during muscle vibration, when all the motoneurons (including those of large size) participate in the response, firing at higher average frequencies would occur in a wider range (132,194-199; cf. 16,18,200). These findings together with the greater ability of large phasic motoneurons to excite R-cells with respect to small tonic motoneurons (61,168,169; cf. 68,107) might explain the higher gain of the R-cell activity induced during vibration as compared to static stretch for increasing frequency of discharge of the Ia afferents.

To test these hypotheses the activity of different size gastrocnemius-soleus motoneurons, classified according to their critical firing level (CFL) by the method described by Clamann et al. (201), was recorded from isolated ventral root filaments of L7 or S1 in decerebrate cats (98; cf. 22). It is known that motoneurons of different size have different critical firing levels; the smaller the motoneuron size, the lower the critical firing level (201). Among 94 gastro-cnemius-soleus motoneurons whose critical firing level varied from 1 to 92%, only 21 (CFL: 2-49%) showed a tonic discharge during maintained stretch. Stretch-evoked responses of motoneurons always occurred in strict order of size, that is, the units with the smallest critical firing level had the lowest thresholds to stretch, while the cells with the largest critical firing level had the highest thresholds (130,131).

In order to study the relationship between afferent and efferent frequencies of the motoneuron pools during the stretch reflex, units were subjected to progressive increases in static stretch of the gastrocnemius-soleus muscle. When the muscle was extended and held at the increased length, the motoneurons fired in a quite narrow frequency range (10.0 imp./sec ± 2.4, S.D.) and except for the

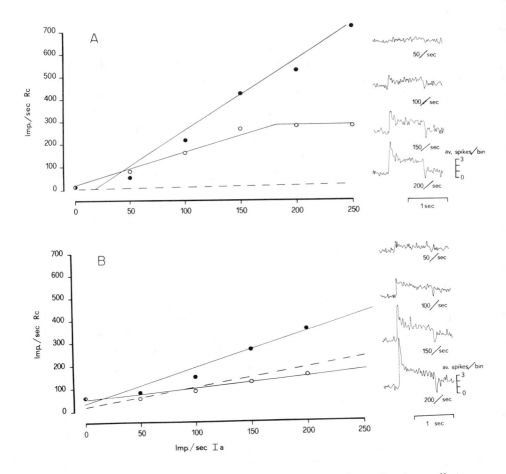

Figure 7 Phasic and tonic components of responses of two Renshaw cells to prolonged vibration of the GS muscle and their relation with the responses induced by static muscle stretch. Experiments performed in decerebrate cat with the de-efferented GS muscle fixed at 8 mm of initial extension. A,B, responses of two different Renshaw cells, disynaptically excited by electrical stimulation of group Ia afferents in GS nerve, during 1-sec vibration at 136 μm amplitude and at different frequencies. Ten trials (A) and 20 trials (B) taken at the repetition rate of 0.1 Hz were accumulated for each of the computer records, using 128 bins with a dwell time of 20 msec per bin. Some of these computer records are illustrated on the right side of the corresponding diagram. The series has been computed once more and the discharge rate of the Renshaw cell (imp./sec Rc) calculated during the "phasic" (dots) and the "tonic" (circles) component of the responses has been plotted in the diagram as a function of the frequency of vibration, that is, of the frequency of discharge of the Ia afferents (imp./sec Ia). The dashed lines in the two diagrams indicate the slope of response of the same cells to static stretch of the

initial recruitment of individual units, virtually no change in frequency occurred for changes in static muscle length (cf. 16,98,118,202-206). Therefore, the estimate of the input-output relationship was 0.15 imp./sec/mm, based on the assumption that the total output frequency of the motoneuron pool was the result of recruitment and not frequency coding and that only a fraction of the pool contributed to the motor output during static stretch (cumulative frequency distribution). Since the average discharge rate of the primary spindle receptors recorded from the de-efferented gastrocnemius-soleus muscle in these experiments corresponded to 2.62 imp./sec/mm of static stretch (96,97; cf. 174,175), the increase in firing rate of the motoneurons during static stretch was converted into an average 0.06 imp./sec of the motoneurons for each imp./sec in the Ia afferents (Fig. 6B, line 1) (98).

In contrast to the findings described previously, all the 94 gastrocnemius-soleus motoneurons (CFL: 1-92%) responded to 1-sec periods of vibration of the homonymous muscle pulled at an average extension of 10 mm (range 8-14 mm). Motoneurons were recruited with increasing amplitude and/or frequency of vibration according to the size principle; however, small-sized motoneurons (CFL: 1-20%) showed a wide scattering in threshold and great differences in firing rate, which varied from 6-34 imp./sec during vibration at standard parameters (1 sec at 150 Hz, 156 μm amplitude), thus covering almost completely the range of values obtained from the whole population of recorded neurons (2-48 imp./sec). However, there was a tendency of large motoneurons to fire at higher rates. Motoneurons which discharged throughout the stimulation period were also subjected to 1-sec periods of muscle vibration at a fixed amplitude, but at increasing frequencies. As soon as the threshold frequency was reached, the mean discharge rate of the tested unit increased with increasing frequency of vibration and above the value of 25-50 Hz, the responses were linearly related to the frequency of vibration, at least up to frequencies of 150-275 Hz. Since the vibration used was of sufficient amplitude to produce driving of all the primary endings of the muscle spindles (170-172), the relationship between the mean afferent and efferent frequencies could be

---

de-efferented GS muscle. The slope was evaluated by recording the response of the Renshaw cells to static stretch of the de-efferented GS muscle from 0 up to 10 mm of initial extension. In particular, 20 periods of about 5-sec duration were accumulated for each of the computer records taken at different initial extensions (0, 2, 4, 6, 8, 10 mm) using 256 bins with a dwell time of 20 msec per bin. The series was computed once more and the resulting values were then expressed in terms of changes of the discharge rate of the Renshaw cell (ordinate) as a function of the frequency of discharge of the Ia afferents (abscissa) evaluated for different mm of initial extensions. Slopes were calculated with the method of the least squares. (From Ref. 97.)

expressed in terms of an average increase in the discharge rate of motoneurons ($imp./sec_\alpha$) per average increase in the discharge rate of the Ia afferents (imp./sec Ia). The gain constant of the frequency transfer curves relating mean afferent and efferent frequencies varied from 0.04 to 0.36 $imp./sec_\alpha$ per imp./sec Ia (mean 0.14, n = 94). The average increase in firing rate of motoneurons per each imp./sec in the Ia afferents during 1-sec periods of muscle vibration (Fig. 6B, line 2) was 2.4 times higher than that evaluated during static stretch. As shown for the R-cells, most of the motoneurons excited by muscle vibration showed a sudden increase in the discharge frequency during the first 100 msec of vibration (phasic response), which reached a steady, albeit lower, level during the last 500 msec of vibration (tonic response). The gain constants for the phasic and the tonic responses corresponded on the average to 0.21 and 0.12 $imp./sec_\alpha$ per imp./sec Ia, respectively (n = 77) (Fig. 6B, lines 3 and 4) (98).

It is of interest that small motoneurons whose critical firing level varied from 1 to 20% showed a great variability in gain constant (0.04–0.22 $imp./sec_\alpha$ per imp./sec Ia). However, the average value (mean 0.11, n = 49) was smaller than that of all motoneurons. Large motoneurons whose critical firing level was higher than 20% also showed great variation in gain constant (0.04–0.36), but the average value (mean 0.17, n = 45) was higher than that of the whole population. In conclusion, with respect to small-sized motoneurons, large-sized motoneurons tended to fire at higher rates during 1-sec periods of vibration with standard parameters and also showed higher gain constants of the linear part of the curve relating output frequency of the motoneurons to the Ia input frequency. The findings that small motoneurons (CFL: 1–20%) showed a wide scattering in thresholds as well as in firing rates to vibration with standard parameters and also a great variability in gain constants of their input–output relation curves (cf. 207,208), indicate that among this population of neurons there are properties that are not entirely dependent on their size (cf. 207,208).

A comparison between the results of these experiments on gastrocnemius-soleus motoneurons and those involving the activity of R-cells recorded during the same experimental conditions support the conclusion that large-sized motoneurons exert more prominent synaptic effects on R-cells than small-sized motoneurons. This conclusion is supported by the results of recent anatomic observations (77) that show that the recurrent collaterals of fast-twitch, fast-fatiguing motoneurons (which are of large size) have more branching and presumably more synaptic endings than those of fast-twitch, fatigue-resistant and slow-twitch, fatigue-resistant motoneurons (which are of smaller size) (Fig. 8) (cf. Sec. III.A). Actually, the number of recurrent collateral end outbulgings (interpreted as synaptic terminals) of a motoneuron correlate as well or better with the type of muscle fiber innervated than with the axonal diameter that is related to cell size. Since R-cells exert a prominent inhibitory influence on small-sized tonic alpha motoneurons (see Sec. IV.A.1), on static gamma motoneurons (see Sec. IV.A.2), as well as on interneurons interposed in the Ia inhibitory pathway (see Sec. IV.A.3), one may postulate that all these effects are more effective during vibration than during static stretch for the same amount of discharge of Ia afferents.

2. Group Ib Muscle Afferents

Group Ib muscle afferents originating from Golgi tendon organs are responsible for autogenetic inhibition of motoneurons innervating homonymous and synergistic muscles (209-214). There are also excitatory connections to motoneurons of antagonists. These effects are mediated by a circuit with one or two interposed interneurons, thus representing a disynaptic or a trisynaptic afferent pathway. Many Ib terminals end in lamina VI (215-217) where they synapse with a well-localized group of interneurons (218) that may in turn project directly to motoneurons. It is of interest that selective activation of group Ia muscle spindle afferents of triceps surae and plantaris muscles may slightly inhibit the motoneurons of homonymous and synergistic muscles and thereby contribute to the effects of Ib afferents (219,220; cf. 212,221). This Ia nonreciprocal inhibition leads to small inhibitory postsynaptic potentials that occur with di- and trisynaptic latencies. It was postulated that the corresponding interneurons are located in Rexed's laminae V-VI (58,159,160,222). Interneurons located in these laminae can, in fact, be monosynaptically excited by both group Ia and Ib afferents (223; cf. 224,225). These interneurons are unaffected by conditioning stimulation of the ventral roots and therefore are not inhibited by R-cells (58,222), in contrast to the interneurons of the Ia inhibitory pathway to motoneurons of antagonistic muscles, which are located in Rexed's lamina VII and that are inhibited by R-cells (58,222,226,227) (Fig. 2D; see Sec. IV.A.3).

The effects of stimulation of Ib afferents on the recurrent inhibitory pathway have been studied by Pompeiano et al. (97). They recorded the activity of individual R-cells coupled with gastrocnemius-soleus motoneurons and compared the amplitude of the response of these R-cells to muscle vibration with the response elicited by electrical stimulation of group I afferents. Vibration of the de-efferented gastrocnemius-soleus muscle at 200 Hz with a peak-to-peak amplitude sufficient to produce driving of all the primary endings of muscle spindles produced a response of R-cells that was always higher than that induced by repetitive electrical stimulation of all the group I afferents in the gastrocnemius-soleus nerve at the same frequency (200 Hz) with an intensity of stimulation lower than or corresponding to 2T (Fig. 3C,D). While muscle vibration selectively excites the primary muscle spindle receptors with little if any excitation of Golgi tendon organs in the de-efferented muscle (170-172), no threshold discrimination between the group Ia and the Ib afferents occurs on electrical stimulation of the gastrocnemius-soleus nerve. It was postulated that in this condition the autogenetic excitation of the homonymous motoneurons induced by

A

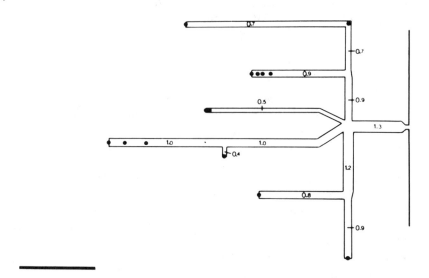

B

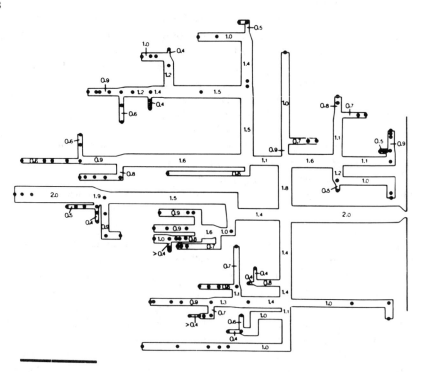

the group Ia volleys was partially depressed by autogenetic inhibition of the same motoneurons elicited by co-stimulation of the Ib afferents and led to a reduced discharge of R-cells. In view of the weak excitatory influence of the Ia afferents on the Ib inhibitory interneurons (cf. 219,220), it is likely that under the latter experimental condition the Ia afferents support the autogenetic inhibition of motoneurons from the Ib afferents. In conclusion, it appears that the group Ib effects on R-cells, similarly to the group Ia effects, are mediated via the corresponding alpha motoneurons.

3. Group II Muscle Afferents

Experiments in which groups I and II fibers were excited by electrical stimuli have indicated that at the segmental level group II fibers inhibit extensor moto-neurons and excite flexor motoneurons irrespective of their muscle of origin (211,228-233; cf. 234); these effects, however, were negligible in the decere-brate cat (cf. 234). Inhibition of extensor motoneurons was also obtained during stretch of the homonymous or synergic muscle after selective blockade of con-duction in the corresponding Ia afferents (235-240; cf., however, 241).

In contrast with these findings, however, the results of several experiments have indicated that the secondary endings of muscle spindles in extensor muscles contribute to autogenetic excitation of the Ia afferents on the homonymous motoneurons. This hypothesis originated from the observation of Matthews (179,242,243) that the tension developed in the soleus muscle during the stretch reflex was much higher, when expressed in terms of tension/imp./sec in the primary endings of the muscle spindles, than the tension/imp./sec that resulted from vibration. To explain this discrepancy he postulated that the secondary endings, which are stimulated during static stretch but not during vibration, contributed excitation to the stretch reflex rather than the classically described inhibition. Moreover, he observed that the reflex elicited by stretch failed to occlude that produced by vibration in the manner expected if they both entirely depended upon the same afferent pathways (192,242,243).

The conclusions of these studies have been criticized on the grounds that the reflex response to a stretch may have been obscured by the length-tension relationship of the contracting muscle (204,244,245) and arguments related to

---

Figure 8. Schematic drawings of two different axon collateral systems, one having a limited number of branches (A), while the other is more extensively developed (B). The numbers indicate the mean axonal diameters (in μm) for each collateral branch as determined from measurements at 10 μm intervals. The dots show the locations of axon collateral swellings interpreted as possibly being synaptic terminals. Scales (100 μm) apply only to the lengths of the axon collateral branches. (From Ref. 75.)

this problem have been further developed to support (150,239,246-249) or disprove (206,250,251) the original hypothesis (cf. 252)

The possibility that electrically induced group II afferent volleys may produce excitation in extensor motoneurons has been reported from time to time (13,134,135,232-234,253-256). Latency measurements actually indicate that some extensor motoneurons may receive a disynaptic excitation from group II afferents (233; see also 241), and that the corresponding spinal interneurons can be monosynaptically excited by group II fibers in the gastrocnemius nerve (257). Interneurons receiving terminals from group II afferents have been reported to be located in two separate regions, one in laminae IV-VI, and the other in the ventral horn, in laminae VII and IX (241,257-259).

The use of the spike-triggered averaging technique to study the connections of group II fibers from muscle spindles has demonstrated the existence in spinal cats of a monosynaptic excitatory projection to homonymous extensor moto-neurons and the probable existence of polysynaptic projections to motoneurons from the same fibers (153,155,260-264; see also 154). In spite of this evidence, the amount of monosynaptic action from secondary endings has been considered to be marginal (cf. 233,265), and it has been maintained that in decerebrate cats the only significant excitatory action contributing to the stretch and the vibration reflexes of the soleus muscle originates from Ia afferents (251).

Independent of the excitatory influence of the secondary endings of muscle spindles on homonymous motoneurons, we postulated that the differences in the gain of the stretch reflex obtained during maintained stretch and that obtained during vibration might depend upon the different amounts of autogenetic inhibition elicited by the two methods of activating Ia afferents. In addition, there is evidence that presynaptic inhibition of Ia fibers originating from homonymous and the synergistic muscles (180,266,267; cf. 268) was preferentially elicited by muscle vibration when compared with that elicited by static muscle stretch (267). Furthermore, an additional mechanism may explain the lower gain of the proprioceptive reflex during vibration than during static stretch. Although it has been shown that R-cells that belong to the pool of gastrocnemius-soleus motoneurons may respond to both static stretch and vibration of the homonymous muscle, the average rate of increase of R-cell discharge with increasing frequency of discharge of primary spindle endings was about 4.3 times greater during vibration than during static stretch of the gastrocnemius-soleus muscle (see Sec. III.B.1). These effects have been attributed in part at least to the fact that large-sized phasic motoneurons that are particularly recruited by muscle vibration are more effective in influencing R-cells than small-sized tonic neurons that represent the main population of motoneurons influenced by static stretch. An additional possibility to be taken into consideration is that group II afferents reduce the gain of the R-cell discharge obtained during static stretch compared to that obtained during vibration for the same frequency of discharge of the Ia afferents.

Several authors considered the possibility that secondary spindle afferents exert an inhibitory influence on R-cells that may not be mediated through motoneurons. These workers found that the activity of R-cells, disynaptically excited by electrically induced group Ia volleys from the ipsilateral gastrocnemius-soleus muscle, was depressed when high-threshold groups II and III muscle afferents were recruited by the stimulus (cf. 31,88,164,269). Figure 4 shows an example in which an increase in intensity (from 2 to 10–20T) of the stimulus applied to the gastrocnemius-soleus nerve reduced the R-cell discharge elicited disynaptically by single shock stimulation of group I afferents. The reduction of the unit discharge did not involve the early component of the response, but only the late component and appeared for stimulus intensities higher than 4–5T, that is, when group III muscle afferents were recruited by the stimulus. However, when repetitive stimulation of the gastrocnemius-soleus nerve was used, the threshold for this depression decreased—a finding that indicates that group II (as well as group Ib) afferents from the gastrocnemius-soleus muscle contributed to it (97,164). In line with these observations are the results of experiments performed by Fromm et al. (249,270) that demonstrated that the amount of recurrent inhibition of tonic extensor gastrocnemius-soleus motoneurons elicited by repetitive electrical stimulation of ventral root filaments was greater during a maximal selective input from the Ia afferents induced by vibrating the triceps surae (100 μm amplitude) than during repetitive electrical stimulation of the gastrocnemius-soleus nerve with stimulus intensities corresponding to or > 1.8T, intensities that recruited group II afferents. Similar results were also obtained by Wand et al. (271).

The decrease of recurrent inhibition by group II input could partly explain the increase in firing rate of tonic motoneurons and the recruitment of more phasic motoneurons that may occur when the group II afferents are recruited by electrical (134,135,255,256) or by mechanical stimuli, such as large amplitudes of vibration that exceed 100 μm (131,132,176,191–193). The reduced discharge of R-cells elicited by electrical stimulation of the gastrocnemius-soleus nerve cannot by itself be attributed to activation of the secondary endings of muscle spindles, since the group II spectrum contains afferents originating from receptor organs in addition to spindles (cf. 18 for ref.). Therefore, attempts have been made to study the effects of natural stimulation of secondary endings of muscle spindles on the R-cell discharge. In a first group of experiments (164), the activity of R-cells coupled with gastrocnemius-soleus motoneurons was tested for increasing amplitudes of muscle vibration. It was found that the secondary endings of the muscle spindles recruited by increasing the amplitude of vibration from 70–80 μm to 300 μm (172) did not modify the response of the R-cells to the group Ia volleys driven by small amplitudes of vibration. This finding, however, is difficult to evaluate, since for the amplitude of vibration used the group II mediated effect was probably not strong enough to overcome the powerful excitation of the R-cells elicited by the group Ia volleys via the monosynaptic reflex discharge of the homonymous motoneurons. The hypothesis that the secondary endings of gastrocnemius-soleus muscle spindles may depress the activity of R-cells coupled with the gastrocnemius-soleus motoneuronal pool is supported by the fact that the responses of these R-cells to static stretch, as well as to muscle vibration (97,164), is progressively increased by pulling the homonymous muscle up to 8 mm, but there is no further increase and actually a slight decrease in the response when the muscle is extended to 10–12 mm. This slight depression can, in part at least, be caused by recruitment of the secondary endings that occurs for large initial extension of the muscle. Benecke et al. (272; cf. 118) provided further evidence for an inhibitory effect of the secondary endings on R-cells. It is known that asynchronous afferent discharges restricted to primary and secondary muscle spindle afferents can be induced by intravenous injection of succinylcholine (SCh). These authors found that in decerebrate cats spontaneous activity of R-cells belonging to the gastrocnemius-soleus pool was usually enhanced or induced after application of SCh which produced reflex discharges of alpha motoneurons. However, in cats deeply anesthetized with pentobarbital and usually lacking spontaneous R-cell activity, no reflex discharges of alpha motoneurons were induced by similar doses of SCh. In these latter preparations the early response of R-cells to antidromic stimulation of ventral root L7 or S1 was reversibly decreased by SCh for several minutes. Apparently, under these conditions no effect of Ia spindle afferents on R-cells could appear because these afferents failed to induce motoneuronal discharges. Therefore, it was concluded that the secondary spindle endings exert an inhibitory influence on R-cells that might be hidden in the decerebrate state. The secondary muscle spindle endings may then disinhibit extensor alpha motoneurons by reducing this natural Renshaw inhibition. The neuronal pathway involved in the inhibitory influence of the group II muscle spindle afferents on R-cells still remains to be identified.

4. Cutaneous and High-Threshold Muscle Afferents

Apart from the influences originating from muscle spindle and Golgi tendon organ afferents, R-cells can be excited or inhibited by electrical or natural stimulation of other segmental afferents (6,13,27,31,36,86,88,97,138,164,241,249, 269,270,273,274). In particular, both cutaneous and high-threshold muscle afferents whose stimulation may elicit the ipsilateral flexor reflex and the crossed extensor reflex, the so-called flexion reflex afferents (FRA: 232,275), contribute to the responses. Central latencies between 3 and 20 msec have been measured for such responses. The observed changes in firing rate of R-cells is only partially dependent upon parallel changes of the corresponding motoneurons. This finding has led some authors to postulate the existence of polysynaptic pathways common to R-cells and to motoneurons (138). It is of interest that in addition to the classic early flexor and crossed extensor reflex, cutaneous and high-threshold muscle afferents may evoke a late long-lasting flexor and crossed extensor reflex after intravenous injection of DOPA (274, 276). DOPA presumably acts by liberating transmitter from a descending noradrenergic pathway. This adrenergic system inhibits transmission in the short-latency reflex pathway, thereby releasing transmission through the long-latency reflex pathway. Activation of the long-latency flexor reflex produces a very effective inhibition of transmission in the recurrent pathway to moto-neurons. In fact, intravenous injection of 100 mg/kg DOPA in unanesthetized spinal cats produced a long-lasting (0.5 sec) depression of both recurrent inhibitory postsynaptic potentials in motoneurons and R-cell discharges caused by stimulation of the flexion reflex afferents (274). The latter events are of interest in view of the relation of these late reflexes to the generation of locomotion. There is, in fact, evidence that these long-latency reflex pathways are organized with mutual reciprocal inhibitory connections between interneurons trans-mitting excitation to flexor and extensor motoneurons (277), much as postu-lated by Graham Brown in his half-center hypothesis (278). These interneuronal pathways could, therefore, provide a centrally programmed alternating activa-tion of flexor and extensor motoneurons—a pattern presumably required for stepping (277,279). The suppression of Renshaw inhibition during activation of the interneuronal pools of the long-latency flexor reflex has been considered as a segmental control system, allowing the entire Ia reflex pattern (including con-siderable heteronymous Ia excitation and reciprocal Ia inhibition from muscles other than the strict antagonist) to contribute to regulation of gait. Studies on R-cell activity during locomotion are, however, still conflicting (see Sec. III.C.2).

C. Supraspinal Descending Systems

R-cells are under the control of several supraspinal systems that can modify transmission in the recurrent pathway (116,280–287). In particular, excitatory and/or inhibitory effects have been evoked by electrical stimulation of the cerebral cortex (282,283), the internal capsule (286), the red nucleus (287), the vestibular nuclear complex (284), the cerebellum (116,281,284,285), the reticular formation (280,281,283,284), and the thalamus (283). There is also evidence that recurrent inhibition of alpha motoneurons is more potent in the decerebrate than in the spinal state (288) and that transmission in recurrent pathways is enhanced by activation of bulbospinal noradrenergic pathways (276). Supraspinal descending volleys may operate on R-cells, either directly or indirectly via alpha motoneurons as shown by the fact that either reciprocal or parallel activity can be observed during stimulation of individual structures.

   Although very little is known about the types of motor activity that utilize descending control systems acting on R-cells, there is now evidence that these systems intervene during the macular labyrinthine reflexes, locomotion and scratch reflex, and voluntary movements.

1. Activity of Renshaw Cells During Macular Labyrinthine Reflexes

During static or dynamic tilts the labyrinthine reflexes may act asymmetrically on limb extensors. Side-down tilt of the head (after eliminating neck reflexes) (289) or side-down rotation about the longitudinal axis of the whole animal (290, 290a) produces contraction, whereas side-up tilt results in extensor relaxation. These responses have been attributed in part to activity of neurons located in the lateral vestibular nucleus of Deiters (LVN). Descending vestibulospinal projections from the lateral vestibular nucleus exert a monosynaptic and/or a disynaptic excitatory influence on ipsilateral extensor motoneurons, including those innervating the hindlimb extensors (291; cf. 292 for ref.). Experiments performed in decerebrate cats have, in fact, shown that most of the lateral vestibular nucleus units tested at standard parameters of sinusoidal tilt (0.026 Hz, $\pm 10°$ peak amplitude) respond preferentially to the direction of orientation of the angular stimulus, that is, to animal position. The predominant pattern is characterized by an increase in the firing rate during side-down tilt and by a decrease in the firing rate during side-up tilt (α-response) (293–295). Similar results have also been reported for the responses to tilt of the majority of otolith receptors in the utriculus, a finding in apparent agreement with the morphologic polarization of the receptors (cf. 293 for refs.).

Recent experiments performed in decerebrate cats have shown that presumably inhibitory reticulospinal neurons collaborate with excitatory vestibulospinal neurons to the motoneuronal output controlling limb extensor activity during labyrinthine reflexes. In fact, reticulospinal neurons, antidromically activated by spinal cord stimulation at T12–L1 and histologically located in the ventromedial aspect of the medullary reticular formation (i.e., in that area that upon stimulation produced inhibitory postsynaptic potentials in ipsilateral hindlimb motoneurons [296–299; cf. 300]), responded to sinusoidal tilt of the animal (301). However, their predominant pattern of response was characterized by a decrease in firing rate during side-down tilt and an increase during side-up tilt (β-response)—this response being the opposite of that found in the lateral vestibulospinal neurons.* Indeed, this finding supports the conclusion that the medullary reticulospinal neurons responding to tilt exert an inhibitory influence on ipsilateral hindlimb extensor motoneurons, in contrast to the vestibulospinal neurons, which are excitatory in function. Therefore, during side-down tilt the motoneurons innervating the ipsilateral limb extensors would not only be excited by the increased discharge of vestibulospinal neurons, but also disinhibited by the reduced discharge of reticulospinal neurons (cf. 301a).

---

*The macular input of one side is actually transmitted to the contralateral medullary reticular formation by the lateral vestibulospinal tract acting on neurons of the crossed spinoreticular pathway (cf. 302,303 for refs.).

It is of interest that medullary reticulospinal neurons responding to animal tilt had a very low resting discharge rate when decerebrate rigidity was present, but this activity greatly increased when the rigidity was reduced by intravenous injection of an anticholinesterase (eserine sulfate, 0.05–0.1 mg/kg) (304). This state-dependent behavior of the units shows that they exert an inhibitory influence on the extensor musculature. The experimental evidence further indicates that this medullary reticulospinal system is under the excitatory control of a cholinergic system, located in the pontine reticular formation, which becomes tonically active following injection of an anticholinesterase (305). In contrast with these findings, the lateral vestibulospinal neurons responding to tilt had a relatively high resting discharge rate in the decerebrate cat, which was mainly maintained by the ipsilateral labyrinthine input and was not significantly affected by the anticholinesterase (306).

With respect to the control situation, the increased resting discharge of the reticulospinal neurons following injection of an anticholinesterase would lead to a greater disinhibition of hindlimb extensor motoneurons during side-down tilt, thus increasing the response gain of the corresponding extensor muscles to the same parameters of animal displacement. This hypothesis has been fully confirmed by recording the electromyographic responses of the gastrocnemius-soleus muscle to animal tilt before and after injection on an anticholinesterase (306a).

The reticulospinal influences on the gastrocnemius-soleus motoneurons during tilt are mediated by R-cells. Pompeiano et al. (307) have shown that in normal decerebrate cats R-cells disynaptically excited by group Ia volleys from the gastrocnemius-soleus nerve either did not respond to labyrinthine stimulation, as obtained by sinusoidal tilt of the head at the standard parameters after bilateral neck deafferentation, or if it did so, showed α-responses (Fig. 9, upper trace). Since in these preparations, the electromyographic activity of the gastrocnemius-soleus muscle either was not modulated or showed only a slight increase during side-down tilt (α-responses), the effects described previously were attributed to the activity of vestibulospinal neurons, whose increased discharge during side-down tilt would exert a weak excitatory influence on gastrocnemius-soleus motoneurons and through their recurrent collaterals on the related R-cells (coactivation of alpha motoneurons and their target R-cells). The most striking finding, however, was that after intravenous injection of eserine sulfate the R-cells coupled with the gastrocnemius-soleus motoneurons responded to standard parameters of tilt, but now all the tested units showed an increased discharge during side-up tilt (β-responses), that is, a response pattern similar to that displayed by the reticulospinal neurons (Fig. 9, middle trace). Correspondingly, in normal decerebrate cats the electromyographic modulation of the gastrocnemius-soleus muscle induced by standard parameters of tilt greatly increased (cf. 306a).

It appears, therefore, that following injection of an anticholinesterase the R-cells linked with the gastrocnemius-soleus motoneurons escape the control of

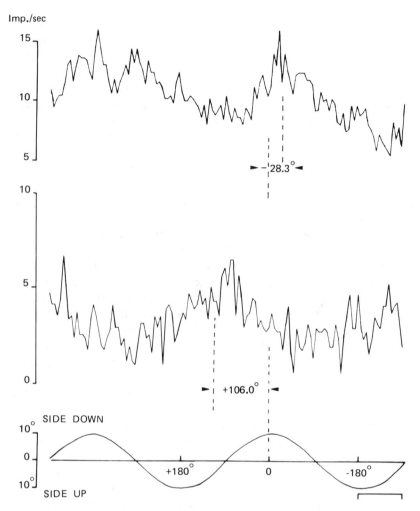

Figure 9 Response patterns of two R-cells coupled with GS motoneurons during stimulation of labyrinthine receptors, as obtained by sinusoidal tilt of the head after bilateral neck deafferentation. Experiments performed in decerebrate cats with GS muscle de-efferented on the left side. The corresponding hindlimb was fixed with the knee and the ankle bent to 90°. The R-cells were monosynaptically excited by ventral root stimulation of L7 and disynaptically excited by single shock stimulation of the intact GS nerve. Upper record, SPDH showing the response of a R-cell to sinusoidal head rotation at 0.026 Hz, ± 10°. Eight sweeps were accumulated using 128 bins with a dwell time of 0.6 sec per bin. The unit increased its firing rate during side-down tilt (α-response); in particular, the response showed a gain of 0.24 imp./sec/deg, a sensitivity of 2.15% of the base frequency per degree and a phase lag of –28.3° with respect to the peak of

the lateral vestibulospinal pathway, thus being decoupled from their input moto-neurons and undergo the most efficient control of the reticulospinal pathway (Fig. 10). In particular, while in normal decerebrate cats the increased discharge of R-cells during side-down tilt would *limit the gain* of response of the gastro-cnemius-soleus muscles to labyrinthine stimulation, after injection of anticholin-esterase the reduced discharge of R-cells for the same direction of animal orien-tation would *enhance the gain* of response of the gastrocnemius-soleus muscle to the same labyrinthine input. Surprisingly, the reduced activity of R-cells during side-down tilt induced by the reticulospinal system counteracts the in-creased discharge of the motor axon collaterals originating from the gastro-cnemius-soleus motoneurons. It is likely that in this experimental condition the small tonic motoneurons, which are more powerfully affected by recurrent inhibition (see Sec. IV.A.1), are more easily disinhibited during side-down tilt. If this is the case, one must assume that the reticulospinal pathway produces a higher density of excitatory synaptic contacts on the cell body and/or the proximal dendrites of R-cells than do the recurrent collaterals of the small tonic gastrocnemius-soleus motoneurons. Finally, it should be mentioned that the lateral vestibular nucleus produces not only monosynaptic and disynaptic excita-tion of ipsilateral extensor motoneurons, but also disynaptic inhibition of the antagonistic flexor motoneurons (Fig. 10) (291). This effect is caused by mono-synaptic excitation exerted by the lateral vestibulospinal tract on interneurons of the Ia inhibitory pathway from the extensor musculature to flexor moto-neurons (308). It would be of interest to know whether in normal decerebrate cats these Ia inhibitory interneurons are excited during side-down tilt at the standard parameters of stimulation, and whether this excitation increases fol-lowing injection of the anticholinesterase; one may expect that under this experimental condition the reduced discharge of R-cells produces less recurrent inhibition of the Ia inhibitory interneurons, which would then mediate a more efficient reciprocal Ia inhibition, just at the time in which the response gain of the gastrocnemius-soleus muscle to tilt is increased.

---

the side-down displacement of the animal, indicated by 0°. Middle record, SPDH showing the response of another R-cell during sinusoidal head rotation at 0.15 Hz, ± 10° performed 21 min after i.v. inspection of an anticholinesterase (0.1 mg/kg of eserine sulfate). Forty-eight sweeps were accumulated using 128 bins with a dwell time of 0.1 sec per bin. The unit increased its firing rate during side-up tilt (β-response) and showed a response gain of 0.12 imp./sec/deg, a sensitivity of 3.37%/deg, and a phase lead of +106.0° with respect to 0°. This unit was unresponsive to the same parameters of tilt before eserine injec-tion. Lower record, head's position. Time calibration: 10 sec for the upper trace, 2 sec for the middle trace. (From Ref. 307.)

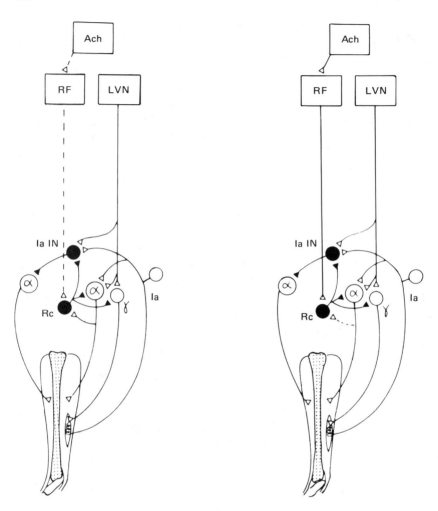

Figure 10 Schematic illustration of vestibulospinal and reticulospinal projections to the lower segments of the spinal cord. The interneuronal connections in the spinal cord are the same as illustrated in Figure 1. Vestibulospinal neurons originating from the lateral vestibular nucleus (LVN) monosynaptically (and also disynaptically) excite alpha and gamma motoneurons to synergistic hindlimb extensors (for instance, the GS muscle); the same neurons also monosynaptically excite interneurons of the Ia inhibitory pathway from the GS muscle to antagonistic motoneurons, IaIN (291,308; cf. 292). On the other hand, reticulospinal neurons originating from the lower part of the medullary reticular formation (RF) excite Renshaw cells (Rc) coupled with the GS motoneurons (it is not known whether this effect is induced mono- or polysynaptically). During animal tilt, LVN neurons undergo an increase in firing rate during side-down tilt, α-responses (292–295), while RF

2. Activity of Renshaw Cells During Locomotion and Scratch Reflex

Recurrent inhibition of motoneurons has been tested during locomotion in mesencephalic cats (309-311). The ability of a train of antidromic volleys in motor axons to inhibit alpha motoneurons and Ia inhibitory interneurons was reduced during treadmill locomotion. It was inferred, therefore, that R-cells are inhibited during locomotion, a finding well in keeping with the postulated importance of the full excitatory and inhibitory Ia pathways in the regulation of gait (279,312) (see Sec. III.B.4). This conclusion, however, has been challenged by several authors (313-315) who have postulated an active role of recurrent inhibition during locomotion. In particular, these workers have observed rhythmical R-cell activity in parallel with the activity of the corresponding motoneurons during fictive locomotion. R-cells would then limit the activity of motoneurons and control the depth of their reciprocal inhibition during rhythmic movements by means of an inhibition of Ia interneurons.

Information concerning the possible role of R-cells in rhythmical movements has been obtained by Deliagina and Feldman (316,317). These workers recorded the activity of R-cells during the fictive scratch reflex, that is, during rhythmical activity in muscle efferents evoked in decerebrate curarized cats by the same stimulus (tactile stimulation of the pinna) that elicits natural scratching before immobilization. The hindlimb ipsilateral to the side of the recorded

---

neurons show a decrease in firing rate, β-responses (301); therefore, for this direction of animal orientation GS motoneurons are excited by LVN, but are disinhibited by RF neurons. In normal decerebrate cats (left side) this disinhibition is negligible, due to the low level of activity of the reticulospinal inhibitory system (dashed line). Therefore, only a small number of GS motoneurons are excited by the descending vestibulospinal volleys during side-down tilt; correspondingly, the gain of the EMG response of the GS muscle to tilt is low. In this condition, the R-cells either are unresponsive or show an α-response, indicating that they are driven by vestibulospinal volleys acting through GS motoneurons and their recurrent collaterals. Activation of a cholinergic system, Ach (right side), which increases the background discharge of the RF but not of the LVN neurons (cf. 305,306), enhances the amount of disinhibition of GS motoneurons during side-down tilt. The R-cells coupled with these motoneurons, which were either unresponsive or showed an α-response to tilt before injection, now show a β-response, indicating that they are driven by reticulospinal volleys; correspondingly, the gain of the EMG response of the GS muscle to the same parameters of tilt greatly increases. In other words, the R-cells escape the recurrent control of the alpha motoneurons (dashed line) activated by the vestibulospinal system and are under enhanced control of the reticulospinal system. The decrease in firing rate of R-cells during side-down tilt occurs in spite of the increased discharge of the related GS motoneurons. For further details, see the text.

R-cells was usually deafferented. The duration of the cycle was about 250 msec, with a short period of extensor activity of about 50 msec (S phase) and a longer period of flexor activity of about 200 msec (L phase). The appearance of rhythmical bursts of discharges was preceded by tonic flexor activity (tonic phase of scratching). Discharges of R-cells were recorded in parallel with the discharges recorded in the gastrocnemius-soleus nerve. During the tonic phase of the scratch reflex, R-cells coupled with flexor motoneurons decreased their activity. No change in activity of R-cells coupled with extensor motoneurons was observed.

During the rhythmical phases of the scratch reflex the majority of R-cells responded phasically with a burst of 50–100 msec duration. In particular, extensor-coupled R-cells reached maximal activity during the S phase, that is, when extensor motoneurons were recruited (cf. 318). This fact is compatible with the hypothesis that motoneurons are the main modulators of R-cell activity. However, some R-cells stop firing before or at the beginning of the S phase, when an increasing number of gastrocnemius-soleus motoneurons are recruited (318). In contrast, flexor-coupled R-cells discharged mainly at the end of the L phase and during the S phase, that is, when the flexor motoneurons terminated their activity. This finding should be related to the observation that the tibialis anterior (and sartorius) alpha motoneurons are most active during the L phase and completely terminate their activity during the second half of this phase. It appears, therefore, that the population of R-cells coupled with flexor motoneurons works reciprocally with their target motoneurons. Thus, R-cells activated antidromically from flexor motoneurons have their main peak of activity after that of the flexor motoneurons, and it can be suggested that the chief input to R-cells is from phasically active interneurons rather than from motoneurons. Spinal cord transection at the C1 level did not change the timing of the discharges during the scratch cycle.

The timing of R-cell activity during scratching suggests that R-cells with input from flexors promote a switch in the activity from flexor populations (of alpha and gamma motoneurons and Ia interneurons) to extensor populations, while R-cells with input from extensors bring about the reverse. Cessation of the background discharge of some R-cells with input from flexors in the tonic phase of scratching is likely to promote proper limb positioning by disinhibition of flexor motoneurons.

These findings indicate that the relation between timing and general activity of R-cells and the corresponding motoneurons can be centrally depending on motor tasks.

3. Activity of Renshaw Cells During Voluntary Motor Contractions

It was postulated by Wilson (13) that strong tonic contractions are accompanied by inhibition of R-cells. In relation to this postulate are the results reported by Koehler et al. (286). These workers found that electrical stimulation of the internal capsule often produced an increase of the monosynaptic reflex, together with a decrease of the resulting R-cell activity, that is, a decoupling of R-cells from their input motoneurons.

Recent studies have made it possible to estimate recurrent inhibition of soleus motoneurons in man by means of eliciting paired Hoffmann reflexes (319–321; cf. 165). In particular, the recurrent inhibition brought about by a conditioning H-reflex discharge was estimated by the amplitude of a test H-reflex involving only the soleus motoneurons that fired in response to the conditioning volley. The modifications of the recurrent inhibition during contraction were evaluated by comparing the amplitude of the test H-reflex to the reference H-reflex. Both reflexes received the excitation underlying the voluntary contraction, but only the test H-reflex was subjected to the recurrent inhibition evoked by the conditioning H-reflex discharge. With this method the excitability of R-cells has been studied in human subjects during various tonic and phasic voluntary contractions of the triceps surae (322–324).

During voluntary *tonic* contractions of various forces the weakest contractions were accompanied by a decrease in the size of the test reflex. Temporal summation of motoneuronal after-hyperpolarization and R-cell excitation secondary to voluntary motor discharge could account for this reduction of the test reflex. On the other hand, with greater contraction forces there was no longer an inhibition of the test reflex, but instead a facilitation was observed. This facilitation grew continuously with increased contraction forces. This finding indicated that with increasing contraction force the recurrent inhibition following the conditioning discharge was progressively decreasing. During *ramp* contractions of varying contraction velocities the time courses of the variations of the test and reference H-reflexes were almost inverse. The experimental evidence indicates that these differential time courses were caused by changes in the amount of recurrent inhibition elicited by the conditioning discharge.

The possibility of occlusion in the recurrent pathway must be considered. However, it was concluded that the decrease in the recurrent inhibition elicited by the conditioning discharge was essentially caused by an inhibitory control elicited from supraspinal centers and/or segmentally from various receptors in the limbs involved in soleus contraction. The segmental afferents to be considered include cutaneous afferents activated by foot pressure and group II afferents from the contracting muscle activated by the alpha-gamma linkage (325). Both cutaneous afferents (269) and group II muscle afferents (see Sec. III.B.3 and 4) may cause inhibition of R-cells, and it is conceivable that they contribute to the inhibition of R-cells during voluntary contraction. A significant contribution from cutaneous receptors was excluded, since it was shown that strong pressure on the foot produced by a cuff did not modify the excitability of R-cells at rest (cf. 323). It has therefore been suggested that inhibition of R-cells observed during the voluntary contraction was caused by a supraspinal control exerted either directly on R-cells or indirectly via the γ-loop and group II afferents. This inhibition of R-cells actually counteracts the increasing excitatory input that they receive via motor axon collaterals during increasing tonic contractions or through ramp contractions.

Since R-cells inhibit interneurons of the Ia inhibitory pathway, a decreased firing of R-cells during voluntary movements would produce less recurrent inhibition of these Ia interneurons and in turn would result in more efficient reciprocal inhibition (323). A more efficient reciprocal Ia inhibition is obvious when studying the effect of a voluntary contraction on the antagonistic muscle spindles: During a strong soleus contraction passive stretch of the pretibial muscles causes a discharge of their Ia afferents. This discharge tends to excite pretibial motoneurons and Ia interneurons that inhibit soleus motoneurons. This "undesirable" inhibitory effect is, however, counteracted by the reciprocal Ia inhibition, since the Ia inhibitory interneurons excited by the contracting soleus muscle project to both the motoneurons of the pretibial antagonistic muscles and to the "opposite" Ia inhibitory interneurons excited by the pretibial muscles (see Sec. IV.A.3).

In summary, it appears that the increasing inhibition of R-cells seen with an increasing force of contraction may be related to the increasing voluntary motor discharge by two mechanisms: A direct reduction of the inhibition of the motoneurons through the recurrent pathway and an indirect mechanism that favors reciprocal Ia inhibition to prevent certain inhibitory influences from reaching the motoneurons.

IV. EFFERENT ACTIONS OF RENSHAW CELLS

A. Limb Motoneurons and Related Interneurons

1. Alpha motoneurons

In this section, evidence concerning the distribution of recurrent inhibition among motoneurons will be reviewed. It is known that the action potential in alpha motoneurons is followed by an after-hyperpolarization (AHP), which is the major intrinsic factor regulating cell firing rate (326,327,327a). Recurrent activation of the Renshaw inhibitory circuit further contributes to the depression of the firing rate of the corresponding motoneurons. Activation of motoneurons innervating a given muscle produces recurrent inhibitory postsynaptic potentials that are larger in motoneurons of the same motor nucleus (68), but many other motoneurons are also strongly inhibited (1,2,6,24,68,69,104). The recurrent inhibitory synapses are largely located on the proximal dendrites of motoneurons (328,329). In early attempts to study the pattern of distribution of recurrent inhibition among motoneurons, it was observed that the amplitude of recurrent inhibitory postsynaptic potentials in motoneurons was related to the distance between these recipient neurons and the nuclei from which the R-cells were activated (1,6,67,68,104). In particular, recurrent inhibition was found to be most pronounced among the motor nuclei within the same segments (1,6; cf. 226). It was therefore suggested that the distribution of recurrent inhibition depended mainly on the distance between motoneurons (the proximity hypothesis), and that a generalized suppressor action on motoneurons occurs, regardless of their function (68).

By itself, however, the proximity hypothesis cannot account for the distribution of recurrent inhibitory postsynaptic potentials (67). In fact, the observation that for a given nerve the most pronounced recurrent inhibition is evoked in the motoneurons activated antidromically and in the motor nuclei of close synergistics suggests that its distribution depends on functional factors (1,6,35, 67,68,86,104,161). According to Hultborn et al. (69), the motor nuclei of muscles that are linked in Ia synergism are mutually interconnected by recurrent inhibition regardless of their location in the spinal cord. For example, large recurrent inhibitory postsynaptic potentials were evoked in gracilis motoneurons from the Ia afferents from the synergist semitendinosus and posterior biceps muscles whose motor nuclei are located some segments away. Recurrent inhibition may also be present between antagonists in a wider sense, for example, extensors and flexors (exemplified by the mutual recurrent inhibition between gastrocnemius-soleus and posterior biceps motor nuclei). However, recurrent inhibitory connections have never been found between nuclei supplying muscles acting as strict antagonists at the same joint (69). This rule is valid also when these motor nuclei have a similar segmental location: The recurrent inhibition is, in fact, lacking between the motor nuclei of tibialis anterior and gastrocnemius-soleus (67) and in quadriceps motor nucleus from gracilis (69). The organization of the recurrent pathways in the spinal segments from which the forelimb muscles are innervated (104) is similar to that of the recurrent pathways acting on hindlimb motoneurons (69).

The striking overlap between the distribution of Renshaw inhibition and Ia excitation should not conceal the fact that recurrent inhibition has a more extensive distribution than Ia excitation. It is likely that the additional recurrent connections may link muscles that act in "functional synergisms" in postures and movements not reflected by the Ia input.

An important problem to be considered is that of the distribution of recurrent inhibition within the same motor nucleus. It has been postulated that if the Renshaw circuit mainly subserves a negative feedback of motoneurons one would expect that activity of a given group of motoneurons should act either selectively on themselves or diffusely on all motoneurons innervating the same muscle (23). The case for a diffuse distribution has received support from the results of intracellular studies of triceps surae motoneurons that have suggested that there is a more or less linear relation between the amount of recurrent inhibition and the size of the monosynaptic reflex in both small and large motoneurons (330) (cf., however, Sec. III.B.1). In contrast, earlier experiments have indicated that recurrent inhibition affects some motoneurons more strongly than others. Holmgren and Merton (331) found that large motoneurons with rapidly conducting axons inhibited other motoneurons of higher electrical threshold and more slowly conducting axons. Further investigations demonstrated that small tonic alpha motoneurons were more strongly influenced by recurrent inhibition than were large, phasic motoneurons (68,107,116,134-136, 332-334; cf. 16); moreover, recurrent inhibitory postsynaptic potentials were larger in small motoneurons that innervate the "red" soleus muscle than in large motoneurons that innervate the "pale" lateral gastrocnemius muscle (129).

The differential effect of recurrent inhibition of alpha motoneurons has been investigated by Wand et al. (176). These authors recorded in decerebrate cats the electrical activity of individual gastrocnemius-soleus motoneurons whose size was estimated by measuring their critical firing level following the method described by Clamann et al. (201). In the de-efferented preparation, the electrical activity of 94 gastrocnemius-soleus motoneurons with critical firing levels ranging from 1 to 92% was tested during 1-sec periods of vibration applied with the standard parameters of 150 Hz and a peak-to-peak amplitude of 156 μm, a value reported to be supramaximal for driving all muscle spindle primary endings (170-172). The response of gastrocnemius-soleus motoneurons to standard parameters of vibration was characterized by a sudden increase in discharge rate during the first 100 msec of a 1-sec vibration period (phasic response) that was usually higher than that occurring during the last 500 msec of the same vibration period (tonic response). However, there were motoneurons in which the discharge rate was not greatly modified throughout the vibration period. If we relate now the ratio between the average discharge rate of the gastrocnemius-soleus motoneurons obtained during the early and that obtained during the late component of the response to 1-sec periods of vibration with standard parameters to motoneuron size, it appears that the corresponding value tends to decrease with increasing critical firing level, that is, size of the motoneurons. However, the ratio between the two components of the response showed a great variability, particularly within the population of neurons with critical firing levels lower than 20% (Fig. 11).

The gastrocnemius-soleus motoneurons reported earlier were also subjected to 1-sec periods of vibration at 156-209 μm, but at increasing frequencies. A linear relation was found between the discharge rate of gastrocnemius-soleus motoneurons and frequency of vibration at least from 25 to 50 up to 150 to 275 Hz. The ratio between the gain constants of the corresponding neurons relating frequency of the motoneuronal output to frequency of the vibratory input (i.e., to discharge frequency of the Ia afferents) tended to decrease with

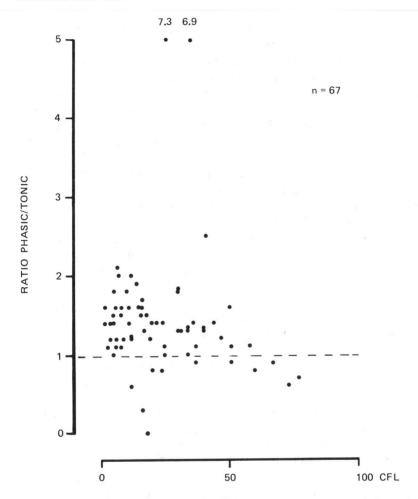

Figure 11 Relation between size of GS alpha motoneurons and the ratio between the average discharge rate obtained during the phasic and that obtained during the tonic component of the response to vibration of the homonymous muscle. The experiments were performed in precollicular decerebrate cats with the de-efferented GS muscle fixed at an average initial extension of 10 mm (range 8–14 mm). For 67 GS motoneurons, the mean discharge rates obtained during the first 100 msec (phasic response) and during the last 500 msec (tonic response) of 1-sec periods of vibration of the homonymous muscle (at 150 Hz, 156 μm amplitude) were evaluated. The ratio of both components (ordinate) was plotted against the size of the motoneurons, expressed in terms of CFL (abscissa). (From Ref. 176.)

increasing critical firing level, that is, size of the motoneurons. Again, there was a great variability within the population of neurons with critical firing levels lower than 20%. In conclusion, different size motoneurons undergo different amounts of autogenetic depression of their firing rate elicited by the orthodromic group Ia volleys during the last 500 msec of a 1-sec vibration period.

Assuming that there is an equal amount of autogenetic presynaptic depolarization affecting the central endings of the group Ia afferents during vibration of the gastrocnemius-soleus muscle (180,266,267), the decreased discharge of the motoneurons may not only depend on postspike after-hyperpolarization or motoneuronal adaptation, but may also depend upon postsynaptic inhibition of the homonymous motoneurons caused by recurrent excitation of R-cells. It is of interest that the firing rate of R-cells that reaches its maximum during the first 100 msec of vibration (phasic response) stabilizes to a lower level (tonic response) during the subsequent part of the vibration period (164). Moreover, the mean discharge rate of the R-cells increased with vibration frequency (164), the gain constant of the phasic response being higher than that of the tonic response (97).

According to the "size principle" the excess of excitation exerted by the Ia afferent volleys on the motoneuron pool is smaller in large-sized motoneurons— since they are the last recruited—than in small-sized motoneurons, which are activated first (cf. 90,335). If the distribution of recurrent inhibition within a motor nucleus were largely uniform and independent of motoneuronal size (131, 330,336,337), one would expect that large motoneurons with their small safety margin would be more sensitive to recurrent inhibition than small motoneurons; the greater safety margin of the latter protects them against recurrent inhibition. This hypothesis is actually supported by the results of ventral root stimulation that show that large motoneurons are more susceptible to recurrent inhibition of stretch-evoked responses than smaller ones (131,152,337). Unfortunately, electrical stimulation of ventral roots does not represent an appropriate tool to investigate R-cell circuitry as antidromic stimulation affects R-cells driven by both agonistic and antagonistic motoneurons. Thus, mutual interactions among different populations of R-cells can hardly be avoided (86).

In the experiments reported previously only R-cells belonging to the gastrocnemius-soleus pool were orthodromically activated during vibration of the homonymous muscle. The ratio between the firing rates (or the gain constants) during the phasic response with respect to the tonic response tended to progressively decrease with increasing critical firing level. This finding indicates that small motoneurons are more sensitive to recurrent inhibition than large motoneurons. The greater sensitivity of small tonic motoneurons to recurrent inhibition does not necessarily indicate a preferential distribution of synaptic contacts of R-cells on these neurons; they can in part be explained by differences in the input resistance of small tonic and large phasic motoneurons (cf. 21). There is, in fact, evidence that in small motoneurons that have higher input resistances than larger motoneurons (186), the same inhibitory input may elicit larger inhibitory postsynaptic potentials than in large motoneurons (68,129).

Apparently, the mechanisms responsible for the steady depression of the motoneuronal discharge during prolonged muscle vibration do not equally affect all the small-sized motoneurons, since the ratio between the phasic and the tonic component of the response of such motoneurons to muscle vibration has great variability. The possibility that the firing rate of small-sized motoneurons can be affected differentially by an inhibitory input is supported by recent work (339). It has therefore been proposed that within the group of small-sized motoneurons there are cell types that either react differentially to the same amount of inhibitory input from R-cells or receive different synaptic densities from this inhibitory source (176). Recent experiments have been performed (340,341) to find out whether the mean amplitude of recurrent inhibitory postsynaptic potentials recorded in cat medial gastrocnemius (MG) alpha motoneurons could be correlated with cell input resistance (i.e., cell size) (342) and/or with motor unit type measured as described in previous studies (343; cf. 188,189,344,345). Motor units were classified as fast twitch, fast fatiguing (FF), fast twitch, fatigue resistant (FR), and slow twitch, fatigue resistant (S) (343,346,347). The amplitude of recurrent inhibitory postsynaptic potentials elicited by stimulation of either the homonymous medial gastrocnemius or heteronymous lateral gastrocnemius-soleus (LGS) muscle nerves were largest in slow-twitch, fatigue-resistant motoneurons, smallest in fast-twitch, fast-fatiguing motoneurons, and intermediate in fast-twitch, fatigue-resistant motoneurons (Fig. 12). Recurrent inhibitory postsynaptic potential amplitude was not critically determined by motoneuron input resistance (cell size), since over a common range of input resistance, recurrent inhibitory postsynaptic potentials were generally larger in slow-twitch, fatigue-resistant than in fast-twitch, fatigue-resistant motoneurons and larger in fast-twitch, fatigue-resistant than in fast-twitch, fast-fatiguing motoneurons.* The relationship between recurrent inhibitory postsynaptic potentials and motor unit type remained significant even after adjusting for any effect of input resistance. These, and other findings that relate recurrent inhibitory postsynaptic potential amplitude

---

*The possibility that the conductance change caused by the inhibitory transmitter may be more important in bringing about inhibitory action than the potential change (338; cf. 131) was disregarded, since somatic conductance measurements revealed no significant change during recurrent inhibition (23, 341; cf. 348). The observed linear summation of recurrent inhibitory postsynaptic potentials and the voltage changes produced by somatic current pulses supports previous studies (329) indicating that the inhibitory effect of the recurrent inhibitory postsynaptic potentials is largely due to its hyperpolarization action rather than to the conductance change that must accompany it.

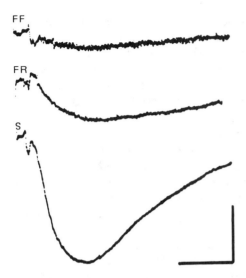

Figure 12 Representative recurrent IPSPs recorded in type-identified medial gastrocnemius motoneurons, following supramaximal electrical stimulation of the lateral gastrocnemius-soleus muscle. Calibration: FF and FR, 0.5 mV, 10 msec; S, 1 mV, 10 msec. (From Ref. 341.)

with maximum tetanic tension produced by the motor units, support the hypothesis that the number of R-cells projecting to a given motoneuron and/or the number of synaptic terminations made on a given motoneuron by an individual R-cell increases in the order FF < FR < S. This hypothesis is in agreement with the result of previous experiments which indicate that: (1) recurrent inhibition most strongly affects motoneurons with lower recruitment thresholds (cf. 16); (2) recurrent inhibition is greater in tonic than in phasic motoneurons (35,68, 107,129,134-136,168,193,331,332,334,349); (3) recurrent inhibitory postsynaptic potentials are larger in motoneurons innervating red muscles than in those innervating pale muscles (129); finally, (4) the autogenetic depression in firing rate during muscle vibration is more prominent in small tonic motoneurons than in large motoneurons, although a wide scatter of this response property has been found in small-sized motoneurons (176).

Recently, van Keulen (127) has used the spike-triggered averaging technique to record recurrent inhibitory postsynaptic potentials generated by single R-cells in cat alpha motoneurons. The effect of an individual R-cell on a motoneuron was very weak (average IPSP amplitude 12.7 μV, range 1.5-54.0 μV, n = 12) in comparison to the compound recurrent inhibitory postsynaptic potentials found in motoneurons after activation of the entire respective motoneuron pool (average 1.5 mV, range 0.6-2.4 mV; ref. 68). Thus, it appears that the amplitude difference of recurrent inhibitory postsynaptic potentials among motor unit types is largely related to a different density of synaptic contacts. Although van Keulen's sample was small (127), the author was able to find that in five cases a motoneuron received recurrent inhibitory postsynaptic potentials from a R-cell activated by its own axon collateral, in two cases a motoneuron excited R-cells but failed to receive recurrent inhibitory postsynaptic potentials, and in seven cases a motoneuron received recurrent inhibitory postsynaptic potentials from R-cells that could not be activated by that motoneuron.

The observation that small tonic alpha motoneurons are subjected to a more effective recurrent inhibition then are the large phasic alpha motoneurons is relevant to the finding that individual R-cells are more powerfully excited by the recurrent collaterals of large phasic alpha motoneurons than by collaterals of the small tonic motoneurons (cf. Secs. III.A and III.B.1). The organization scheme of the inputs to and outputs from the R-cell pool presented by Pompeiano et al. (97,169) (Fig. 13), can be considered valid in the sense that fast-twitch, fast-fatigue motoneurons have the greatest output to the R-cell pool, but the smallest recurrent inhibitory postsynaptic potentials, while slow-twitch, fatigue-resistant motoneurons have the least output to the R-cell pool, but the largest recurrent inhibitory postsynaptic potentials. Fast-twitch, fatigue-resistant motoneurons are intermediate in both input and output relations with the Renshaw pool (cf. 340,341).

2. Gamma Motoneurons

Gamma motoneurons have cell bodies and axons of smaller diameter than alpha motoneurons. In contrast to the conclusion by Sprague (350) that gamma moto-neurons might be located in the ventral part of the region now described as lamina VII of Rexed (39-41), there is evidence that the gamma motoneurons lie in the same region of the spinal cord as the alpha motoneurons (38,89,351-355). The structure of the gamma motoneurons located in the cat lumbosacral spinal cord has been investigated following intracellular injection of HRP (78,105,106). The dendritic trees of the gamma motoneurons extended as far as those of the alpha motoneurons. However, their complexity and the total surface area of each cell were clearly related to axonal conduction velocity and to cell body size (78). As reported previously (see Sec. III.A), most of the injected gamma motoneu-rons did not show recurrent collaterals; this finding, however, does not exclude the possibility that gamma motoneurons are subjected to recurrent inhibition.

The firing rate of gamma motoneurons is similar to that of alpha moto-neurons in that it is regulated by both an after-hyperpolarization as well as by recurrent inhibition. It was claimed by Kemm and Westbury (356) that most gamma motoneurons in the cat lumbar spinal cord lacked an after-hyperpolariza-tion. However, experiments in which the after-hyperpolarization duration, and to a certain extent the amplitude, was estimated by an extracellular technique

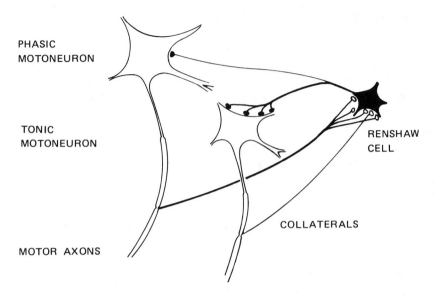

Figure 13 Diagram of the recurrent inhibitory pathways to small tonic and large phasic GS motoneurons. Recurrent collaterals of small tonic and large phasic GS motoneurons synapse on the same Renshaw cell. In turn, the Renshaw cell axon inhibits both types of motoneurons. Recurrent collaterals and axonal branches of the Renshaw cell may have different effectiveness as indicated by their relative thickness. It is postulated that Renshaw cells which are known to affect mainly small tonic motoneurons, are in their turn more powerfully excited by the recurrent collaterals originating from large phasic motoneurons. Excitatory synapses are drawn as empty structures; inhibitory synapses are filled in. (From Ref. 169.)

that used the antidromic latency method, indicate that all gamma motoneurons have a long-lasting after-hyperpolarization with a duration varying from 50 to 150 msec. These long durations would allow for regular firing at frequencies as low as 7-20 imp./sec, that is, similar to that in alpha motoneurons (357).

For years, gamma motoneurons were thought to lack recurrent inhibition (107,351,357a,358). However, Eccles et al. (351) recorded from one gamma motoneuron with quite definite recurrent inhibition produced by single shock stimulation of the ventral root. Later studies have firmly established the presence of recurrent inhibition in gamma motoneurons (359-363) and showed that it may be evoked by ventral root volleys evoked by currents at threshold for activation of alpha motor axons (362).

A recurrent inhibitory circuit from alpha to gamma motoneurons could operate during static and dynamic muscle stretches. Hunt (364) was the first to describe the inhibition of fusimotor extensor neurons that occurs during stretch of the muscle with intact afferents. Since this observation, evidence has accumulated that indicates the existence in the decerebrate preparation of an autogenetic inhibition of gamma motoneurons that arises from stretch-sensitive proprioceptors within the homonymous and heteronymous synergic muscle of the triceps (see 150 for review). In particular, it was found that the slope of the frequency-extension curve of muscle spindle afferents increases after deafferentation (365-367). This effect was attributed to release from inhibition of fusimotor activity that would have been present during stretch with afferents intact (cf. 364). Such inhibition of fusimotor neurons was found in response to muscle stretch (195,368), as well as in response to selective activation of group Ia afferents by vibration (195). In most of these experiments gamma efferents were identified on the basis of relative spike amplitude.

The hypothesis that autogenetic inhibition of gamma motoneurons occurs following activation of homonymous and synergistic alpha motoneurons during the stretch reflex was clearly demonstrated by Fromm et al. (369). These workers found that in decerebrate cats extension of the triceps surae muscle to a length of 8 mm or > decreased the resting discharge of 9 out of 25 gamma efferents in the medial gastrocnemius nerve. Fromm and Noth (370,371) also showed that gamma motoneurons were inhibited during muscle vibration. In both groups of experiments the same gamma efferents were found to receive recurrent inhibition by repetitive antidromic stimulation of the ventral root or the homonymous muscle nerve. These findings suggested that the inhibition of fusimotor neurons was at least partly mediated by the recurrent collaterals of the alpha motoneurons activated by muscle stretch or vibration (cf. 195). It also seems likely that some gamma motoneurons resemble small tonic alpha motoneurons in that they are presumably inhibited by the recurrent collaterals of larger alpha motoneurons (359,360). However, no control recordings of the type of efferent axons excited by vibration were reported in these studies.

It should be mentioned that autogenetic inhibition of spontaneously discharging fusimotor neurons was present in decerebrate (364,369) but not in spinal cats (357a); this finding suggests that autogenetic inhibition affects static fusimotor neurons (cf. 372-374). Inhibition from recurrent collaterals of alpha motoneurons actually affected dynamic as well as static gamma motoneurons (361,362; cf., however, 374a), but it appeared not to be evenly distributed; some motoneurons were not inhibited at all, while others were affected to a variable extent (362). It is known that alpha motoneurons receive recurrent inhibition mainly from motoneurons of homonymous and closely synergistic muscles (see Sec. IV.A.1); as far as has been investigated, the distribution of recurrent inhibition to gamma motoneurons is similar (362).*

A final problem concerns the relative degree to which the alpha and the gamma motoneurons are inhibited by the recurrent loop. Recurrent inhibition of gamma motoneurons was not found as frequently as that of alpha motoneurons (359,361-363), although no direct comparison of numbers of motoneurons was made in these studies. Moreover, repetitive antidromic volleys did not completely silence gamma motoneurons (363,369), even when the volley was maximal for alpha axons in a muscle nerve (cf. 108,109).

In order to assess the relative strength of recurrent inhibition on the tonic firing of gastrocnemius-soleus and gamma motoneurons, Ellaway and Murphy (109) studied these two populations of neurons under similar conditions in decerebrate cats. They found that 91% of alpha and 54% of gamma motoneurons could be inhibited by antidromic volleys in alpha motoneuron axons. In this study, alpha motoneurons with low thresholds for tonic firing in response to stretch were recorded. These low-threshold alpha motoneurons are the small tonic units (349), which are found to be inhibited more frequently than large phasic motoneurons (107,332). Although some gamma motoneurons were inhibited as strongly as alpha motoneurons, they generally received less inhibition. Irrespective of the type of motoneurons, the duration of the inhibition was

---

*Not all gamma motoneurons were inhibited by the group Ia afferents excited by muscle vibration or brief stretches of the homonymous muscle. In fact, some were excited (369-371,375-378). The reflex is polysynaptic in comparison with the prominent monosynaptic spindle primary (Ia) action on alpha motoneurons. In addition to this autogenetic excitation of fusimotor neurons produced by selective stimulation of muscle spindle primary endings, there is evidence that the group Ib afferents from tendon organs might have autogenetic inhibitory connections to fusimotor neurons (373,376,379,380). These findings indicate that fusimotor neurons have reflex connections from group I afferents supplying muscle spindle receptors and Golgi tendon organs similar to the corresponding homonymous alpha motoneurons. However, these conditions do not exist for all fusimotor cells and the proprioceptive inputs appear to be weaker than those of the alpha motoneuron counterparts. Finally, discharge of secondary spindle endings may facilitate gamma motoneurons of the dynamic type (381,382; cf. 383). It is of interest that Ia autogenetic inhibition of gamma motoneurons following small muscle stretch, which are below threshold for Ib afferents (378) appeared with minimal segmental latencies (1.7 msec) similar to those in alpha motoneurons. These minimal latencies would be clearly within ranges for stretch-evoked disynaptic inhibitory postsynaptic potentials (220). It has been postulated that the early autogenetic inhibition of gamma motoneurons is evoked by the same interneurons that mediate the nonreciprocal Ia inhibition of alpha motoneurons rather than via R-cells (371). R-cells activated secondarily to excitation of alpha motoneurons could contribute only to later responses.

shown to be dependent upon the frequency of firing. Alpha and gamma motoneurons tended to have the same duration of recurrent inhibition if their discharge rates were comparable. However, since gamma motoneurons are able to
fire at higher rates than alpha motoneurons, the duration of recurrent inhibition
was generally longer (20-50 msec) for alpha motoneurons than for gamma
motoneurons (5-40 msec). Future experiments are required to find out whether
beta motoneurons, which innervate both skeletomotor and fusimotor fibers
(110a) are subjected to recurrent inhibition.

3.   Interneurons of the Group Ia Inhibitory Pathway

The Ia pathway, which supplies monosynaptic excitation to motoneurons innervating their own synergistic muscles, also gives rise to reciprocal inhibition of
motoneurons of muscles acting as antagonists at the same joint (228-230,401,
402). This reciprocal inhibition is not a "direct inhibition," but utilizes an interneuron—the Ia inhibitory interneuron; the details of this pathway are fully
discussed in another chapter (384). Reciprocal Ia inhibition is particularly efficient in small tonic alpha motoneurons, also when their high input resistance was
compensated for (385). While the terminations of R-cells responsible for recurrent inhibitory postsynaptic potentials are located largely on the proximal
dendrites of motoneurons, the terminations of the interneurons generating Ia
inhibitory postsynaptic potentials appear to be closer to or on the cell bodies
(227,328,329,348,385a). Moreover, there is evidence that opposite Ia inhibitory
interneurons (i.e., interneurons monosynaptically connected to antagonistic
muscles) mutually inhibit each other (58,226,386). If so, an increased activity in
Ia afferents from one muscle should secure an increased excitability of homonymous motoneurons, not only by direct monosynaptic excitation, but also by
releasing them from a possible reciprocal Ia inhibition (386).

Electrophysiologic experiments have indicated that Ia inhibitory interneurons are located in the ventral horn, dorsomedial to motor nuclei (large filled
circles in the drawings of the spinal gray matter in Fig. 2D). Their location is
different from that in which the R-cells are located, since they were found more
dorsally in lamina VII with respect to R-cells (46,51,58; cf. also 88). The Ia inhibitory interneurons are not identical with the Ia excited interneurons located in
the intermediate region, which originally were proposed to mediate Ia reciprocal
inhibition to motoneurons (15,62). In fact, these latter interneurons (points in
Fig. 2D), which are monosynaptically excited by Ia afferents, lack recurrent
inhibition and presumably project to some other neurons than motoneurons
(58; cf. 387). It is of interest that the Ia-excited interneurons that are responsible either for primary afferent depolarization in Ia afferent terminals (226) or
for the Ia inhibitory postsynaptic potential evoked in certain Ib ventral spinocerebellar tract neurons (387) are not affected by ventral root volleys.

Antidromic impulses in ventral roots or peripheral nerves effectively depress
transmission in the Ia inhibitory pathway to alpha motoneurons (226; cf. 388-
390, for review). In particular, the inhibitory postsynaptic potentials evoked by Ia

afferent volleys were effectively decreased when preceded by antidromic impulses in motor axons. This effect has been found for Ia inhibitory postsynaptic potentials in almost all tested motoneurons, including those that supply different flexor and extensor muscles of the hindlimb. This effect seems, therefore, to be a general property of Ia inhibitory pathways to hindlimb motoneurons. Since the depression occurred without any concomitant conductance change in the membrane of the recorded motoneurons and without excitability change in the group Ia primary afferents attributable to primary afferent depolarization, the observed effect is thought to be caused by inhibition of the Ia inhibitory pathway. By varying the interval between the conditioning and the testing volleys it was found that the depression occurred at an interval corresponding to a disynaptic linkage from motor axons to the Ia inhibitory interneurons. Furthermore, the time course of the depression was similar to that of the recurrent inhibition of motoneurons (1,6). These findings led to the conclusion that the recurrent depression of the Ia inhibitory postsynaptic potential was caused by postsynaptic inhibition of the Ia inhibitory interneurons evoked through alpha motor axon collaterals and R-cells (58,226,391). Indeed, large recurrent inhibitory postsynaptic potentials were seen during intracellular recording from Ia inhibitory interneurons (58,386,391a,392).

The relative contribution of different efferent nerves to the depression of transmission in Ia inhibitory pathways to different species of motoneurons has also been investigated (68,69). The depression of Ia inhibitory postsynaptic potentials in a given species of motoneuron was found to be mediated via axon collaterals of motoneurons supplying antagonists rather than those innervating synergists. In other words, in all motor nuclei investigated the strongest depression of Ia inhibitory postsynaptic potentials was evoked from motor fibers in those muscle nerves whose Ia afferents produced the inhibitory postsynaptic potentials. For example, the Ia inhibitory postsynaptic potential from the knee extensors recorded in motoneurons to a knee flexor was most effectively depressed by antidromic stimulation of motor fibers to the knee extensors. The depression of Ia inhibitory postsynaptic potentials from other nerves, if found at all, was always much weaker than that evoked from the nerve whose efferents elicited the Ia inhibitory postsynaptic potentials. The observation that recurrent collaterals from motoneurons activate R-cells that in turn inhibit the interneurons of the Ia inhibitory pathway has been confirmed and extended by several authors (58,69,88,226,388,389,391,393,394–400).

Since alpha motoneurons and Ia inhibitory interneurons that receive the same Ia connections may often act together, it was of interest to compare the origin of the recurrent inhibition of these two groups of neurons. It turned out that the distribution of recurrent effects are very similar, with the corresponding neurons always inhibited from the same efferent motor fibers (69). This parallelism appeared to be even more striking when the amplitudes of the recurrent inhibitory postsynaptic potentials in motoneurons were compared with the amount of inhibition of the corresponding Ia inhibitory interneurons (69). The great similarity between recurrent inhibition of alpha motoneurons and Ia inhibitory interneurons suggests that the same population of R-cells mediates effects to alpha motoneurons and to Ia inhibitory interneurons.*

It would be of interest to know the extent to which an increased Ia excitation of the Ia inhibitory interneurons would be counteracted by recurrent inhibition from motor axon collaterals. In an attempt to elucidate this problem, reciprocal inhibition of flexor motoneurons has been investigated during the tonic stretch reflex in the extensor muscles (403; cf. 404). With increasing stretch of extensor (quadriceps or triceps surae) muscle, there was first a linear augmentation of reciprocal inhibition, but concomitant with the stretch reflex in the extensor, a plateau appeared in the inhibition of the flexor, although the extensor stretch reflex increased with further stretching. Since the depth of reciprocal Ia inhibition depends on the activity in the Ia inhibitory interneurons, the results suggest that their firing frequency during the initial stage of extension increased in direct relation to the increased firing rate in the Ia afferents from the extended muscle. After the onset of the stretch reflex, their firing rate stabilized, mainly because the incrementing Ia excitation was now counteracted by increasing recurrent inhibition.

It has been proposed that recurrent inhibition of Ia inhibitory interneurons may serve a segmental autoregulatory mechanism that prevents excessive reciprocal Ia inhibition during increased alpha–gamma–linked excitation of agonists. The recurrent control of the Ia inhibitory interneurons therefore resembles that of small tonic alpha motoneurons, since in both cases the discharge frequency is stabilized by the stretch reflex. The effects of static and dynamic muscle stretches on the discharge of R-cells linked with the motoneurons innervating the stretched muscle have been described in Section III.B.1. The recurrent inhibitory action on Ia inhibitory interneurons was also investigated during static and dynamic muscle stretches. In particular, Benecke and Henatsch (405) have recorded in decerebrate or anesthetized cats the activity of Ia inhibitory interneurons during ramp stretches of the triceps surae. Ia inhibitory interneurons, monosynaptically activated from the gastrocnemius-soleus nerve, showed an increased firing during stretch as long as motoneuronal reflex responses were

*It has been reported previously (page 511) that Ia inhibitory interneurons projecting to antagonistic motoneurons mutually inhibit each other. In fact, interneurons that mediate reciprocal Ia inhibition to motoneurons also receive disynaptic Ia inhibitory postsynaptic potentials, namely, from nerves to antagonist muscles of those supplying Ia excitation to the interneurons (58,226,388–390). These Ia inhibitory postsynaptic potentials are also depressed by ventral root volleys (388,389).

absent. If, however, the stretch led to pronounced reflex responses of alpha motoneurons, a strong inhibitory influence on the Ia inhibitory interneurons via the R-pathway occurred; total blockage of firing was usually seen during the dynamic state of stretch synchronously with the burstlike firing of R-cells (399, 406). However, during the static phase of stretch, the Ia inhibitory interneuronal activity usually remained unaffected. Since the recurrent inhibition of the Ia interneurons depends upon the discharge of R-cells, these findings further support the conclusion that orthodromic activation of R-cells is predominantly linked to rapid phasic rather than to slow tonic motoneuronal firing (97,169). It is of interest that the increase in firing rate of individual Ia inhibitory interneurons (monosynaptically activated from the gastrocnemius-soleus nerve) during ramp stretch of the triceps surae was greatly enhanced after administration of dihydro-β-erythroidine, a substance that blocks cholinergic excitation of R-cells by motor axon collaterals (406).

Movements often depend on a coactivation of alpha and gamma motoneurons (16,150). To produce well-coordinated movements it is important that the neuronal pathways that evoke alpha-gamma-linked movements achieve a coupling between excitation of agonists and inhibition of antagonists by exciting not only alpha and gamma motoneurons to agonists but also Ia inhibitory interneurons impinging on motoneurons to antagonists (407,408). In this scheme the servo-assistance given by the γ-loop (cf. 150) will support not only the contraction of agonists but also the relaxation of antagonists (cf. also 409). This has been demonstrated during activation of macular labyrinthine reflexes (unpublished observations), during locomotion (311), and also during voluntary movements in man (410). In these experimental conditions the firing of the Ia inhibitory neurons coincided with the activation of the muscle that supplied their Ia afferent input. Moreover, experiments performed on de-efferented hindlimb, that is, where the γ-loop was broken, have indicated that the normal activation of the interneurons was due to convergent excitation from both the group Ia afferents as well as the central nervous structures that generated postural changes (unpublished observations) or stepping movements (311). There is also evidence that supraspinal descending systems acting directly on R-cells may not only modify the transmission in the recurrent pathway to motoneurons, but they may also change the sensitivity of the recurrent regulation of Ia inhibition (cf. 388).

Before concluding this section we should refer to a particular example of a spinal reflex pathway utilizing interneurons inhibited by recurrent inhibition. By intracellular recording from motoneurons in the lower sacral (S2–S3) segments of the spinal cord in cats, Jankowska et al. (72) analyzed the neuronal organization evoked in these motoneurons from contralateral afferents. Stimulation of the lowest threshold afferents of contralateral dorsal roots elicited inhibitory postsynaptic potentials in tail motoneurons with latencies similar to those of disynaptic inhibitory postsynaptic potentials evoked from group Ia muscle spindle afferents in ipsilateral limb motoneurons. The crossed disynaptic inhibitory postsynaptic potentials in sacral motoneurons were found to be mediated by interneurons that were themselves inhibited by R-cells, these interneurons and R-cells being activated from the dorsal and ventral roots, respectively, on the side of the body opposite to the location of the inhibited motoneurons. Furthermore, in unanesthetized decerebrate preparations crossed recurrent facilitation of sacral motoneurons was evoked with a time course similar to that of recurrent facilitation of lumbar motoneurons. This finding suggested a tonic inhibition of sacral motoneurons by interneurons responsible for their crossed disynaptic inhibition, and a disinhibition following stimulation of contralateral ventral roots. Crossed disynaptic inhibition of tail motoneurons under recurrent inhibitory control would indicate that the activity of the left and right side tail muscles may be as closely related as that of the strict antagonists operating at the same joint of a limb.

4. Interneurons of the Flexion Reflex Afferent Pathway

In addition to the efficient recurrent depression of Ia inhibitory postsynaptic potentials in motoneurons, Hultborn et al. (226) reported that some inhibitory postsynaptic potentials evoked from the ipsilateral flexion reflex afferents were also slightly depressed by volleys in ventral roots. On the other hand, inhibitory postsynaptic potentials from Ib afferents were not affected. The recurrent depression of the flexion reflex afferent inhibitory postsynaptic potentials was tentatively explained by a convergence of excitatory effects from the flexion reflex afferents on the Ia inhibitory interneurons, which were assumed to mediate at least part of the flexion reflex afferent inhibitory postsynaptic potential recorded in the motoneurons (226,408). If this interpretation is correct, then it would be expected that volleys in afferents that evoke an inhibitory postsynaptic potential susceptible to recurrent depression should also facilitate transmission in the Ia inhibitory pathway. Fedina and Hultborn (394; cf. 388) have indeed shown that Ia inhibitory postsynaptic potentials in flexors as well as in extensor motoneurons are facilitated by flexion reflex afferents (cutaneous and high-threshold muscle and joint afferents) and also through a separate neuronal pathway from low-threshold cutaneous afferents. It was postulated that the Ia inhibitory interneurons received excitatory actions from the ipsilateral flexion reflex afferents and through a separate pathway from low-threshold cutaneous afferents.*

The recurrent effects from motor axon collaterals were investigated on inhibitory transmission to motoneurons from different afferents. A strong positive correlation was found between the susceptibility of flexion reflex

---

*Flexion reflex afferents may also produce inhibitory postsynaptic potentials in Ia inhibitory interneurons (58,391a).

afferent inhibitory postsynaptic potentials to recurrent depression and the ability of flexion reflex afferent volleys to facilitate the transmission in the Ia inhibitory pathway to motoneurons. Likewise, the susceptibility of inhibitory postsynaptic potentials evoked in motoneurons from different descending systems (cortico-, rubro-, and vestibulospinal tracts as well as a presumed reticulospinal pathway descending in the medial longitudinal fasciculus) to recurrent depression correlated well with the ability of these systems to facilitate transmission in the Ia inhibitory pathway (388,396,397). All these findings indicate that the recurrent effects on motoneurons evoked either from primary afferents or from descending tracts are restricted to inhibition of the interneurons in the reciprocal Ia inhibitory pathway (226; cf. 388). Similar results were also obtained in an investigation of recurrent depression of inhibitory postsynaptic potentials from the contralateral flexion reflex afferents and effects from these afferents on the transmission in the Ia inhibitory pathways (411). In summary, it appears that the recurrent depression of inhibitory postsynaptic potentials from different primary afferents is restricted to the Ia inhibitory interneurons that mediate at least part of the inhibitory postsynaptic potentials evoked in the motoneurons from these afferents.

5. Renshaw Cells

Impulses in motor axons can give rise not only to recurrent inhibition, but also in some instances to recurrent facilitation of motoneurons (1). This effect, which can be elicited in some motoneurons following stimulation of other motor nuclei, has been attributed to disinhibition, that is, to recurrent inhibition from motor axon collaterals through R-cells of some tonically active inhibitory interneurons that evoke a steady hyperpolarization of the motoneurons (67,412–415; cf. 13). Interneurons inhibited from motor axon collaterals were studied by many investigators, although without identification of their excitatory afferent connections (36,44,280,415–418; cf. 17 for ref.).

Some of the interneurons inhibited during recurrent facilitation of motoneurons are Renshaw cells. Although first reported by Renshaw (2), mutual inhibition between R-cells was often doubted (6,269), but convincing evidence for its existence has been obtained by Ryall and coworkers (59,86–88,103). In particular, Ryall (86) has found that antidromic volleys in some deafferented motor nerve fibers in anesthetized cats can evoke a postsynaptic inhibition of R-cells without causing prior excitation. The brief latency of this inhibition, which is compatible with a disynaptic linkage, the similarity between the time course of the inhibition and that of the early discharge of R-cells, and the blocking action of dihydro-β-erythroidine indicate that other R-cells were responsible for the inhibition. The projections of R-cells to other R-cells has been found to extend ipsilaterally over distances up to 5.5 mm (59). No evidence of contralateral projections was obtained in this study.

The pattern of distribution of this inhibition was originally established by Renshaw (1) and Wilson et al. (67). Ryall (100–102; cf. 86) studied both the patterns of recurrent excitation and mutual inhibition of R-cells to antidromic volleys in motor axons in cats anesthetized with chloralose. While populations of R-cells received convergent excitation from motoneurons supplying functionally synergistic muscles (see Sec. III.A), mutual inhibition of R-cells was most effective when activated by antagonistic motoneurons. In particular, two major types of mutual inhibitory interactions were observed in which R-cells activated via axon collaterals of flexor or extensor motoneurons were inhibited by R-cells activated by the antagonistic motoneurons. It seems likely that one function of mutual inhibition could be to suppress liminal excitation of R-cells so as to sharpen the focus of convergent excitation and improve the selectivity of excitatory transmission to the R-cells.

Mutual inhibition may follow the excitation evoked by stimulation of a single motor nerve (59,86). The significance of mutual inhibition within a particular motor nucleus is unknown, but it may be quite different from the proposed significance of mutual inhibition between different motor nuclei (for instance, it may shorten the duration of the recurrent inhibition within a given motor pool).

Volleys in recurrent motor axon collaterals that inhibit the tonically active (58) interneurons interposed in the reciprocal Ia inhibitory pathway (cf. Sec. IV.A.3) may well contribute to the recurrent facilitation of motoneurons. Hultborn et al. (69) have investigated the pattern of recurrent inhibition of Ia inhibitory postsynaptic potentials in motoneurons. Although the motor nerves stimulated were different than those used in Ryall's (102) experiments, the pattern was superficially similar to that found for the mutual inhibition. In fact, the depression of Ia inhibitory postsynaptic potentials was evoked mainly from antagonists as was mutual inhibition in the Ryall study (102). In conclusion, the mutual inhibition of R-cells, together with recurrent inhibition of group Ia interneurons, may explain the phenomenon of recurrent facilitation of motoneurons. Although it has been reported that the inhibitory interaction between R-cells is very weak (419), the relative contribution of the two inhibitory mechanisms in determining the recurrent facilitation remains unknown.

6. Ventral Spinocerebellar Tract Neurons

Ventral spinocerebellar tract neurons receive monosynaptic excitation from Golgi tendon organ (Ib) afferents (420–423; cf. 424). The vast majority of neurons, however, receive strong polysynaptic effects, mainly inhibitory from the flexion reflex afferents (cf. 424). The cell bodies of the Ib ventral spinocerebellar tract neurons have been found scattered in a region located dorsomedially to the motor nuclei (425; cf. 46). Cells along the lateral border of the ventral horn, apparently identical with the "spinal border cells" of Cooper and

Sherrington (426), also contribute to the ventral spinocerebellar tract (427, 428). However, a number of these cells are monosynaptically excited from large muscle spindle (Ia) afferents, while Ib-excited cells are only occasionally encountered in this region (429). Furthermore, many of the "spinal border cells" are not monosynaptically excited by primary afferents (429,430; cf. 422,423). These data suggest that ventral spinocerebellar tract neurons can be divided into three main groups (see 390 for review) depending on whether they receive monosynaptic excitation from either Ia or Ib or are without monosynaptic excitation from primary afferents (387,421,422,429–431). A fourth smaller group of ventral spinocerebellar tract neurons seems to receive convergence of monosynaptic excitation from both Ia and Ib afferents (387,422,429–431).

a. *Recurrent inhibition of ventral spinocerebellar tract neurons.* Lindström and Schomburg (431) reported that a small proportion of ventral spinocerebellar tract neurons received recurrent inhibition upon antidromic stimulation of ventral roots. The inhibitory postsynaptic potentials were evoked by alpha fibers, had segmental latencies indicating a disynaptic linkage from the motor axons to the ventral spinocerebellar tract neurons, and had a duration of about 50 msec, that is, similar to the time course of the recurrent inhibitory postsynaptic potentials in motoneurons and Ia inhibitory interneurons (cf. 6,122). All the recurrently inhibited ventral spinocerebellar tract neurons received monosynaptic excitation from Ia afferents as do alpha motoneurons and Ia inhibitory interneurons. Moreover, the ventral roots giving rise to inhibition in a given ventral spinocerebellar tract cell were the same as those which produce recurrent inhibition in alpha motoneurons and in Ia inhibitory interneurons excited by Ia afferents of the same muscle as the ventral spinocerebellar tract cell (226). The results indicate that the same R-cells that project to alpha motoneurons and to Ia inhibitory interneurons also send collaterals to ventral spinocerebellar tract neurons. However, only a small proportion of Ia-excited ventral spinocerebellar tract neurons received recurrent inhibition (431). Other ventral spinocerebellar tract neurons received Ia excitation or Ia excitation together with effects from the descending systems known to affect Ia inhibitory interneurons (or motoneurons) without any recurrent inhibition. These findings indicate a high degree of selectivity of the connections to individual ventral spinocerebellar tract neurons. If the cerebellum compares the output from two similarly Ia-excited ventral spinocerebellar tract cells with and without recurrent inhibition, the difference in firing frequency between these two cells may give a measure of the strength of the recurrent inhibition of alpha motoneurons and Ia inhibitory interneurons (cf. 432).

b. *Recurrent inhibition of interneurons of the Ia inhibitory pathway to ventral spinocerebellar tract neurons.* Disynaptic Ia inhibitory postsynaptic potentials similar to those in motoneurons are evoked in all categories of ventral spinocerebellar tract neurons from nerves to hip and knee muscles, most frequently from the nerve to the knee extensor quadriceps (387,422,429,430). The hypothesis that the Ia inhibition of ventral spinocerebellar tract neurons is produced by activation of collateral connections from the interneurons that relay reciprocal Ia inhibition to motoneurons has been tested by Gustafsson and Lindström (430). These authors compared the pattern of synaptic convergence of Ia inhibitory interneurons to ventral spinocerebellar tract neurons and to motoneurons starting with one premise that Ia inhibitory interneurons to the latter cells are selectively inhibited from recurrent motor axon collaterals through R-cells (58,226,388). If the Ia inhibition of the ventral spinocerebellar tract cells is relayed through the same interneurons, then the Ia inhibitory postsynaptic potential in ventral spinocerebellar tract neurons should be depressed by conditioning antidromic impulses in ventral roots (cf. 226). If no such effect occurs, then the Ia inhibition of the ventral spinocerebellar tract must be mediated by interneurons other than those relaying Ia inhibition to motoneurons. Recurrent inhibition through motor axon collaterals and R-cells depressed not only the Ia inhibitory postsynaptic potentials on motoneurons (58,226), but also inhibitory postsynaptic potentials in ventral spinocerebellar tract neurons. Ia inhibitory postsynaptic potentials in ventral spinocerebellar tract cells excited from Ia afferents and those without group Ia excitation were particularly susceptible to recurrent depression elicited by volleys in motor axon collaterals (430,433), while the Ia inhibitory postsynaptic potentials in a considerable proportion of the ventral spinocerebellar tract cells excited from Ib afferents and in all the Ia/Ib cells were unaffected (387). Summing up, there are apparently two populations of Ia inhibitory interneurons producing Ia inhibitory postsynaptic potentials in ventral spinocerebellar tract neurons—one with, and one without, recurrent inhibition evoked from motor axon collaterals through R-cells.

It is of interest that disynaptic Ia inhibitory postsynaptic potentials were evoked in Ia ventral spinocerebellar tract neurons either from the same nerve as the one supplying monosynaptic Ia excitation to the cell or from the nerve to the antagonist muscle of the one supplying the Ia excitation (429). In both instances, the Ia inhibitory postsynaptic potentials were susceptible to recurrent depression (430).

The recurrent depression of Ia inhibitory postsynaptic potentials in ventral spinocerebellar tract neurons occurred without any recurrent inhibitory effect on the ventral spinocerebellar tract cells themselves (431). The latencies and time courses of this depression were similar to those seen in motoneurons (cf. 226, 430). Further, the effect was evoked from alpha efferents and inhibitory postsynaptic potentials from quadriceps were depressed from the L5 and L6 ventral roots, but not from the L7 and S1 ventral roots, while inhibitory postsynaptic potentials from the posterior biceps-semitendinosus nerve were depressed from the L7 and S1 ventral roots, but not from the L5 and L6 ventral roots (387,430).

The striking correspondence between the recurrent effects on Ia inhibitory post-synaptic potential in ventral spinocerebellar tract neurons and in motoneurons (226) is in accordance with the idea that the Ia inhibition in ventral spinocere-bellar tract neurons is evoked through collateral connections of the interneurons that relay Ia inhibition to motoneurons. The other explanation of the findings—namely, two parallel Ia inhibitory pathways, one directed to the ventral spino-cerebellar tract neurons and the other to motoneurons, and both being recur-rently controlled—is extemely unlikely (430).*

The results of recurrent stimulation on inhibitory postsynaptic potentials elicited from afferent systems other than the Ia afferents are entirely in accord-ance with the findings from motoneurons (387,430). Thus, Ib inhibitory post-synaptic potentials were reported to be unaffected by ventral root volleys, while inhibitory postsynaptic potentials evoked by stimulation of ipsilateral and contralateral flexion reflex afferents were depressed in some cells. It is note-worthy that recurrent depression of flexion reflex afferent inhibitory postsyn-aptic potentials were found only in ventral spinocerebellar tract cells with Ia inhibitory postsynaptic potentials susceptible to recurrent depression and not in the large sample of ventral spinocerebellar tract neurons lacking such inhibi-tion. In cells with recurrently affected flexion reflex afferent inhibitory post-synaptic potentials it was possible to facilitate the Ia inhibitory postsynaptic potentials from the flexion reflex afferents—a situation similar to that found in motoneurons. In addition, some disynaptic descending inhibitory postsynaptic potentials were recurrently depressed in cells with Ia inhibitory postsynaptic potentials. In unanesthetized preparations recurrent facilitatory potentials similar to those seen in motoneurons were evoked in ventral spinocerebellar tract neurons with Ia inhibitory postsynaptic potentials, but only from the ventral roots that depressed the Ia inhibitory postsynaptic potentials in the latter cells. Since all these effects were observed in cells lacking recurrent inhibition from motor axon collaterals, the recurrent effects on interneuronal transmission in the case of ventral spinocerebellar tract neurons can also be explained by a selec-tive action on the Ia inhibitory interneurons.

The results reported in this section are in agreement with the hypothesis formulated by Lundberg (432), namely, that ventral spinocerebellar tract cells monitor transmission in inhibitory pathways to motoneurons by comparing the output from last-order inhibitory interneurons to the excitatory input to the motoneurons. With respect to the ventral spinocerebellar tract neurons receiving

---

*Disynaptic Ia inhibitory postsynaptic potentials were also evoked in dorsal spinocerebellar tract (DSCT) neurons with monosynaptic excitation from group I muscle afferents (434,435). However, these inhibitory postsynaptic potentials were not sensitive to recurrent depression from motor axon collaterals (436).

monosynaptic excitation and/or disynaptic inhibition from Ia afferents, Lundberg (432) suggested that the Ia excitation of ventral spinocerebellar tract cells was related to the excitation of Ia inhibitory interneurons from these same afferents and that the corresponding inhibition of the ventral spinocerebellar tract was evoked through collateral connections from the Ia inhibitory interneurons. Ventral spinocerebellar tract cells with Ia excitation and inhibition from the same nerve could thus be considered as input–output comparators for this pathway. Other Ia-excited ventral spinocerebellar tract neurons may receive only the synaptic effects converging onto the Ia inhibitory interneurons or a fraction of these effects. These cells may in a wider sense contribute to the comparator function of the ventral spinocerebellar tract by providing the cerebellum with a reference for the input-output comparing cells. The hypothesis that the ventral spinocerebellar tract conveys information about transmission in segmental inhibitory pathways to motoneurons should be considered in relation to the extensive convergence from different segmental and descending sources onto the interneurons interrelated in such reflex pathways (cf. 58,99,408,437). It has been suggested that higher centers may need feedback information from these interneurons in order to achieve an accurate control of movements.

B. Respiratory Motoneurons

Although recurrent inhibition of motoneurons is a widespread phenomenon, it is neither uniformly nor universally present (see Sec. III.A). In the case of respiratory motoneurons, neither Gill and Kuno (84,85), who studied phrenic motoneurons, nor Sears (438), who investigated internal and external intercostal motoneurons, observed inhibitory postsynaptic potentials following antidromic volleys in motor axons. Sears (438) did, however, observe R-cell–like discharges in the ventral horn of the thoracic cord following stimulation of the intercostal nerves. Despite the equivocal nature of the evidence, intercostal motoneurons have been cited as examples of motoneurons that lack recurrent inhibition (226,362,439,440). Hultborn et al. (226) used these data to support their contention that the recurrent inhibition of motoneurons is strongly linked with the recurrent inhibition of Ia inhibitory interneurons. They argued that since intercostal motoneurons seem to be without Ia reciprocal inhibition, it made sense that they also lacked recurrent inhibition.

That the inspiratory and the expiratory muscles supplied by the intercostal nerves are not strict antagonists is shown by the observation that stimulation of low-threshold afferents in the internal intercostal nerve produces monosynaptic excitatory postsynaptic potentials in all the motoneurons supplying the internal intercostal nerve of the same segment, some motoneurons suppling the internal nerve of the adjacent segments, and 70% of the external intercostal nerve motoneurons of the same segment. On the other hand, monosynaptic excitation from external intercostal spindle afferents has been shown to occur in 70% of the external motoneurons of the same segment and some of the external intercostal motoneurons of adjacent segments (438,441,442). Moreover, no equivalent of the Ia inhibitory pathway, which is such an important feature of hindlimb reflex organization, has been demonstrated for intercostal motoneurons. The results reported by Kirkwood et al. (433,444) are at some variance with those of Hultborn et al. (226) in that the former workers demonstrated a reasonably strong Renshaw effect where reciprocal Ia inhibition does not seem to be an important factor. In particular, the external and internal intercostal nerves of a single intercostal space were stimulated in anesthetized paralyzed cats with the corresponding dorsal roots transected. Extracellular recording in the ventral horn revealed single units that fired in high-frequency bursts with a short latency to stimulation of either or both of the two nerves at stimulus strengths appropriate to the activation of alpha motor axons. The bursts could thus be attributed to activation of R-cells. Small (0.1–0.2 mV) hyperpolarizing potentials with a duration of up to 50 msec were also recorded intracellularly in both inspiratory and expiratory motoneurons of the same segment. Latencies and thresholds were appropriate for disynaptic inhibitory postsynaptic potentials evoked by collaterals of alpha motor axons. Finally, by studying the changes in the probability of firing of inspiratory alpha motoneurons following stimulation of the nerves of the corresponding segment or of other segments, a period of reduced probability of firing of up to 24 msec duration (corresponding to disynaptic inhibition from alpha motor axon collaterals) was seen in the segment stimulated and up to three segments distant. This finding implies a spread of the effect to six or seven segments following stimulation of one nerve. Either nerve could evoke such inhibition. However, the strongest effects on external intercostal motoneurons were seen following volleys in the internal intercostal nerve, while only a weak effect occurred by stimulating the external intercostal nerve. It is of interest that the length of the axons of R-cells related to intercostal motoneurons (up to 30 mm according to Kirkwood et al., 444) was longer than that measured by Jankowska and Smith (70) for R-cells related to hindlimb motoneurons (up to 11–13 mm), but both types of R-cell axons had comparable conduction velocities (14 m/sec). It was concluded that recurrent inhibition utilizing R-cells is present in intercostal motoneurons. Inspiratory or expiratory gamma discharges were inhibited less than the alphas in the same segment for stimulus strength that was appropriate for alpha motoneurons axons. According to Kirkwood et al. (443,444), all external intercostal motoneurons should be regarded as part of one motor nucleus (12 segments in length), but with partitioned reflex inputs illustrated by the restricted monosynaptic connections (three segments for any one afferent). The internal intercostal motor nucleus could be similarly defined and because of the monosynaptic connections to external intercostal nerve motoneurons, at least some of the muscles supplied by the internal intercostal nerve would have to be regarded as weak synergists of the external intercostal muscle. In these terms, then, it is quite consistent with published work on the limbs (6,68,104,226) that there should be a relatively strong recurrent effect on external intercostal motoneurons from stimulating the internal intercostal nerve, even with only a weak effect from stimulating the external intercostal nerve. Further experiments are required to find out whether the recurrent inhibition revealed on intercostal motoneurons is related more to respiratory function or to other functions of the intercostal musculature, such as those involved in posture.

C. Sympathetic and Parasympathetic Preganglionic Neurons

The problem of the recurrent inhibition in the intermediolateral sympathetic preganglionic neuron pool (B_2-SPN according to the classification of Lebedev et al., 445) should now be considered. The observation that one fourth of B_2-SPNs neurons submitted to pairs of antidromic stimuli could not generate a second antidromic spike at interstimulus intervals shorter than 20 msec, that is, at intervals far exceeding the likely duration of the absolute refractory period of the somata and axons of these neurons, has led to the suggestion that these neurons are subjected to recurrent inhibition from their neighbors (446).

However, Kirchner et al. (446-449) have expressed the opinion that B_2-SPNs lack recurrent inhibition. They attributed the prolonged lack of antidromic responsiveness in the wake of a test antidromic spike to prolonged subnormality or postfiring depression of the axons of SPNs.

In recent experiments performed in anesthetized, immobilized cats, Lebedev et al. (450) found that 32.5% of the B_2-SPN neurons in T3, T8-9 and L2 spinal segments could be reexcited antidromically by repeated stimuli only at very long interstimulus intervals (16 msec or more)—intervals that considerably exceed the refractoriness of the soma and axon of these neurons. In this group of neurons orthodromic spikes effectively inhibited the generation of antidromic ones for a period that was substantially longer than the possible collision time. The preceding antidromic activation of a fraction of the B_2-SPN segmental pool partly inhibited the orthodromic reactions of the other neurons in the same segment elicited by stimulation of segmental afferent fibers or of spinal descending pathways. These data definitely indicate that some of the B_2-SPN group have a recurrent inhibitory mechanism. It is of interest that this inhibition reached its maximum 5-7 msec after the arrival of the antidromic impulses at the spinal cord. The transmission of the inhibitory influences to B_2-SPNs could be performed disynaptically as shown for motoneurons (6). In fact, the discharge latency of R-cells after ventral root stimulation was about 1.2-2.0 msec and the rise time of recurrent inhibitory postsynaptic potentials was as long as 3-5 msec. Thus, the sum of these values is about the same as the maximum duration of inhibition of the B_2-SPNs. The neuronal elements that transmit the recurrent inhibitory influences to B_2-SPNs still remain to be identified.

In addition to sympathetic preganglionic neurons, recurrent inhibition may also affect parasympathetic preganglionic neurons (451,452). No crossed recurrent inhibition has so far been reported except for preliminary observations of Ishikawa (453); however, such inhibition of parasympathetic neurons is apparently mediated by a group of cells different from the typical R-cells (451,452).

V. FUNCTIONAL CONSIDERATIONS

The demonstration that hindlimb extensor motoneurons show a low resting discharge during the stretch reflex has been taken as evidence that recurrent inhibition acts as a negative feedback system that would serve the dual function of *stabilizing* and *limiting* the discharge frequency of strongly activated alpha motoneurons, without compromising recruitment of motoneurons that were not firing (6,10,11,16,19,68,107,116,137,204,331,333,454); cf., however, 455). In addition, it has been proposed on the basis of theoretical models that recurrent inhibition reduces the sensitivity of motoneurons to disturbances (456) and increases the speed of response of the motoneuronal discharge while increasing the stability of the system (457).

Recurrent inhibition affects not only the homonymous, but also and more prominently, the heteronymous motoneurons, that is, the motor nuclei of muscles linked in Ia synergism. This finding has led to the suggestion that recurrent inhibition may control the *spatial pattern* of the motor output by inhibiting surrounding groups of motoneurons (surround inhibition), thus focusing action on a given pool of alpha motoneurons. This would enhance the motor contrast (16,37,118,458,459; cf. 19), just as sensory contrast is sharpened by lateral (460–463) and afferent (464) inhibition.

After the demonstration that recurrent inhibition from motor axon collaterals involves not only the alpha motoneurons to synergistic muscles, but also the interneurons of the Ia inhibitory pathway to antagonistic muscles, the hypothesis of recurrent control of the spatial pattern of motor activity has been formulated in more specific terms (69). In particular, a decreased discharge of R-cells would act to suppress recurrent inhibition of both motoneurons and Ia inhibitory interneurons. This suppression would thus permit the development of the full pattern of Ia action, including heteronymous excitation and reciprocal inhibition. In contrast, an increased discharge of R-cells would spatially restrict the extent of excitatory effects on heteronymous motoneurons and prevent a concomitant reciprocal inhibition of motoneurons to antagonists. This would permit a more selective control of individual muscles via the γ-loop and would allow complex movements or postures involving cocontraction of extensors and flexors at the same joints. Appropriate experiments are required to verify this hypothesis.

In addition to spatial patterns, the *temporal pattern* of motoneuronal activity can be affected by recurrent inhibition. In fact, it has been suggested that recurrent inhibition may prevent the synchronized firing of motoneurons that might otherwise be evoked, together with tremor, when a strong excitatory input impinges on a motoneuron pool (465-470; cf. 471,472).

The hypotheses formulated previously are grounded on the assumption that R-cells are exclusively controlled by alpha motoneurons via their recurrent collaterals. In this situation, a coactivation of alpha motoneurons and their target R-cells occurs during the tonic stretch reflex and the vibration reflex (cf. 20,22) and during fictive locomotion (313-315). During the vibration reflex the increase in frequency of discharge of the Ia input was actually accompanied by a parallel increase in activity of the corresponding alpha motoneurons (98) and the related R-cells (97); in other words, the gain of the input-output curve relating the frequency of discharge of the Ia afferents to the frequency of discharge of the motoneurons (output) increased in spite of the increase in gain of response of the R-cells to the same excitatory input.

The demonstration, however, that R-cells are subjected to direct excitatory and inhibitory influences originating from certain peripheral or supraspinal sources suggests that under given conditions the amount of motoneuronal activity and the related muscular force may be determined by the amount of R-cell activity. There are in fact instances in which the activity of the two populations of alpha motoneurons and their target R-cells changes reciprocally as shown during stimulation of either the group II muscle afferents (249,270-272) or the cerebellar interpositus nucleus (285) and the internal capsule (286). Therefore, it has been postulated that the gain of the input-output curve relating the excitatory input to the activity of the pool of motoneurons (output) would increase when the R-cells are inhibited, but would decrease when the R-cells are facilitated (cf. 124). In this way, the recurrent inhibition may act a *variable gain regulator* at the motoneuronal level (473). In agreement with this hypothesis are the results of experiments reported in Sec. III.C. During the postural adjustments evoked by stimulation of macular labyrinthine reflexes in cat (307) as well as during voluntary movements in man (321,323), weak muscle contractions were accompanied by an increased discharge of R-cells. Conversely, strong muscle contractions were associated with a reduced discharge of R-cells which would reduce the gain of the recurrent loop, and thus enhance the motoneuronal discharge. The facilitation of R-cells during weak muscle contractions was apparently caused by the activity of a small number of alpha motoneurons through their recurrent collaterals, although a facilitation by supraspinal volleys acting directly on R-cells could not be excluded. On the other hand, a reduced discharge of R-cells, leading to strong muscle contractions, was attributed either to the reduced activity of a supraspinal excitatory pathway (307) or to the increased discharge of supraspinal or segmental inhibitory pathways (321, 323) acting on R-cells . In these instances, R-cells would be uncoupled from the corresponding alpha motoneurons. It should be mentioned that postural muscle contractions as well as voluntary movements may involve parallel and balanced excitation of alpha and gamma motoneurons of a muscle, as well as of the interneurons inhibiting its antagonists; therefore, all three groups of neurons have been considered together as forming an output stage of the motor system (Fig. 1; cf. 473). Since the same R-cells probably inhibit alpha motoneurons, gamma motoneurons, and Ia inhibitory interneurons, they could serve as a variable gain regulator at the level of this output stage (473).

The hypotheses discussed previously concerning the function of recurrent inhibition of alpha motoneurons via motor-axon collaterals and R-cells are based on the assumption that (1) all motoneurons contribute equally to the excitation of R-cells (cf. 91,330), and (2) recurrent inhibition within a pool is diffusely distributed among motoneurons and independent of motoneuronal size or type (131,300,336,337; cf. 90). The experimental evidence reviewed in this chapter, however, points to another type of organization in that recurrent inhibition is produced mainly by large phasic motoneurons that are recruited late, that is, at high tensions and that is received mainly by small tonic motoneurons activated with the weakest contractions (cf. Secs. III.B.1 and IV.A.1). The first aspect of this hypothesis, based on competition between phasic and tonic motoneurons to drive the recurrent inhibitory pathway, was largely supported by the results of physiologic experiments that showed that small tonic motoneurons activated during static stretch were only slightly effective in exciting the corresponding R-cells, while large phasic motoneurons, recruited during dynamic stretches (vibration), strongly excited the same R-cells for comparable discharge frequencies of the muscle spindle primary endings (cf. 20,22). These findings were later confirmed by the results of anatomic observations that showed that the diameter of central axons of alpha motoneurons, which correlates with the motoneuronal size, was strictly related to both size of their axon collaterals and number of their axon end branches (75,77). As to the second aspect of this hypothesis, physiologic experiments have demonstrated that recurrent inhibition acts more powerfully on small tonic than on large phasic motor units (340,341). Thus, these results support the conclusion that as more fast-contracting units are recruited—as in forceful phasic movements— slow motor unit activity may be subjected to recurrent inhibition from fast motoneurons.

Autogenic inhibition which acts asymmetrically from large phasic to small tonic motoneurons by utilizing R-cells may play an important role during fast movements. It is known that when large-sized motoneurons are recruited, small tonic motoneurons fire with a greater safety margin than do the bigger ones. The more prominent inhibitory influences of R-cells on small-sized motoneurons during recruitment of large-sized motoneurons would be particularly useful to counteract the safety margin that protects the small motoneurons against recurrent inhibition. This does not mean that recurrent inhibition driven by recruitment of large phasic alpha motoneurons during fast movements should be so strong as to switch off the activity of small tonic motoneurons. However, under certain conditions, this differential inhibitory influence may suppress tonic functions during fast movements—functions that might hinder the rapid movements (cf. 68,107,474). Such a relationship would appear to be advantageous under certain conditions, since slow motor units may require more than 100 msec to reach peak tension, and hence would compromise vigorous phasic movements.

The hypothesis that large motoneurons may suppress the activity of small-sized motoneurons has been opposed by Henneman and Mendell (90) who postulated that recruitment of motoneurons always occurs according to the size principle for both fast and for slow movements. Studies of slow and fast extensor motor-unit recruitment in freely moving cats performing a wide range of movements have indeed shown that slow units were actively involved in all movements, including powerful phasic movements such as maximal vertical jumps (475). Nevertheless, recent studies have demonstrated that reversal of the "usual" recruitment order with a selective recruitment of fast motor units and suppression of slow motor units may occur under certain conditions (476,477). These authors (476,477) suggested that preferential derecruitment of slow motor units occurs under conditions where the usual recruitment order is disadvantageous, such as rapid alternating or ballistic movements (but see 337). Demonstration of a differential recurrent inhibitory input related to size and/or type of motoneurons supports the hypothesis that the recurrent inhibitory system may play a role in such a derecruitment.

The pronounced asymmetry in the distribution of recurrent inhibition within a given motor nucleus should be taken into account while considering the hypothesis that the R-cells may serve as an adjustable gain regulator at the motoneuronal level (473). Actually, the presence of segmental or supraspinal pathways acting directly on R-cells by increasing or decreasing their activity should not uniformly modify the activity of all the alpha motoneurons, but namely, that of small tonic motoneurons. For instance, command signals for increased muscular force acting through separate, but parallel, channels both by exciting alpha motoneurons and reducing the discharge rate of R-cells, will obviously lead not only to recruitment and excitation of larger size agonist motoneurons following the size principle (cf. 90), but also to release from recurrent inhibition of small tonic motoneurons to the same agonist muscle. As a result of these changes, one should expect an increase in the force of muscle contraction, but a decrease in the velocity at which fast motor units contract. Disinhibition of small alpha motoneurons (and probably also of static gamma motoneurons) might also be associated with disinhibition of the Ia inhibitory interneurons to antagonistic motoneurons and thus lead to an increase in reciprocal inhibition. On the other hand, command signals for increasing muscular force exciting both alpha motoneurons as well as the related R-cells should lead to recruitment and excitation of larger size motoneurons, but now the small tonic motoneurons to the same agonist muscle would be subjected to a different amount of recurrent inhibition. In these conditions, the time to reach peak tension during vigorous phasic movements will not be compromised. Inhibition of small alpha motoneurons (and probably static gamma motoneurons) might also be coupled with inhibition of the Ia inhibitory interneurons to antagonistic motoneurons, thus reducing reciprocal inhibition.

Further experiments are required in order to define the modalities of operation of the recurrent inhibitory circuit when an increased muscular force is required during postural adjustments and slow ramp movements or during fast ballistic movements. It is reasonable to believe that R-cells and the related feedback mechanism from motor outflow may display a high degree of flexibility, thus playing crucial and subtle roles in the final control of different postural and motor tasks.

REFERENCES

1. Renshaw, B. (1941). Influence of discharge of motoneurons upon excitation of neighboring motoneurons. *J. Neurophysiol. 4*:167–183.

2. Renshaw, B. (1946). Central effects of centripetal impulses in axons of spinal ventral roots. *J. Neurophysiol. 9*:191–204.

3. Golgi, C. (1886). *Sulla Fina Anatomia degli Organi Centrali del Sistema Nervoso*, Hoepli, Milano.

4. Golgi, C. (1903). *Opera Omnia*, vol. II, Hoepli, Milano.

5. Cajal, S. R. y (1909). *Histologie du Système Nerveux de l'Homme et des Vertébrés*, vol. 1, Maloine Paris.

6. Eccles, J. C., Fatt, P., and Koketsu, K. (1954). Cholinergic and inhibitory synapses in a pathway from motor-axon collaterals to motoneurones. *J. Physiol. (Lond.) 126*:524–562.

7. Eccles, J. C. (1957). *The Physiology of Nerve Cells*, Johns Hopkins Press, Baltimore.

8. Eccles, J. C. (1961). Inhibitory pathways to motoneurons. In *Nervous Inhibition*, E. Florey (Ed.), Pergamon Press, Oxford, pp. 47–60.

9. Eccles, J. C. (1961). The synaptic mechanism for postsynaptic inhibition. In *Nervous Inhibition*, E. Florey (Ed.), Pergamon Press, Oxford, pp. 71–86.

10. Granit, R. (1961). Regulation of discharge rate by inhibition especially by recurrent inhibition. In *Nervous Inhibition*, E. Florey (Ed.), Pergamon Press, Oxford, pp. 61–70.

11. Granit, R. (1963). Recurrent inhibition as a mechanism of control. *Prog. Brain Res. 1*:23–37.
12. Eccles, J. C. (1964). *The Physiology of Synapses*, Springer-Verlag, Berlin.
13. Wilson, V. J. (1966). Regulation and function of Renshaw cell discharge. In *Muscular Afferents and Motor Control*, R. Granit (Ed.), Alqvist and Wiksell, Stockholm, pp. 317–329.
14. Eccles, J. C. (1969). Central cholinergic transmission and its behavioral aspects: Historical introduction. *Fed. Proc. 28*:90–94.
15. Eccles, J. C. (1969). *The Inhibitory Pathways of the Central Nervous System*, Charles C Thomas, Springfield, Illinois.
16. Granit, R. (1970). *The Basis of Motor Control*, Academic Press, New York.
17. Willis, W. D. (1971). The case for the Renshaw cell. *Brain, Behav. Evol. 4*:5–52.
18. Granit, R. (1972). *Mechanisms Regulating the Discharge of Motoneurons*, Liverpool University Press, Liverpool.
19. Haase, J., Cleveland, S., and Ross, H.-G. (1975). Problems of postsynaptic autogenous and recurrent inhibition in the mammalisn spinal cord. *Rev. Physiol. Pharmacol. 73*:74–129.
20. Pompeiano, O., and Wand, P. (1976). The relative sensitivity of Renshaw cells to static and dynamic changes in muscle length. *Prog. Brain Res. 44*: 199–222.
21. Burke, R. E., and Rudomín, P. (1977). Spinal neurons and synapses. In *Handbook of Physiology*, Sect. 1, *The Nervous System*, vol. I, *Cellular Biology of Neurons*, Part 1, E. R. Kandel (Ed.), American Physiological Society, Bethesda, pp. 877–944.
22. Wand, P., and Pompeiano, O. (1979). Contribution of different size motoneurons to Renshaw cell discharge during stretch vibration reflexes. *Prog. Brain Res. 50*:45–60.
23. Baldissera, F., Hultborn, H., and Illert, M. (1981). Integration in spinal neuronal systems. In *Handbook of Physiology*, Sect. 1, *The Nervous System*, vol. II, *Motor Control*, Part I, V. B. Brooks (Ed.), American Physiological Society, Bethesda, pp. 509–595.
24. Eccles, J. C., Eccles, R. M., and Fatt, P. (1956). Pharmacological investigations on a central synapse operated by acetylcholine. *J. Physiol. (Lond.) 131*:154–169.
25. Curtis, D. R., and Eccles, R. M. (1958). The excitation of Renshaw cells by pharmacological agents applied electrophoretically. *J. Physiol. (Lond.) 141*:435–445.
26. Curtis, D. R., and Eccles, R. M. (1958). The effect of diffusional barriers upon the pharmacology of cells within the central nervous system. *J. Physiol. (Lond.) 141*:446–463.
27. Curtis, D. R., Phillis, J. W., and Watkins, J. C. (1961). Cholinergic and noncholinergic transmission in the mammalian spinal cord. *J. Physiol. (Lond.) 158*:296–323.

28. Ryall, R. W., Stone, N. E., Curtis, D. R., and Watkins, J. C. (1964). Action of acetylcholine extracted from brain on spinal Renshaw cells. *Nature (Lond.) 201*:1034-1035.

29. Curtis, D. R., and Ryall, R. W. (1966). The excitation of Renshaw cells by cholinomimetics. *Exp. Brain Res. 2*:49-65.

30. Curtis, D. R., and Ryall, R. W. (1966). The acetylcholine receptors of Renshaw cells. *Exp. Brain Res. 2*:66-80.

31. Curtis, D. R., and Ryall, R. W. (1966). The synaptic excitation of Renshaw cells. *Exp. Brain Res. 2*:81-96.

32. Kuno, M., and Rudomín, P. (1966). The release of acetylcholine from the spinal cord of the cat by antidromic stimulation of motor nerves. *J. Physiol. (Lond.) 187*:177-193.

33. Krnjević, K. (1974). Chemical nature of synaptic transmission in vertebrates. *Physiol. Rev. 54*:418-540.

34. Cullheim, S., and Kellerth, J.-O. (1981). Two kinds of recurrent inhibition of cat spinal α-motoneurones as differentiated pharmacologically. *J. Physiol. (Lond.) 312*:209-224.

35. Eccles, J. C., Eccles, R. M., Iggo, A., and Lundberg, A. (1961). Electrophysiological investigations on Renshaw cells. *J. Physiol. (Lond.) 159*:461-478.

36. Frank, K., and Fuortes, M. G. F. (1956). Unitary activity of spinal interneurones of cats. *J. Physiol. (Lond.) 131*:424-435.

37. Brooks, V. B., and Wilson, V. J. (1959). Recurrent inhibition in the cat's spinal cord. *J. Physiol. (Lond.) 146*:380-391.

38. Willis, W. D., Skinner, R. D., and Weir, M. A. (1969). Field potentials of alpha and gamma motoneurons and Renshaw cells in response to activation of motor axons. *Exp. Neurol. 25*:57-69.

39. Rexed, B. (1952). The cytoarchitectonic organization of the spinal cord in the cat. *J. Comp. Neurol. 96*:415-466.

40. Rexed, B. (1954). A cytoarchitectonic atlas of the spinal cord in the cat. *J. Comp. Neurol. 100*:297-379.

41. Rexed, B. (1964). Some aspects of the cytoarchitectonics and synaptology of the spinal cord. *Prog. Brain Res. 11*:58-92.

42. Willis, W. D., and Willis, J. C. (1964). Location of Renshaw cells. *Nature 204*:1214-1215.

43. Thomas, R. C., and Wilson, V. J. (1965). Precise localization of Renshaw cells with a new marking technique. *Nature 206*:211-213.

44. Willis, W. D., and Willis, J. C. (1966). Properties of interneurons in the ventral spinal cord. *Arch. Ital. Biol. 104*:354-386.

45. Willis, W. D., Jr. (1969). The localization of functional groups of interneurons. In M. A. B. Brazier (Ed.), *The Interneuron*, UCLA Forum in Medical Sciences, No. 11, University of California Press, Berkeley, pp. 267-287.

46. Jankowska, E., and Lindström, S. (1972). Morphology of interneurones mediating 1a reciprocal inhibition of motoneurones in the spinal cord of the cat. *J. Physiol. (Lond.) 226*:805-823.

47. Jankowska, E. (1979). Identification and projections of Renshaw cells. *Neurosci. Lett. (Suppl.)3*:S312.

48. Jankowska, E., and Lindström, S. (1971). Morphological identification of Renshaw cells. *Acta Physiol. Scand. 81*:428–430.

49. van Keulen, L. C. M. (1971). Identification des cellules de Renshaw par l'injection intracellulaire, de la substance fluorescente "procion yellow." *J. Physiol. (Paris) 63*:131A.

50. van Keulen, L. C. M. (1971). Morphology of Renshaw cells. *Pflügers Arch. 328*:235–236.

51. Jankowska, E., and Lindström, S. (1973). Procion yellow staining of functionally identified interneurons in the spinal cord of the cat. In *Intracellular Staining Techniques in Neurobiology*, S. B. Kater and C. Nicholson (Eds.), Springer-Verlag, New York, pp. 199–209.

52. van Keulen, L. C. M. (1979). Axon trajectories of Renshaw cells in the lumbar spinal cord of the cat, as reconstructed after intracellular staining with horseradish peroxidase. *Brain Res. 167*:157–162.

53. Lagerbäck, P.-Å., Ronnevi, L.-O., Cullheim, S., and Kellerth, J.-O. (1981). An ultrastructural study of the synaptic contacts of α_1-motoneuron axon collaterals. II. Contacts in lamina VII. *Brain Res. 222*:29–41.

54. Lagerbäck, P.-Å., and Ronnevi, L.-O. (1982). An ultrastructural study of serially sectioned Renshaw cells. I. Architecture of the cell body, axon hillock, initial axon segment and proximal dendrites. *Brain Res. 235*:1–15.

55. Holmqvist, B. (1961). Crossed spinal reflex actions evoked by volleys in somatic afferents. *Acta Physiol. Scand. 52(Suppl. 181)*:1–67.

56. Scheibel, M. E., and Scheibel, A. B. (1964). Are there Renshaw cells? *Anat. Rec. 148*:332.

57. Scheibel, M. E., and Scheibel, A. B. (1966). Spinal motoneurons, interneurons and Renshaw cells. A Golgi study. *Arch. Ital. Biol. 104*:328–353.

58. Hultborn, H., Jankowska, E., and Lindström, S. (1971). Recurrent inhibition of interneurones monosynaptically activated from group Ia afferents. *J. Physiol. (Lond.) 215*:613–636.

59. Ryall, R. W., Piercey, M. F., and Polosa, C. (1971). Intersegmental and intrasegmental distribution of mutual inhibition of Renshaw cells. *J. Neurophysiol. 34*:700–707.

60. Scheibel, M. E., and Scheibel, A. B. (1971). Inhibition and the Renshaw cell. A structural critique. *Brain, Behav. Evol. 4*:53–93.

61. Ryall, R. W., Piercey, M. F., Polosa, C., and Goldfarb, J. (1972). Excitation of Renshaw cells in relation to orthodromic and antidromic excitation of motoneurons. *J. Neurophysiol. 35*:137–148.

62. Eccles, J. C., Fatt, P., and Landgren, S. (1956). The central pathway for the direct inhibitory action of impulses in the largest afferent nerve fibers to muscle. *J. Neurophysiol. 19*:75–98.

63. Testa, C. (1964). Functional implications of the morphology of spinal ventral horn neurons of the cat. *J. Comp. Neurol. 123*:425–433.

64. Erulkar, S. D., Nichols, C. W., Popp, M. B., and Koelle, G. B. (1968). Renshaw elements. Identification and acetylcholinesterase content. *J. Histochem. Cytochem.* 16:128–135.

65. Weight, F. (1968). Cholinergic mechanisms in recurrent inhibition of motoneurons. In *Psychopharmacology: A Review of Progress, 1957–1967*, Public Health Service Pub. No. 1856, pp. 69–75.

66. Szentágothai, J. (1967). Synaptic architecture of the spinal motoneuron pool. *EEG Clin. Neurophysiol. (Suppl.)* 25:4–19.

67. Wilson, V. J., Talbot, W. H., and Diecke, F. P. J. (1960). Distribution of recurrent facilitation and inhibition in cat spinal cord. *J. Neurophysiol.* 23:144–153.

68. Eccles, J. C., Eccles, R. M., Iggo, A., and Ito, M. (1961). Distribution of recurrent inhibition among motoneurones. *J. Physiol. (Lond.)* 159: 479–499.

69. Hultborn, H., Jankowska, E., and Lindström, S. (1971). Relative contribution from different nerves to recurrent depression of Ia IPSPs in motoneurones. *J. Physiol. (Lond.)* 215:637–664.

70. Jankowska, E., and Smith, D. O. (1973). Antidromic activation of Renshaw cells and their axonal projections. *Acta Physiol. Scand.* 88:198–214.

71. Romanes, G. J. (1951). The motor cell columns of the lumbo-sacral spinal cord of the cat. *J. Comp. Neurol.* 94:313–363.

72. Jankowska, E., Padel, Y., and Zarzecki, P. (1978). Crossed disynaptic inhibition of sacral motoneurones. *J. Physiol. (Lond.)* 285:425–444.

73. Prestige, M. C. (1966). Initial collaterals of motor axons within the spinal cord of the cat. *J. Comp. Neurol.* 126:123–135.

74. Cullheim, S., and Kellerth, J.-O. (1976). Combined light and electron microscopic tracing of neurons, including axons and synaptic terminals, after intracellular injection of horseradish peroxidase. *Neurosci. Lett.* 2: 307–313.

75. Cullheim, S., and Kellerth, J. O. (1978). A morphological study of the axons and recurrent axon collaterals of cat sciatic α-motoneurons after intracellular staining with horseradish peroxidase. *J. Comp. Neurol.* 178: 537–558.

76. Cullheim, S., and Kellerth, J.-O. (1978). A morphological study of the axons and recurrent axon collaterals of cat α-motoneurons supplying different hind-limb muscles. *J. Physiol. (Lond.)* 281:285–299.

77. Cullheim, S., and Kellerth, J.-O. (1978). A morphological study of the axons and recurrent axon collaterals of cat α-motoneurones supplying different functional types of muscle unit. *J. Physiol. (Lond.)* 281:301–313.

78. Westbury, D. R. (1982). A comparison of the structures of α- and γ-spinal motoneurones of the cat. *J. Physiol. (Lond.)* 325:79–91.

79. Cullheim, S., Kellerth, J.-O., and Conradi, S. (1977). Evidence for direct synaptic interconnections between cat spinal α-motoneurons via the recurrent axon collaterals: A morphological study using intracellular injection of horseradish peroxidase. *Brain Res.* 132:1–10.

80. Evinger, C., Baker, R., and McCrea, R. A. (1979). Axon collaterals of cat medial rectus motoneurones. *Brain Res. 174*:153–160.

81. Lagerbäck, P.-Å., Ronnevi, L.-O., Cullheim, S., and Kellerth, J.-O. (1978). Ultrastructural characteristics of a central cholinergic synapse in the cat. *Brain Res. 148*:197–201.

82. Lagerbäck, P.-Å., Ronnevi, L.-O., Cullheim, S., and Kellerth, J.-O. (1981). An ultrastructural study of the synaptic contacts of α-motoneurone axon collaterals. I. Contacts in lamina IX and with identified α-motoneurone dendrites in lamina VII. *Brain Res. 207*:247–266.

82a. Eggar, M. D., Freeman, N. C. G., and Proshansky, E. (1980). Morphology of spinal motoneurones mediating a cutaneous spinal reflex in the cat. *J. Physiol. (Lond.) 306*:349–363.

83. Sasaki, K. (1963). Electrophysiological studies on oculomotor neurons of the cat. *Jpn. J. Physiol. 13*:287–302.

84. Gill, P. K., and Kuno, M. (1963). Properties of phrenic motoneurones. *J. Physiol. (Lond.) 168*:258–273.

85. Gill, P. K., and Kuno, M. (1963). Excitatory and inhibitory actions on phrenic motoneurones. *J. Physiol. (Lond.) 168*:274–289.

86. Ryall, R. W. (1970). Renshaw cell mediated inhibition of Renshaw cells: Patterns of excitation and inhibition from impulses in motor axon collaterals. *J. Neurophysiol. 33*:257–270.

87. Ryall, R. W., and Piercey, M. (1970). Excitatory and inhibitory convergence onto Renshaw cells from motor axon collaterals. *Fed. Proc. 29*:391.

88. Ryall, R. W., and Piercey, M. F. (1971). Excitation and inhibition of Renshaw cells by impulses in peripheral afferent nerve fibers. *J. Neurophysiol. 34*:242–251.

89. Burke, R. E., Strick, P. L., Kanda, K., Kim, C. C., and Walmsley, B. (1977). Anatomy of medial gastrocnemius and soleus motor nuclei in cat spinal cord. *J. Neurophysiol. 40*:667–680.

90. Henneman, E., and Mendell, L. M. (1981). Functional organization of motoneuron pool and its inputs. In *Handbook of Physiology*, Sect. 1, *The Nervous System*, vol. II, *Motor Control*, Part 1, V. B. Brooks (Ed.), American Physiological Society, Bethesda, pp. 423–507.

91. Kato, M., and Fukushima, K. (1974). Effect of differential blocking of motor axons on antidromic activation of Renshaw cells in the cat. *Exp. Brain Res. 20*:135–143.

92. Eccles, J. C., and Sherrington, C. S. (1930). Numbers and contraction-values of individual motor-units examined in some muscles of the limb. *Proc. R. Soc. Lond. (Biol.) 106*:326–357.

93. Gilliatt, R. W. (1966). Axon branching in motor nerves. In *Control and Innervation of Skeletal Muscle*, B. L. Andrew (Ed.), Livingston, Edinburgh, pp. 53–63.

94. Ebel, H. C., and Gilman, S. (1969). Estimation of errors in conduction velocity measurements due to branching of peripheral nerve fibers. *Brain Res. 16*:273–276.

95. Copack, P. B., Felman, E., Lieberman, J. S., and Gilman, S. (1975). Differences in proximal and distal conduction velocities of efferent nerve fibers to the medial gastrocnemius muscle. *Brain Res. 91*:147–150.
96. Pompeiano, O., Wand, P., and Sontag, K.-H. (1974). A quantitative analysis of Renshaw cell discharges caused by stretch and vibration reflexes. *Brain Res. 66*:519–524.
97. Pompeiano, O., Wand, P., and Sontag, K.-H. (1975). The relative sensitivity of Renshaw cells to orthodromic group Ia volleys caused by static stretch and vibration of extensor muscles. *Arch. Ital. Biol. 113*:238–279.
98. Wand, P., Pompeiano, O., and Fayein, N. A. (1980). The relative sensitivity of different size motoneurons to group Ia volleys caused by static stretch and vibration of extensor muscles. *Arch. Ital. Biol. 118*:243–269.
99. Lundberg, A. (1966). Integration in the reflex pathway. In *Muscular Afferents and Motor Control*, R. Granit (Ed.), Almqvist and Wiksell, Stockholm, pp. 275–305.
100. Ryall, R. W. (1972). Excitatory convergence on Renshaw cells. *J. Physiol. (Lond.) 226*:69P–70P.
101. Ryall, R. W. (1979). Excitation and mutual inhibition of Renshaw cells. *Neurosci. Lett. (Suppl.) 3*:S315.
102. Ryall, R. W. (1981). Patterns of recurrent excitation and mutual inhibition of cat Renshaw cells. *J. Physiol. (Lond.) 316*:439–452.
103. Ryall, R. W., Piercey, M. F., and Polosa, C. (1972). Strychnine-resistant mutual inhibition of Renshaw cells. *Brain Res. 41*:119–129.
104. Thomas, R. C., and Wilson, V. J. (1967). Recurrent interactions between motoneurons of known location in the cervical cord of the cat. *J. Neurophysiol. 30*:661–674.
105. Cullheim, S., and Ulfhake, B. (1979). Observations on the morphology of intracellularly stained γ-motoneurons in relation to their axon conduction velocity. *Neurosci. Lett. 13*:47–50.
106. Westbury, D. R. (1979). The morphology of four gamma motoneurones examined by horseradish peroxidase histochemistry. *J. Physiol. (Lond.) 292*:25P–26P.
107. Granit, R., Pascoe, J. E., and Steg, G. (1957). The behaviour of tonic α and γ motoneurones during stimulation of recurrent collaterals. *J. Physiol. (Lond.) 138*:381–400.
108. Ellaway, P. H., and Murphy, P. R. (1980). A quantitative comparison of recurrent inhibition of alpha and gamma motoneurones in the cat. *J. Physiol. (Lond.) 301*:55P–56P.
109. Ellaway, P. H., and Murphy, P. R. (1980). A comparison of the recurrent inhibition of α- and γ-motoneurones in the cat. *J. Physiol. (Lond.) 315*:43–58.
110. Westbury, D. R. (1980). Lack of a contribution from gamma motoneurone axons to Renshaw inhibition in the cat spinal cord. *Brain Res. 186*:217–221.
110a. Emonet-Denand, F., and Laporte, Y. (1975). Proportion of muscle spindles supplied by skeleto-fusimotor axons (β-axons) in the peroneus brevis muscle of the cat. *J. Neurophysiol. 38*:1390–1394.

111. Willis, W. D., Grace, R. R., and Skinner, R. D. (1967). Ventral root afferent fibres and the recurrent inhibitory pathway. *Nature 216*:1010–1011.

112. Longo, V. G., Martin, W. R., and Unna, K. R. (1960). A pharmacological study on the Renshaw cell. *J. Pharmacol. Exp. Ther. 129*:61–68.

113. Curtis, D. R., and Duggan, A. W. (1969). On the existence of Renshaw cells. *Brain Res. 15*:597–599.

114. Walmsley, B., and Tracey, D. J. (1981). An intracellular study of Renshaw cells. *Brain Res. 223*:170–175.

115. Curtis, D. R., Game, C. J. A., Lodge, D., and McCullock, R. M. (1976). A pharmacological study of Renshaw cell inhibition. *J. Physiol. (Lond.) 258*: 227–242.

116. Granit, R., Haase, J., and Rutledge, L. T. (1960). Recurrent inhibition in relation to frequency of firing and limitation of discharge rate of extensor motoneurones. *J. Physiol. (Lond.) 154*:308–328.

117. Granit, R., and Renkin, B. (1961). Net depolarization and discharge rate of motoneurones, as measured by recurrent inhibition. *J. Physiol. (Lond.) 158*:461–475.

118. Meyer-Lohmann, J., Henatsch, H.-D., Benecke, R., and Hellweg, C. (1976). Muscle stretch and chemical muscle spindle excitation: Effects on Renshaw cells and efficiency of recurrent inhibition. *Prog. Brain Res. 44*:223–233.

119. Haase, J. (1963). Die Transformation des Entladungsmusters der Renshaw-Zellen bei tetanischer antidromer Reizung. *Pflügers Arch. 276*:471–480.

120. Ross, H.-G., Cleveland, S., and Haase, J. (1975). Response of Renshaw cells to minimal antidromic input at various frequencies. *Pflügers Arch. (Suppl.) 355*:R91.

121. Ross, H.-G. (1976). *Experimentelle Untersuchungen und Modellvorstellungen zur quantitativen Charakterisierung der rekurrenten Inhibition spinaler Alpha-Motoneurone*, Habilitationsschrift, Düsseldorf.

122. Ross, H.-G., Cleveland, S., and Haase, J. (1976). Quantitative relation between discharge frequencies of a Renshaw cell and an intracellularly depolarized motoneuron. *Neurosci. Lett. 3*:129–132.

123. Cleveland, S., Kuschmierz, A., and Ross, H.-G. (1981). Static input–output relations in the spinal recurrent inhibitory pathway. *Biol. Cybern. 40*: 223–231.

124. Hultborn, H., and Pierrot-Deseilligny, E. (1979). Input–output relations in the pathway of recurrent inhibition to motoneurones in the cat. *J. Physiol. (Lond.) 297*:267–287.

125. Ross, H.-G., Cleveland, S., and Haase, J. (1975). Contribution of single motoneurones to Renshaw cell activity. *Neurosci. Lett. 1*:105–108.

126. van Keulen, L. C. M. (1979). Relations between individual motoneurones and individual Renshaw cells. *Neurosci. Lett. (Suppl.) 3*:S313.

127. van Keulen, L. C. M. (1981). Autogenetic recurrent inhibition of individual spinal motoneurones of the cat. *Neurosci. Lett. 21*:297–300.

128. Granit, R., Phillips, C. G., Skoglund, S., and Steg, G. (1957). Differentiation of tonic from phasic alpha ventral horn cells by stretch, pinna and crossed extensor reflexes. *J. Neurophysiol. 20*:470–481.

129. Kuno, M. (1959). Excitability following antidromic activation in spinal motoneurones supplying red muscles. *J. Physiol. (Lond.) 149*:374–393.

130. Henneman, E., Somjen, G., and Carpenter, D. O. (1965). Functional significance of cell size in spinal motoneurons. *J. Neurophysiol. 28*:560–580.

131. Henneman, E., Somjen, G., and Carpenter, D. O. (1965). Excitability and inhibitability of motoneurons of different sizes. *J. Neurophysiol. 28*:599–620.

132. Anastasijević, R., Anojčic, M., Todorović, B., and Vučo, J. (1968). The differential reflex excitability of alpha motoneurons of decerebrate cats caused by vibration applied to the tendon of the gastrocnemius medialis muscles. *Brain Res. 11*:336–346.

133. Anastasijević, R., Cvetković, M., and Vučo, J. (1971). The effect of short-lasting repetitive vibration of the triceps muscle and concomitant fusimotor stimulation on the reflex response of spinal alpha motoneurones in decerebrated cats. *Pflügers Arch. 325*:220–234.

134. Tan, Ü. (1971). Changes in firing rates of extensor motoneurones caused by electrically increased spinal inputs. *Pflügers Arch. 326*:35–47.

135. Tan, Ü. (1972). The role of recurrent and presynaptic inhibition in the depression of tonic motoneuronal activity. *Pflügers Arch. 337*:229–239.

136. Tan, Ü., Yörükan, S., and Ridvanağaoğlu, A. Y. (1972). A quantitative analysis of the motoneuronal depression produced by increasing the stimulus parameters of afferent tetanization. *Pflügers Arch. 333*:240–257.

137. Granit, R. (1962). Quantitative aspects of control of the discharge frequency of nerve cells. *Proceedings XXII International Congress of Physiological Sciences, Leiden*, I, part 1:22–27.

138. Piercey, M. F., and Goldfarb, J. (1974). Discharge patterns of Renshaw cells evoked by volleys in ipsilateral cutaneous and high-threshold muscle afferents and their relationship to reflexes recorded in ventral roots. *J. Neurophysiol. 37*:294–302.

139. Lloyd, D. P. C. (1943). Conduction and synaptic transmission of the reflex response to stretch in spinal cats. *J. Neurophysiol. 6*:317–326.

140. Eccles, J. C., Eccles, R. M., and Lundberg, A. (1957). The convergence of monosynaptic excitatory afferents on to many different species of alpha motoneurones. *J. Physiol. (Lond.) 137*:22–50.

141. Eccles, J. C., Eccles, R. M., and Lundberg, A. (1960). Types of neurone in and around the intermediate nucleus of the lumbosacral cord. *J. Physiol. (Lond.) 154*:89–114.

142. Tsukahara, N., and Ohye, C. (1964). Polysynaptic activation of extensor motoneurones from group Ia fibres in the cat spinal cord. *Experientia 20*:628–629.

143. Cook, W. A., Jr., Neilson, D. R., Jr., and Brookhart, J. M. (1965). Primary afferent depolarization and monosynaptic reflex depression following succinylcholine administration. *J. Neurophysiol. 28*:290–311.

144. Decandia, M., Gasteiger, E. L., and Mann, M. D. (1971). Excitability changes of extensor motoneurons and primary afferent endings during prolonged stimulation of flexor afferents. *Exp. Brain Res.* *12*:150–160.
145. Kanda, K. (1972). Contribution of polysynaptic pathways to tonic vibration reflex. *Jpn. J. Physiol.* *22*:367–377.
146. Homma, S., and Kanda, K. (1973). Impulse decoding process in stretch reflex. In *Motor Control*, A. A. Gydikov, N. T. Tankov, and D. S. Kosarov (Eds.), Plenum, New York, pp. 45–64.
147. Homma, S., Kanda, K., and Mizote, M. (1973). Role of mono- and polysynaptic reflex arcs during the stretch reflex. *EEG Clin. Neurophysiol.* *34*: 799.
148. Hultborn, H., Wigström, H., and Wängberg, B. (1975). Prolonged activation of soleus motoneurones following a conditioning train in soleus Ia afferents—A case for a reverberating loop? *Neurosci. Lett.* *1*:147–152.
149. Hultborn, H., and Wigström, H. (1980). Motor response with long latency and maintained duration evoked by activity in Ia afferents. In *Spinal and Supraspinal Mechanisms of Voluntary Motor Control and Locomotion*, J. E. Desmedt (Ed.), Karger, Basel, *Prog. Clin. Neurophysiol.* *8*:99–115.
150. Matthews, P. B. C. (1972). *Mammalian Muscle Receptors and Their Central Actions*, Edward Arnold, London.
151. Pacheco, P., and Guzman-Flores, C. (1969). Intracellular recording in extensor motoneurones of spastic cats. *Exp. Neurol.* *25*:472–481.
152. Mendell, L. M., and Henneman, E. (1971). Terminals of single Ia fibers: Location, density, and distribution within a pool of 300 homonymous motoneurons. *J. Neurophysiol.* *34*:171–187.
153. Stauffer, E. K., Watt, D. G. D., Taylor, A., Reinking, R. M., and Stuart, D. G. (1976). Analysis of muscle receptor connections by spike-triggered averaging. 2. Spindle group II afferents. *J. Neurophysiol.* *39*:1393–1402.
154. Taylor, A., Watt, D. G. D., Stauffer, E. K., Reinking, R. M., and Stuart, D. G. (1976). Use of afferent triggered averaging to study the central connections of muscle spindle afferents. *Prog. Brain Res.* *44*:171–181.
155. Watt, D. G. D., Stauffer, E. K., Taylor, A., Reinking, R. M., and Stuart, D. (1976). Analysis of muscle receptor connections by spike-triggered averaging. 1. Spindle primary and tendon organ afferents. *J. Neurophysiol.* *39*:1375–1392.
156. Schomburg, E. D., and Behrends, H. B. (1978). The possibility of phase-dependent monosynaptic and polysynaptic Ia excitation to homonymous motoneurones during fictive locomotion. *Brain Res.* *143*:533–537.
157. Munson, J. B., and Sypert, G. W. (1979). Properties of single central Ia afferent fibres projecting to motoneurons. *J. Physiol. (Lond.)* *296*:315–327.
158. Jankowska, E., McCrea, D., and Mackel, R. (1981). Oligosynaptic excitation of motoneurones by impulses in group Ia muscle spindle afferents in the cat. *J. Physiol. (Lond.)* *316*:411–425.

159. Czarkowska, J., Jankowska, E., and Sybirska, E. (1981). Common inter-
     neurones in reflex pathways from group Ia and Ib afferents of knee flexors
     and extensors in the cat. *J. Physiol. (Lond.) 310*:367–380.
160. Jankowska, E., Johannisson, T., and Lipski, J. (1981). Common inter-
     neurones in reflex pathways from group Ia and Ib afferents of ankle ex-
     tensors in the cat. *J. Physiol. (Lond.) 310*:381–402.
161. Haase, J., and Vogel, B. (1971). Die Erregung der Renshaw-Zellen durch
     reflektorische Entladungen der α-Motoneurone. *Pflügers Arch. 325*:
     14–27.
162. Ross, H.-G., Cleveland, S., and Haase, J. (1972). Quantitative relation of
     Renshaw cell discharge to monosynaptic reflex height. *Pflügers Arch. 332*:
     73–79.
163. Pompeiano, O., Wand, P., and Sontag, K.-H. (1974). Excitation of Renshaw
     cells by orthodromic group Ia volleys following vibration of extensor
     muscles. *Pflügers Arch. 347*:137–144.
164. Pompeiano, O., Wand, P., and Sontag, K.-H. (1975). Response of Renshaw
     cells to sinusoidal stretch of hindlimb extensor muscles. *Arch. Ital. Biol.
     113*:205–237.
165. Hultborn, H., Pierrot-Deseilligny, E., and Wigström, H. (1979). Recurrent
     inhibition and afterhyperpolarization following motoneuronal discharge
     in the cat. *J. Physiol. (Lond.) 297*:253–266.
166. Ross, H.-G., Cleveland, S., Wolf, E., and Haase, J. (1973). Changes in the
     excitability of Renshaw cells due to orthodromic tetanic stimuli. *Pflügers
     Arch. 344*:299–307.
167. Benecke, R., Hellweg, C., and Meyer-Lohmann, J. (1974). Activity and
     excitability of Renshaw cells in nondecerebrate and decerebrate cats. *Exp.
     Brain Res. 21*:113–124.
168. Hellweg, C., Meyer-Lohmann, J., Benecke, R., and Windhorst, U. (1974).
     Responses of Renshaw cells to muscle ramp stretch. *Exp. Brain Res. 21*:
     353–360.
169. Pompeiano, O., Wand, P., and Sontag, K.-H. (1975). The sensitivity of
     Renshaw cells to velocity of sinusoidal stretches of the triceps surae
     muscle. *Arch. Ital. Biol. 113*:280–294.
170. Bianconi, R., and Van der Meulen, J. P. (1963). The response to vibration
     of the end organs of mammalian muscle spindles. *J. Neurophysiol. 26*:
     177–190.
171. Brown, M. C., Engberg, I., and Matthews, P. B. C. (1967). The relative
     sensitivity to vibration of muscle receptors of the cat. *J. Physiol. (Lond.)
     192*:773–800.
172. Stuart, D. G., Mosher, C. G., Gerlach, R. L., and Reinking, R. M. (1970).
     Selective activation of Ia afferents by transient muscle stretch. *Exp. Brain
     Res. 10*:477–487.
173. Granit, R., Henatsch, H.-D. (1956). Gamma control of dynamic properties
     of muscle spindles. *J. Neurophysiol. 19*:356–366.
174. Granit, R. (1958). Neuromuscular interaction in postural tone of the cat's
     isometric soleus muscle. *J. Physiol. (Lond.) 143*:387–402.

175. Matthews, P. B. C., and Stein, R. B. (1969). The sensitivity of muscle spindle afferents to small sinusoidal changes of length. *J. Physiol. (Lond.)* 200:723–743.

176. Wand, P., Pompeiano, O., and Fayein, N. A. (1980). Impulse decoding process in extensor motoneurones of different size during the vibration reflex. *Arch. Ital. Biol.* 118:205–242.

177. Hagbarth, K.-E., and Eklund, G. (1966). Motor effects of vibratory muscle stimuli in man. In *Muscular Afferents and Motor Control*, R. Granit (Ed.), Almqvist and Wiksell, Stockholm, pp. 177–186.

178. Matthews, P. B. C. (1966). The reflex excitation of the soleus muscle of the decerebrate cat caused by vibration applied to its tendon. *J. Physiol. (Lond.)* 184:450–472.

179. Matthews, P. B. C. (1967). Vibration and the stretch reflex. In *Myotatic, Kinesthetic and Vestibular Mechanisms*, Ciba Foundation Symposium, A. V. S. de Reuck and J. Knight, (Eds.), Churchill, London, pp. 40–50.

180. Barnes, C. D., and Pompeiano, O. (1970). Presynaptic and postsynaptic effects in the monosynaptic reflex pathway to extensor motoneurons following vibration of synergic muscles. *Arch. Ital. Biol.* 108:259–294.

181. Noske, W., Ross, H.-G., Cleveland, S., and Haase, J. (1974). Decrease of antidromic inhibition due to orthodromic tetanic stimuli. *Pflügers Arch.* 350:223–230.

182. Cleveland, S., and Ross, H.-G. (1977). Dynamic properties of Renshaw cells: Frequency response characteristics. *Biol. Cybern.* 27:175–184.

183. Van Meter, W. G. (1978). Temporal analysis of post tetanic depression of antidromically activated Renshaw cells. *Soc. Neurosci. Abstr.* 4:572.

184. Cleveland, S., and Ross, H.-G. (1981). Antidromic inhibition of spinal motoneurons reflects the response properties of Renshaw cells. *Pflügers Arch. (Suppl.)* 389:R33.

185. Ross, H.-G., Cleveland, S., and Kuschmierz, A. (1982). Dynamic properties of Renshaw cells: Equivalence of responses to step changes in recruitment and discharge frequency of motor axons. *Pflügers Arch.* 394:239–242.

186. Kernell, D. (1966). Input resistance, electrical excitability, and size of ventral horn cells in cat spinal cord. *Science* 152:1637–1640.

187. Burke, R. E. (1967). Motor unit types of cat triceps surae muscle. *J. Physiol. (Lond.)* 193:141–160.

188. Burke, R. E. (1968). Group Ia synaptic input to fast and slow twitch motor units of cat triceps surae. *J. Physiol. (Lond.)* 196:605–630.

189. Burke, R. E. (1968). Firing patterns of gastrocnemius motor units in the decerebrate cat. *J. Physiol. (Lond.)* 196:631–654.

190. Burke, R., and ten Bruggencate, G. (1971). Electrotonic characteristics of alpha motoneurones of varying size. *J. Physiol. (Lond.)* 212:1–20.

191. Westbury, D. R. (1971). The response of α-motoneurones of the cat to sinusoidal movements of the muscles they innervate. *Brain Res.* 25:75–86.

192. Westbury, D. R. (1972). A study of stretch and vibration reflexes of the cat by intracellular recording from motoneurones. *J. Physiol. (Lond.)* 226:37–56.

193. Anastasijević, R., Stanojević, M., and Vučo, J. (1976). Patterns of motoneuronal units discharge during naturally evoked afferent input. *Prog. Brain Res.* 44:267–278.

194. Homma, S., Ishikawa, K., and Watanabe, S. (1967). Optimal frequency of muscle vibration for motoneuron firing. *J. Chiba Med. Soc.* 43:190–196.

195. Brown, M. C., Lawrence, D. G., and Matthews, P. B. C. (1968). Reflex inhibition by Ia afferent input of spontaneously discharging motoneurons in the decerebrate cat. *J. Physiol. (Lond.)* 198:5P–7P.

196. Homma, S., Ishikawa, K., and Stuart, D. G. (1970). Motoneuron responses to linearly rising muscle stretch. *Am. J. Phys. Med.* 49:290–306.

197. Homma, S., Kobayashi, H., and Watanabe, S. (1970). Vibratory stimulation of muscles and stretch reflex. *Jpn. J. Physiol.* 20:309–319.

198. Homma, S., Kanda, K., and Watanabe, S. (1971). Monosynaptic coding of group Ia afferent discharges during vibratory stimulation of muscle. *Jpn. J. Physiol.* 21:405–417.

199. Homma, S., Kanda, K., and Watanabe, S. (1972). Preferred spike intervals in the vibration reflex. *Jpn. J. Physiol.* 22:421–432.

200. Eccles, J. C., Eccles, R. M., and Lundberg, A. (1958). The action potentials of the alpha motoneurones supplying fast and slow muscles. *J. Physiol. (Lond.)* 142:275–291.

201. Clamann, H. P., Gillies, I. D., Skinner, R. D., and Henneman, E. (1974). Quantitative measures of output of a motoneuron pool during monosynaptic reflexes. *J. Neurophysiol.* 37:1328–1337.

202. Denny-Brown, D. (1929). On the nature of postural reflexes. *Proc. R. Soc. (Biol.)* 104:252–301.

203. Meyer-Lohmann, J., and Henatsch, H.-D. (1966). Die Bedeutung der natürlichen recurrenten Hemmung (NRH) für die Frequenz tonisch entladender Extensor-α-Motoneurone. *Pflügers Arch. (Suppl.)* 291:R3.

204. Grillner, S., and Udo, M. (1971). Motor unit activity and stiffness of the contracting muscle fibres in the tonic stretch reflex. *Acta Physiol. Scand.* 81:422–424.

205. Grillner, S., and Udo, M. (1971). Recruitment in the tonic stretch reflex. *Acta Physiol. Scand.* 81:571–573.

206. Grillner, S. (1973). A consideration of stretch and vibration data in relation to the tonic stretch reflex. In *Advances in Behavioral Biology, Control of Posture and Locomotion*, vol. 7, R. B. Stein, K. B. Pearson, R. S. Smith, and J. B. Redford (Eds.), Plenum, New York, pp. 397–405.

207. Henneman, E., and Harris, D. (1976). Identification of fast and slow firing types of motoneurones in the same pool. *Prog. Brain Res.* 44:377–380.

208. Harris, D. A., and Henneman, E. (1977). Identification of two species of alpha motoneurons in cat's plantaris pool. *J. Neurophysiol.* 40:16–25.

209. Granit, R. (1950). Reflex self-regulation of the muscle contraction and autogenetic inhibition. *J. Neurophysiol.* 13:351–372.

210. Hunt, C. C. (1952). The effect of stretch receptors from muscle on the discharge of motoneurones. *J. Physiol. (Lond.)* 117:359–379.

211. Laporte, Y., and Lloyd, D. P. C. (1952). Nature and significance of the reflex connections established by large afferent fibers of muscular origin. *Am. J. Physiol. 169*:609–621.

212. Eccles, J. C., Eccles, R. M., and Lundberg, A. (1957). Synaptic actions on motoneurones in relation to the two components of the group I muscle afferent volley. *J. Physiol. (Lond.) 136*:527–546.

213. Eccles, J. C., Eccles, R. M., and Lundberg, A. (1957). Synaptic actions on motoneurones caused by impulses in Golgi tendon organ afferents. *J. Physiol. (Lond.) 138*:227–252.

214. Paintal, A. S. (1960). Functional analysis of group III afferent fibres of mammalian muscles. *J. Physiol. (Lond.) 152*:250–270.

215. Willis, W. D., Núñez, R., and Rudomín, P. (1976). Excitability changes of terminal arborizations of single Ia and Ib afferent fibers produced by muscle and cutaneous conditioning volleys. *J. Neurophysiol. 39*:1150–1159.

216. Brown, A. G., and Fyffe, R. E. W. (1978). The morphology of group Ib muscle afferent fiber collaterals. *J. Physiol. (Lond.) 277*:44P–45P.

217. Hongo, T., Ishizuka, N., Mannen, H., and Sasaki, S. (1978). Axonal trajectory of single group Ia and Ib fibers in the cat spinal cord. *Neurosci. Lett. 8*:321–328.

218. Lucas, M. E., and Willis, W. D. (1974). Identification of muscle afferents which activate interneurons in the intermediate nucleus. *J. Neurophysiol. 37*:282–293.

219. Fetz, E. E., Jankowska, E., Johannisson, T., and Lipski, J. (1979). Autogenetic inhibition of motoneurones by impulses in group Ia muscle spindle afferents. *J. Physiol. (Lond.) 293*:173–195.

220. Jankowska, E., McCrea, D., and Mackel, R. (1981). Pattern of "nonreciprocal" inhibition of motoneurones by impulses in group Ia muscle spindle afferents in the cat. *J. Physiol. (Lond.) 316*:393–409.

221. Lundberg, A., Malmgren, K., and Schomburg, E. D. (1977). Cutaneous facilitation of transmission in reflex pathways from Ib afferents to motoneurones. *J. Physiol. (Lond.) 265*:763–780.

222. Jankowska, E., and McCrea, D. (1980). Evidence that the nonreciprocal inhibition of spinal motoneurones by Ia muscle spindle afferents and by Ib tendon organ afferents is mediated by the same interneurones. *Acta Physiol. Scand. 109*:18A.

223. Hongo, T., Jankowska, E., and Lundberg, A. (1966). Convergence of excitatory and inhibitory action on interneurones in the lumbosacral cord. *Exp. Brain Res. 1*:338–358.

224. Czarkowska, J., Jankowska, E., and Sybirska, E. (1976). Axonal projections of spinal interneurones excited by group I afferents in the cat, revealed by intracellular staining with horseradish peroxidase. *Brain Res. 118*:115–118.

225. Jankowska, E. (1979). New observations on neuronal organization of reflexes from tendon organ afferents and relation to reflexes evoked from muscle spindle afferents. *Prog. Brain Res. 50*:29–36.

226. Hultborn, H., Jankowska, E., and Lindström, S. (1971). Recurrent inhibition from motor axon collaterals of transmission in the Ia inhibitory pathway to motoneurones. *J. Physiol. (Lond.)* 215:591–612.

227. Jankowska, E., and Roberts, W. J. (1972). Synaptic actions of single interneurones mediating reciprocal Ia inhibition of motoneurones. *J. Physiol. (Lond.)* 222:623–642.

228. Lloyd, D. P. C. (1943). Reflex action in relation to pattern and peripheral source of afferent stimulation. *J. Neurophysiol.* 6:111–120.

229. Lloyd, D. P. C. (1943). Neuron patterns controlling transmission of ipsilateral hind limb reflexes in cat. *J. Neurophysiol.* 6:293–315.

230. Lloyd, D. P. C. (1946). Facilitation and inhibition of spinal motoneurones. *J. Neurophysiol.* 9:421–438.

231. Hunt, C. C. (1954). Relation of function to diameter in afferent fibers of muscle nerves. *J. Gen. Physiol.* 38:117–131.

232. Eccles, R. M., and Lundberg, A. (1959). Synaptic actions in motoneurones by afferents which may evoke the flexion reflex. *Arch. Ital. Biol.* 97:199–221.

233. Lundberg, A., Malmgren, K., and Schomburg, E. D. (1975). Characteristics of the excitatory pathway from group II muscle afferents to alpha motoneurones. *Brain Res.* 88:538–542.

234. Lundberg, A. (1964). Supraspinal control of transmission in reflex paths to motoneurones and primary afferents. *Prog. Brain Res.* 12:197–221.

235. Laporte, Y., and Bessou, P. (1959). Modification d'excitabilité de motoneurones homonymes provoquées par l'activation physiologique de fibres afférentes d'origine nusculaire du groupe II. *J. Physiol. (Paris)* 51:897–908.

236. Cook, W. A., Jr., and Duncan, C. C., Jr. (1971). Contribution of group I afferents to the tonic stretch reflex of the decerebrate cat. *Brain Res. 33:* 509–513.

237. Cangiano, A., and Lutzemberger, L. (1972). The action of selectively activated group II muscle afferent fibers on extensor motoneurons. *Brain Res.* 41:475–478.

238. Emonet-Dénand, F., Jami, L., Joffry, M., and Laporte, Y. (1972). Absence de réflexe myotatique après blocage de la conduction dans les fibres du groupe I. *C. R. Acad. Sci. (Paris)* 274:1542–1545.

239. Kanda, R., and Rymer, W. Z. (1977). An estimate of the secondary spindle receptor afferent contribution to the stretch reflex in extensor muscles of the decerebrate cat. *J. Physiol. (Lond.)* 264:63–87.

240. Chapman, C. E., Michalski, W. J., and Séguin, J. J. (1979). The effects of cold-induced muscle spindle secondary activity on monosynaptic and stretch reflexes in the decerebrate cat. *Can. J. Physiol. Pharmacol. 57:* 606–614.

241. Kato, M., and Fukushima, K. (1976). Selective activation of group II muscle afferents and its effects on cat spinal neurones. *Prog. Brain Res.* 44:185–196.

242. Matthews, P. B. C. (1969). Evidence that the secondary as well as the primary endings of muscle spindles may be responsible for the tonic stretch reflex of the decerebrate cat. *J. Physiol. (Lond.)* 204:365-393.

243. Matthews, P. B. C. (1970). The origin and functional significance of the stretch reflex. In *Excitatory Synaptic Mechanisms*, P. Andersen and J. K. S. Jansen (Eds.), Universitetsforlaget, Oslo, pp. 301-315.

244. Grillner, S. (1970). Is the tonic stretch reflex dependent upon group II excitation? *Acta Physiol. Scand.* 78:431-432.

245. Grillner, S., and Udo, M. (1970). Is the tonic stretch reflex dependent on suppression of autogenetic inhibitory reflexes? *Acta Physiol. Scand.* 79: 13A-14A.

246. Matthews, P. B. C. (1970). A reply to criticism of the hypothesis that the group II afferents contribute excitation to the stretch reflex. *Acta Physiol. Scand.* 79:431-433.

247. McGrath, G. J., and Matthews, P. B. C. (1973). Evidence from the use of vibration during procaine nerve block that the spindle group II fibres contribute excitation to the tonic stretch reflex of the decerebrate cat. *J. Physiol. (Lond.)* 235:371-408.

248. Matthews, P. B. C. (1973). A critique of the hypothesis that the spindle secondary endings contribute excitation to the stretch reflex. In *Advances in Behavioral Biology, Control of Posture and Locomotion*, vol. 7, R. B. Stein, K. G. Pearson, R. S. Smith, and J. B. Redford (Eds.), Plenum, New York, pp. 227-243.

249. Fromm, C., Haase, J., and Wolf, E. (1977). Depression of the recurrent inhibition of extensor motoneurones by the action of group II afferents. *Brain Res.* 120:459-468.

250. Grillner, S. (1973). Muscle stiffness and motor control-forces in the ankle during locomotion and standing. In *Motor Control*, A. A. Gydikov, N. T. Tankov, and D. S. Kosarov (Eds.), Plenum, New York, pp. 195-215.

251. Jack, J. J. B., and Roberts, R. C. (1978). The role of muscle spindle afferents in stretch and vibration reflexes of the soleus muscle of the decerebrate cat. *Brain Res.* 146:366-372.

252. Alnaes, E., and Jansen, J. K. S. (1970). Summary of the discussion on the stretch reflex. In *Excitatory Synaptic Mechanisms*, P. Andersen and J. K. S. Jansen (Eds.), Universitetsforlaget, Oslo, pp. 323-325.

253. Wilson, V. J., and Kato, M. (1965). Excitation on extensor motoneurons by group II afferent fibers in ipsilateral muscle nerves. *J. Neurophysiol.* 28:545-554.

254. Lund, S., and Pompeiano, O. (1970). Electrically induced monosynaptic and polysynaptic reflexes involving the same motoneuronal pool in the unrestrained cat. *Arch. Ital. Biol.* 108:130-153.

255. Tan, Ü. (1979). The effects of electrically stimulated group I and II extensor afferents on agonist motoneurons. *Neurosci. Lett. (Suppl.)* 3:S102.

256. Wand, P., Pompeiano, O., and Fayein, N. A. (1981). Effects of repetitive stimulation of group I and group II muscle afferents on homonymous motoneurons. *Arch. Ital. Biol.* 119:52-75.

257. Fukushima, K., and Kato, M. (1975). Spinal interneurons responding to group II muscle afferent fibers in the cat. *Brain Res. 90*:307–312.

258. Fu, T. C., Santini, M., and Schomburg, E. D. (1974). Characteristics and distribution of spinal focal synaptic potentials generated by group II muscle afferents. *Acta Physiol. Scand. 91*:298–313.

259. Fu, T. C., and Schomburg, E. D. (1974). Electrophysiological investigation of the projection of secondary muscle spindle afferents in the cat spinal cord. *Acta Physiol. Scand. 91*:314–329.

260. Kirkwood, P. A., and Sears, T. A. (1974). Monosynaptic excitation of motoneurones from secondary endings of muscle spindles. *Nature 252*: 243–244.

261. Kirkwood, P. A., and Sears, T. A. (1975). Monosynaptic excitation of motoneurones from muscle spindle secondary endings of intercostal and triceps surae muscles in the cat. *J. Physiol. (Lond.) 245*:64P–66P.

262. Lüscher, H.-R., Ruenzel, P., Fetz, E., and Henneman, E. (1979). Postsynaptic population potentials recorded from ventral roots perfused with isotonic sucrose: Connections of groups Ia and II spindle afferent fibers with large populations of motoneurons. *J. Neurophysiol. 42*:1146–1164.

263. Lüscher, H.-R., Ruenzel, P., and Henneman, E. (1980). Topographic distribution of terminals of Ia and group II fibers in spinal cord, as revealed by postsynaptic population potentials. *J. Neurophysiol. 43*:968–985.

264. Sypert, G. W., Fleshman, J. W., and Munson, J. B. (1980). Comparison of monosynaptic actions of medial gastrocnemius group Ia and group II muscle spindle afferents on triceps surae motoneurons. *J. Neurophysiol. 44*:726–738.

265. Lundberg, A., Malmgren, K., and Schomburg, E. D. (1977). Comments on reflex actions evoked by electrical stimulation of group II muscle afferents. *Brain Res. 122*:551–555.

266. Magherini, P. C., Pompeiano, O., and Thoden, U. (1972). The relative significance of presynaptic and postsynaptic effects on monosynaptic extensor reflexes during vibration of synergic muscles. *Arch. Ital. Biol. 110*:70–89.

267. Thoden, U., Magherini, P. C., and Pompeiano, O. (1972). Evidence that presynaptic inhibition may decrease the autogenetic excitation caused by vibration of extensor muscles. *Arch. Ital. Biol. 110*:90–116.

268. Pompeiano, O. (1975). Autogenetic excitation and presynaptic inhibition during vibration of extensor muscles. In *Sensory Organization of Movements*, A. S. Batuev (Ed.), Izdatelstvo "Nauka," Leningrad, pp. 164–173.

269. Wilson, V. J. Talbot, W. H., and Kato, M. (1964). Inhibitory convergence upon Renshaw cells. *J. Neurophysiol. 27*:1063–1079.

270. Fromm, C., Haase, J., and Wolf, E. (1975). Decrease of the recurrent inhibition of extensor motoneurons due to group II afferent input. *Pflügers Arch. (Suppl.) 359*:R78.

271. Wand, P., Pompeiano, O., and Fayein, N. A. (1978). Recurrent inhibition of the motoneuronal discharge elicited by mechanical or electrical stimulation of the group I afferents. *Pflügers Arch. (Suppl.) 373*:R70.

272. Benecke, R., Meyer-Lohmann, J., and Henatsch, H.-D. (1976). Evidence for an inhibitory action from secondary muscle spindle endings on Renshaw cells. *III. International Symposium on Motor Control*, pp. 26–29.

273. Wilson, V. J., and Talbot, W. H. (1963). Integration at an inhibitory interneurone: Inhibition of Renshaw cells. *Nature 200*:1325–1327.

274. Bergmans, J., Burke, R., and Lundberg, A. (1969). Inhibition of transmission in the recurrent inhibitory pathway to motoneurones. *Brain Res. 13*:600–602.

275. Holmqvist, B., and Lundberg, A. (1961). Differential supraspinal control of synaptic actions evoked by volleys in the flexion reflex afferents in alpha motoneurones. *Acta Physiol. Scand. 54(Suppl. 186)*:1–51.

276. Andén, N.-E., Jukes, M. G. M., Lundberg, A., and Vyklický, L. (1966). The effect of DOPA on the spinal cord. 1. Influence on transmission from primary afferents. *Acta Physiol. Scand. 67*:373–386.

277. Jankowska, E., Jukes, M. G. M., Lund, S., and Lundberg, A. (1967). The effect of DOPA on the spinal cord. 5. Reciprocal organization of pathways transmitting excitatory action to alpha motoneurones of flexors and extensors. *Acta Physiol. Scand. 70*:369–388.

278. Brown, T. G. (1911). The intrinsic factors in the act of progression in the mammal. *Proc. R. Soc. Lond. (Biol.) 84*:308–319.

279. Engberg, I., and Lundberg, A. (1969). An electromyographic analysis of muscular activity in the hindlimb of the cat during unrestrained locomotion. *Acta Physiol. Scand. 75*:614–630.

280. Koizumi, K., Uschiyama, J., and Brooks, C. McC. (1959). A study of reticular formation action on spinal interneurones and motoneurones. *Jpn. J. Physiol. 9*:282–303.

281. Haase, J., and Van der Meulen, J. P. (1961). Effects of supraspinal stimulation on Renshaw cells belonging to extensor motoneurones. *J. Neurophysiol. 24*:510–520.

282. Henatsch, H.-D., Kaese, H.-J., Langrehr, D., and Meyer-Lohmann, J. (1961). Einflüsse des motorischen Cortex der Katze auf die Renshaw-Rückkoppelungshemmung der Motoneurone. *Pflügers Arch. 274*:51–52.

283. MacLean, J. B., and Leffman, H. (1967). Supraspinal control of Renshaw cells. *Exp. Neurol. 18*:94–104.

284. Haase, J., and Vogel, B. (1971). Direkte und indirekte Wirkungen supraspinaler Reizungen auf Renshaw-Zellen. *Pflügers Arch. 325*:334–346.

285. Benecke, R., Meyer-Lohmann, J., and Guntau, J. (1976). Inverse changes in the excitability of Renshaw cells and α-motoneurones induced by interpositus stimulation. *Pflügers Arch. (Suppl.) 365*:R40.

286. Koehler, W., Windhorst, U., Schmidt, J., Meyer-Lohmann, J., and Henatsch, H.-D. (1978). Diverging influences on Renshaw cell responses and monosynaptic reflexes from stimulation of capsula interna. *Neurosci. Lett. 8*:35–39.

287. Windhorst, U., Ptok, M., Meyer-Lohmann, J., and Schmidt, J. (1978). Effects of conditioning stimulation of the contralateral n. ruber on antidromic Renshaw cell responses and monosynaptic reflexes. *Pflügers Arch. (Suppl.) 373*:R70.

288. Holmqvist, B., and Lundberg, A. (1959). On the organization of the supraspinal inhibitory control of interneurones of various spinal reflex arcs. *Arch. Ital. Biol. 97*:340-356.

289. Lindsay, K. W., Roberts, T. D. M., and Rosenberg, J. R. (1976). Asymmetric tonic labyrinth reflexes and their interaction with neck reflexes in the decerebrate cat. *J. Physiol. (Lond.) 261*:583-601.

290. Schor, R. H., and Miller, A. D. (1981). Vestibular reflexes in neck and forelimb muscles evoked by roll tilt. *J. Neurophysiol. 46*:167-178.

290a. Manzoni, D., Pompeiano, O., Srivastava, U. C., and Stampacchia, G. (1983). Responses of forelimb extensors to sinusoidal stimulation of macular labyrinth and neck receptors. *Arch. Ital. Biol. 121*:205-214.

291. Lund, S., and Pompeiano, O. (1968). Monosynaptic excitation of alphamotoneurones from supraspinal structures in the cat. *Acta Physiol. Scand. 73*:1-21.

292. Pompeiano, O. (1975). Vestibulo-spinal relationships. In *The Vestibular System*, R. F. Naunton (Ed.), Academic Press, New York, pp. 147-180.

293. Boyle, R., and Pompeiano, O. (1980). Reciprocal responses to sinusoidal tilt of neurons in Deiters' nucleus and their dynamic characteristics. *Arch. Ital. Biol. 118*:1-32.

294. Boyle, R., and Pompeiano, O. (1981). Convergence and interaction of neck and macular vestibular inputs on vestibulospinal neurons. *J. Neurophysiol. 45*:852-868.

295. Schor, R. H., and Miller, A. D. (1982). Relationship of cat vestibular neurons to otolith-spinal reflexes. *Exp. Brain Res. 47*:137-144.

296. Llinás, R., and Terzuolo, C. A. (1964). Mechanisms of supraspinal actions upon spinal cord activities. Reticular inhibitory mechanisms on alphaextensor motoneurons. *J. Neurophysiol. 27*:579-591.

297. Llinás, R., and Terzuolo, C. A. (1965). Mechanisms of supraspinal actions upon spinal cord activities. Reticular inhibitory mechanisms upon flexor motoneurons. *J. Neurophysiol. 28*:413-422.

298. Jankowska, E., Lund, S., Lundberg, A., and Pompeiano, O. (1968). Inhibitory effects evoked through ventral reticulospinal pathways. *Arch. Ital. Biol. 106*:124-140.

299. Peterson, B. P., Pitts, N. G., and Fukushima, K. (1979). Reticulospinal connections with limb and axial motoneurons. *Exp. Brain Res. 36*:1-20.

300. Magoun, H. W., and Rhines, R. (1946). An inhibitory mechanism in the bulbar reticular formation. *J. Neurophysiol. 9*:165-171.

301. Manzoni, D., Pompeiano, O., Stampacchia, G., and Srivastava, U. C. (1983). Responses of medullary reticulospinal neurons to sinusoidal stimulation of labyrinth receptors in decerebrate cat. *J. Neurophysiol. 50*:1059-1079.

301a. Pompeiano, O. (1984). A comparison of the response characteristics of vestibulospinal and medullary reticulospinal neurons to labyrinth and neck inputs. In *Brainstem Control of Spinal Cord Function*, C. D. Barnes (Ed.), Academic Press, New York, pp. 87-140.

302. Pompeiano, O. (1975). Macular input to neurons of the spinoreticulocerebellar pathway. *Brain Res. 95*:351–368.
303. Pompeiano, O. (1979). Neck and macular labyrinthine influences on the cervical spino-reticulocerebellar pathway. *Prog. Brain Res. 50*:501–514.
304. Srivastava, U. C., Manzoni, D., Pompeiano, O., and Stampacchia, G. (1982). State-dependent properties of medullary reticular neurons involved during the labyrinth and neck reflexes. *Neurosci. Lett. (Suppl.) 10*:S461.
305. Pompeiano, O. (1980). Cholinergic activation of reticular and vestibular mechanisms controlling posture and eye movements. In *The Reticular Formation Revisited*, J. A. Hobson and M. A. B. Brazier (Eds.), Raven, New York, pp. 473–512.
306. Thoden, U., Magherini, P. C., and Pompeiano, O. (1972). Cholinergic mechanisms related to REM sleep. II. Effects of an anticholinesterase on the discharge of central vestibular neurons in the decerebrate cat. *Arch. Ital. Biol. 110*:260–283.
306a. Pompeiano, O., Manzoni, D., Srivastava, U. C., and Stampacchia, G. (1983). Cholinergic mechanism controlling the response gain of forelimb extensor muscles to sinusoidal stimulation of macular labyrinth and neck receptors. *Arch. Ital. Biol. 121*:285–303.
307. Pompeiano, O., Wand, P., and Srivastava, U. C. (1983). Effects of Renshaw cell activity on the response gain of limb extensors to sinusoidal labyrinth stimulation. *Neuroscience Lett., (Suppl.) 14*:S289.
308. Grillner, S., Hongo, T., and Lund, S. (1966). Interaction between the inhibitory pathways from the Deiters' nucleus and Ia afferents to flexor motoneurones. *Acta Physiol. Scand. 68(Suppl. 277)*:61.
309. Severin, F. V., Orlovsky, G. N., and Shik, M. L. (1968). Recurrent inhibitory effects on single motoneurones during an electrically evoked locomotion. *Bull. Exp. Biol. Med. USSR 66*:3–9.
310. Severin, F. V., Orlovsky, G. N., and Shik, M. L. (1968). Reciprocal influences on work of single motoneurones during controlled locomotion. *Bull. Exp. Biol. Med. USSR 66*:713–716.
311. Feldman, A. G., and Orlovsky, G. N. (1975). Activity of interneurons mediating reciprocal Ia inhibition during locomotion. *Brain Res. 84*: 181–194.
312. Lundberg, A. (1969). Reflex control of stepping. *The Nansen Memorial Lecture V*, Universitetsforlaget, Oslo, pp. 5–42.
313. McCrea, D. A., and Jordan, L. M. (1976). Recurrent inhibition during locomotion. *Soc. Neurosci. Abstr. 2*:754.
314. McCrea, D. A., Pratt, C. A., and Jordan, L. M. (1980). Renshaw cell activity and recurrent effects on motoneurons during fictive locomotion. *J. Neurophysiol. 44*:475–488.
315. Pratt, C. A., and Jordan, L. M. (1980). Recurrent inhibition of motoneurons in decerebrate cats during controlled treadmill locomotion. *J. Neurophysiol. 44*:489–500.
316. Deliagina, T. G., and Feldman, A. G. (1978). Modulation of activity of Renshaw cells during scratching. *Neurophysiologia 10*:209–211.
317. Deliagina, T. G., and Feldman, A. G. (1981). Activity of Renshaw cells during fictive scratch reflex in the cat. *Exp. Brain Res. 42*:108–115.

318. Berkinblit, M. B., Deliagina, T. G., Orlovsky, G. N., and Feldman, A. G. (1980). Activity of motoneurons during fictitious scratch reflex in the cat. *Brain Res. 193*:427–438.

319. Pierrot-Deseilligny, E., and Bussel, B. (1975). Evidence for recurrent inhibition by motoneurones in human subjects. *Brain Res. 88*:105–108.

320. Pierrot-Deseilligny, E., Bussel, B., Held, J. P., and Katz, R. (1976). Excitability of human motoneurones after discharge in a conditioning reflex. *EEG Clin. Neurophysiol. 40*:279–287.

321. Bussel, B., and Pierrot-Deseilligny, E. (1977). Inhibition of human motoneurones, probably of Renshaw origin, elicited by an orthodromic motor discharge. *J. Physiol. (Lond.) 269*:319–339.

322. Pierrot-Deseilligny, E., Morin, C., Katz, R., and Bussel, B. (1977). Influence of voluntary movement and posture on recurrent inhibition in human subjects. *Brain Res. 124*:427–436.

323. Hultborn, H., and Pierrot-Deseilligny, E. (1979). Changes in recurrent inhibition during voluntary soleus contractions in man studied by an H-reflex technique. *J. Physiol. (Lond.) 297*:229–251.

324. Pierrot-Deseilligny, E., and Morin, C. (1980). Evidence for supraspinal influences on Renshaw inhibition during motor activity in man. In *Spinal and Supraspinal Mechanisms of Voluntary Motor Control and Locomotion*, J. E. Desmedt (Ed.), Karger, Basel, *Prog. Clin. Neurophysiol. 8*:142–169.

325. Vallbo, Å. B. (1974). Afferent discharge from human muscle spindles in non-contracting muscles. Steady state impulse frequency as a function of joint angle. *Acta Physiol. Scand. 90*:303–318.

326. Kernell, D., Sjöholm, H. (1973). Repetitive impulse firing: Comparisons between neuron models based on "voltage clamp equations" and spinal motoneurones. *Acta Physiol. Scand. 87*:40–56.

327. Baldissera, F., and Gustafsson, B. (1974). Firing behaviour of a neurone model based on the afterhyperpolarization conductance time course and algebraical summation. Adaptation and steady state firing. *Acta Physiol. Scand. 92*:27–47.

327a. Gustafsson, B. (1974). Afterhyperpolarization and the control of repetitive firing in spinal neurones of the cat. *Acta Physiol. Scand. 92 (Suppl. 416)*:1–47.

328. Burke, R. E., Fedina, L., and Lundberg, A. (1968). Differential chloride reversal of IPSPs from group Ia afferents and motor axon collaterals. *Acta Physiol. Scand. 73*:3A–4A.

329. Burke, R. E., Fedina, L., and Lundberg, A. (1971). Spatial synaptic distribution of recurrent and group Ia inhibitory systems in cat spinal motoneurones. *J. Physiol. (Lond.) 214*:305–326.

330. Hultborn, H., Pierrot-Deseilligny, E., and Wigström, H. (1978). Distribution of recurrent inhibition within a motor nucleus. *Neurosci. Lett. (Suppl.) 1*:S97.

331. Holmgren, B., and Merton, P. A. (1954). Local feedback control of motoneurones. *J. Physiol. (Lond.) 123*:47P–48P.

332. Henatsch, H.-D., and Shulte, F. J. (1958). Reflexerregung und Eigen-hemmung tonischer und phasischer Alpha-Motoneurone während chem-ischer Dauererregung der Muskelspindeln. *Pflügers Arch. 268*:134–147.

333. Granit, T., and Rutledge, L. T. (1960). Surplus excitation in reflex action of motoneurones as measured by recurrent inhibition. *J. Physiol. (Lond.) 154*:288–307.

334. Tan, Ü. (1975). Post-tetanic changes in the discharge pattern of the ex-tensor alpha motoneurones. *Pflügers Arch. 353*:43–57.

335. Henneman, E. (1977). Functional organization of motoneuron pools: The size principle. *Proceedings XXVII International Congress Physiological Sciences, Paris,* XII:50.

336. Hennemann, E., Clamann, H. P., Gillies, I. D., and Skinner, R. D. (1974). Rank order of motoneurons within a pool: Law of combination. *J. Neuro-physiol. 37*:1338–1349.

337. Clamann, H. P., Gillies, I. D., and Hennemann, E. (1974). Effects of inhibi-tory inputs on critical firing level and rank order of motoneurones. *J. Neurophysiol. 37*:1350–1360.

338. Fatt, P., and Katz, B. (1953). The effect of inhibitory nerve impulses on a crustacean muscle fibre. *J. Physiol. (Lond.) 121*:374–389.

339. Harris, D. A., and Hennemann, E. (1979). Different species of alpha moto-neurons in same pool: Further evidence from effects of inhibition on their firing rates. *J. Neurophysiol. 42*:927–935.

340. Friedman, W. A., Sypert, G. W., Munson, J. B., and Fleshman, J. W. (1980). Recurrent inhibition of type-identified motoneurons. *Soc. Neurosci. Abstr. 6*:714.

341. Friedman, W. A., Sypert, G. W., Munson, J. B., and Fleshman, J. W. (1981). Recurrent inhibition in type-identified motoneurons. *J. Neurophysiol. 46*: 1349–1359.

342. Barrett, J. N., and Crill, W. E. (1974). Specific membrane properties of cat motoneurones. *J. Physiol. (Lond.) 239*:301–324.

343. Fleshman, J. W., Munson, J. B., and Sypert, G. W. (1981). Homonymous projection of individual group Ia-fibers to physiologically characterized medial gastrocnemius motoneurons in the cat. *J. Neurophysiol. 46*:1339–1348.

344. Burke, R. E. (1973). On the central nervous system control of fast and slow twitch motor units. In *New Developments in Electromyography and Clinical Neurophysiology,* J. E. Desmedt (Ed.), Karger, Basel, *3*:69–94.

345. Burke, R. E. (1981). Motor units: Anatomy, physiology and functional organization. In *Handbook of Physiology,* Sect. 1, *The Nervous System,* vol. II, *Motor Control,* Part 1, E. R. Kandel (Ed.), American Physiological Society, Bethesda, pp. 345–422.

346. Burke, R. E., Levine, D. N., Tsairis, P., and Zajac, F. E. (1973). Physio-logical types and histochemical profiles in motor units of the cat gastro-cnemius. *J. Physiol. (Lond.) 234*:723–748.

347. Fleshman, J. W., Munson, J. B., Sypert, G. W., and Friedman, W. A. (1981). Rheobase, input resistance, and motor-unit type in medial gastrocnemius motoneurons in the cat. *J. Neurophysiol. 46*:1326–1338.

348. Smith, T. G., Wuerker, R. B., and Frank K. (1967). Membrane impedance changes during synaptic transmission in cat spinal motoneurons. *J. Neurophysiol. 30*:1072–1096.

349. Granit, R., Henatsch, H.-D., and Steg, G. (1957). Tonic and phasic ventral horn cells differentiated by post-tetanic potentiation in cat extensors. *Acta Physiol. Scand. 37*:114–126.

350. Sprague, J. M. (1951). Motor and propriospinal cells in the thoracic and lumbar ventral horn of the Rhesus monkey. *J. Comp. Neurol. 95*:103–124.

351. Eccles, J. C. Eccles, R. M., Iggo, A., and Lundberg, A. (1960). Electrophysiological studies on gamma motoneurones. *Acta Physiol. Scand. 50*:32–40.

352. Nyberg-Hansen, R. (1965). Anatomical demonstration of gamma motoneurons in the cat's spinal cord. *Exp. Neurol. 13*:71–81.

353. Van Buren, J. M., and Frank, K. (1965). Correlation between the morphology and potential field of a spinal motor nucleus in the cat. *EEG Clin. Neurophysiol. 19*:112–126.

354. Bryan, R. N., Trevino, D. L., and Willis, W. D. (1972). Evidence for a common location of alpha and gamma motoneurons. *Brain Res. 38*:193–196.

355. Pellegrini, M., Pompeiano, O., and Corvaja, M. (1977). Identification of different size motoneurons labeled by the retrograde axonal transport of horseradish peroxidase. *Pflügers Arch. 368*:161–163.

356. Kemm, R. E., and Westbury, D. R. (1978). Some properties of spinal γ-motoneurones in the cat determined by micro-electrode recording. *J. Physiol. (Lond.) 282*:59–71.

357. Gustafsson, B., and Lipski, J. (1979). Do γ-motoneurones lack a long-lasting afterhyperpolarization? *Brain Res. 172*:349–353.

357a. Hunt, C. C., and Paintal, A. S. (1958). Spinal reflex regulation of fusimotor neurones. *J. Physiol. (Lond.) 143*:195–212.

358. Voorhoeve, P. E., and van Kanten, R. W. (1962). Reflex behaviour of fusimotor neurones of the cat upon electrical stimulation of various afferent fibres. *Acta Physiol. Pharmacol. Neerl. 10*:391–407.

359. Brown, M. C., Lawrence, D. G., and Matthews, P. B. C. (1968). Antidromic inhibition of presumed fusimotor neurones by repetitive stimulation of the ventral root in the decerebrate cat. *Experientia 24*:1210–1211.

360. Ellaway, P. H. (1968). Antidromic inhibition of fusimotor neurones. *J. Physiol. (Lond.) 198*:39P–40P.

361. Grillner, S. (1969). The influence of DOPA on the static and dynamic fusimotor activity to the triceps surae of the spinal cat. *Acta Physiol. Scand. 77*:490–509.

362. Ellaway, P. H. (1971). Recurrent inhibition of fusimotor neurons exhibiting background discharges in the decerebrate and the spinal cat. *J. Physiol. (Lond.) 216*:419–439.

362a. Ellaway, P. H. (1972). The variability in discharge of fusimotor neurones in the decerebrate cat. *Exp. Brain Res. 14*:105–117.

363. Noth, J. (1971). Recurrente Hemmung der Extensor-Fusimotoneurone? *Pflügers Arch. 329*:23–33.

364. Hunt, C. C. (1951). The reflex activity of mammalian small-nerve fibres. *J. Physiol. (Lond.) 115*:456–469.

365. Eldred, E., Granit, R., and Merton, P. A. (1953). Supraspinal control of the muscle spindles and its significance. *J. Physiol. (Lond.) 122*:498–523.

366. Fromm, C., and Haase, J. (1970). Positionsempfindlichkeit und fusimotorische Aktivierung prätibialer Muskelspindelendigungen vor und nach Deafferentierung. *Pflügers Arch. 321*:242–252.

367. Proske, U., and Lewis, D. M. (1972). The effects of muscle stretch and vibration on fusimotor activity in the lightly anaesthetised cat. *Brain Res. 46*:55–69.

368. Diete-Spiff, K., and Pascoe, J. E. (1959). The spindle motor nerves to the gastrocnemius muscle of the rabbit. *J. Physiol. (Lond.) 149*:120–134.

369. Fromm, C., Haase, J., and Noth, J. (1974). Length-dependent autogenetic inhibition of extensor γ-motoneurones in the decerebrate cat. *Pflügers Arch. 346*:251–262.

370. Fromm, C., and Noth, J. (1975). Vibration-induced autogenetic inhibition of gamma motoneurons. *Brain Res. 83*:495–497.

371. Fromm, C., and Noth, J. (1976). Reflex responses of gamma motoneurones to vibration of the muscle they innervate. *J. Physiol. (Lond.) 256*:117–136.

372. Grillner, S. (1969). Supraspinal and segmental control of static and dynamic γ-motoneurones in the cat. *Acta Physiol. Scand. 77 (Suppl. 327)*:1–34.

373. Grillner, S., Hongo, T., and Lund, S. (1969). Descending monosynaptic and reflex control of γ-motoneurones. *Acta Physiol. Scand. 75*:592–613.

374. Fromm, C., and Noth, J. (1974). Autogenetic inhibition of γ-motoneurones in the spinal cat uncovered by Dopa injection. *Pflügers Arch. 349*:247–256.

374a. Voorhoeve, P. E., and Rey, J. G. (1972). Inhibition récurrente des décharges fusimotrices, présumées statiques, chez le chat. *J. Physiol. (Paris) 65*: 314A–315A.

375. Trott, J. R. (1975). Reflex responses of fusimotor neurones during muscle vibration. *J. Physiol. (Lond.) 247*:20P–22P.

376. Ellaway, P. H., and Trott, J. R. (1976). Reflex connections from muscle stretch receptors to their own fusimotor neurones. *Prog. Brain Res. 44*: 113–122.

377. Trott, J. R. (1976). The effect of low amplitude muscle vibration on the discharge of fusimotor neurones in the decerebrate cat. *J. Physiol. (Lond.) 255*:635–649.

378. Ellaway, P. H., and Trott, J. R. (1978). Autogenetic reflex action on to gamma motoneurones by stretch of triceps surae in the decerebrated cat. *J. Physiol. (Lond.) 276*:49–66.

379. Ellaway, P. H., and Trott, J. R. (1976). Inhibition of fusimotor neurones on eliciting contraction of the homonymous muscle. *J. Physiol. (Lond.) 256*:52P–53P.

380. Ellaway, P. H., Murphy, P. R., and Trott, J. R. (1979). Inhibition of gamma motoneurone discharge by contraction of the homonymous muscle in the decerebrate cat. *J. Physiol. (Lond.) 291*:425–441.

381. Appelberg, B., Johansson, H., and Kalistratov, G. (1977). The influence of group II muscle afferents and low threshold skin afferents on dynamic fusimotor neurones to the triceps surae of the cat. *Brain Res. 132*:153–158.

382. Noth, J., and Thilmann, A. (1980). Autogenetic excitation of extensor γ-motoneurones by group II muscle afferents in the cat. *Neurosci. Lett.* *17*:23–26.

383. Noth, J. (1981). Autogenetic and antagonistic group II effects on extensor gamma motoneurons of the decerebrated cat. In *Muscle Receptors and Movement*, A. Taylor and A. Prochazka (Eds.), Macmillan, London, pp. 207–213.

384. Davidoff, R. A., and Hackman, J. C. (1984). Spinal inhibition. In *Handbook of the Spinal Cord*, vols. 2 and 3, *Anatomy and Physiology*, R. A. Davidoff (Ed.), Marcel Dekker, New York, pp. 385–459.

385. Burke, R. E., Rymer, W. Z., and Walsh, J. V., Jr. (1976). Relative strength of synaptic input from short-latency pathways to motor units of defined type in cat medial gastrocnemius. *J. Neurophysiol. 39*:447–458.

385a. Curtis, D. R., and Eccles, J. C. (1959). The time courses of excitatory and inhibitory synaptic actions. *J. Physiol. 145*:529–546.

386. Hultborn, H., Illert, M., and Santini, M. (1976). Convergence on interneurones mediating the reciprocal Ia inhibition of motoneurones. I. Disynaptic Ia inhibition of Ia inhibitory interneurones. *Acta Physiol. Scand. 96*:193–201.

387. Lindström, S., and Schomburg, E. D. (1974). Group I inhibition in Ib excited ventral spinocerebellar tract neurones. *Acta Physiol. Scand. 90*: 166–185.

388. Hultborn, H. (1972). Convergence on interneurones in the reciprocal Ia inhibitory pathway to motoneurones. *Acta Physiol. Scand. 85(Suppl. 375)*:1–42.

389. Hultborn, H. (1972). On the control of transmission in the reciprocal Ia inhibitory pathway to motoneurones. In *Mechanisms of Neuronal Integration in Nerve Centers, Kiev*.

390. Lindström, S. (1973). Recurrent control from motor axon collaterals of Ia inhibitory pathways in the spinal cord of the cat. *Acta Physiol. Scand. 89(Suppl. 392)*:1–43.

391. Hultborn, H., Jankowska, E., and Lindström, S. (1968). Recurrent inhibition from motor axon collaterals in interneurones monosynaptically activated from Ia afferents. *Brain Res. 9*:367–369.

391a. Hultborn, H., Illert, M., and Santini, M. (1976). Convergence on interneurones mediating the reciprocal Ia inhibition of motoneurones. II. Effects from segmental flexor reflex pathways. *Acta Physiol. Scand. 96*:351–367.

392. Hultborn, H., Illert, M., and Santini, M. (1976). Convergence on interneurones mediating the reciprocal Ia inhibition of motoneurones. III. Effects from supraspinal pathways. *Acta Physiol. Scand. 96*:368–391.

393. Cleveland, S., Haase, J., Ross, H.-G., and Wand, P. (1972). Antidromic conditioning of reciprocally inhibited monosynaptic extensor and flexor reflexes in decerebrate cats. *Pflügers Arch. 337*:219–228.

394. Fedina, L., and Hultborn, H. (1972). Facilitation from ipsilateral primary afferents of interneuronal transmission in the Ia inhibitory pathway to motoneurones. *Acta Physiol. Scand. 86*:59–81.

395. Hultborn, H., and Udo, M. (1972). Convergence in the reciprocal Ia inhibitory pathway of excitation from descending pathways and inhibition from motor axon collaterals. *Acta Physiol. Scand. 84*:95–108.

396. Hultborn, H., and Udo, M. (1972). Convergence of large muscle spindle (Ia) afferents at interneuronal level in the reciprocal Ia inhibitory pathway to motoneurones. *Acta Physiol. Scand.* *84*:493-499.
397. Hultborn, H., and Udo, M. (1972). Recurrent depression from motor axon collaterals of supraspinal inhibition in motoneurones. *Acta Physiol. Scand.* *85*:44-57.
398. Benecke, R., and Böttcher, U. (1973). Recurrent facilitation of monosynaptic flexor reflexes during dynamic stretch of triceps surae muscle. *Pflügers Arch.(Suppl.)343*:R74.
399. Benecke, R., and Meyer-Lohmann, J. (1973). Discharge patterns of single Ia inhibitory interneurones during ramp stretch of triceps surae muscle. *Pflügers Arch.(Suppl.)339*:R74.
400. Belcher, G., Davies, J., and Ryall, R. W. (1976). Glycine-mediated inhibitory transmission of group Ia-excited inhibitory interneurones by Renshaw cells. *J. Physiol. (Lond.) 256*:651-662.
401. Lloyd, D. P. C. (1941). A direct central inhibitory action of antidromically conducted impulses. *J. Neurophysiol. 4*:184-190.
402. Lloyd, D. P. C. (1946). Integrative pattern of excitation and inhibition in two-neuron reflex arcs. *J. Neurophysiol. 9*:439-444.
403. Fu, T.-C., Hultborn, H., Larsson, R., and Lundberg, A. (1978). Reciprocal inhibition during the tonic stretch reflex in the decerebrate cat. *J. Physiol. (Lond.) 284*:345-369.
404. Hultborn, H., and Lundberg, A. (1972). Reciprocal inhibition during the stretch reflex. *Acta Physiol. Scand. 85*:136-138.
405. Benecke, R., and Henatsch, H.-D. (1974). Some physiological aspects of inhibitory action on Ia inhibitory interneurones. *Proceedings XXVI International Congress Physiological Sciences, New Delhi, XI*:153.
406. Benecke, R., Böttcher, U., Henatsch, H.-D., Meyer-Lohmann, J., and Schmidt, J. (1975). Recurrent inhibition of individual Ia inhibitory interneurones and disinhibition of their target α-motoneurones during muscle stretches. *Exp. Brain Res. 23*:13-28.
407. Hongo, T., Jankowska, E., and Lundberg, A. (1969). The rubrospinal tract. II. Facilitation of interneuronal transmission in reflex paths to motoneurones. *Exp. Brain Res. 7*:365-391.
408. Lundberg, A. (1970). The excitatory control of the Ia inhibitory pathway. In *Excitatory Synaptic Mechanisms*, P. Andersen and J. K. S. Jansen (Eds.), Universitetsforlaget, Oslo, pp. 333-340.
409. Hultborn, H. (1976). Transmission in the pathway of reciprocal Ia inhibition to motoneurones and its control during the tonic stretch reflex. *Prog. Brain Res. 44*:235-255.
410. Tanaka, R. (1976). Reciprocal Ia inhibition and voluntary movements in man. *Prog. Brain Res. 44*:291-302.
411. Fedina, L., Hultborn, H., and Illert, M. (1975). Facilitation from contralateral primary afferents of interneuronal transmission in the Ia inhibitory pathway to motoneurones. *Acta Physiol. Scand. 94*:198-221.

412. Wilson, V. J. (1959). Recurrent facilitation of spinal reflexes. *J. Gen. Physiol.* 42:703-713.

413. Wilson, V. J., Diecke, F. P. J., and Talbot, W. H. (1960). Action of tetanus toxin on conditioning of spinal motoneurons. *J. Neurophysiol.* 23:659-666.

414. Wilson, V. J., and Burgess, P. R. (1962). Disinhibition in the cat spinal cord. *J. Neurophysiol.* 25:392-404.

415. Wilson, V. J., and Burgess, P. R. (1962). Effects of antidromic conditioning on some motoneurons and interneurons. *J. Neurophysiol.* 25:636-650.

416. Hunt, C. C., and Kuno, M. (1959). Background discharge and evoked responses of spinal interneurones. *J. Physiol. (Lond.)* 147:364-384.

417. Biscoe, T. J., and Krnjevíc, K. (1963). Chloralose and the activity of Renshaw cells. *Exp. Neurol.* 8:395-405.

418. Smerdlov, S. M., and Maksimova, E. V. (1965). Effects of antidromic impulses on spontaneous activity of interneurons in cat spinal cord. *Fiziol. Zh. SSSR* 57:717-719. In *Fed. Proc.* (1966), 25(transl. Suppl.): 419-422.

419. Hultborn, H., Jankowska, E., Lindström, S., and Roberts, W. (1971). Neuronal pathway of the recurrent facilitation of motoneurones. *J. Physiol. (Lond.)* 218:495-514.

420. Oscarsson, O. (1956). Functional organization of the ventral spino-cerebellar tract in the cat. I. Electrophysiological identification of the tract. *Acta Physiol. Scand.* 38:145-165.

421. Oscarsson, O. (1957). Functional organization of the ventral spino-cerebellar tract in the cat. II. Connections with muscle, joint, and skin nerve afferents and effects on adequate stimulation of various receptors. *Acta Physiol. Scand.* 42(Suppl. 146):1-107.

422. Eccles, J. C., Hubbard, J. I., and Oscarsson, O. (1961). Intracellular recording from cells of the ventral spino-cerebellar tract. *J. Physiol. (Lond.)* 158:486-516.

423. Lundberg, A., and Oscarsson, O. (1962). Functional organization of the ventral spinocerebellar tract in the cat. IV. Identification of units by antidromic activation from the cerebellar cortex. *Acta Physiol. Scand.* 54: 252-269.

424. Oscarsson, O. (1965). Functional organization of the spinocerebellar tracts. *Physiol. Rev.* 45:495-522.

425. Hubbard, J. I., and Oscarsson, O. (1962). Localization of the cell bodies of the ventral spino-cerebellar tract in lumbar segments of the cat. *J. Comp. Neurol.* 118:199-204.

426. Cooper, S., and Sherrington, C. S. (1940). Gower's tract and spinal border cells. *Brain* 63:123-134.

427. Jankowska, E., and Lindström, S. (1970). Morphological identification of physiologically defined neurones in the cat spinal cord. *Brain Res.* 20: 323-326.

428. Burke, R., Lundberg, A., and Weight, F. (1971). Spinal border cell origin of the ventral spinocerebellar tract. *Exp. Brain Res. 12*:283–294.

429. Lundberg, A., and Weight, F. (1971). Functional organization of connexions to the ventral spinocerebellar tract. *Exp. Brain Res. 12*:295–316.

430. Gustafsson, B., and Lindström, S. (1973). Recurrent control from motor axon collaterals of Ia inhibitory pathways to ventral spinocerebellar tract neurones. *Acta Physiol. Scand. 89*:457–481.

431. Lindström, S., and Schomburg, E. D. (1973). Recurrent inhibition from motor axon collaterals of ventral spinocerebellar tract neurones. *Acta Physiol. Scand. 88*:505–515.

432. Lundberg, A. (1971). Function of the ventral spinocerebellar tract—a new hypothesis. *Exp. Brain Res. 12*:317–330.

433. Gustafsson, B., and Lindström, S. (1970). Depression of Ia IPSP in spinal border cells by impulses in recurrent motor axon collaterals. *Acta Physiol. Scand. 80*:13A–14A.

434. Curtis, D. R., Eccles, J. C., and Lundberg, A. (1958). Intracellular recording from cells in Clarke's column. *Acta Physiol. Scand. 43*:303–314.

435. Eccles, J. C., Oscarsson, O., and Willis, W. D. (1961). Synaptic action of group I and II afferent fibres of muscle on the cells of the dorsal spinocerebellar tract. *J. Physiol. (Lond.) 158*:517–543.

436. Lindström, S., and Takata, M. (1972). Monosynaptic excitation of dorsal spinocerebellar tract neurones from low threshold joint afferents. *Acta Physiol. Scand. 84*:430–432.

437. Lundberg, A. (1969). Convergence of excitatory and inhibitory action on interneurones in the spinal cord. In *The Interneuron*, M. A. B. Brazier (Ed.), UCLA Forum in Medical Sciences, No. 11, University of California Press, Los Angeles, pp. 231–265.

438. Sears, T. A. (1964). Some properties and reflex connections of respiratory motoneurons of the cat's thoracic spinal cord. *J. Physiol. (Lond.) 175*:386–403.

439. Eklund, G., von Euler, C., and Rutkowski, S. (1964). Spontaneous and reflex activity of intercostal gamma motoneurones. *J. Physiol. (Lond.) 171*:139–163.

440. Davson, H., and Segal, M. B. (1978). *Introduction to Physiology*, vol. 4, Academic Press, London.

441. Sears, T. A. (1964). Investigations on respiratory motoneurones of the thoracic spinal cord. *Prog. Brain Res. 12*:259–273.

442. Kirkwood, P. A., and Sears, T. A. (1980). Comparisons between unitary excitatory post-synaptic potentials and cross correlation histograms for intercostal motoneurones. *J. Physiol. (Lond.) 305*:39P–40P.

443. Kirkwood, P. A., Sears, T. A., and Westgaard, R. H. (1980). Recurrent inhibition of external (inspiratory) intercostal motoneurones. *Neurosci. Lett. (Suppl.) 5*:S226.

444. Kirkwood, P. A., Sears, T. A., and Westgaard, R. H. (1981). Recurrent inhibition of intercostal motoneurones in the cat. *J. Physiol. (Lond.) 319*: 111-130.

445. Lebedev, V. P., Petrov, V. I., and Skobelev, V. A. (1976). Antidromic discharges of sympathetic preganglionic neurones located outside of the spinal cord lateral horns. *Neurosci. Lett. 2*:325-329.

446. Fernandez de Molina, A., Kuno, M., and Perl, E. R. (1965). Antidromically evoked responses from sympathetic preganglionic neurones. *J. Physiol. (Lond.) 180*:321-335.

447. Kirchner, F., Kirchner, D., and Polosa, C. (1975). Spinal organization of sympathetic inhibition by spinal afferent fibers. *Brain Res. 87*:161-170.

448. Polosa, C. (1967). The silent period of sympathetic preganglionic neurones. *Can. J. Physiol. Pharmacol. 45*:1033-1045.

449. Réthelyi, M. (1972). Cell and neuropil architecture of the intermediolateral (sympathetic) nucleus of cat spinal cord. *Brain Res. 46*:203-213.

450. Lebedev, V. P., Petrov, V. I., and Skobelev, V. A. (1980). Do sympathetic preganglionic neurones have a recurrent inhibitory mechanism? *Pflügers Arch. 383*:91-97.

451. De Groat, W. C. (1976). Mechanisms underlying recurrent inhibition in the sacral parasympathetic outflow to the urinary bladder. *J. Physiol. (Lond.) 257*:503-513.

452. De Groat, W. C., and Ryall, R. W. (1968). Recurrent inhibition in sacral parasympathetic pathways to the bladder. *J. Physiol. (Lond.) 196*:579-591.

453. Ishikawa, T. (1961). Recurrent inhibition in the lower sacral segment. *Kobe J. Med. Sci. 7*:378-385.

454. Bracchi, F., Decandia, M., and Gualtierotti, T. (1966). Frequency stabilization in the motor centers of spinal cord and caudal brain stem. *Amer. J. Physiol. 210*:1170-1177.

455. Redman, S. J., and Lampard, D. G. (1967). Monosynaptic stochastic stimulation of spinal motoneurones in the cat. *Nature 216*:921-922.

456. Taylor, W. K. (1965). A model of learning mechanisms in the brain. *Prog. Brain Res. 17*:369-397.

457. Wenstøp, F., and Rudjord, T. (1971). Recurrent Renshaw inhibition studied by digital stimulation. In *Proceedings of the First European Biophysics Congress*, vol. 5, E. Broda, A. Locker, and H. Springer-Lederer (Eds.), Verlag der Wiener Medizinischen Akademie, Wien, pp. 365-369.

458. Brooks, V. B., and Wilson, V. J. (1958). Localization of stretch reflexes by recurrent inhibition. *Science 127*:472-473.

459. Brooks, V. B. (1959). Contrast and stability in the nervous system. *Trans. N.Y. Acad. Sci. 21*:387-394.

460. Ratliff, F., Miller, W. H., and Hartline, H. K. (1958). Neural interaction in the eye and the integration of receptor activity. *Ann. N.Y. Acad. Sci. 74*: 210-222.

461. Hartline, H. K., Ratliff, F., and Miller, W. H. (1961). Inhibitory interaction in the retina and its significance in vision. In *Nervous Inhibition*, E. Florey (Ed.), Pergamon Press, Oxford, pp. 241–284.

462. Ratliff, F., Hartline, H. K., and Miller, W. H. (1963). Spatial and temporal aspects of retinal inhibitory interaction. *J. Opt. Soc. Am. 53*:110–120.

463. Ratliff, F. (1965). *Mach Bands: Quantitative Studies on Neural Networks in the Retina*, Holden-Day, San Francisco.

464. Mountcastle, V. B. (1957). Modality and topographic properties of single neurons of cat's somatic sensory cortex. *J. Neurophysiol. 20*:408–434.

465. Gelfand, I. M., Gurfinkel, V. S., Kots, Y. M., Tsetlin, M. L., and Shik, M. L. (1963). Synchronization of motor units and associated model concepts. *Biofizika 8*:475–486.

466. Gelfand, I. M., Gurfinkel, V. S., Kots, Y. M., Krinskii, V. I., Tsetlin, M. L., and Shik, M. L. (1964). Investigation of postural activity. *Biofizika 9*: 710–717.

467. Elble, R. J., and Randall, J. E. (1976). Motor-unit activity responsible for 8- to 12-Hz component of human physiological finger tremor. *J. Neurophysiol. 39*:370–383.

468. Mori, S., and Ishida, A. (1976). Synchronization of motor units and its stimulation in parallel feedback system. *Biol. Cybern. 21*:107–111.

469. Adam, D., Windhorst, U., and Inbar, G. F. (1978). The effects of recurrent inhibition on the cross-correlated firing patterns of motoneurones (and their relation to signal transmission in the spinal cord-muscle channel). *Biol. Cybern. 29*:229–235.

470. Windhorst, U., Adam, D., and Inbar, G. F. (1978). The effects of recurrent inhibitory feedback in shaping discharge patterns of motoneurones excited by phasic muscle stretches. *Biol. Cybern. 29*:221–227.

471. Sears, T. A., and Stagg, A. (1976). Short-term synchronization of intercostal motoneurone activity. *J. Physiol. (Lond.) 263*:357–381.

472. Kirkwood, P. A., and Sears, T. A. (1978). The synaptic connexions to intercostal motoneurones as revealed by the average common excitation potential. *J. Physiol. (Lond.) 275*:103–134.

473. Hultborn, H., Lindström, S., and Wigström, H. (1979). On the function of recurrent inhibition in the spinal cord. *Exp. Brain Res. 37*:399–403.

474. Denny-Brown, D. (1928). *On the Essential Mechanism of Mammalian Posture*, Ph.D. dissertation, University of Oxford, England.

475. Walmsley, B., Hodgson, J. A., and Burke, R. E. (1978). Forces produced by medial gastrocnemius and soleus muscles during locomotion in freely moving cats. *J. Neurophysiol. 41*:1203–1216.

476. Kanda, K., Burke, R. E., and Walmsley, B. (1977). Differential control of fast and slow twitch motor units in the decerebrate cat. *Exp. Brain Res. 29*:57–74.

477. Smith, J. L., Betts, B., Edgerton, V. R., and Zernicke, R. F. (1980). Rapid ankle extension during paw shakes: Selective recruitment of fast ankle extensors. *J. Neurophysiol. 43*:612–620.

12
MAMMALIAN MUSCLE RECEPTORS

Ziaul Hasan and Douglas G. Stuart   *Department of Physiology, College of Medicine, University of Arizona Health Sciences Center, Tucson, Arizona*

I. INTRODUCTION

A great deal of effort has been devoted in the twentieth century to the study of muscle receptors. (For a detailed historical account see Ref. 1, and subsequent reviews 2-5). Much of this research has been concerned with the muscle spindle, which is a receptor of complex morphology. The attention given to the structurally more simple Golgi tendon organ and "other" muscle receptors has been much less than what would be expected from their relative abundance. For none of the receptors, complex or simple, has the available knowledge proved amenable to summarization in the form of clear and definitive conceptions of the internal operation and response characteristics. Such conceptions, however, do exist for restricted conditions, though it is not clear which of them would be important for further generalization.

In this chapter, we strive to present the current understanding of the distribution, structure, and response characteristics of mammalian muscle receptors. A nonhistorical framework of presentation was chosen in order to emphasize the logical connections that we have been able to extract from the various experimental observations, old and new. In the case of the spindle, which has been the subject of intense experimental assault, this strategy has obliged us to be extremely selective with regard to the literature. This selectivity reflects our attempt to incorporate the observations in the picture we present, and it should not be construed as a judgment of merit. On the other hand, our handling of the material concerning Golgi tendon organs and other receptors has been influenced by our estimation of the importance of these receptors. Consequently, we give extended attention to the limited amount of available material.

The gaps in the current understanding include some basic issues that appear to have gotten lost on the way. We point out some of the issues that are derserving of attention, in the hope of stimulating further studies. We hope also to rectify certain ideas, no longer valid, that continue to be promulgated in many textbooks. (As examples, one may cite the following incorrect statements: tendon organs are found primarily in tendons; they are high-threshold receptors; spindle afferent response is the sum of components proportional to position and to velocity of movement.) To some extent, the survival of misconceptions may have been fostered by the lack of simple alternatives. Unfortunately, we are still a long way from achieving simplicity in our understanding of muscle receptors, but we have made considerable progress toward outgrowing the false assurance of having achieved it.

II. NUMBER AND DISTRIBUTION OF RECEPTORS

A. Spindles and Tendon Organs

The number of muscle spindles (and to a far lesser extent, tendon organs) has been determined for a wide variety of muscles in several mammalian species (6-9), including the human (10). A generalization that emerges from these studies is that both spindles and tendon organs are plentiful in striated somatic muscles that (1) operate on a joint (thereby excluding, for example, certain facial muscles), (2) develop relatively substantial force (excluding, for example, tendon organs in cat tenuissimus), and (3) are subject to unpredictable inertial loads (excluding, for example, jaw-opening muscles). In 149 human muscles that meet these criteria the number of spindles range from six in the small (1.2 g) stylohyoideus muscle to 1306 in the largest (1.5 kg) muscle complex in the body—the quadriceps femoris (10). Spindle densities (number/g muscle weight) tend to be higher in small muscles. These densities also correspond to some degree with the presumed role of the muscle in the control of postural stability and/or in fine movements. For example, spindles are exceptionally dense in muscles interlinking cervical vertebrae and relatively sparse in large muscles like the gluteus maximus that are presumably used primarily for powerful and relatively coarse movements.

Spindles are usually found where the major intramuscular nerve trunks branch into finer divisions (6). Superficial spindles are also prominent near aponeuroses of origin and insertion. In contrast, tendon organs are restricted to lining these aponeuroses (6), *with few in the tendon(s) proper.* However, tendon organs are also found deep in some muscles, provided an aponeurosis extends there.

A striking features of the distribution of these receptors is the close association between spindles and select muscle fibers that connect with tendon organs (i.e., the "dyad" arrangement; see 7). The receptors tend also to be closely associated with "oxidative" (low-force, low-functional threshold) muscle fibers, particularly in "compartmentalized" muscles in which the oxidative fibers are concentrated in a limited receptor-rich portion of the muscle and "glycolytic" (high-force, high-threshold) fibers are concentrated in a receptor-poor portion (7).

B. Other Receptors

In most muscles, there are few receptors with clearly differentiated endings and end organs, other than spindles and tendon organs. When present, these other differentiated receptors are usually supplied with group II afferent fibers (11), but they are sometimes supplied by group III and even group I as well (12). One or more paciniform corpuscles are usually found in each muscle (several only rarely). When present, they are always in close association with tendon organs (12). Pacinian corpuscles and receptors with Ruffini endings are much rarer.

Undifferentiated receptors (free nerve endings) are even more plentiful than spindles and tendon organs. They are supplied predominantly by groups III and IV afferents (12,13) and perhaps by group II (14). Indeed, *the majority of receptors in muscle are innervated by groups III and IV afferents.* For example, as reported by Kniffki et al. (13), in the chronically sympathectomized hindlimb of the cat, the nerves to the gastrocnemius and soleus contain some 1200 myelinated afferents and efferents together with 1000 unmyelinated (group IV) afferents. Of the myelinated axons, 480 are afferents (groups I-III) and 175 of these are group III.

The distributions of undifferentiated receptors innervated by group III or IV afferents are difficult to study systematically. Stacey (12) found them widely distributed, innervating all types of intramuscular tissue except the capillary network. It remains for the future to determine if intramuscular receptors with free nerve endings demonstrate an ultrastructural diversity that correlates with their location, as has recently been found for such receptors in the Achilles tendon of the cat (15).

The anatomic work has demonstrated the wealth of receptors with which a muscle is supplied, above and beyond spindles and tendon organs. As reviewed in Sec. VI, they subserve not only nociception but also appear to be involved in thermoreception and in cardiovascular and respiratory adjustments during exercise ("ergoreceptive" function), and some might even contribute to kinesthesis and motor control.

Summary. Most muscles are richly supplied with spindles and tendon organs. Spindles are often located deep in the muscle, while tendon organs are usually found at the musculotendinous junctions. Within a muscle, the receptors tend to be more plentiful where there are more oxidative fibers.

The majority of afferent axons in a muscle nerve innervate receptors other than spindles and tendon organs. Most of these other receptors are undifferentiated, free nerve endings.

III. MUSCLE SPINDLES

A. Structure

Although the complexity of the muscle spindle approaches that of the eye, the essential components of its structure can be enumerated rather simply as follows (16). (1) A bundle of several (2-12) specialized muscle fibers, called "intrafusal" fibers, that are shorter and more slender compared to ordinary, "extrafusal," muscle fibers with which they lie in parallel.* (2) Various types of afferent and efferent nerve endings associated with the intrafusal fibers; these endings arise from several (8-25) axons. (3) A connective tissue capsule that overlies the middle portion of the intrafusal fibers and contains gelatinous material. The capsule gives the spindle the fusiform appearance responsible for its name.

The middle portion of an intrafusal fiber is unusual compared to its extrafusal counterpart in that it contains many nuclei and is deficient or lacking in striations (1,17). This portion is enveloped by one or more mechanoreceptive afferent nerve endings. Efferent axons to the spindle terminate on striated portions of intrafusal fibers and are referred to as "fusimotor" axons. Contractions resulting from fusimotor activity tend to *elongate* the middle portion. Elongation of the middle portion occurs also when the length of the whole intrafusal fiber is increased, as in the case of muscle stretch. This elongation, arising from either mechanism, is sensed by the mechanoreceptive afferent nerve endings.

1. Intrafusal Fibers

The recognition of *three* different types of intrafusal muscle fibers has given coherence to a large number of anatomic and physiologic findings. These types

---

*Some authors prefer the terms "fusimotor" to "intrafusal," and "skeletomotor" to "extrafusal." While granting that the term extrafusal leaves much to be desired, the usage we adopt here has the advantage of allowing us to distinguish intrafusal muscle fibers from the fusimotor nerve axons that innervate them. Our use of the term fusimotor includes those axons, sometimes referred to as "skeletofusimotor," or "beta," axons, whose collaterals innervate extrafusal muscle fibers.

are distinguishable on grounds that include morphology, ultrastructure, and histochemistry (18) as well as mechanical properties (19). They are referred to as "bag 1," "bag 2," and "chain" fibers. The terminology (bag and chain) reflects the arrangement of nuclei in the middle portion of the intrafusal fiber, but it is not indicative of the shape of the fiber (1), contrary to the depictions in many textbooks. Factors that distinguish bag 2 from bag 1 fibers include the abundance of associated elastic strands (20) and alkali-resistant adenosine triphosphatase (ATPase) activity (18).

Maintenance of intrafusal fiber types is compromised by deafferentation (21,22). Afferent innervation also seems to play a major role in spindle ontogeny, since differentiation of intrafusal fibers commences after afferent innervation, before there are any fusimotor endings (23). However, the completion of the process of differentiation may well be contingent upon fusimotor innervation (23,24). The chain fibers are the last to differentiate (23), and these fibers also exhibit more atrophy upon de-efferentation (21).

Spindles in cat hindlimb muscles typically contain one bag 1, one bag 2, and four chain fibers, although there is considerable variation (16). Bag fibers are somewhat less than 10 mm long, the bag 2 fiber being often longer than the bag 1, and chain fibers are approximately half as long as bag fibers (25). Typical diameters are 30 μm for bag fibers and 14 μm for chain fibers (1). Some spindles lack the bag 1 fiber and may share a bag 2 fiber with another spindle (26,27). Such tandem and complex arrangements are quite common in neck muscles (28), but their significance is unknown.

Surprisingly, it is not clear exactly how the intrafusal fibers are attached to the aponeuroses, although there is no doubt that muscle stretch is transmitted to all intrafusal fibers. The extension of the middle portion, however, is related in a complex manner to the elongation of the whole fiber because of nonuniformity of mechanical properties along the length of the fiber (29). The nonuniformity may be related to the deficit of myofibrils in the middle region. Little is known about how the myofibrils terminate in this region.

2. Afferent Innervation

There are two distinct types of afferent nerve endings, called "primary" and "secondary" (see refs. 16 and 26 for reviews). The *primary* ending consists of a number of spirals, one for each intrafusal fiber of a spindle, enveloping their middle portions. The spirals are branches of an axon, usually one per spindle, whose conduction velocity (CV) in the nerve trunk is in the group I range. The *secondary* ending often takes the form of spirals located adjacent to the spirals of the primary ending but confined to the chain fibers; however, a considerable degree of variation is exhibited, including nonspiral ("flower spray") terminations on chain fibers and also on bag fibers. There are 0-5 afferent axons

(average = 1.6) per spindle that form secondary endings; their conduction velocities are in the group II range. The groups I and II axons associated with spindles
will be referred to as Ia and spII afferents, respectively, in order to distinguish
them from nonspindle afferents with similar conduction velocities.

3. Efferent Innervation

Fusimotor axons terminate in motor end-plates on the striated portions of
intrafusal fibers. Unlike the extrafusal case, a mature intrafusal fiber often has
more than one end-plate, sometimes from more than one fusimotor axon. A
fusimotor axon may terminate in a spray of small end-plates along the fiber,
which is called a "trail ending" (16).

A fusimotor axon that innervates a bag 1 fiber rarely branches to innervate
other fibers in the same spindle. On the other hand, bag 2 and chain fibers in a
spindle are often innervated by branches of the same fusimotor axons (25). A
particular axon of the latter type may terminate on different combinations of
bag 2 and chain fibers in different spindles (30).

The majority of fusimotor axons have conduction velocities between 10 and
50 m/sec (i.e., in the Aγ range) and are called γ axons (1). Their cell bodies lie
in the ventral horn intermingled with the much larger alpha motoneurons. In
addition, a significant minority (sometimes 30%) of spindle efferents are, in fact,
branches of some of the alpha motor axons that innervate extrafusal muscle
(31). These efferents are referred to as "skeletofusimotor" axons (31), but the
term "β fibers" is prevalent despite the fact that these axons do not form a
distinct group on the criterion of conduction velocity (5).

There is evidence for innervation of intrafusal fibers as well as of the spindle
capsule by axons of the autonomic nervous system (32). The significance of this
innervation is unknown (but see 33). The capsule itself, a continuation of the
perineural epithelium, may be more than a simple protective covering, since it
contains dephosphorylating enzymes (34).

Summary. A spindle contains three types of intrafusal fibers (bag 1, bag 2,
and chain) and two types of afferent nerve endings (primary and secondary).
The afferent endings are located in a position where they can be responsive
simultaneously to stretch of the spindle and to intrafusal contraction. A primary
ending arises from a Ia axon and innervates all intrafusal fibers, while a
secondary ending arises from a spII axon and innervates preferentially the chain
fibers. Efferent or fusimotor axons, for the most part, can be categorized into
those that innervate bag 1 fibers only, and those that innervate bag 2 and chain
fibers.

B. Functional Properties

Spindle afferent discharge is altered when there is a change in muscle length or in
the discharge rate of fusimotor axons. Study of the afferent response to these

two kinds of stimuli is complicated by the fact that the effect of either kind of stimulus is modified by the other kind. The respective effects and their interaction have been studied in three categories of experiment.

1. The length of a living, isolated spindle is manipulated and fusimotor axons are stimulated while the spindle is visualized and afferent discharge is recorded.

2. The discharge of an afferent axon from an unseen spindle embedded in a muscle is monitored while muscle length is controlled. Intrafusal state is either controlled by electrical stimulation of fusimotor axons or is allowed to be determined "spontaneously," as, for example, in the case of a decerebrate animal.

3. Discharge of an afferent axon from an embedded spindle is recorded during active and passive movements in an essentially intact animal or human while muscle length is monitored. In this type of experiment fusimotor activity is usually not directly accessible.

All three approaches to spindle function have provided valuable information.

1. Isolated Spindles

A living spindle may be teased out from one of the small muscles of the tail (35) or from the ribbonlike tenuissimus muscle of the cat (29,36) and studied in vitro. In these studies, deterioration of neuromuscular activity can be minimized by the presence of certain amino acids. Alternatively, a spindle in the tenuissimus can be visualized without removal from the muscle while the appropriate afferent and efferent axons are accessed in filaments of spinal roots (37,38).

Deformation of the spindle capsule is not thought to play a role in the response properties of spindle afferents (cf. 39), since work on in vitro spindles has revealed that the responses to longitudinal stretch are unaltered after removal of the capsule (29,40).

The most commonly employed mechanical stimulus consists of stretch at constant velocity followed by maintenance of length in the elongated condition ("ramp-and-hold" stretch). As regards the response, attention has been focused upon the "instantaneous discharge rate," that is, the reciprocal of each interspike interval graphed against time. This serves as the relevant measure arising from the pattern of afferent action potentials.

a. Transducing properties. The process of transduction from extension of the afferent terminations to increase in the rate of afferent discharge can be studied profitably, much as in other kinds of receptors, without the need to consider the peculiarities of fusimotor innervation of the spindle. The ionic basis of the receptor potential of the primary ending has been investigated by Hunt et al. (40) who recorded, after tetrodotoxin blockade of action potentials, what may be called a "compound" receptor potential elicited by the elongation of the spiral terminations of a Ia axon. This receptor potential (in the direction of depolarization) is due largely to inward movement of Na^+. However, Ca^{2+} (and Li^+) can substitute for Na^+ to some extent. Concomitantly, there is a voltage-dependent increase in K^+ conductance that is susceptible to tetraethyl-ammonium (TEA) blockade. Since this increase outlasts the voltage change, it confers some dynamic properties to the response. When maintained stretch of the afferent ending is reduced, the receptor potential, as expected, is of the opposite sign, but its ionic basis is not clear. (There may be a decrease in permeability to Na^+ and/or an increase in permeability to K^+ through channels that are not susceptible to total blockade by TEA.)

In the more normal situation when action potentials are not blocked, the interactions between currents associated with action potentials, with electrogenic pumping, and with permeability changes due to deformation of the terminals, are likely to be complicated. Suffice it to say that when the situations before and after impulse blockade are compared, the rate of impulse discharge appears to be proportional to the recorded receptor potential and, to some extent, to the rate of change of that potential (35).

Since an afferent axon branches to form terminations on several intrafusal fibers, the question arises as to whether the rate of impulse discharge reflects a combination of the processes taking place in the various terminations, or there are multiple sites of spike initiation (i.e., pacemakers), one of which, at a given moment, dominates the discharge. There is circumstantial evidence (41) that seems to favor the concept of multiple pacemakers, in line with the results obtained more directly in amphibian spindles (42,43).

Summary. Increased permeability that allows movement of Na^+ underlies the depolarization of the afferent terminals upon stretch, but other ions also play a role in determining the dynamic changes in the membrane potential. The rate of afferent discharge is probably dominated by one of several sites of spike initiation associated with the afferent branches. But when the passive spindle is stretched, the rate of discharge can be described to a first approximation as proportional to the depolarization and to its rate of change.

b. Mechanical properties in the absence of fusimotor activity. The transformation of spindle stretch to extension of afferent terminals is governed by the mechanical properties of intrafusal fibers. In what follows, the consequences of some simple assumptions about the mechanical properties are compared qualitatively with observations.

Let it be assumed that the portion of an intrafusal fiber enveloped by the afferent nerve ending behaves as a simple spring, while the rest of the fiber exhibits viscous friction and, therefore, cannot change in length instantaneously. It follows that a sudden increase in the length of the intrafusal fiber will cause immediate extension of the afferent ending, followed in time by a slow process of elongation of the rest of the intrafusal fiber and concomitant reduction in extension of the nerve ending. In other words, the extension of the nerve ending will show an overshoot followed by slow adaptation. This discussion illustrates how the nonuniformity of mechanical properties along the length of an intrafusal fiber can have a profound effect on the dynamic properties of afferent response. In fact, Boyd and Ward (44) report in a qualitative study using stretch of unstimulated, isolated spindles that "when the stretching ceased the polar regions of the nuclear bag fibers continued to extend slowly, with consequent shortening of the equatorial [middle] zone of time course similar to the adaptation of the [primary ending] discharge which is thus largely mechanical in origin." However, from this description one cannot conclude that the simple assumptions made above are valid ones. It follows from these assumptions that if the stretch amplitude were doubled the tension response would also double. Such is very far from being the case; it has been observed (45) that changes in tension and in length of the spindle are proportional only for extremely small variations, that is, 10 μm in length or 1 μN in force. This and other facts suggest that the frictional property is not the same as viscosity, but it may be more akin to "dry" or "static" friction (cf. 46).

The zone of afferent termination does indeed appear to behave much like a spring whose stiffness remains unchanged when the spindle is stretched to different lengths (29). But the mechanical properties of the other zones are clearly quite complicated and await systematic study. Of special interest is the case of the "sluggish" bag 1 fiber that can under certain circumstances exhibit stretch-activation (47); this phenomenon is not normally observed in other types of striated mammalian muscle.

Afferent endings on chain fibers do not exhibit pronounced overshoot and adaptation after a stretch, which helps explain the less prominent dynamic response of secondary endings (44). Chain fibers may be more uniform mechanically along their lengths and/or the frictional property may be less pronounced in their case.

Summary. The difference in mechanical properties of unstimulated intrafusal muscle fibers of different types is such as to give rise to the observed difference between dynamic responsiveness of primary and secondary endings, at least in a qualitative sense. The striated portions of a bag 1 fiber seem especially sluggish in changing their length, a phenomenon that is reminiscent of friction. As a result, the Ia termination on the bag 1 fiber takes the brunt of a sudden stretch of the spindle, but it relaxes or adapts subsequently. These mechanical events confer a large measure of dynamic responsiveness to the primary ending.

c. Fusimotor effects. When all the intrafusal fibers of a spindle are contracting maximally, the total active force is only a few mg wt, which makes a negligible contribution to muscle force, yet it is sufficient to elongate the primary ending spirals by approximately 20% (48). A comparable extension of the spirals by muscle stretch in the absence of fusimotor activity would require the muscle to be stretched maximally to its physiologic limit. Thus, in relation to their respective physiologic ranges, *muscle stretch and fusimotor activity are of comparable "potency" in eliciting afferent discharge.*

The effects of contraction of identified intrafusal fibers upon Ia discharge rate are summarized on the basis of Boyd's observations (49). Contraction of the bag 1 fiber has a small effect when the spindle is held at constant length, but there is a very pronounced facilitatory effect upon the afferent discharge rate when the spindle is being stretched. Also, in the latter situation, the adaptation of afferent discharge rate after stretch plateau is much prolonged owing to the mechanical creep of the bag 1 fiber (50), which attests to an increase in the effective viscosity upon contraction. These influences of bag 1 contraction upon Ia response to stretch can be described as "dynamic" in nature, since they assert themselves most conspicuously in the context of dynamic changes in spindle length. In contrast, the effects of bag 2 or chain fiber contraction can be described as "static" even though these effects are not identical to each other but because both are markedly different from the dynamic effects. To wit, bag 2 contraction increases significantly the Ia discharge rate at all lengths of the spindle, whether the length is changing or not, while chain fiber contraction tends to synchronize the Ia discharge to the unfused twitches in a one-to-one fashion almost regardless of spindle length.

The contrast between the dynamic effects of bag 1 contraction and the static effects of bag 2 or chain fiber contraction has its counterpart in two classes of fusimotor axons. "Dynamic" and "static" fusimotor axons are those whose activity results in the corresponding effects on Ia discharge. In other words, the activity of dynamic fusimotor axons enhances the Ia response *during* spindle stretch and retards the decrease (i.e., adaptation) of the response after completion of the stretch; this activity has only a small effect on the afferent discharge rate if spindle length is maintained constant for some time. The most conspicuous effect of static fusimotor activity, on the other hand, is a substantial increase in afferent discharge rate at maintained length; concomitantly, the sensitivity of afferent discharge to stretch may be decreased.

A variety of evidence, collected painstakingly, has led to the conclusion that dynamic fusimotor axons innervate bag 1 fibers, and static fusimotor axons innervate bag 2 and/or chain fibers (5). However, the dichotomy between the dynamic and static systems may not be perfect, as evidenced by the existence of intermediate types of effects (51), glycogen depletion in bag 1 fibers by static fusimotor stimulation (52), and chance observation of innervation of a bag 2 fiber by a dynamic fusimotor axon (53). It has been suggested that perhaps 5% of fusimotor axons break the rule of separation of dynamic and static systems (20).

Stimulation of dynamic fusimotor axons results in nonpropagating junctional potentials in the intrafusal muscle fiber (53). In view of the ultrastructural specializations of the bag 1 fiber it is possible that a rigorlike state of stiffness is produced locally without much overt shortening. If so, the Ia response to spindle stretch will be increased (because the stiff region resists elongation), but there will not be a significant effect on the discharge rate at constant spindle length (since there is little shortening upon activation). These effects are indeed the hallmark of dynamic action (5).

The bag 2 fibers also show junctional potentials, although action potentials are observed occasionally, while chain fibers have all-or-none propagated action potentials (53). Nevertheless, unfused twitches in chain fibers rarely synchronize secondary ending discharge with or without stretch, but only increase the discharge rate (49), which is perhaps an indication of the lesser sensitivity of the receptor mechanism associated with secondary endings. Effects of bag fiber contraction on secondary endings are usually small (49) even though the contact area of their terminals with bag fibers is significant (26). Some of these apparent discrepancies between anatomic and physiologic findings may be related to shifts among pacemaker sites in the living spindle that was alluded to earlier.

Summary. There are two fairly distinct systems of fusimotor axons and intrafusal fibers innervated by them, which have quite different effects on the afferent response. Activity of the "dynamic" system produces an increase in afferent sensitivity to stretch when spindle length is changing. Activity of the "static" system results in increase of the afferent discharge rate at all lengths, whether or not the length is changing, and may decrease the sensitivity to stretch. Dynamic fusimotor axons innervate bag 1 fibers and can thus exert their effects on the primary ending, while static fusimotor axons innervate bag 2 and chain fibers and are in a position to influence the primary as well as the secondary ending.

2. Embedded Spindles in Reduced Preparations

The bulk of the information concerning the response properties of spindle receptors has been provided by the technique of recording afferent activity identified as originating from a selected muscle (1).

a. Experimental technique. The test muscle is usually dissected free and attached to a pulling device for external control of muscle length, leaving intact the innervation and the blood supply. Use of wire-hook electrodes in contact with an isolated, fine filament of an appropriate dorsal root is the preferred method for monitoring single afferents owing to the relative ease with which these filaments can be teased out and repeatedly split lengthwise. In order to decrease the number of active axons in a dorsal root filament other than those from the test muscle much of the rest of the receptive field of the dorsal root is often sacrificed by extensive denervation.

Afferent identification. Two criteria are commonly employed to distinguish spindle afferents from other afferents.

1. When a muscle twitch is elicited by stimulation of the muscle nerve at a strength that is well below the threshold for gamma axons, spindle afferents

usually decrease or cease their activity during the period that the muscle length is decreasing, unlike tendon organ afferents that typically increase their activity during the same period owing to the increase in muscle force. It may be noted that even under ostensibly isometric conditions muscle twitch inevitably results in some ("internal") shortening that is often sufficient to briefly silence spindle afferent discharge. Some often ignored problems with the use of this criterion are as follows. A spindle afferent may be mistaken for a tendon organ afferent if (1) the spindle lies in series with extrafusal fibers (54), or (2) the muscle action potential is "ephaptically" coupled to the afferent axon (1,55). A tendon organ afferent may be mistaken for a spindle afferent if the contraction is uneven in different regions of the muscle, so that a strong contraction in one region may unload the tendon organs in another region (cf. 55). Despite these limitations the criterion of afferent silence during twitch contraction of the muscle is probably adequate in a majority of cases.

2. The measurement of the axonal conduction velocity is used to distinguish spindle afferents from groups III and IV afferents (see Sec. III.A.2), although not from tendon organ afferents (group Ib). However, the existence of nonspindle muscle afferents in the group II or even group I range (12,14) might on occasion confound the identification. The measurement of conduction velocity is also relied upon for distinguishing between Ia and spII afferents, the dividing line being placed at a conduction velocity of 72 m/sec. This hard and fast distinction is perhaps less justified the nearer the conduction velocity lies to the dividing line (1).

Taken together, these criteria enable the experimenter to quickly identify the type of afferent whose activity is being monitored, although the possibility of occasional errors cannot be ruled out. In certain situations, the use of succinylcholine, an agent that causes contraction of bag fibers (cf. 56), can be an aid to identification (cf. 57; see, however, 58). Although intrafusal and extrafusal fibers are affected differentially by curare (59) or by dantrolene (60), these agents have not found practical use for purposes of identification.

Stimulus and response. Ramp-and-hold stretch of the muscle is employed commonly, although sinusoidal changes in length have also been utilized to a significant extent, especially when studying the responsiveness to small amplitudes of length change. Other types of mechanical stimuli, such as triangular, parabolic, or random changes in muscle length, have found use in some studies (61,62). The assessment of response is based upon the instantaneous discharge rate; but in the case of sinusoidal stretch, the modulation of the rate of discharge is often determined by measuring the probability of an afferent spike in each phase of the stretch cycle (63).

Summary. Despite some exceptions, a pause in discharge of an afferent axon during muscle twitch is an identifying characteristic of a spindle afferent. Ia and spII afferents can be distinguished on the basis of their axonal conduction velocities. The stimulus often consists of controlled stretch of the receptor-bearing muscle by a certain extent and velocity. Response is assessed by the instantaneous discharge rate.

b. De-efferented spindles. Sectioning the appropriate ventral roots leaves the response of spindle afferents to be determined exclusively by changes in muscle length. If one manipulates muscle length and monitors the discharge of primary and secondary endings in turn, it is easy to perceive a characteristic difference in the responsiveness of the two types of ending: The primary ending appears far more "sensitive" than the secondary. However, the quantification of this difference has turned out to be a nontrivial matter, as discussed in the following paragraphs.

Static and dynamic responses. The two types of afferent endings increase their discharge rates by comparable amounts when muscle length is increased and the discharge rates settle, that is, they cease to vary with time (1,64). (However, this increase in discharge rate is slightly larger for secondary endings and the difference is statistically significant [65].) In other words, the static responses of the two types of endings to a change in muscle length are of the same order of magnitude. (Static response is defined as the maintained increase in discharge rate elicited by a maintained increase in muscle length. It may be noted that static response has no a priori relation with static fusimotor effects.)

The much greater responsiveness of primary compared to secondary endings is brought out under dynamic conditions, that is, while muscle length is changing (66). Lest it be inferred that the two types of endings differ in a component of response that depends on velocity of stretch, it is important to point out that the greater response of the primary compared to the secondary endings is found to persist even when the velocity of stretch verges on zero (67,68).

Figure 1A is a diagrammatic depiction of the responses of typical primary and secondary endings to ramp-and-hold stretches at two different velocities. The increments in response (above prestretch levels) *during* constant velocity stretch are replotted in Figure 1B as functions of *muscle length* in order to illustrate the following points. (1) The static length-sensitivities (slopes of the dotted lines) are comparable for the two types of endings. (2) The primary ending shows greater response during constant velocity stretch than does the secondary. (3) For either type of ending, increasing the stretch velocity by a factor of four results in only an approximately 1.5-fold increase in the response (68). (4) The slopes of these graphs are not simply an expression of the static length-sensitivity, since they depend on stretch velocity (69). In fact, these slopes as well as the corresponding intercepts can be described to a good approximation by assuming that the velocity-dependence of the response is multiplicative (rather than additive) to the length-dependence, and that the former varies as a small power of stretch velocity for either type of ending (68).

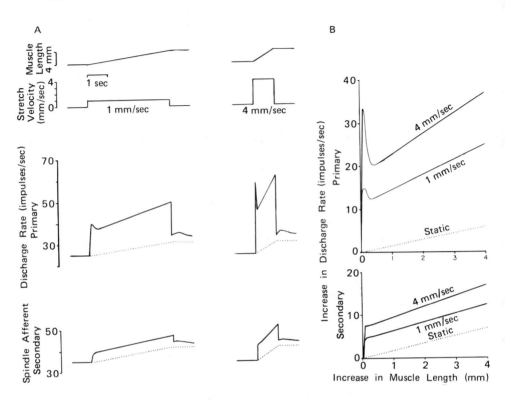

Figure 1 A, Diagrammatic depiction of responses of a primary and a secondary ending to ramp-and-hold stretch of the muscle. The abscissa represents time. Two velocities of stretch are indicated in the two columns. The dotted lines represent static responses, i.e., the discharge rates that would be obtained at each muscle length if that length were to be held constant for a long period. Dynamic response is the difference between the total response (shown by full lines) and the static response. B, The responses during constant-velocity stretch shown in A are graphed against muscle length rather than against time. The increase in discharge (above the level obtaining before ramp stretch), for any particular increase in muscle length, increases with stretch velocity but not in proportion to it. (For further details, see the text.)

In order to avoid apparent paradoxes that arise if dynamic response is considered synonymous to velocity response, it is useful to define the term "dynamic response" as simply that component of the response that is over and above the static response. (Note that dynamic response should not be confused with dynamic fusimotor effects.) With this definition it is possible to state without contradiction that (1) for any particular stretch velocity the dynamic response is greater for the primary than for the secondary ending, but (2) if the stretch velocity is increased, the dynamic responses of the two types of ending increase by approximately the same factor.

The greater dynamic response of the primary ending arises during the initial period of the ramp stretch (64,70) and a good part of it persists while the stretch continues. With respect to the initial change in length, a greater stretch responsiveness of primary compared to secondary endings has also been demonstrated using small ramp or sinusoidal stretches (67,70–72). Use of the latter stimulus shows that the phase difference between cycles of stretch and response is comparable for the two types of endings over a large range of stretch frequencies. This and other observations made with small variations in length demonstrate that the greater responsiveness of primary compared to secondary endings to these stimuli is a feature that is almost independent of velocity of movement.

The sensitivity of primary endings to small (e.g., $< 100 \ \mu$m) stretch of the muscle, even when the stretch is applied over a long duration (e.g., 1 min; see 67), is often 100 times greater than the static length-sensitivity measured with millimeter stretches. The high sensitivity to small stretch is manifested (66) as a transient peak ("initial burst") following onset of large stretch (Fig. 1A). This burst of action potentials does not represent a specific response to acceleration; in fact, it is quite dependent on prior history of movement and of fusimotor activity (46,61). However, the transient burst may well provide information related to sudden change in stretch velocity during an otherwise smooth movement (68).

Summary. When muscle stretch is small the primary ending responds with very high sensitivity to change in muscle length, while the secondary ending is rather less sensitive. (Both sensitivities increase in an essentially parallel manner as stretch velocity is increased.) When the stretch is large the sensitivity of both types of endings is reduced, but the reduction is more pronounced for the primary ending. With large ramp stretch the response of either type of ending to the initial part, that is, the response to a necessarily small stretch, persists to some extent, especially during continuing stretch. Consequently, the primary ending exhibits a greater response to large ramp stretch than does the secondary ending. (However, this greater response of the primary ending, during constant-velocity stretch, scales with stretch velocity in a manner comparable to that of the secondary ending.) Under static conditions, when the response to the initial part of the stretch has had ample time to decay, the sensitivities of the two types of endings are of the same order.

Adequate stimulus. The pronounced and persistent response of primary endings (and to a lesser extent of secondary endings) to the initial part of the stretch when the ramp stretch is initiated after holding muscle length constant for some time, is a feature that suggests that the adequate stimulus for spindle afferents is "motion" per se rather than the velocity and/or extent of the movement (68). In a more realistic situation when muscle length is not held rigidly constant for any length of time, the high responsiveness to small changes in length can be interpreted as the detection of minute irregularities of movement or of postural regulation (see later on). The response to the extent of movement is likely to be overshadowed in natural conditions by the responses to small irregularities, at least during slow movements. It therefore becomes problematic to view the primary ending as a transducer that reports the extent and velocity of movement to the central nervous system, even when the spindle is not under fusimotor control. However, if movement is proceeding smoothly, the average afferent discharge rate of spindles during stretch of a passive muscle can be expected to indicate a multiplicative combination of muscle length and velocity of movement. It is not known whether the conscious perception of position during a nonsmooth movement is affected by the irregularities of movement.

Summary. The primary ending is so highly responsive to small movements that it is difficult to see how it can serve to monitor the extent and velocity of a large movement, unless muscle stretch is free of small irregularities. The secondary ending may be more suited for this role.

c. Activation of single fusimotor axons. A filament of ventral root containing a single fusimotor axon can be stimulated electrically, while the discharge of a spindle afferent influenced by it is recorded simultaneously from a dorsal root filament. Dynamic and static fusimotor effects, as described in Sec. III.B.1.c, can be distinguished on the basis of how the stimulation of the efferent axon alters Ia discharge during dynamic changes in muscle length. A simple test for making this distinction consists of measuring the extent of adaptation of afferent discharge during a period of 0.5 sec after stretch plateau, following a constant-velocity stretch. This measure, the "dynamic index," is enhanced (reduced) in the event of stimulation of dynamic (static) fusimotor axons, compared to the case without stimulation (73).

The use of a single measure to distinguish dynamic and static fusimotor effects is a useful but somewhat "insensitive guide" (51). The essential sign of dynamic fusimotor action is the slow adaptation (related to mechanical creep) of discharge rate on the plateau of ramp stretch, while static fusimotor action is most clearly manifested when the afferent discharge does not cease during muscle shortening (51). Certainly, any number of measures can be invented to help distinguish the two types of fusimotor effects, but it is noteworthy that specific effects on the dynamic and static components of the response cannot be used as reliable criteria (5,72).

The very significant transition in sensitivity of the de-efferented primary ending, which occurs in going from small to large stretch, can be "softened" by either type of fusimotor activity, though in quite different ways. Dynamic fusimotor activity tends to preserve the sensitivity even as the stretch amplitude is increased, although there is a slight reduction in the sensitivity to small stretch (72). Static fusimotor activity, on the other hand, results in marked reduction of the sensitivity to small stretch (72); this too softens the transition, and renders the primary ending response similar to that of the secondary ending.

Since the spindle is presumably influenced by both types of fusimotor activity in its normal operation, it is of interest to examine the interactions that result when static and dynamic fusimotor axons are stimulated in conjunction. Two findings stand out (74,75): (1) If at a given phase of movement, the Ia discharge rate produced by static fusimotor stimulation is higher than that produced by dynamic fusimotor stimulation, the former effect occludes the latter when both fusimotor axons are stimulated. As an example, during muscle shortening, the effect of static, or static plus dynamic, fusimotor stimulation is the same. (2) When dynamic fusimotor stimulation gives rise to a higher rate of afferent discharge than does the static, the effect of combined stimulation is essentially a summation of the effects, that is, there is little occlusion. The mechanistic basis of these two phenomena is under investigation (cf. 41).

Some fusimotor axons when stimulated produce effects that resemble the effects of combined stimulation of static and dynamic fusimotor axons. These "intermediate" types are presumably the ones that violate the dichotomous innervation patterns of intrafusal fibers (51). Secondary endings, as is to be expected from their morphology, are subject to static fusimotor effects (76); there also are reports of dynamic fusimotor effects on some of them (77).

Fusimotor axons, either dynamic or static, are not only of the gamma variety, which are anatomically distinct from the alpha motor axons. Some of them are, in fact, branches of motor axons that innervate extrafusal muscle. Among these so-called beta axons, the dynamic ones supply slow-twitch extrafusal fibers, while the static ones innervate fast-contracting fibers (see 52 for a synopsis). Since dynamic betas would be expected to be recruited before static betas (Chapter 13), it is possible that there is a similar order among gamma fusimotor axons as well.

Summary. The Ia response to muscle stretch is affected in characteristic ways by stimulation of dynamic or static fusimotor axons, in line with the findings for isolated spindles. Combined stimulation of the two fusimotor types can result in occlusion or summation of the effects, depending upon whether the individual effects of static or dynamic fusimotor stimulation predominate in the particular conditions. The amplitude dependence of the stretch sensitivity of de-efferented primary endings can be rendered less conspicuous by fusimotor activity; specifically, dynamic stimulation enhances the sensitivity to large stretch and static stimulation reduces the sensitivity to small stretch.

d. Spontaneous fusimotor activity. The relative degree of activity of the dynamic and static fusimotor systems under natural conditions is not known, although it is known that the balance between them can be altered supraspinally

(78). The spontaneously occurring fusimotor activity in unanesthetized, decerebrate cats may be considered somewhat representative of natural conditions, to the extent that this preparation has long been regarded as a useful one for the study of spinal mechanisms.

In the decerebrate preparation compared to the de-efferented one, the afferent discharge rate at constant muscle length is (1) elevated (79), (2) much more irregular from one interpulse interval to the next (80), and (3) quite labile from one trial to the next (64). In addition, the dynamic response to constant-velocity stretch is greater than in the de-efferented case (68). These differences bespeak of a mixture of static and dynamic fusimotor activity in the decerebrate preparation. It appears that both gamma and beta systems are involved (81).

The variability of discharge can be averaged out over several trials, applying an identical stretch each time. The properties of response thus revealed in the decerebrate cat are similar, in qualitative terms, to those described in the section on de-efferented spindles (see Sec. III.B.2.b), although there are quantitative differences (68). For example, the nonlinearity is less conspicuous (64).

Summary. In the decerebrate cat, the response of spindle afferents to muscle stretch is more variable than in the de-efferented case or with controlled fusimotor activation. The augmentation of discharge rate and the increase in dynamic response are symptomatic of the combined actions of the static and dynamic fusimotor systems.

3. Spindle Discharge During Natural Movements

During a natural movement, a spindle afferent responds simultaneously to change in muscle length and in fusimotor activity. It has not yet proved possible to separate unequivocally the contributions of the two kinds of stimuli. Attention has been focused on the question of whether or not the fusimotor system is coactivated in an obligatory fashion with the alpha motor axons, a question that is outside the purview of this chapter. If one asks the question of which events are signaled by the spindle afferents to the central nervous system, an important finding is that in many conditions the discharge rate of a spindle afferent increases while the parent muscle is *shortening*, caused no doubt by fusimotor activity.

a. Animal studies. Spindle afferent discharge has been recorded in a variety of preparations that exhibit rhythmic, stereotyped motor activity (see 82 for a review). In one such study (83) concerning the scratching movement of the cat, the same afferents were monitored while the parent muscle was held under isometric or isotonic conditions. Spindle afferents from a flexor muscle were found to increase their discharge rate during increase of muscle force or during shortening, whichever was allowed. This rendered muscle length almost irrelevant as a stimulus to the spindle. In contrast, spindles in an extensor muscle under isotonic conditions increased their discharge when the muscle was lengthening passively but not when it was shortening actively. However, in the case of the extensor spindles, rhythmic fusimotor activity was present in sufficient degree to ensure increase in afferent discharge during increase of force under isometric conditions despite whatever internal shortening may have occurred.

Similarly, during active jaw movements, spindle afferents from the masseter muscle respond to both fusimotor and muscle-length stimuli (84). During this movement, not only is rhythmical fusimotor activity present in putative static axons, there are putative dynamic fusimotor axons that show a sustained increase in discharge that could preserve or even enhance the response to muscle length during the epochs that the static fusimotor axons may be silent.

Recording of afferents from dorsal roots (or dorsal root ganglia) using chronically implanted electrodes in fully conscious animals has not simplified this picture of diversity. During movement at different speeds the discharge of spindle afferents exhibits various patterns. Seeking a generalization from this variety, one group has concluded that fusimotor activity dominates spindle discharge during unobstructed movements as long as the speed of muscle shortening is slower than 0.2 muscle rest-lengths per sec (85). At faster speeds the change in muscle is the dominant stimulus. However, another group (cf. 86) has disputed this claim and has offered a different tentative generalization; namely, the spindles in muscles (or portions of muscles) that undergo lengthening contraction during locomotion (in the support, or stance, phase) respond primarily to muscle length, while the spindles in the muscles (or portions thereof) that shorten during contractions (in the transfer, or swing, phase) respond primarily to the fusimotor drive. Since these two categories to a certain extent can be identified with extensors and flexors, respectively, the results quoted previously for the scratching movement are supportive of this tentative generalization. It is not clear, however, whether the dynamic and static fusimotor systems are preferentially active in relation to these two categories of muscle. The technique of selective blockade of gamma axons by application of local anesthetic (87) may help resolve these issues. However, even if a simplifying rule could be established for locomotion, there is no guarantee that the same rule will apply to other hindlimb movements, or to movements of other body parts.

   b. Human studies. It is possible to record muscle afferent discharge in conscious humans by inserting a microelectrode in a peripheral nerve. But the extent of movement has to be curtailed drastically (in comparison with the animal experiments), in order not to dislodge the electrode. Results obtained with the use of this technique point to the dominant influence of the fusimotor system in that spindle afferent discharge can increase during contraction (88). Nevertheless, the spindle afferents, particularly Ia axons, remain sensitive to minute irregularities of movement (89). The discharge rate is very sensitive to lack of smoothness of the movement, although it gives little information about absolute muscle length. If the muscle is stretched forcibly, the Ia afferents exhibit a segmented pattern of discharge that presumably reflects mechanical oscillations in the muscle (90).

During parkinsonian tremor, as indeed during rhythmical voluntary movement in normal subjects, the discharge of Ia afferents is linked to muscle stretch as well as to muscle contraction. In contrast, during clonus in spastic patients, Ia discharge occurs as a result of passive stretch on the falling phase of contraction, presumably without significant fusimotor involvement (91).

In view of the findings that have been obtained in more or less natural conditions it is difficult to ascribe to spindle afferents from a contracting muscle the role of signaling muscle length. Nevertheless, a length-related signal with emphasis on small changes appears to be contained in the afferent discharge. The unknown pattern of fusimotor activity is a complicating factor in the interpretation of the afferent discharge. The response of spindle afferents may be more amenable to interpretation in the case of muscles that are stretched passively during movement. There has been insufficient emphasis on the role that spindle afferents from passive antagonists may play (but see 92,93). Also, there are few reported instances of information obtained from reduced preparations concerning the response properties of spindle afferents with various degrees of fusimotor activity in *shortening* muscle (e.g., 94). The difficulty of interpretation of afferent responses during active movement underscores the need for further investigations of response properties under controlled conditions.

Summary. In natural movements, spindle afferent discharge often increases during active shortening of the receptor-bearing muscle. Knowledge of the activity patterns of the two fusimotor systems in this situation is rudimentary at present. It appears that fusimotor activity may vary depending upon the muscle or the task. However, the discharge rate of spindle afferents from actively shortening muscle does contain length-related information, and it is especially sensitive to small irregularities in the profile of change in muscle length. It remains to be elucidated how the relatively complex pattern of afferent response from active muscles, and the simpler pattern of response from spindles in muscles that are stretched passively during movement, can together be interpreted to yield information about the state of the muscle and about external impediments.

C. Modeling of Spindle Responses

It is a sobering fact that despite the great volume of studies of response properties of spindle afferents, there does not yet exist a method for predicting the discharge of an afferent, even of a suitably idealized one, when muscle length and fusimotor activity vary with time. Assuming that such a method were proposed, it would still be problematic to test it against available data, since these data highlight the range of effects on many afferents in each chosen condition rather than the effects on each afferent across conditions.

A point of departure for modeling of spindle responses is, nevertheless, available. There are several quantitative summarizations of experimental data concerning select features of spindle afferent responses, albeit restricted to particular conditions and particular forms of muscle stretch (63,68,69,71). These summarizations are sometimes referred to as "models," even though the claim has not been made that they can be used profitably with other forms of muscle stretch and in other conditions. A model, properly so called, should not only account for the known responses of the receptor to the "standard" time courses of the stimulus, it should be capable of predicting the responses to nonstandard ones as well. It is the experimental testability of predictions that provides the *raison d'etre* for a model.

These quantitative summarizations of data have the further disadvantage that they are restricted to the situation where fusimotor activity is either absent or at least does not vary with time. There is insufficient quantitative information on the transient effects of change in fusimotor rate, either alone or in conjunction with change in muscle length (but see 95,96). Also, the available data concerning the effects of fusimotor stimulation span different rates of stimulation in different experiments. Perhaps the proposal, in the future, of a comprehensive model will help streamline the data base.

If attention is confined to the situation where fusimotor activity is absent or is constant, there are several features of the response to muscle stretch that are noteworthy because they present a special challenge to a modeler. One such feature is the frictionlike property in intrafusal elements mentioned earlier. A related feature is the phenomenon that the high sensitivity to small stretch is not specific to any particular muscle length; therefore, if muscle length is altered, the region of high sensitivity is obliged to start resetting, which is bound to have profound consequences on the response during large stretch. Furthermore, the relation between increments of response and of muscle length is more markedly nonlinear just after ramp plateau than it is during ramp stretch (70). This last observation indicates that the nonlinearity of response is not a matter of simple saturation, since the nonlinearity is more manifest, in this instance, when the discharge rate happens to be lower.

A model of afferent responses to muscle stretch has recently been proposed by one of us (97). This model accounts for the features mentioned earlier, on the basis of the assumption that the frictionlike property of striated portions of intrafusal muscle is similar to a property observed for amphibian extrafusal muscle and attributed to myofibrillar interactions (98). An additional assumption in the model is that the rate of afferent discharge depends not only on the elongation of the afferent termination, but also on its time derivative (see Sec. III.B.1.a). There is quantitative agreement between predictions of the model for stretch responses of de-efferented primary and secondary endings and the corresponding observations for small as well as large muscle stretch. Other predictions based on the model are also amenable to experimental testing; these include the time course of adaptation of response after ramp plateau, as well as responses to nonstandard forms of stretch. In the model, the effects of fusimotor stimulation at constant rate are mimicked qualitatively, again, for both small and large stretch. However, no attempt has been made to encompass the transient effects of change in fusimotor activity.

Based on these modeling studies that deal with the details of the nonlinearities, a characteristic property of spindle afferent response emerges to the fore, though this property is implicit in the various reported observations. Namely, *the receptor possesses exquisitely high sensitivity, but unlike many man-made transducers of high sensitivity, the range of operation of the receptor (in terms of muscle length) is not sacrificed in consequence*. Instead, the region of high sensitivity is "portable"; it is dissolved and reestablished continually as muscle length changes. Dynamic fusimotor activity can be seen as slowing down this process of resetting, while static fusimotor activity, in addition to augmenting the discharge rate, speeds up this process. The process of resetting makes the spindle quite unlike most transducing devices used in engineering practice, although an analogy can be drawn with the Dolby system of sound recording (R. S. Wilkinson, personal communication).

Summary. There is no comprehensive model of spindle afferent response that could account for all the known facts and be capable of making testable predictions. There are some quantitative summarizations of select features of responses under particular conditions, but these have little predictive power. However, when fusimotor activity is absent or is constant, the features of response can be captured in a model, properly so called, which is based on the assumption of frictionlike properties of intrafusal elements. The characteristic property of spindle afferents that emerges is that the high-sensitivity region of the receptor is continually being reset as muscle length changes. This property allows spindles to possess high sensitivity for small perturbations, without sacrificing the range of operation, as muscle length varies widely.

D. Summary

The structure of a spindle is essentially comprised of three specialized types of intrafusal muscle fibers, enveloped in their middle regions by two types of mechanoreceptive afferent nerve endings, and innervated in the more highly striated regions by two types of efferent axons. The discharge of a spindle afferent axon depends upon longitudinal stretch of the spindle, whether applied directly to an isolated spindle or indirectly by way of muscle stretch, and also depends upon efferent activity. The effects of these two kinds of stimuli have been examined in turn and also in conjunction.

Stretch alone brings out a difference in the responsiveness of the two afferent types, Ia and spII. When the stretch is small, the discharge rates of Ia afferents are more sensitive to the stretch compared to the case of spII afferents.

If stretch continues, there is a reduction in the sensitivities of both types of afferents to additional stretch, and the reduction is more pronounced for Ia afferents. However, in this situation of continuing stretch, the Ia response remains elevated above the spII response. After the stretching is terminated and the length is maintained constant for some time, the final, static increment in discharge rate is relatively modest and is comparable for the two afferent types. High sensitivity to small stretch is reestablished at the new length. In this manner, a region of high sensitivity is retained without sacrificing the range of operation of the receptor in terms of muscle length.

The activation of spindle efferent axons at constant spindle length results in increase of afferent discharge. The increase is small in the case of "dynamic" efferents and substantial for "static" efferents.

Activity of the two types of efferents has characteristic effects on the afferent response to spindle stretch. Dynamic efferent activity enhances considerably the response to a large stretch, but it also causes a slight reduction in the response to a small stretch. These actions result in softening the transition in sensitivity of the Ia discharge in response to increasing stretch. In addition, the period of adaptation of discharge rate after stretch plateau is prolonged considerably. There is little effect of dynamic efferent activity on spII afferents. In contrast, static efferents affect both types of afferents, and the result of their activity, in addition to augmentation of afferent discharge rate at all lengths of the spindle, may be a reduction in responsiveness to small as well as large stretches.

The properties of afferent responsiveness described previously are consistent with the observed mechanical effects of stretch and/or activation of identified intrafusal muscle fibers. These properties can be mimicked by a mathematical model in which it is assumed that a frictional effect arises as a result of myofibrillar interactions that enables the region of high sensitivity to be dissolved and reestablished gradually as spindle length is changed, even in the absence of efferent activity. An additional assumption in the model, consistent with observations, is that the rate of afferent discharge depends not only on the elongation of the afferent termination, but also on the rate of change of the elongation.

In natural conditions, neither muscle length nor spindle efferent activity is held constant. No model exists currently that can enable one to infer the pattern of spindle efferent activity from measurements of muscle length and afferent discharge. Nevertheless, these measurements have been interpreted to imply that the activation of spindle efferents commences at about the same time as the activation of the efferents that innervate the ("extrafusal") muscle itself. Spindle afferent discharge during natural movements is influenced so strongly by spindle efferents that it is difficult to see how the afferent signal can be interpreted to yield muscle length or its derivatives, although the effect of minute irregularities of the change in muscle length during slow movements may be readily discernible.

IV. GOLGI TENDON ORGANS

A. Structure and Intramuscular Relationships

Tendon organs consist largely of collagenous fascicles and nerve endings, encased in a spindle-shaped connective tissue capsule, similar in fine structure to that of the muscle spindle (4).

The capsule dimensions vary little from muscle to muscle (6), but they may show some species dependency. For example, Bridgman (99) found tendon organs in the rat extensor digitorum brevis muscle to be somewhat smaller (length = 640 μm, width at midsection = 47 μm) than those of the cat, whereas human receptors were found to be larger (1600 and 120 μm, respectively).

The capsular lumen is divided into discrete compartments by several transverse septa of different size that extend inward from the capsule wall. At one end, the collagenous fascicles within each compartment connect with an aponeurosis of origin or insertion. (Recall that there are few tendon organs in the tendon proper.) At the other end, these fascicles connect with 5-25 muscle fibers (mean ca. 10), which can be considered as directly "in-series" with the receptor, adjacent fibers being "in-parallel."

At the midsection, the collagenous fascicles are sufficiently separate to permit entry of two sensory axons. The first of these is the heavily myelinated Ib fiber, which sometimes supplies a second and, even rarer, a third tendon organ (100); the second axon (not always present) is a small, thinly myelinated group III fiber whose function is still unknown.

There are several functional implications to the anatomic relationships within the tendon organ capsule and between each capsule and surrounding intramuscular structures. The intracapsular association between collagen bundles and Ib axonal branches (reviewed in 4) appears to optimize the possibility of microlengthening (straightening) of the collagen strands, perhaps resulting in the physical distortion (lengthening, twisting, and pinching) of a relatively large surface area of the axonal branches. This distortion can be considered as the "adequate stimulus" for activation of the Ib's terminals. It is readily achieved by contraction of muscle fibers inserting directly into the capsule. In contrast, muscle stretch must accomplish little collagen lengthening, unless the in-series fibers are in active contraction. Thus, stretch of the passive muscle should be a relatively ineffective stimulus. Contraction of in-parallel muscle fibers immediately adjacent to the receptor might provide an "unloading" effect.

At a grosser structural level, it should be kept in mind that the territory of single motor units is relatively widespread throughout a limited cross section of the muscle (101). In a matrix of 10 adjacent fibers (the number typically clasped by a single receptor) there is rarely more than one fiber belonging to a single motor unit. As a result, the in-series fibers providing the force input to the receptor should typically belong to different motor units, some of whose other fibers are no doubt contributing an unloading (in-parallel) stimulus to the receptor. In mixed muscles, these 10-fiber matrices include fibers belonging to units of different type and functional threshold (101). Even in compartmentalized muscles featuring a close association between muscle receptors and oxidative muscle fibers belonging to low-threshold motor units, the oxidative compartment typically contains 20–25% glycolytic fibers belonging to high-threshold units (e.g., 102). As a result, the anatomy suggests that the fibers clasped by each single tendon organ provide the receptor with a random sample of forces from the different motor-unit types.

Finally, the intracapsular arrangement between muscle fibers and collagen strands suggests the possibility of a different mechanical advantage between each single fiber and a limited number of Ib axon branches within each intracapsular collagenous compartment (discussed later).

Summary. The tendon organ capsule contains collagenous fascicles that are connected at one end to an aponeurosis and at the other end to a number (ca. 10) of muscle fibers. The force exerted by these muscle fibers via the fascicles causes distortion of the terminations of a mechanoreceptive Ib afferent axon. The muscle fibers in series with a particular receptor belong, typically, to different motor units.

B. Functional Properties

1. Isolated Tendon Organs

Fukami and Wilkinson have shown that single or pairs of tendon organs, with or without muscle fibers attached, can be isolated from cat tail muscles and maintained in vitro for several hours in good functional state (100,103–105). They have studied the firing patterns of Ib afferents supplying isolated receptors during short stimulation epochs in which the axon's impulse initiation site(s) was activated by either a constant depolarizing current applied near the point of nerve entry into the receptor capsule or by mechanical perturbations resulting from manual deformation with a fine probe, controlled ramp-and-hold and sinusoidal stretches, and even by contraction of the inserting muscle fibers. It was also possible to study graded receptor potentials by blocking impulse activity with tetrodotoxin. These potentials are thought to be generated within the capsule itself and conducted decrementally to the nearby recording site along the Ib axon.

As with other mechanoreceptors, sensory transduction in embedded tendon organs involves: (1) transmission of force (active and/or passive) to the receptor and its subsequent mechanical deformation; (2) generation of a receptor potential in the sensory ending(s); and (3) impulse initiation in the afferent nerve. Fukami and Wilkinson's virtuosic experiments give insight into all three of these stages.

a. Receptor deformation and mechanical properties. When different tendon organs are subjected to a stress (measured as force/cross section), their subsequent strain (measured as change of length/total length), and hence elastic stiffness, can vary over 10-fold. (Experimentally, this measurement is actually made in reverse; that is, stress measured in response to strain.) The stiffest of the receptors have a Young's modulus (stress/strain index) apparently greater than even the tendon itself. The relationship between stress and strain is approximately linear up to 5% strain, the physiologic maximum before permanent deformation of the collagen macromolecules occurs. The stiffness is relatively rate independent, at least between 0.1 and 80.0 Hz. By way of comparison, muscle spindles are an order of magnitude less stiff (i.e., more compliant) than tendon organs and their stress-strain relations are considerably more dependent on rate.

b. Transducing properties. Fukami and Wilkinson (103) showed that the amplitude of the "steady-state" receptor potential in isolated receptors is graded in proportion to applied static tension. An initial dynamic component was present that increased with increasing velocity of stretch. The extent of accommodation was more difficult to assess owing largely to the failure of the isolated preparations to maintain a sustained discharge lasting for more than 30 sec. (This failure was attributed to a combination of the lack of blood supply and the low [25°C] temperature at which the measurements were taken.) Analysis of responses (both receptor potential and action potential) to constant stimulating currents of various intensities and combined electrical and mechanical stimulation suggested that a single impulse initiation site was involved, probably within the capsule itself (but see 106).

In Fukami and Wilkinson's initial work (103), Ib firing patterns appeared to be more highly correlated with strain of the receptor capsule than with stress. Subsequently (105), they proposed that the tension may have two components, one lengthening individual collagen fibers and one "rearranging" them. As a result, the sensory terminals would be subjected to both a microlengthening and a twisting and pinching by the collagen fibers. These mechanical events appear to underlie the tendon organs' steady-state response to static forces. The dynamic responsiveness of the receptor appears to arise more from ionic processes within the sensory terminals. In contrast, both the dynamic and static length-responsiveness of muscle spindles appear to arise from a combination of mechanical and ionic events (discussed previously).

The response modulation, R (in imp./sec), of the average isolated tendon organ to applied modulation of tension (T) fits the power relation ($R \approx T^{0.87}$) that, as with other mechanoreceptors, reveals the capability of the receptor to compress the range of its output in response to a wide range of force inputs. However, for tendon organs, this compression is small (i.e., the power relation approaches linearity) as compared to that of isolated spindles' responses to displacement modulation, D (see 45), average values for Ia and spII afferents being $R \approx D^{0.5}$ and $D^{0.67}$, respectively. For example, as reported by Wilkinson and Fukami (105), a change in impulse rate of two orders of magnitude (e.g., from 1 to 100 imp./sec) encodes a 10,000-fold change in muscle length for Ia and 1000-fold for spII afferents, whereas the corresponding change in force for Ib afferents is only 200-fold.

Finally, isolated tendon organs bear one striking similarity to isolated muscle spindles. Just as spindles have a low threshold to lengthening perturbations, Fukami and Wilkinson's work has provided direct evidence of the low-force threshold of isolated tendon organs to in-series force. For sustained afferent discharge, this absolute (active + passive) force was found to be about 8-170 mg wt at 24°C. It was also demonstrated that the contraction of a single muscle fiber could initiate impulse discharge from the receptor with the absolute dynamic force threshold being 4.5-14.0 mg wt. These static and dynamic thresholds might be even lower at normal muscle temperature. Thus, *these direct measurements show irrefutably that the tendon organ is a particularly low-threshold force receptor.*

Summary. The stress-strain relation in the physiologic range for a tendon organ is approximately linear and rate-independent. The deformation (strain) of the nerve ending is presumably proportional to the applied force, without the complication of dynamic properties. However, the ionic processes underlying the receptor potential do confer a measure of dynamic responsiveness to the receptor. Modulation of discharge rate is not exactly proportional to modulation of force, but the range compression due to nonlinearity is modest.

The threshold force necessary to elicit afferent discharge is sufficiently small so that the contractile force of only one of the in-series muscle fibers can exceed it.

2. Embedded Tendon Organs in Reduced Preparations

As with muscle spindles, the favored approach throughout the twentieth century for the study of tendon organs has extended on the classic work of B. H. C. Matthews (107) by analyzing the responses of Ib afferents supplying embedded tendon organs in reduced preparations. Until 1964, the tendon organ "languished in relative obscurity" (108), largely because it was viewed as a high-threshold force detector, not concerned with the moment-to-moment reflex control of muscle. Subsequently, the reports of Jansen and Rudjord (109; see also 110), and, particularly those of Houk and Henneman (111), emphasized the low-threshold responsiveness of tendon organs. This finding was soon repeatedly confirmed in Houk's and other laboratories (e.g., 112-115), but it has been surprisingly slow to find its way into the textbooks.

The key change in the experimental approach introduced by Houk and Henneman (111) was to study responses of tendon organs to contraction of single and small groups of motor units. Prior to their work, only responses to the stretch or contraction of the whole muscle had been studied, an approach that is not particularly revealing because of the structural relationships outlined earlier (i.e., it does not take into account the mechanical arrangement of tendon organs within the muscle). Nonetheless, some aspects of Ib responses to whole-muscle perturbations are still worthy of note.

    a. Response to stretch of passive muscle. At one stage, controversy centered around whether or not tendon organs can discharge steadily within the physiologic range of passive muscle stretch (111,112,116). Interest in this issue subsided when it became obvious that the passive force responsiveness of these receptors depends not only on the muscle under study but also on the relationship between the intramuscular location of each receptor and the muscle's "line-of-pull." Probably the most interesting analysis to emerge from the argument was one in which Houk and his collaborators provided an indirect estimate of the threshold force for a sustained tendon organ response. If it is accepted that two thirds of the passive tension in muscle is supported by connective tissue (117) and that there are approximately 24,000 muscle fibers in soleus (118), of which 10 are attached to each tendon organ (119), then Houk et al. (112) reasoned that passive tension exerted on the receptor can be estimated as passive force at the tendon $\times$ 1/3 $\times$ (10/24,000). Applying this calculation to their experimental results showing sustained Ib afferent discharge to a passive tension in soleus of 200 g wt, they arrived at an absolute static-force threshold of 28 mg wt.

    b. Responses to motor-unit contraction. As emphasized previously, the preferred in situ technique for studying the tendon organ involves noting its responses to contraction of single and small groups of motor units. However, following Houk and Henneman's (111) unequivocal demonstration of this point, there have been few reports from other laboratories that have extended upon their original approach (see 4,108 for reviews). Six features of tendon organ responses to motor-unit contractions deserve special emphasis.

    Low force threshold. Houk and Henneman (111) showed the tendon organs in the cat soleus muscle can be provoked into sustained discharge by the tetanic force of a single motor unit. Since only 4–15 motor units were shown to activate a single receptor, they reasoned that the threshold of activation for a tendon organ must be less than the maximum force produced by one or two muscle fibers that insert into the receptor's capsule. Their estimate of 28 mg wt for the absolute (active + passive) steady-state force threshold (112) was followed by an estimate of 4 mg wt for the absolute threshold required to elicit a single action potential during twitch of a single muscle fiber belonging to a single motor unit (115). Recall that these indirect estimates have subsequently been confirmed by measurements on isolated receptors (103,104). Binder et al. (115) argued that a dynamic force threshold of 4 mg wt was considerably less than the force produced by the twitch of a single muscle fiber in the cat soleus. Their conclusion that "the force threshold of every tendon organ is less than the force produced by any muscle fiber connected to it" has not been confirmed directly. However, given the close anatomic intramuscular association between oxidative low-threshold fibers and tendon organs, the conclusion seems inescapable that the sensitivity of tendon organs ensures that even the smallest of forces that develop in a muscle will be reflected in a population of Ib afferent impulses projecting to the spinal cord. From this perspective, the sensitivity of tendon organs to muscle force is at least on par with the sensitivity of muscle spindles to muscle length, within their respective physiologic ranges.

Motor unit type and recruitment order. As another extension of Houk and Henneman's (111) observations, study has been made of the neuromechanical properties of groups of motor units whose contraction excites a single tendon in the "mixed" cat medial gastrocnemius muscle (4,114,120). It was shown that units of each group exhibit a wide range of contractile properties, in keeping with previous and subsequent motor unit studies (see 101 for a review) showing that in any matrix of adjacent fibers in a mixed muscle, the number (5-25) that could conceivably be clasped by a tendon organ will contain an admixture of the muscle's different fiber types, with each single fiber belonging to a different single motor unit. This arrangement provides each single tendon organ with the possibility of providing the nervous system with an approximate indication of whole-muscle force, even though each receptor samples but a minute sample of the force of a small number of motor units.

Henneman's "size principle" of orderly motor unit recruitment (121) suggests that, in general, the graded development of muscle force is brought about by motor units producing small amounts of force being recruited before those producing large forces, a recruitment pattern that is generally accompanied by an elevation in the firing rate of the active motor units. The fibers whose forces are sampled by a single tendon organ are representative not only of the different fiber and motor unit types in the muscle but also of their recruitment order. Thus, the possibility exists that each single tendon organ can provide information about the *full* range of force development.

In-series and in-parallel relationships. One possible explanation for the erroneous impression that tendon organs are in the tendon proper and the slow acceptance of the low-force threshold of tendon organs has been the widespread belief that while spindles have essentially an in-parallel relationship with the surrounding muscle fibers, tendon organs are in-series with the *whole* muscle. This concept was first proposed by Fulton and Pi-Suñer (122) in 1928, and, unfortunately, it was quickly supported by the experimental work of B. H. C. Matthews (107) in which the analysis of afferent responses was limited to stretch and contraction of the whole muscle. It remained for Houk and Henneman (111) to note that tendon organs are in-series with but a minute number of muscle fibers and in-parallel with the remainder. What now remains to be determined is the relative effectiveness of this in-parallel force, particularly when the receptor is responding to in-series force. This dual stimulation of the tendon organ can conceivably occur during the contraction of even a single motor unit.

The experience of Houk and Henneman (111) and of Gregory and Proske (123) was that the response of a tendon organ to the contraction of a strongly excitatory motor unit or small group of units is not attenuated by contraction of in-parallel units or even contraction of all motor units having little or no excitatory action on the receptor. In contrast, Stuart et al. (113) provided examples of the response of the tendon organ to contraction of a small group of in-series units being obviated by the cocontraction of another group of in-parallel units. Subsequently, Binder (124) provided evidence showing that the response of a tendon organ to stimulation of a group of excitatory units is attenuated by the cocontraction of all the motor units in the muscle.

A further complication is that in experiments of this kind, it is not uncommon to find a Ib's response to contraction of a low-force motor unit being of greater magnitude than to contraction of a high-force unit (114,120,123). It has been argued that this is explainable by different mechanical advantages between single muscle fibers and intracapsular compartments of the receptor (120,123). However, in Fukami's work on isolated tendon organs (104) the contraction of each fiber inserting on a receptor was of equal potency. He argued that in embedded preparations, the possibility exists that the relative balance between in-series and in-parallel force development by single units can explain those instances in which weaker units seem to elicit stronger responses from tendon organs.

The case for tendon organs being in-series with but a small number of muscle fibers is now unequivocal, as established both physiologically and anatomically. However, more remains to be learned about the functional significance of in-parallel force.

Ensemble Ib discharge. Ensemble analyses of Ib input have been undertaken to test Houk and Henneman's (111) proposition that it is the collective (ensemble) discharge rather than the discharge of any single tendon organ that provides the central nervous system with the most accurate assessment of total muscle force. To date, these ensemble analyses have involved noting the pattern of response of several Ib afferents to the individual contraction of several single motor units and then summing the discharges of Ib afferents as a function of the sum of the forces of all the motor units studied. This approach is far from the naturally occurring ensemble situation, of course. Nonetheless, its use has served to emphasize two issues requiring further work.

First, the relationship between the collective tendon organ discharge and force developed at the tendon depends on the order in which the motor unit–tendon organ responses are summed. When the units are added in order of increasing tension, there is at first a relatively large increase in total tendon organ response that then tends to increase less rapidly as more units are added. If, as is likely, this situation is representative of normal tendon organ–motor unit behavior, then it suggests that during weak contractions the collective tendon organ discharge from the muscle is *relatively* stronger than during larger contractions (120).

Second, if in addition, the force of the exciting motor units is varied, either by fatiguing them or taking advantage of their individual length-tension properties (125), then the relationship between the collective tendon organ discharge and force developed at the tendon reveals that changes in the force of contraction of *single* motor units result in relatively small changes in ensemble Ib firing. Rather, the receptor is far more responsive to changes in the number of motor units active at any one time.

Low dynamic sensitivity. The tendon organ exhibits a small dynamic response to stretch of the passive muscle (e.g., 126) and to contractions of a single unit or the whole muscle under isometric as well as ramp-and-hold conditions (e.g., 111,125,127,128). Surprisingly, this finding is downplayed in the experimental literature, possibly because some investigators have failed to emphasize how weak is the dynamic response, again particularly when compared to that of Ia and even spII afferents. However, the response to stimulation of high-force motor units shows a significant dynamic response (123).

Responses to two or more units. Houk and Henneman (111) showed that the combined stimulation of two or more motor units elicits less than the expected sum of responses of an excited Ib afferent. This finding has also been extended upon. For example, Gregory and Proske (123) compared the individual and summed responses of a Ib afferent to eight "exciting" motor units in the cat medial gastrocnemius. They showed that the motor unit tension summed almost algebraically (total sum predicted from individual tensions 1043 g wt; tension reached 890 g wt), whereas the increase in Ib firing rate was much less than expected (peak rate 240 imp./sec; expected peak 523 imp./sec) (cf. 124). When they artificially summed Ib responses in the order of the increasing tension of each motor unit, the plot of firing rate against tension suggested a negatively accelerating function (123,129). It would be of interest to extend this type of analysis to muscles in which the tendon organs are restricted to a portion of the muscle that is rich in oxidative muscle fibers that are known to be of lower recruitment threshold (121). In this instance, the tendon organ response to cumulative force development might become even more curvilinear.

Another observation by these workers (130) was that the response of a tendon organ to contraction of a motor unit could show adaptation of discharge if preceded by a conditioning contraction of another motor unit. A mechanical model was proposed to account for such a "cross-adaptation." The muscle fiber from each motor unit is envisioned to pull on a collagen strand that supports one of the receptor terminals. The nonlinear summation of responses on combinated stimulation and the phenomenon of cross-adaptation were accounted for by mechanical cross-links between collagen strands such that one muscle fiber would pull on more than one receptor terminal. At this time, it is difficult to reconcile this interesting model with the previously described data on isolated tendon organs and the current understanding of the intracapsular structure of tendon organs. However, the model is thought provoking and should provide an effective stimulus for further anatomic and physiologic studies on the receptor.

 c. Responses to spontaneous force development. Responses of embedded tendon organs have also been noted to force development in unanesthetized decerebrate cats, a preparation that provides the possibility of substantial experimental interventions. One study on the homogeneous (type SO fiber) cat soleus muscle (131) revealed: (1) the responses of most tendon organs are illustrative of a relatively linear relation between averaged near steady-state force development and Ib firing rate; and (2) a few receptors respond to steady-state force with steplike increases in rate that are not matched by comparable changes in total muscle force, as if to suggest the receptors are especially sensitive to the recruitment of new motor units. It will be of interest to compare these results to those obtained from heterogeneous muscles in which the possibility exists that more responses of the second type might be encountered (cf. 132).

 Another approach with the decerebrate cat has been to record from Ib afferents during "controlled" treadmill locomotion, evoked by continuous electrical stimulation of the brain stem (133). The published observations emphasize that tendon organs exhibit low passive force responsiveness during stepping and, at slow speeds, are not necessarily activated unless presumably "in-line" with active muscle fibers. Furthermore, the peak Ib discharge is not necessarily at the peak of muscle force development, an observation also reported (but without comment) for Ib discharge from the diaphragm in the anesthetized cat (134).

 Summary. Stretch of passive muscle results in a small increase in muscle force, of which only a minute fraction is exerted through any particular tendon organ. Consequently, the force-threshold of Ib response is not reached without substantial stretch if the muscle is passive.

 The low force-threshold of tendon organ response is brought out unequivocally when single motor units are stimulated. The receptors can respond to even the smallest of forces developed in the muscle. A particular receptor seems to be responsive to a sample of forces developed by different types of motor units; the sample is essentially random and, therefore, possibly representative of the muscle as a whole. In the soleus muscle of the decerebrate cat, the responses of most tendon organs are illustrative of a linear relation between Ib discharge rate and spontaneously generated whole muscle force, at least up to a certain level. The dynamic component of Ib response to change in force is marginal, except possibly when high-force motor units are stimulated.

The combined stimulation of two or more motor units elicits less than the sum of individual responses; the interaction effects are presumably due to mechanical cross-links between fascicles in a receptor capsule. Another type of interaction between the effects of stimulation of motor units results from the fact that the contraction of muscle fibers that are not in series with a particular receptor may tend to unload the receptor, thus decreasing its discharge rate. The ensemble of Ib discharges from a muscle, compared to the discharge of a single Ib afferent, may be less affected by these local phenomena. In fact, during artificial recruitment of motor units in order of increasing tension, an ensemble of Ib discharges has been found to be a monotonically increasing (though not linear) function of whole-muscle force.

3. Tendon Organ Discharge During Natural Movements

In intact subjects, the identification of a Ib afferent spike train is considerably more difficult than that for a spindle afferent. Possibly for this reason, much less is known about the tendon organ than spindle behavior during the unrestrained movements of conscious humans and experimental animals.

a. Animal studies. The few published observations on tendon organ behavior during normal movements have focused on either unrestrained stepping (86,135) or a "voluntary" knee flexion against an externally applied extension (136). The stepping studies have provided examples of the lack of *strict* correspondence between whole muscle electromyographic activity and the Ib discharge of single receptors. In addition, the knee-flexion study showed that tendon organs are capable of vigorous discharge during isotonic shortening, a movement which has rarely been studied under the controlled conditions possible in a reduced preparation. Interestingly, the afferents studied had vigorous discharge at muscle shortening velocities exceeding 0.2 resting lengths per second, beyond which rate muscle spindles during controlled, near natural, and natural movements may be silenced (discussed previously). This suggests that in rapid movements, the net input from afferents in shortening muscles to the central nervous system may be dominated by tendon organs.

b. Human studies. It is particularly difficult to identify Ib afferent discharge in conscious humans, because the test muscle must be completely relaxed in order to verify low passive force responsiveness and, further, demonstration is usually not attempted of vigorous discharge in response to *discrete* "in-series" force. Nonetheless, the reports reviewed by Vallbo et al. (132) emphasize that human Ib afferents can have a very low threshold to active force and, further, that the discharge of some units during voluntary contraction is a discontinuous function of total muscle force with steps in impulse frequency suggestive of the progressive recruitment of single motor units.

Summary. The findings to date for natural movements support the notion that tendon organs signal moment-to-moment changes in active force development and that the individual firing patterns give a reasonably if not fully representative picture of whole-muscle force.

C. Modeling of Tendon Organ Responses

Based on the morphologic relation between tendon organs and muscle fibers, it is clear that the input signal for a tendon organ is the force exerted by the muscle fibers that lie in series with it. It is true that the response of the tendon organ can be altered by contraction of fibers that lie in parallel, but this phenomenon can occur only because such contraction shortens the in-series fibers, and consequently, reduces the force sensed by the tendon organ. With this consideration in view, one would expect that a model of the dependence of the response on force should rely exclusively on data obtained with isolated tendon organs, because it is not possible to measure the force exerted on any particular tendon organ while it is embedded in muscle. However, more attention has been paid experimentally to the relation between discharge of an embedded tendon organ and whole-muscle force. Since the latter type of data are often considered to be of greater significance in the context of the ensemble Ib signal to the spinal cord, it is useful also to try to build a model on their basis.

The behavior of isolated tendon organs in response to sinuoisdal stretch is described quantitatively by Wilkinson and Fukami (105). They systematically varied the frequency and amplitude of the sinusoidal stretch as well as the initial tension. Their results concerning the receptor potential, in summary, are as follows. The sensitivity declines somewhat with increasing amplitude (gain compression), and increases with initial tension. The dynamic responsiveness is modest, and the parameters that describe it are nearly independent of amplitude as well as of initial tension. In other words, the nonlinearity and the dynamic responsiveness can be described as arising from separate, sequential transformations, unlike the case for the muscle spindle. Thus, it is possible to view the quantitative summarization of the data as a model, with some confidence that one has not overlooked some interaction between the respective transformations. However, the dynamic process of impulse initiation (encoding) is not captured in this model.

When whole-muscle force and tendon organ discharge are considered to be the input and the output, respectively, the data have not been utilized amply for the characterization of nonlinearity and dynamic response. However, if force is developed by orderly recruitment of motor units, neither of the two properties is particularly conspicuous (131). In fact, Crago et al. (131) showed that the observations in this situation can be described quite well by assuming that the response is governrd by a linear, dynamic transfer function. The dynamic effects are so modest that it is difficult to distinguish between two quite different transfer functions (128,137) that have been proposed.

Summary. In the case of isolated tendon organs, it has been possible to quantify separately the nonlinearity and the dynamic properties of response. Neither phenomenon is particularly conspicuous. A similar conclusion can be drawn from experiments in which the whole-muscle force is considered to be the input variable, although data covering the entire physiologic range of muscle force have not been employed in modeling studies.

D. Summary

A tendon organ consists essentially of mechanoreceptive nerve endings in association with collagenous fascicles through which several muscle fibers exert their forces. The Ib afferent arising from a tendon organ is an exquisitely sensitive monitor of force applied to the receptor organ. The contraction of even a single muscle fiber that inserts through a tendon organ may be sufficient to elicit afferent discharge. As in the case of man-made force gauges, the receptor organ is quite stiff and undamped, and its output signal is related to the force in a more or less linear, nondynamic fashion, at least to a first approximation.

The muscle fibers that insert through a tendon organ belong usually to different motor units, and the sampling appears to be random. Thus, several motor units can excite a particular Ib axon. The intracapsular interactions between the strains due to contractions of different muscle fibers as well as the complications resulting from the fact that many muscle fibers belonging to an "exciting" motor unit lie in-parallel with the receptor organ, preclude a simple description of receptor response to normal activation of the muscle. Tendon organ discharge can signal moment-to-moment changes in localized, intramuscular force, but it is not fully representative of a muscle's total force output. However, the summed responses of all the tendon organs in a muscle should provide a better estimate of total muscle force than the responses of any single receptor.

V. COEXISTENCE OF SPINDLES AND TENDON ORGANS

In this speculative section we address the question of the significance of two different types of mechanoreceptors in skeletal muscle and whether they provide information that is complementary or redundant (cf. 138).

The motor control system evidently contains the machinery for solving problems that one can phrase as problems in Newtonian mechanics, for example, how to move a mass from one specified position to another. Considering that the fundamental entities, between which Newtonian mechanics provides the link, are position and force (and, of course, their derivatives), it seems logical that there are muscle receptors whose responses are related to position and to force. The fact that responses of spindle afferents, even in the absence of fusimotor activity, are related to muscle length only in a dynamic and complicated manner does not detract from the previous consideration, since it seems perfectly possible to reformulate Newtonian mechanics in terms of an appropriate dynamic transform of position. Armed with such a formulation, the motor system could deduce, from the activities of the two types of receptors, the characteristics of the external load (e.g., properties related to elasticity, vicosity, and inertia) and use these to advantage for computing the course of subsequent movement. Indeed, the pattern of muscular activations is found to be affected by the kinetics of movement in ways that suggest that muscles can be utilized for purposes of damping (93) or braking (139) when so warranted by the characteristics of the external load, namely, elasticity or inertia, respectively.

This conceptual harmony between properties of muscle receptors and requirements for determining the nature of the load is, however, jeopardized when the underlying issues are examined more specifically. During the course of a movement, spindles in a passively stretched muscle could provide position-related information, but the tendon organs in that muscle are likely to remain silent for the most part. In an active muscle, the tendon organs would provide a sample of muscle force, but spindle afferents may be very much influenced by fusimotor activity. Indeed, in an active muscle, responses of Ia and Ib afferents begin to resemble each other, the more so if intrafusal and extrafusal contractions go hand-in-hand. The impression of redundancy of these two types of afferents is further fortified if one considers that they share interneurons in their projections in the spinal cord to motoneurons (140). However, what does not seem redundant is the discharge of tendon organs in active muscles and spindles in passive antagonist muscles, which, in conjunction, can be utilized to discern the nature of the load acting on the joint.

Even though Ia and Ib afferents from a muscle exert their effects on homonymous motoneurons partly via shared interneurons, there are differences between their respective synaptic effects; these differences include (but are not limited to) the monosynaptic excitatory connections of Ia afferents (141). This observation weakens the argument for redundancy of the receptor types, even when attention is confined to receptors in one muscle. Moreover, despite the broad similarity of spindle and tendon organ responses from a muscle during natural, unobstructed movement, it is not unreasonable to suppose that spindle afferents, in comparison with tendon organ afferents, convey nonredundant information of the following categories. (1) The extent to which fusimotor activity is decoupled from alpha motoneuron activity, for example, rhythmicity in spindle afferent discharge preceding rhythmicity in muscle activity (83). (2) Differences in contractile properties of intrafusal and extrafusal muscle. This category includes the possibility that when fatigue affects extrafusal but not intrafusal muscle tendon organ afferents would decrease their discharge rate owing to reduced muscular tension, while spindle afferents may increase their discharge because of reduction in speed of muscle shortening; this difference could be a source of information concerning fatigue. (3) Characteristics of an external impediment, discussed in the following paragraph.

The effects of contractile fatigue, which is internal to the muscle, are to be contrasted with the effects of an external obstruction or change. If, for example, the inertia was increased while all else remained the same, the ensuing decrease in speed of muscle shortening would cause elevation of discharge of spindle as well as of tendon organ afferents, the latter because muscles develop more force when shortening at slower speeds. It appears from these examples concerning fatigue and inertia that internal changes can be distinguished from external changes on the basis of afferent discharges of the two types of receptor organ (cf. 138). Moreover, the changes in internal state of the muscle, such as fatigue or history-dependent stiffness, could be compensated for, on the basis of muscle afferent activity, without recourse to a model of muscle mechanics (142). However, there is little evidence for fatigue compensation at the spinal level (cf. 60).

The relatively close association of tendon organs with slow-twitch, oxidative muscle fibers (7) may serve to allow Ib afferents to monitor force even when the muscle is minimally active, because the slow fibers are the first to be recruited and the last to be derecruited (121). The relative concentration of spindles in the same, oxidative portion is in keeping with the possibility that, since local changes in extrafusal activity preferentially affect nearby spindles (143), the information about local changes in length may be utilized in a complementary fashion with the information coming from tendon organs that sample the force generated by the same portion of the muscle. It has been suggested that a small change in extrafusal activation, and the consequent responses of the affected muscle receptors, may serve as a "test" of the state of the muscle and of the load (144), but this remains conjectural.

The utilization of muscle afferent information in conjunction with efference copy for the conscious appreciation of movement, force, and effort has been reviewed by Matthews (145).

Summary. Information related to both position and force can apprise the nervous system of the nature of the external load. Spindles in passive muscles and tendon organs in active muscles are well suited to provide this information. Moreover, spindle and tendon organ responses from the same active muscle, though broadly similar during natural, unobstructed movement, can help distinguish internal changes (e.g., fatigue) from external impediments (e.g., inertia), and may be utilized in compensatory adjustments. In addition, internal changes within a portion of a muscle may be discernible. In view of these considerations, spindles and tendon organs appear to provide complementary rather than redundant information.

VI. OTHER MUSCLE RECEPTORS

Until recently, most other types of muscle receptors have been classified as "pressure-pain" units (e.g., 146,147). However, particularly since Stacey (12) showed how plentiful were these receptors (especially those with free nerve endings) there has been a progressive interest in determining if the population innervated particularly by groups III and IV afferents can be subdivided into more discrete groups (e.g., 13). Since there is much uncertainty as to the relative extent to which these afferents exhibit bi- and polymodal sensitivities, it seems best for the moment to think of their activity as contributing to select functions, rather than classifying them as unimodal receptor types, even though many of them could ultimately be shown to be so. At this stage, it seems reasonable to propose that about 50% of this group (predominantly with group IV innervation) subserve nociceptive function. The remainder (predominantly group III) appear to be activated by non-noxious stimuli that might have thermoregulatory and ergoreceptive (exercise-related) function, and perhaps a small number (possibly supplied by group II) might even subserve kinesthesis and motor control.

A. Nociceptive Function

Nociceptors respond to stimuli that damage or threaten to damage tissue. Many group III and particularly group IV afferents in muscle respond to stimuli that are known to be painful, such as high mechanical pressure and squeezing, or the injection of algesic (pain-producing) agents such as bradykinin (148) or hypertonic saline (147). Perhaps muscle pain may be attributable in part to nociceptive input activated by chemical substances released by cellular injury (13).

B. Thermoreceptive Function

Most muscle receptors (including even spindles) are sensitive to temperature changes, but whether or not they subserve thermoregulation is less certain. For example, it is doubtful that the thermal sensitivity of Ia (increased discharge with warming, decreased with cooling) and of spII (responses in opposite direction) afferents (149) contributes to temperature regulation. It is more likely that the groups III and IV afferents with firing patterns like those of typical cold and warm receptors of the skin (13) have thermoregulatory effects, although this function has yet to be proven.

C. Ergoreceptive Function

It has long been conjectured (150) that muscle afferents might contribute to exercise-related rises in blood pressure and ventilation rate (151; see 13 for a review). Potential candidates for such ergoreceptive function include those receptors (particularly with group III innervation) that respond to non-noxious warming, touch, pressure, and contraction. The latency of their responses to the mechanical stimuli is usually much longer than that of spindles and tendon organs, but such "tardiness" and the tendency for the discharge to outlast the stimulus might have a particular significance during ongoing exercise. There is, however, no evidence for afferents being excited by the metabolites that accumulate in muscle during steady-state exercise, as was once popularly considered. Possibly, metabolic levels during exhaustive exercise can activate nociceptive afferents but, again, this remains to be proven.

D. Kinesthetic and Motor-Control Function

Paciniform corpuscles (usually innervated by group III, but sometimes by I and II afferents) are presumably vibration sensitive like pacinian corpuscles (6,12) and could conceivably contribute to kinesthetic function, along with other group III and a few group IV afferents with free nerve endings that respond to low-threshold pressure (13).

The responses reported to date for most of the groups III and IV afferents that are sensitive to low-threshold mechanical stimuli are too "inconsistent" to suggest a significant role in either kinesthesia or motor control. At this stage then, the case for a *substantial* number of nonspindle group II, group III, and group IV afferents contributing to kinesthesia and motor control does not appear strong. However, it has recently been shown by Rymer et al. (14) that the clasp-knife reflex of an experimental animal model cannot be attributed to inhibitory segmental effects from Ib or spII afferents but rather to nonspindle group II afferents with limited stretch sensitivity (a few of which were encountered in their study) and possibly groups III and IV afferents as well. Perhaps a substantial number of such afferents are not required, provided their segmental inhibitory effects are "amplified" by appropriate interneuronal activity (Chapter 13).

Obviously, it is of great interest to search for groups II–IV afferents with a possible kinesthetic and motor-control function, but for technical reasons, information will accumulate slowly on this issue.

E. Summary

Many of the receptors other than spindles and tendon organs often respond to more than one stimulus modality. A large number are responsive to stimuli that are known to be painful. Some may be involved in temperature regulation and exercise-related rises in blood pressure and ventilation rate.

The long latency and variability of response of most muscle receptors other than spindles and tendon organs have been seen as precluding any role of these other receptors in motor control and kinesthesia. Some recent results, however, would attribute to the activity of these receptors such phenomena as the clasp-knife reaction.

ACKNOWLEDGMENTS

We would like to thank Drs. Marc Binder, Roger Enoka, Thomas Hamm, and W. Zev Rymer for their criticisms of a draft of this chapter.

This work was supported by USPHS grants HL-07249 (to the Department of Physiology), NS-19407 (to Ziaul Hasan), and NS-07888 (to Douglas G. Stuart).

REFERENCES

1. Matthews, P. B. C. (1972). *Mammalian Muscle Receptors and Their Central Actions*, Edward Arnold, London.
2. Stein, R. B. (1974). Peripheral control of movement. *Physiol. Rev. 54*: 215–243.
3. Murthy, K. S. K. (1978). Vertebrate fusimotor neurones and their influences on motor behavior. *Prog. Neurobiol. 11*:249–307.
4. Proske, U. (1981). The Golgi tendon organ. Properties of the receptor and reflex action of impulses arising from tendon organs. In *International Review of Physiology: Neurophysiology IV*, R. Porter (Ed.), University Park Press, Baltimore, pp. 127–171.
5. Matthews, P. B. C. (1981). Evolving views on the internal operation and functional role of the muscle spindle. *J. Physiol. (Lond.) 320*:1–30.
6. Barker, D. (1974). The morphology of muscle receptors. In *Handbook of Sensory Physiology*, vol. III/2, C. C. Hunt (Ed.), Springer, Berlin, 1974, pp. 1–190.
7. Botterman, B. R., Binder, M. D., and Stuart, D. G. (1978). Functional anatomy of the association between motor units and muscle receptors. *Am. Zool. 18*:135–152.
8. Maier, A. (1979). Occurrence and distribution of muscle spindles in masticatory and suprahyoid muscles of the rat. *Am. J. Anat. 155*:483–506.
9. Bakker, D. A., and Richmond, F. J. R. (1982). Muscle spindle complexes in muscles around upper cervical vertebrae in the cat. *J. Neurophysiol. 48*:62–74.
10. Voss, V. H. (1971). Tabelle der absoluten und relativen muskelspindelzahlen der menschlichen skeleffmuskulatur. *Anat. Anz. Bd. 129*:562–572.

11. Boyd, I. A., and Davey, M. R. (1968). *Composition of Peripheral Nerves*, Livingstone, Edinburgh.
12. Stacey, M. J. (1969). Free nerve endings in skeletal muscle of the cat. *J. Anat. 105*:231–254.
13. Kniffki, K. D., Mense, S., and Schmidt, R. F. (1981). Muscle receptors with fine afferent fibres which may evoke circulatory reflexes. *Circ. Res.* (Supp. I) *48*:1–25.
14. Rymer, W. Z., Houk, J. C., and Crago, P. E. (1979). Mechanisms of the clasp-knife reflex studied in an animal model. *Exp. Brain Res. 37*:93–113.
15. Andres, K. H., von Düring, M. Jänig, W., and Schmidt, R. F. (1980). Ultrastructure of fine afferent terminals in the Achilles tendon of the cat. *Pflugers Arch. 384*:R33.
16. Boyd, I. A. (1980). The isolated mammalian muscle spindle. *Trends Neurosci. 3*:258–265.
17. Corvaja, N., Marinozzi, V., and Pompeiano, O. (1969). Muscle spindles in the lumbrical muscle of the adult cat. Electron microscopic observation and functional considerations. *Arch. Ital. Biol. 107*:365–543.
18. Banks, R. W., Harker, D. W., and Stacey, M. J. (1977). A study of mammalian intrafusal muscle fibres using a combined histochemical and ultrastructural technique. *J. Anat. 123*:783–796.
19. Boyd, I. A. (1976). The mechanical properties of dynamic nuclear bag fibres, static nuclear bag fibres and nuclear chain fibres in isolated cat muscle spindles. *Prog. Brain Res. 44*:33–49.
20. Banks, R. W., Barker, D., and Stacey, M. J. (1981). In *Muscle Receptors and Movement*, A. Taylor and A. Prochazka (Eds.), Macmillan, London, pp. 5–16.
21. Boyd, I. A. (1962). The structure and innervation of the nuclear bag muscle fibre system and the nuclear chain muscle fibre system in mammalian muscle spindles. *Philos. Trans. R. Soc. Lond. (Biol.) 245*:81–136.
22. Kucera, J. (1980). Myofibrillar ATPase activity of intrafusal fibers in chronically de-afferented rat muscle spindles. *Histochemistry 66*:221–228.
23. Milburn, A. (1973). The early development of muscle spindles in the rat. *J. Cell Sci. 12*:175–195.
24. Barker, D., and Milburn, A. (1982). Development of cat muscle spindles. *J. Physiol. 325*:85P.
25. Banks, R. W. (1981). A histological study of the motor innervation of the cat's muscle spindle. *J. Anat. 133*:571–591.
26. Banks, R. W., Barker, D., and Stacey, M. J. (1982). Form and distribution of sensory terminals in cat hindlimb muscle spindles. *Philos. Trans. R. Soc. Lond. (Biol.) 299*:329–364.
27. Kucera, J. (1982). One-bag-fiber muscle spindles in tenuissimus muscles of the cat. *Histochemistry 76*:315–328.
28. Bakker, D. A., and Richmond, F. J. R. (1981). Two types of muscle spindles in cat neck muscles: A histochemical study of intrafusal fiber composition. *J. Neurophysiol. 45*:973–986.

29. Poppele, R. E., Kennedy, W. R., and Quick, D. C. (1979). A determination of static mechanical properties of intrafusal muscle in isolated cat muscle spindles. *Neuroscience 4*:401–411.

30. Barker, D., Emonet-Denánd, F., Laporte, Y., Proske, U., and Stacey, M. J. (1973). Morphological identification and intrafusal distribution of the endings of static fusimotor axons in the cat. *J. Physiol. (Lond.) 230*:405–427.

31. Emonet-Dénand, F., Jami, L., and Laporte, Y. (1980). Histophysiological observations on the skeleto-fusimotor innervation of mammalian spindles. *Prog. Clin. Neurophysiol. 8*:1–11.

32. Barker, D., and Saito, M. (1980). Autonomic innervation of cat muscle spindles. *J. Physiol. (Lond.) 301*:24P.

33. Hunt, C. C. (1960). The effect of sympathetic stimulation on mammalian muscle spindles. *J. Physiol. (Lond.) 151*:332–341.

34. Shantha, T. R., Golarz, M. N., and Bourne, G. H. (1968). Histological and histochemical observations on the capsule of the muscle spindle in normal and denervated muscle. *Acta Anat. 69*:632–646.

35. Hunt, C. C., and Ottoson, D. (1975). Impulse activity and receptor potential of primary and secondary endings of isolated mammalian muscle spindles. *J. Physiol. (Lond.) 252*:259–281.

36. Boyd, I. A., and Ward, J. (1975). Motor control of nuclear bag and nuclear chain intrafusal fibres in isolated living muscle spindles from the cat. *J. Physiol. (Lond.) 244*:83–112.

37. Bessou, P., and Pagès, B. (1975). Cinematographic analysis of contractile events produced in intrafusal muscle fibres by stimulation of static and dynamic fusimotor axons. *J. Physiol. (Lond.) 252*:397–427.

38. Boyd, I. A., Gladden, M. H., McWilliam, P. N., and Ward, J. (1977). Control of static and dynamic nuclear bag fibres and nuclear chain fibres by gamma and beta axons in isolated cat muscle spindles. *J. Physiol. (Lond.) 265*:133–162.

39. Bridgman, C. F., and Eldred, E. (1965). Intramuscular pressure changes during contraction in relation to muscle spindles. *Am. J. Physiol. 209*: 891–899.

40. Hunt, C. C., Wilkinson, R. S., and Fukami, Y. (1978). Ionic basis of the receptor potential in primary endings of mammalian muscle spindles. *J. Gen. Physiol. 71*:683–698.

41. Hulliger, M., and Noth, J. (1979). Static and dynamic fusimotor interaction and the possibility of multiple pace-makers operating in the cat muscle spindle. *Brain Res. 173*:21–28.

42. Katz, B. (1950). Action potentials from a sensory nerve ending. *J. Physiol. (Lond.) 111*:248–260.

43. Ito, F., and Komatsu, Y. (1976). Sensory terminal responses of frog muscle spindle recorded across vaseline gap onto intrafusal muscle fibre. *Pflugers Arch. 366*:25–30.

44. Boyd, I. A., and Ward, J. (1969). The response of isolated cat muscle spindles to stretch. *J. Physiol. (Lond.) 200*:104P–105P.

45. Hunt, C. C., and Wilkinson, R. S. (1980). An analysis of receptor potential and tension of isolated cat muscle spindles in response to sinusoidal stretch. *J. Physiol. (Lond.)* 302:241–262.

46. Brown, M. C., Goodwin, G. M., and Matthews, P. B. C. (1969). After effects of fusimotor stimulation on the response of muscle spindle primary afferent endings. *J. Physiol. (Lond.)* 205:677–694.

47. Poppele, R. E., and Quick, D. C. (1981). Stretch-induced contraction of intrafusal muscle in cat muscle spindle. *J. Neurosci.* 1:1069–1074.

48. Boyd, I. A. (1976). The response of fast and slow nuclear bag fibres and nuclear chain fibres in isolated cat muscle spindles to fusimotor simulation, and the effect of intrafusal contraction on the sensory endings. *Q. J. Exp. Physiol.* 61:203–252.

49. Boyd, I. A. (1981). The action of the three types of intrafusal fibre in isolated cat muscle spindles on the dynamic and length sensitivities of primary and secondary sensory endings. In *Muscle Receptors and Movement*, A. Taylor and A. Prochazka (Eds.), Macmillan, London, pp. 17–32.

50. Boyd, I. A. (1976). The mechanical properties of dynamic nuclear bag fibres, static nuclear bag fibres and nuclear chain fibres in isolated cat muscle spindles. *Prog. Brain Res.* 44:33–49.

51. Emonet-Dénand, F., Laporte, Y., Matthews, P. B. C., and Petit, J. (1977). On the sub-division of static and dynamic fusimotor actions on the primary ending of the cat muscle spindle. *J. Physiol. (Lond.)* 268:827–861.

52. Emonet-Dénand, F., Jami, L., Laporte, Y., and Tankov, N. (1980). Glycogen depletion of bag_1 fibres elicited by stimulation of static axons in cat peroneus brevis muscle spindles. *J. Physiol. (Lond.)* 302:311–321.

53. Barker, D., Bessou, P., Jankowska, E., Pagès, B., and Stacey, M. J. (1978). Identification of intrafusal muscle fibres activated by single fusimotor axons and injected with fluorescent dye in cat tenuissimus spindles. *J. Physiol. (Lond.)* 275:149–165.

54. Binder, M. D., and Stuart, D. G. (1980). Responses of Ia and spindle group II afferents to single motor-unit contractions. *J. Neurophysiol.* 43:621–629.

55. Cameron, W. E., Binder, M. D., Botterman, B. R., Reinking, R. M., and Stuart, D. G. (1981). "Sensory partitioning" of cat medial gastrocnemius muscle by its muscle spindles and tendon organs. *J. Neurophysiol.* 46:32–47.

56. Dutia, M. B. (1980). Activation of cat muscle spindle primary, secondary and intermediate sensory endings by suxamethonium. *J. Physiol. (Lond.)* 304:315–330.

57. Prochazka, A., Westerman, R. A., and Ziccone, S. P. (1977). Ia afferent activity during a variety of voluntary movements in the cat. *J. Physiol. (Lond.)* 268:423–448.

58. Dutia, M. B., and Ferrell, W. R. (1980). The effect of suxamethonium on the response to stretch of Golgi tendon organs in the cat. *J. Physiol.* 305:511–518.

59. Carli, G., Diete-Spiff, K., and Pompeiano, O. (1967). Mechanisms of muscle spindle excitation. *Arch. Ital. Biol.* 105:273–289.

60. Rymer, W. Z., and Hasan, Z. (1980). Absence of force-feedback regulation in soleus muscle of the decerebrate cat. *Brain Res. 184*:203–209.

61. Lennerstrand, G., and Thoden, U. (1968). Dynamic analysis of muscle spindle endings in the cat using length changes of different length-time relations. *Acta Physiol. Scand. 73*:234–250.

62. Poppele, R. E. (1981). An analysis of muscle spindle behavior using randomly applied stretches. *Neuroscience 6*:1157–1165.

63. Matthews, P. B. C., and Stein, R. B. (1969). The sensitivity of muscle spindle afferents to sinusoidal stretching. *J. Physiol. (Lond.) 200*:723–748.

64. Houk, J. C., Harris, D. A., and Hasan, Z. (1973). Non-linear behavior of spindle receptors. In *Control of Posture and Locomotion*, R. B. Stein, K. B. Pearson, R. S. Smith, and J. B. Redford (Eds.), Plenum, New York, pp. 147–164.

65. Botterman, B. R., and Eldred, E. (1982). Static stretch sensitivity of Ia and II afferents in the cat's gastrocnemius. *Pflugers Arch. 395*:204–211.

66. Matthews, P. B. C. (1963). The response of de-efferented muscle spindle receptors to stretching at different velocities. *J. Physiol. (Lond.). 168*: 660–678.

67. Hasan, Z., and Houk, J. C. (1975). Analysis of response properties of de-efferented mammalian spindle receptors based on frequency response. *J. Neurophysiol. 38*:663–672.

68. Houk, J. C., Rymer, W. Z., and Crago, P. E. (1981). Dependence of dynamic response of spindle receptors on muscle length and velocity. *J. Neurophysiol. 46*:143–166.

69. Lennerstrand, G. (1968). Position and velocity sensitivity of muscle spindles in the cat. I. Primary and secondary endings deprived of fusimotor activation. *Acta Physiol. Scand. 73*:281–299.

70. Hasan, Z., and Houk, J. C. (1975). The transition in the sensitivity of spindle receptors that occurs when muscle is stretched more than a fraction of a millimeter. *J. Neurophysiol. 38*:673–689.

71. Poppele, R. E., and Bowman, R. J. (1970). Quantitative description of linear behavior of mammalian muscle spindles. *J. Neurophysiol. 33*:59–72.

72. Hulliger, M., Matthews, P. B. C., and Noth, J. (1977). Static and dynamic fusimotor action on the response of Ia fibres to low frequency sinusoidal stretching of widely ranging amplitude. *J. Physiol. (Lond.) 267*:811–838.

73. Crowe, A., and Mathews, P. B. C. (1964). The effects of stimulating static and dynamic fusimotor fibres on the response to stretching of the primary endings of muscle spindles. *J. Physiol. (Lond.) 174*:109–131.

74. Lennerstrand, G. (1968). Position and velocity sensitivity of muscle spindles in the cat. IV. Interaction between two fusimotor fibres converging on the same spindle ending. *Acta Physiol. Scand. 74*:257–273.

75. Hulliger, M., Matthews, P. B. C., and Noth, J. (1977). Effects of combining static and dynamic fusimotor stimulation on the response of the muscle spindle primary ending to sinusoidal stretching. *J. Physiol. (Lond.) 267*:839–856.

76. Jami, L., and Petit, J. (1978). Fusimotor actions on sensitivity of spindle secondary endings to slow muscle stretch in cat peroneus tertius. *J. Neurophysiol.* 41:860-869.

77. Durkovic, R. G., and Preston, J. B. (1974). Evidence of dynamic fusimotor excitation of secondary muscle spindle afferents in soleus muscle of cat. *Brain Res.* 75:320-323.

78. Appelberg, B. (1981). Selective central control of dynamic gamma motoneurones utilized for the functional classification of gamma cells. In *Muscle Receptors and Movement*, A. Taylor and A. Prochazka (Eds.), Macmillan, London, pp. 97-108.

79. Jansen, J. K. S., and Matthews, P. B. C. (1962). The effects of fusimotor activity on the static responsiveness of primary and secondary endings of muscle spindles in the decerebrate cat. *Acta Physiol. Scand.* 55:376-386.

80. Matthews, P. B. C., and Stein, R. B. (1969). The regularity of primary and secondary muscle spindle afferent discharges. *J. Physiol. (Lond.)* 202:59-82.

81. Post, E. M., Rymer, W. Z., and Hasan, Z. (1980). Relation between intrafusal and extrafusal activity in triceps surae muscles of the decerebrate cat: Evidence of β action. *J. Neurophysiol.* 44:383-404.

82. Stuart, D. G., Binder, M. D., and Botterman, B. R. (1979). Features of segmental motor control revealed in single-unit recordings during natural movements. In *Posture and Movement*, R. E. Talbott and D. R. Humphrey (Eds.), Raven, New York, pp. 281-294.

83. Feldman, A. G., Orlovsky, G. N., and Perret, C. (1977). Activity of muscle spindle afferents during scratching in the cat. *Brain Res.* 129:192-196.

84. Taylor, A., Appenteng, K., Morimoto, T. (1981). Proprioceptive input from the jaw muscles and its influence on lapping, chewing, and posture. *Can. J. Physiol. Pharmacol.* 59:636-644.

85. Prochazka, A., Stephens, J. A., and Wand, P. (1976). Muscle spindle discharge in normal and obstructed movements. *J. Physiol. (Lond.)* 287:57-66.

86. Loeb, G. E. (1981). Somatosensory unit input to the spinal cord during normal walking. *Can. J. Physiol. Pharmacol.* 59:627-635.

87. Hoffer, J. A., and Loeb, G. E. (1983). A technique for reversible fusimotor blockade during chronic recording from spindle afferents in walking cats. *Exp. Brain Res. Supp.* 7:272-279.

88. Burke, D. (1980). Muscle spindle function during movement. *Trends Neurosci.* 3:251-253.

89. Vallbo, Å. (1981). Basic patterns of muscle spindle discharge in man. In *Muscle Receptors and Movement*, A. Taylor and A. Prochazka (Eds.), Macmillan, London, pp. 263-275.

90. Hagbarth, K. E., Hägglund, J. V., Wallin, E. U., and Young, R. R. (1981). Grouped spindle and electromyographic responses to abrupt wrist extension movements in man. *J. Physiol. (Lond.)* 312:81-96.

91. Hagbarth, K. E., Wallin, B. G., and Löfstedt, L. (1975). Muscle spindle activity in man during voluntary fast alternating movements. *J. Neurol. Neurosurg. Psychiat.* 38:625-635.

92. Capaday, C., and Cooke, J. D. (1980). The effects of muscle vibration on the attainment of intended final position during voluntary human arm movements. *Exp. Brain Res. 42*:228–230.

93. Ghez, C., and Martin, J. H. (1982). The control of rapid limb movement in the cat. III. Agonist-antagonist coupling. *Exp. Brain Res. 45*:115–125.

94. Appenteng, K., Prochazka, A., Proske, U., and Wand, P. (1982). Fusimotor stimulation can maintain cat soleus Ia firing even during very rapid muscle shortening. *J. Physiol. (Lond.) 326*:51P.

95. Hulliger, M. (1979). The responses of primary spindle afferents to fusimotor stimulation at constant and abruptly changing rates. *J. Physiol. (Lond.) 294*:461–482.

96. Emonet-Dénand, F., and Laporte, Y. (1981). Muscle stretch as a way of detecting brief activation of bag_1 fibres by dynamic axons. In *Muscle Receptors and Movement*, A. Taylor and A. Prochazka (Eds.), Macmillan, London, pp. 67–76.

97. Hasan, Z. (1983). A model of spindle afferent response to muscle stretch. *J. Neurophysiol. 49*:989–1006.

98. Hill, D. K. (1968). Tension due to interaction between the sliding filaments in resting striated muscle. The effect of stimulation. *J. Physiol. (Lond.) 199*:637–684.

99. Bridgman, C. F. (1970). Comparisons in structure of tendon organs in the rat, cat and man. *J. Comp. Neurol. 138*:369–372.

100. Fukami, Y. (1980). Interaction of impulse activities originating from individual Golgi tendon organs innervated by branches of a single axon. *J. Physiol. (Lond.) 298*:483–499.

101. Burke, R. E. (1981). Motor units: Anatomy, physiology, and functional organization. In *Handbook of Physiology*, Sect. 1, *The Nervous System*, Vol. 2, *Motor Control*, V. B. Brooks (Ed.), American Physiological Society, Bethesda, Maryland, pp. 345–422.

102. Gonyea, W. J., and Ericson, G. C. (1977). Morphological and histochemical organization of the flexor carpi radialis muscle in the cat. *Am. J. Anat. 148*:329–344.

103. Fukami, Y., and Wilkinson, R. S. (1977). Responses of isolated Golgi tendon organs of the cat. *J. Physiol. (Lond.) 265*:673–689.

104. Fukami, Y. (1981). Responses of isolated Golgi tendon organs of the cat to muscle contraction and electrical stimulation. *J. Physiol. (Lond.) 318*:429–443.

105. Wilkinson, R. S., and Fukami, Y. (1983). Responses of isolated Golgi tendon organs of cat to sinusoidal stretch. *J. Neurophysiol. 49*:976–988.

106. Proske, U., and Gregory, J. E. (1976). Multiple sites of impulse initiation in a tendon organ. *Exp. Neurol. 50*:515–520.

107. Matthews, B. H. C. (1933). Nerve endings in mammalian muscle. *J. Physiol. (Lond.) 78*:1–53.

108. Binder, M. D., Houk, J. C., Nichols, T. R., Rymer, W. Z., and Stuart, D. G. (1982). Properties and segmental actions of mammalian muscle receptors: An update. *Fed. Proc. 41*:2907–2918.

109. Jansen, J. K. S., and Rudjord, T. (1964). On the silent period and Golgi tendon organs of the soleus muscle of the cat. *Acta Physiol. Scand. 62*: 364–379.

110. Green, D. G., and Kellerth, J. O. (1967). Intracellular autogenetic and synergistic effect of muscular contraction on flexor motoneurones. *J. Physiol. (Lond.) 193*:73–94.

111. Houk, J. C., and Henneman, E. (1967). Responses of Golgi tendon organs to active contractions of the soleus muscle of the cat. *J. Neurophysiol. 30*:466–481.

112. Houk, J. C., Singer, J. J., and Henneman, E. (1971). Adequate stimulus for tendon organs with observations on mechanics of ankle joint. *J. Neurophysiol. 34*:1051–1065.

113. Stuart, D. G., Mosher, C. G., Gerlach, R. L., and Reinking, R. M. (1972). Mechanical arrangement and transducing properties of Golgi tendon organs. *Exp. Brain Res. 14*:274–292.

114. Jami, L., and Petit, J. (1976). Frequency of tendon organ discharges elicited by the contraction of motor units in cat leg muscles. *J. Physiol. (Lond.) 261*:633–645.

115. Binder, M. D., Kroin, J. S., Moore, G. P., and Stuart, D. G. (1977). The response of Golgi tendon organs to single motor unit contractions. *J. Physiol. (Lond.) 271*:337–349.

116. Stuart, D. G., Mosher, C. G., and Gerlach, R. L. (1972). Properties and central connections of Golgi tendon organs with special reference to locomotion. In *Research in Muscle Development and the Muscle Spindle*, B. Q. Banker, P. J. Przybylski, J. P. van der Meulen, and M. Victor (Eds.), Excerpta Medica, Amsterdam, pp. 437–462.

117. Houk, J. C. (1967). A viscoelastic interaction which produces a component of adaptation in responses of Golgi tendon organs. *J. Neurophysiol. 30*:1482–1493.

118. Clark, D. A. (1931). Muscle counts of motor units—A study in innervation ratios. *Am. J. Physiol. 96*:296–304.

119. Barker, D. (1967). The innervation of mammalian skeletal muscle. In *Myotatic, Kinesthetic and Vestibular Mechanisms*, A. V. S. de Reuck and J. Knight (Eds.), Little, Brown, Boston, pp. 3–15.

120. Reinking, R. M., Stephens, J. A., and Stuart, D. G. (1975). The tendon organs of cat medial gastrocnemius: Significance of motor unit type and size for the activation of Ib afferents. *J. Physiol. (Lond.) 250*:491–512.

121. Henneman, E., and Mendell, L. M. (1981). Functional organization of motoneuron pool and its inputs. In *Handbook of Physiology*, Sec. 1, *The Nervous System*, Vol. 2, *Motor Control*, V. B. Brooks (Ed.), American Physiological Society, Bethesda, Maryland, pp. 423–508.

122. Fulton, J. F., and Pi-Suñer, J. (1928). A note concerning the probable function of various afferent end-organs in skeletal muscle. *Am. J. Physiol. 83*:554–562.

123. Gregory, J. E., and Proske, U. (1979). The responses of Golgi tendon organs to stimulation of different combinations of motor units. *J. Physiol. 295*:251–262.

124. Binder, M. D. (1981). Further evidence that the Golgi tendon organ monitors the activity of a discrete set of motor units within a muscle. *Exp. Brain Res. 43*:186-192.

125. Stephens, J. A., Reinking, R. M., and Stuart, D. G. (1975). Tendon organs of cat medial gastrocnemius: Responses to active and passive forces as a function of muscle length. *J. Neurophysiol. 38*:1217-1231.

126. Goslow, G. E., Stauffer, E. K., Nemeth, W. C., and Stuart, D. G. (1973). The cat step cycle: Responses of muscle spindles and tendon organs to passive stretch within the locomotor range. *Brain Res. 60*:35-54.

127. Stauffer, E. K., and Stephens, J. A. (1975). The tendon organs of cat soleus: Static sensitivity to active force. *Exp. Brain Res. 23*:279-291.

128. Anderson, J. H. (1974). Dynamic characteristics of Golgi tendon organs. *Brain Res. 67*:531-537.

129. Proske, U., and Gregory, J. E. (1980). The discharge rate: tension relation of Golgi tendon organs. *Neurosci. Lett. 16*:287-290.

130. Gregory, J. E., and Proske, U. (1981). Motor unit contractions initiating impulses in a tendon organ in the cat. *J. Physiol. (Lond.) 313*:251-262.

131. Crago, P. E., Houk, J. C., and Rymer, W. Z. (1982). Sampling of total muscle force by tendon organs. *J. Neurophysiol. 47*:1069-1083.

132. Vallbo, Å. B., Hagbarth, K. E., Torebjörk, H. E., and Wallin, B. G. (1979). Somatosensory, proprioceptive and sympathetic activity in human peripheral nerves. *Physiol. Rev. 59*:919-957.

133. Severin, F. V., Orlovsky, G. N., and Shik, M. L. (1967). Work of the muscle receptors during controlled locomotion. *Biophysics 12*:575-586.

134. Corda, M., von Euler, C., and Lennerstrand, G. (1965). Proprioceptive innervation of the diaphragm. *J. Physiol. (Lond.) 178*:161-178.

135. Prochazka, A., Westerman, R. A., and Ziccone, S. P. (1976). Discharges of single hindlimb afferents in the freely moving cat. *J. Neurophysiol. 39*: 1090-1104.

136. Prochazka, A., and Wand, P. (1980). Tendon organ discharge during voluntary movements in cats. *J. Physiol. (Lond.) 303*:385-390.

137. Houk, J. C., and Simon, W. (1967). Responses of Golgi tendon organs to forces applied to muscle tendon. *J. Neurophysiol. 30*:1466-1481.

138. Binder, M. D., and Stuart, D. G. (1980). Motor unit–muscle receptor interactions: Design features of the neuromuscular control system. *Prog. Clin. Neurophysiol. 8*:72-98.

139. Lestienne, F. (1979). Effects of inertial load and velocity on the braking process of voluntary limb movements. *Exp. Brain Res. 35*:407-418.

140. Jankowska, E., Johannisson, T., and Lipski, J. (1981). Common interneurones in reflex pathways from group Ia and Ib afferents of ankle extensors in the cat. *J. Physiol. (Lond.) 310*:381-402.

141. Watt, D. G. D., Stauffer, E. K., Taylor, A., Reinking, R. M., and Stuart, D. G. (1976). Analysis of muscle receptor connections by spike-triggered averaging. 1. Spindle primary and tendon organ afferents. *J. Neurophysiol. 39*:1375-1392.

142. Houk, J. C. (1979). Regulation of stiffness by skeletomotor reflexes. *Ann. Rev. Physiol. 41*:99–114.
143. Cameron, W. E., Binder, M. D., Botterman, B. R., Reinking, R. M., and Stuart, D. G. (1980). Motor unit–muscle spindle interactions in active muscles of decerebrate cats. *Neurosci. Lett. 19*:55–60.
144. Allum, J. H. J. (1975). Responses to load disturbances in human shoulder muscles: The hypothesis that one component is a true pulse test information signal. *Exp. Brain Res. 22*:307–326.
145. Matthews, P. B. C. (1982). Where does Sherrington's 'muscular sense' originate? Muscles, joints, corollary discharges? *Ann. Rev. Neurosci. 5*: 189–218.
146. Paintal, A. S. (1960). Functional analysis of group III afferent fibres of mammalian muscles. *J. Physiol. (Lond.) 152*:250–270.
147. Iggo, A. (1961). Non-myelinated afferent fibres from mammalian skeletal muscle. *J. Physiol. (Lond.) 155*:52P–53P.
148. Franz, M., and Mense, S. (1975). Muscle receptors with group IV afferent fibres responding to application of bradykinin. *Brain Res. 92*:369–383.
149. Mense, S. (1978). Effects of temperature on the discharges of muscle spindles and tendon organs. *Pflugers Arch. 374*:159–166.
150. Paterson, W. D. (1928). Circulatory and respiratory changes in response to muscular exercise in man. *J. Physiol. (Lond.) 66*:323–345.
151. McCloskey, D. I., and Mitchell, J. H. (1972). Reflex cardiovascular and respiratory responses originating in exercising muscle. *J. Physiol. (Lond.) 224*:173–186.

13
SPINAL MECHANISMS FOR CONTROL OF MUSCLE LENGTH AND TENSION

William Z. Rymer   *Northwestern University Medical School, Chicago, Illinois*

I. INTRODUCTION

A. General Principles and Definitions

It is convenient to begin an analysis of spinal cord mechanisms involved in the control of muscular contraction with a consideration of the possible types of motor operations that are performed by the spinal cord. In particular, spinal neural elements are responsible for regulatory and control functions, for synergic relations, and for pattern generation. By regulatory functions, we mean those actions of spinal neurons that act to preserve or maintain the commanded state of a muscle or group of muscles. Regulatory functions depend upon the sensory information that is provided to spinal circuits by sensory receptors in muscle. Control functions are those in which the commanded state is varied, either as a consequence of a descending command, carried via some long spinal pathways, or as a result of input from some regional pattern generator. Synergic relations are the spatial patterns of muscle activation that are used during reflexive or voluntary movements. Pattern generators are neural circuits, typically regionally located, which are capable of mediating rhythmical or oscillatory movements, such as locomotion, breathing, or mastication. These pattern generators are described in more detail in the companion chapter by Stein (Chap. 14)

609

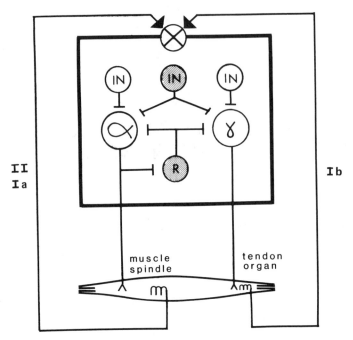

II
Ia   Ib

Figure 1 Elements involved in regulation of muscle contraction include muscle spindle receptors giving rise to group Ia and II fibers, and tendon organs, giving rise to Ib fibers. Afferent fibers synapse with α and γ motoneurons, and a variety of inhibitory and excitatory interneurons.

B. Definition of the Motor Servo

The functional relations between these various motor operations are illustrated in Figure 1, which also serves to introduce the concept of the *motor servo*, the functional unit responsible for regulation of the single muscle (1,2). The motor servo consists of the muscle and its afferent and efferent innervation, together with interneuronal circuits responsible for the processing of afferent information from muscle. The motor servo is the final common pathway for processing motor commands to muscle, playing a role somewhat analogous to the more traditional role of the motor neuron as the "final common pathway" of motor output on a more microscopic scale. The motor servo can be conceived as acting in a regulatory capacity when the input from descending pathways is unchanging, and in a controller capacity when inputs from descending pathways or pattern generators are varying. For example, regulatory functions would arise during the response of limbs to external perturbations, or to changes in muscle contractile force (such as those arising in fatigue), while control functions would arise during voluntary movement or during locomotion. In either instance, command signals address the appropriate spinal neurons as a functionally integrated group, rather than as isolated entities. While this approach remains somewhat hypothetical at present, it represents a potentially simple but important unifying step in approaching the apparently overwhelming complexity of spinal reflex circuity.

II. AUTOGENETIC REGULATION: THE SINGLE MUSCLE

A. The Physical Plant

Increases in spinal motoneuronal discharge rate induce contraction of skeletal muscle, resulting in increased force being exerted on the skeleton and associated load. If the force change is sufficient to exceed the load force, motion will result. The physical characteristics of muscle and its response to neural discharge are therefore of major importance in the neural control of movement. In this section, some of the important mechanical properties of muscle will be described.

1. Length-Tension Relations

A major determinant of the tension magnitude elicited in response to motoneuronal excitation is the length at which the muscle held. For a given level of neural excitation, increasing static muscle length is associated with increasing tension, with the tension reaching a maximum at or near the maximum naturally occurring length, or "rest length" of the muscle. Changes in tension of whole muscle are associated with comparable changes in the length-tension relations of individual sarcomeres (3,4). An increase in tension with increasing muscle length amounts to springlike behavior of muscle, an important mechanical feature for movement regulation.

Strictly speaking, the relation between length and tension is not quite analogous to a simple spring, in that the relation often shows considerable curvature (5). The form of this curvature in the length-tension relation depends upon the level of activation of the muscle, which is determined, in turn, by the rate of stimulation of the motor axons (5). Increasing stimulus rates induce both an increase in the slope of the length-tension relation (which amounts to an increase in stiffness or spring constant of our biologic spring) and a leftward shift in the length intercept (which amounts to a reduction in the set point of this biologic spring). In spite of the curvature, the length-tension relation can be described conveniently by the equation of an hypothetical spring, in which both the spring stiffness, K_s, and the intercept, X_s, are functions of the stimulus rate, s

$$F = K_s (X - X_s)$$

where F is the isometric force, and X is the muscle length.

While the static length-tension relation conditions shows consistent curvature (convex upward at high rates, concave upward at low rates), the slope of the length-tension relation recorded during slow stretch becomes much more linear (6), making the parameter K_s more akin to the spring constant of a simple linear spring.

2. Force-Velocity Relations

A second important dynamic characteristic of muscle is the property that the maximum shortening velocity is determined by the load supported by the muscle (7). (The inverse relation also holds true, in that the maximum tension that can be generated by a muscle is determined by the velocity of muscle shortening.) The relation (between shortening velocity and load) is described, approximately, by an hyperbolic relation that has the effect that the development of even a very small shortening velocity is accompanied by a sharp decline in tension output. As was shown for the static length-tension relation, force-velocity relations appear to show a dependence upon muscle activation level (defined again in terms of the stimulus rate applied to the motor axons).

In contrast, the relation between force and velocity during forced muscle lengthening is much less readily quantified. This is because the shape of the relation depends quite critically upon the rate of neural activation. For the particular case of the cat gastrocnemius muscles (8) examined at low rates of activation, and after a constant stretch amplitude has been reached, the force produced may even fall below isometric values at some velocities, or maintain values relatively comparable to those shown under isometric conditions. At higher rates of activation, the force measured at the same length and stretch velocity may be somewhat higher than that seen at low rates, but the tension increase is usually relatively modest (8). The net outcome of these comparisons is that velocity relations are quite asymmetric for shortening versus lengthening muscle. A note of caution is warranted, however. In shortening muscle, the muscle is acting on the load and muscle properties determine force output and shortening velocity. In forcible lengthening, on the other hand, the interaction with load is less readily defined, since the force produced may have no subsequent effect on the time-course of muscle lengthening. (Consider, for example, the situation in which a muscle is being elongated by a position-regulated muscle stretcher.) It follows that the shortening and lengthening states are not analogous. In spite of these differences, the two forms of muscle activation have several obvious and important physiologic parallels.

For example, movement typically requires active muscle shortening, so that muscle force must exceed load magnitude. In some other important instances, however, muscle is forcibly lengthened, such as during the early stance phase of walking, in which soleus and gastrocnemius muscles are active before heel strike, and are used to slow the rate of ankle dorsiflexion.

3. Relation Between Neural Input and Muscle Tension

A third important property of muscle is the relation between motoneuronal discharge and muscle tension. Under isometric conditions, muscle acts approximately as a low-pass filter of the incoming neural input, which is to say that high-frequency components of the stimulus train are attenuated (9). Thus, a step change in stimulus rate, which would arise for example at the onset of a tetanic stimulus train applied to the muscle nerve, produces a smoothed, rather gradual increase in muscle tension which may take several hundred milliseconds to reach a steady tension level.

The relation between neural input and isometric tension has been modeled as a linear, critically damped second-order system, with specified natural frequency, low-frequency gain, and damping ratio (10). These three parameters differ for different muscles, and they also differ for a given muscle under different stimulus conditions, such as during variations in initial muscle length and mean stimulus rate (5,11). These parametric dependencies mean that simple linear descriptions of muscular response to neural input are useful if they are applied to specific response regions, such as for a specific initial length, nerve stimulus frequency, and limited range of rate variation. In spite of these limitations, the linear systems approach is quite useful for modeling muscle contributions in complex regulatory systems, and it imposes important constraints on modeling muscular contraction at the molecular level (12).

4. Nonlinear Features of Muscular Response

An important aspect of muscular behavior, especially relevant to the neural control of muscle contraction, is the complex nonlinear dependence of muscle tendon on both the amplitude and rate of applied length change and on the rates and patterns of motoneuronal discharge. Figure 2a illustrates the marked changes in tension that arise during stretch of electrically activated soleus muscle in the cat (8,13,14). The tension rises steeply over the first few hundred micrometers of stretch, then drops abruptly before increasing again during the continued dynamic phase of stretch. There is a second, later decline in tension at ramp end, at the point of transition from movement to a new stationary length. The initial steep rise in tension has been termed the "short-range stiffness" (8,14), while the abrupt decline in tension has been called the muscle "yield" (8,14). These phenomena clearly represent nonlinear behavior, in that scaled variations in stretch amplitude are not accompanied by comparably scaled tension changes.

In contrast, tension recorded during symmetric muscle shortening displays a much smoother trajectory, following the time-course of imposed length change somewhat more closely than is the case during stretch. The yielding of tension during stretch is almost certainly a consequence of stretch-induced disruption of actomyosin cross bridges, linking thick and thin filaments of the muscle sarcomere (8). As such, it might be predicted that the characteristics of the short-range stiffness and the yield depend upon the level of activation of the muscle, and this turns out to be correct (14). Thus, at low stimulus rates, the yield is quite prominent, while at higher stimulus rates, the yield may be largely obscured, apparently compensated by the high rate of new cross bridge formation.

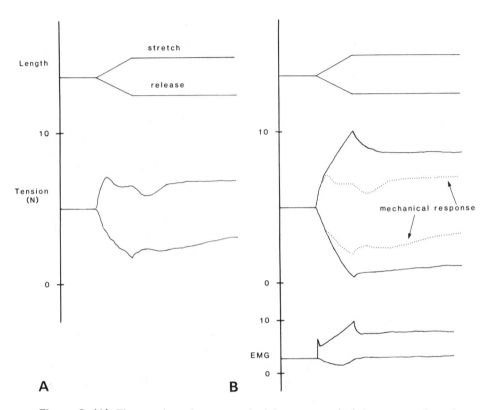

Figure 2 (A) The tension changes evoked by symmetrical 2-mm stretch and release of the active cat soleus muscle are quite asymmetrical. Muscle is activated here by asynchronous electrical stimulation of several ventral root fascicles. (B) Stretch reflex responses of the cat soleus, elicited in the decerebrated preparation. Tension changes are now quite symmetrical, but the associated changes in EMG, recorded from within the muscle, show asymmetry opposite to that of the muscle "mechanical response."

While the changes in tension recorded during constant-velocity stretch are quite complex, and also show strong dependence on both the parameters of the stretch and on the initial force level, variations in the tension profile are rather easily predicted, once the "template" or time-course of response is established for a given initial force and initial length (14). Thus, if a given tension record is observed in response to a stretch of a particular velocity and amplitude, then tension records observed during responses initiated at different forces can be shown to scale simply in proportion to the changes in initial force level, especially when the force is varied simply by varying the initial level of motoneuron recruitment. This approach, which can be achieved experimentally by varying the number of ventral root motor axons that are activated, works well because recruitment simply adds parallel muscular elements, whose net contribution can be estimated by simple linear summation of the response of each motor unit (14). The tension response recorded during stretch can also be predicted by similar scaling procedures even when initial tension is modified by variations in stimulus rate rather than by changes in recruitment level. These scaling techniques are then somewhat less accurate, especially when the effects of widely disparate rates of stimulation are compared.

A further nonlinear characteristic of the muscle tension response to imposed length change can be observed by comparing the response of electrically stimulated muscle to symmetric stretch and release, of constant amplitude and velocity (Fig. 2a). The tension responses to such symmetric length changes are typically markedly asymmetric, suggesting that correspondingly asymmetric neural compensatory signals are required in normally innervated, active muscle if these rather complex mechanical properties are to be compensated.

A number of additional, rather more subtle nonlinear types of behavior also arise in relation to the response of muscle to neural input. For example, the isometric tension evoked by a tetanic stimulus train is not accurately predicted from the response of muscle to a single twitch (15). If the twitch response is equated to the impulse response of a linear, critically damped second-order system, then the tetanic tension magnitude should be predictable simply through linear summation of the individual impulse responses. In fact, the actual tension recorded is typically much less during unfused tetani, presumably because internal motion of each sarcomere helps to degrade tension output of muscle sarcomeres.

Another important nonlinearity is the so-called "catch property," in which a pair of closely spaced stimulus pulses, termed a "doublet," produces a disproportionate increase in isometric muscle tension, which may be maintained long after the doublet stimulus is applied (16,17).

To conclude this description of muscle, it is perhaps important to note that many key features of muscle remain incompletely characterized, largely because normally occurring behaviors are associated with simultaneously occurring changes in muscle length, movement velocity, stimulus rate, and fractional recruitment, conditions not replicated easily in the laboratory.

B. Afferent Input

The responses of muscle receptor afferents to various types of muscle stimulation are discussed in Chapter 12 (this volume). In this section, we will highlight those aspects of autogenetic afferent input that are important in understanding the functional characteristics of stretch reflex action, as well as the characteristics of a second important autogenetic reflex, the clasp-knife reflex.

1. Muscle Spindle Receptors

Primary and secondary muscle spindle endings give rise to groups Ia and II afferent fibers, respectively. Figure 3 shows schematically the response of a primary and secondary ending from the same muscle to ramp and hold stretch and to ramp and hold release of comparable magnitude and velocity. Several key features warrant emphasis. First, the response of the Ia afferent (originating in the primary ending) is very large during the ramp or dynamic velocity phase of the stretch before subsiding to a rather modest discharge rate during the

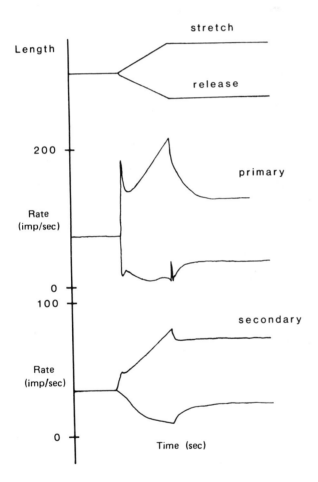

Figure 3 Responses of primary and secondary spindle receptor afferents to symmetrical stretch and release, recorded in soleus muscle of the decerebrate cat. Muscle spindles are receiving substantial spontaneous fusimotor input, both static and dynamic in type.

"hold" or static phase of the stretch. There is some dynamic increase in the discharge rate of the secondary ending during the ramp phase, but this effect is much less prominent than that shown by the primary ending. The rate increase recorded during the dynamic phase of stretch is usefully called the "dynamic response," and it has been traditionally treated as reflecting velocity sensitivity of the primary ending. However, as shown in Chapter 12 (this volume), the dynamic response increases relatively little with substantial increases in stretch velocity; a hundredfold increase in stretch velocity gives rise to only a two- to threefold increase in the size of the dynamic response. The proposed sensitivity to velocity is probably better regarded as a sensitivity to motion, rather than to velocity per se. The velocity dependence of secondary endings is quantitatively similar to that of primary endings, but since the size of the dynamic response is so much less prominent, the secondary ending is reasonably regarded as signaling information about muscle length.

A second important issue is evident in the comparison of primary ending response to symmetric stretch and release. As shown in Figure 3a, the primary ending shows a substantial dynamic response during ramp stretch, but a much smaller rate diminution during muscle shortening. In the absence of static fusimotor input to the muscle spindle, the response asymmetry is typically associated with silencing of spindle afferent discharge during the shortening phase. (Here the asymmetry is partly attributable to the fact that the initial discharge rate is not usually sufficiently high to permit symmetric rate increases and decreases.) However, the asymmetry is not simply an outcome of the absence of fusimotor input. The asymmetry is actually enhanced in the presence of high levels of static and dynamic fusimotor input (18). At moderate stretch velocities, muscle shortening may evoke little or no reduction in discharge rate when static fusimotor input is high, whereas muscle stretch may induce very high discharge rates, especially when dynamic fusimotor input is strong. The net outcome is that under normal conditions, in which static and dynamic fusimotor activity presumably coexist, the response asymmetry would be even greater than that recorded in de-efferented spindles, or in spindles showing low levels of fusimotor activity.

Although this discussion of fusimotor effects has centered on the effects of gamma input, the effects of beta or skeletofusimotor innervation of muscle spindles seem to be essentially comparable to those of gamma fibers (see Chapter 12, this volume).

2. Tendon Organs

Tendon organs are accurate transducers of muscle tension (see Chapter 12, this volume). Although each receptor receives direct mechanical input from a rather limited sample of the total muscle fibers in its general area (12-16 fibers out a local population of several hundred), the tendon organ still appears able to provide a rather good estimate of net muscle tension, as measured at the tendon.

Tendon organ discharge appears to reflect primarily the instantaneous tension magnitude, together with a small component reflecting the rate of change of muscle tension. It must be acknowledged, however, that the range of different muscles examined to this point is still rather limited, so that this rather simple view of tendon organ response may not be accurate when extended to other muscles located in different preparations.

There are also several nonlinearities in the tendon organ response to naturally occurring tension increase. These nonlinearities are especially evident at low-tension levels when few motor units are active (19,20), and there may be departures from linearity at high-tension levels. On the whole, the tendon organ is a surprisingly accurate transducer of net muscle tension.

3. Free Nerve Endings

By far the most numerous receptors in muscle are free nerve endings. These endings appear to be specialized to show sensitivity to a particular stimulus type, including mechanical, thermal, pH, nociceptive, and chemical stimuli (21-26). A given free nerve ending may show sensitivity to several types of stimuli, but apparently shows preferential responsiveness to one stimulus type. Muscle free nerve ending afferent fibers may be myelinated or unmyelinated. While the myelinated fibers are typically slowly conducting, a significant fraction may be quite large, and conduct with conduction velocities comparable to those shown by spindle and tendon organ afferents (23). These more rapidly conducting fibers may be responsible, at least in part, for the apparent complexity of the synaptic actions evoked by electrical stimulation of different muscle nerves.

Free nerve ending afferents may be responsible for muscle pain sensation, for the respiratory and circulatory response to exercise, and for important spinal reflexes, especially in pathologic neural states such as spasticity, An exemplary pathologic reflex will be addressed in a later section.

C. Autogenetic Synaptic Connections of Muscle Afferents

In this section, we will survey the important synaptic connections of muscle afferents, with a view toward establishing a possible wiring diagram of muscle-related neuronal circuitry, upon which hypotheses about functional roles of muscle afferents might reasonably be based. For the most part, details about synaptic mechanisms and putative transmitters are described in other chapters of this series. The object of this section is to present a succinct overview.

1. Ia Afferents

Ia afferent fibers make dense and widespread monosynaptic connections with autogenetic motoneurons, so that a given spindle primary afferent projects essentially to all motoneurons of a given motoneuron pool (see Chap. 9). There are also dense monosynaptic projections to close synergists, less dense projections to more remote motoneuron pools belonging to functional synergists, and occasional projections to motoneurons of functional antagonists. While the patterns of convergence and divergence of muscle primary spindle afferents are quite complex, the patterns of connectivity support the view that reflex actions of Ia afferents promote excitation of autogenetic and close synergist motoneurons.

There is also strongly suggestive, if inconclusive, evidence that Ia afferents make polysynaptic excitatory connections with homonymous motoneurons, and perhaps with motoneurons of close synergists as well. The evidence here is indirect, but cumulatively quite strong (27-34). For example, complex excitatory postsynaptic potentials (EPSPs) with disynaptic and longer latencies can be elicited in spinal motoneurons of cats showing fictive locomotion (30). Repetitive stimulation of Ia afferents evokes long-lasting depolarization of motoneurons, which far outlasts the duration of the stimulus train (27,31-33). Longitudinal vibration of cat hindlimb extensor muscles provokes depolarization that continues well beyond the cessation of the vibratory stimulus (31-33). Finally, the tonic reflex contraction evoked by tendon vibration (the tonic vibration reflex) continues well after cessation of the vibratory stimulus, and is effectively eliminated by small doses of barbiturate that are insufficient to reduce the size of the monosynaptic excitatory postsynaptic potential (34). These lines of evidence, while important, should not be allowed to obscure the fact that the existence of such a group of Ia excitatory neurons has yet to be verified by direct recording.

2. The Ib Afferent Pathway

Ib fibers, derived from tendon organ receptors, have been thought to mediate autogenetic inhibition via a di- or trisynaptic projection (35). The evidence for this claim is based largely upon intracellular recordings from spinal motoneurons, during synchronous electrical stimulation of homonymous and heteronymous muscle nerves, at intensities slightly above group I threshold (35). Inhibitory postsynaptic potentials were recorded at stimulus intensities appropriate to excite Ib fibers. While the autogenetic projection of Ia fibers in extensor muscles is potent, the analogous projection of the Ib fibers is apparently much weaker. Instead, Ib fibers appear to project quite diffusely and perhaps preferentially to some rather remote motoneuron pools, innervating muscles crossing other joints (35).

The existence of inhibitory projections from tendon organs onto motoneurons from the same muscle raises the possibility of a closed-loop force-regulating system. However, as will be addressed in a later section, the existence of a significant force-feedback loop has been difficult to verify in readily accessible animal preparations. Moreover, there are now a number of observations that indicate that attempts to understand the functions of tendon organ projections in isolation, without considering the effects of simultaneous spindle afferent are likely to be in error (36). These observations indicate that the "Ib" inter-neuron acts as a point of convergence for many different sensory and descend-ing projections. For example, many "Ib" interneurons appear to receive input from regional Ia afferents, as well as from cutaneous, joint, and high-threshold muscle afferents (37). These interneurons also receive inhibitory input from other interneurons and they are strongly excited by several descending path-ways. It is evident that an exclusive emphasis on Ib inputs to such neurons may be misplaced.

There are relatively few studies in which putative Ib interneurons have been sought directly. One major study was that of Lucas and Willis (38), who described the extracellular responses of a group of Ib interneurons in the inter-mediate gray matter of the lumbosacral cord of the anesthetized cat. These interneurons were implicated as being Ib because although group I input was discernible, it was not of a low-threshold type (and therefore did not originate in Ia fibers). On the other hand, a substantial response was evident when stimuli were sufficiently intense to activate Ib afferent fibers. In spite of this apparent clear indication of selective Ib input, intracellular recordings from a small number of these interneurons revealed convergence from Ia and Ib afferents in the same muscle, a finding which has since been confirmed and extended in Jankowska's laboratory (Fetz et al., 36).

3. Group II Inputs

Secondary spindle afferent fibers form the most numerous and best-studied source of group II fibers in muscle nerves; however, there is now good reason to believe that muscle afferents with group II diameter are heterogenous in both their receptor origin and in their central projections (39). As discussed earlier, some free nerve endings may give rise to group II afferents. This dichotomy of fiber source is also likely to be reflected in the pattern of central projections, although this prediction remains formally unverified at this time.

Secondary spindle afferent fibers are now known to make excitatory mono-synaptic connections with homonymous (40–42) and presumably heteronymous motoneurons, although the strength of these connections is apparently consider-ably less than that of Ia afferents from the same muscle (see Chap. 13 and Ref. 43). Collateral fiber projections also extend to reach more lateral portions of intermediate gray matter (44) and dorsal gray, and presumably synapse with interneurons in these regions. Nonspindle afferents are likely to follow similar projection patterns to those shown by groups III and IV fibers, which synapse superficially in the dorsal horn.

4. Groups III and IV Muscle Afferents

The central projection sof fine myelinated and unmyelinated muscle fibers are apparently similar to those of nociceptive afferents from skin and deeper tissues of the limb (44).

D. Regulation of Motor Output

Synaptic excitation of spinal motoneurons may give rise to activation of previously silent motoneurons (termed recruitment), or to rate augmentation of previously active motoneurons (termed rate modulation). As discussed by Lewis (Chap. 8, this volume), recruitment of motoneurons typically occurs in a reliable order, which is correlated broadly with motor unit type. Slow-twitch units before fast-twitch units, and fatigue-resistant before fatigue-sensitive units. Within motor unit type, recruitment rank order correlates closely with motoneuron size, although size per se may not be the most important causal factor.

From the standpoint of spinal regulation of muscle contraction, an important outcome is that the tension increment evoked by recruitment of each new motor unit is initially quite small, but rises progressively as new motor units are recruited in rank order. Expressed somewhat differently, the number of motor units recruited for each unitary increase in muscle tension (1 newton, for example) is very large initially, then falls swiftly with each subsequent unitary increment in tension (45). The relation between unit number and tension increment is well described by an exponential function of the form:

$$N = K e^{-Bf}$$

where N is the number of new motor units recruited in each 1 newton force increment, f is the isometric tension magnitude, and B and K are constants.

As a result of this relation, the increment in tension evoked by recruitment of each new motor unit is a constant proportion of the total tension measured at the tendon, displaying a relation broadly comparable to the Weber-Fechner law of sensory psychophysics. (This law relates just noticeable sensory differences to differences to the background stimulus intensity.) In the present context, this means that the tension increment generated by the recruitment of each new motor unit is a constant fraction of background tension, allowing the system to maintain a constant fractional sensitivity over a wide dynamic range of motor output.

The effects of rate modulation are best understood by examining isometric stimulus-tension functions, relating rates of electrical stimulation of the motor axon, or naturally occurring discharge rates of the motoneuron, to the resultant motor unit tension. The form of the relation between motor unit discharge rate and the resultant tension is sigmoidal, indicating that the tension generated is initially modest when motor units are stimulated at rates below their fusion frequency; however, when rates sufficient to induce partial fusion are reached, tension begins to climb steeply, ultimately reaching a plateau when tetanic fusion is complete.

Under normal conditions, the contributions of rate modulation are superimposed upon those of recruitment. As more motor units are recruited, the contribution of rate modulation to total tension output increases until eventually, rate modulation assumes the dominant role. For the particular case of the human first dorsal interosseus muscle (a well-studied system) the tension at which rate modulation effects equaled those of recruitment was estimated to be at 50% of maximum (45). It is worth noting that this point may well be quite different for different muscles, depending on the profile of motor unit recruitment, and the way in which motor unit rate modulation varies with motor unit type and recruitment rank order (35,36).

The relation between motor unit discharge rate and isometric muscle tension does not appear to vary systematically with recruitment order in the human first dorsal interosseus (48), or in the cat medial gastrocnemius (49). However, plots of motor unit discharge against elbow torque in human biceps muscle show systematic, although modest, increases in the slope of the relation between discharge rate and torque for motor units higher in the recruitment rank order (46). It appears that some differences in rate modulation characteristics may occur in different types of motor units within the one muscle.

To summarize, increases in muscle tension are generated by orderly increases in motor unit discharge rate, superimposed upon orderly recruitment of motor units that occurs in a reliable rank order.

E. Performance of the Closed Loop

1. Introduction

While the regulation and control functions of the spinal cord and higher centers are probably never imposed exclusively upon a single muscle, it is convenient to begin our analysis using autogenetic regulatory functions as our model system. These autogenetic functions are embodied in the concept of the motor servo, described in the introduction to this chapter.

Regulation of muscle contraction is dependent upon receptors that provide information about muscle state. The major encapsulated receptors (muscle spindle receptors and tendon organs) reviewed earlier, provide information about muscle length, the velocity of length change, and muscle tension. It follows that the sensory information available for neural regulation includes muscle length, muscle tension, and perhaps their time derivatives (such as velocity, rate of tension change) or some combinations of these variables (see later). For a variety of reasons, both experimental and circumstantial, the role of length sensors was most strongly emphasized initially, and we will begin by briefly reviewing classic approaches toward the regulation of muscle length.

2. Length Servo

The advent of control theory during the 1940s provided a potent stimulus toward evaluating neural regulation of muscle contraction in terms of this newly developed framework. While the existence of tendon organs was well known, they were thought to be rather insensitive to muscle tension change, responding adequately only at very high forces. (This view, which is now known to be erroneous, was based upon recordings made in passive muscle [50].) Muscle spindle receptors were considered to be the most important receptors for regulation of muscle contraction under normal conditions.

In 1951, Merton (51) reported that electromyographic activity in isometric human thumb muscles was silenced briefly by an electrically delivered muscle twitch. This observation was interpreted by Merton to suggest that spindle receptors were sensitive to the small internal length changes that arise during an ostensibly isometric contraction, and that these receptors might therefore be sufficiently sensitive to perform regulation of muscle length during more substantial lengthening perturbations (52).

A second, related hypothesis, based on the observation by Eldred et al. (54) that gamma efferent innervation of the muscle spindle could be modulated by central neural pathways, was that the spindle receptor apparatus could also be used to command changes in muscle length. This motor command was thought to be introduced by varying the discharge of gamma efferent fibers, which then altered spindle afferent discharge, resulting in appropriate changes in motoneuronal discharge and in muscle tension.

In the first example, that of electrical muscle stimulation, the command to the muscle is unchanging, and the system is then said to be acting to regulate muscle length. In the second condition, that of variation in efferent command to the spindle, the system is said to be controlling muscle length. A physiologic analogy for this distinction is the difference between posture and movement. In postural states, joint angle, and, therefore, muscle length is maintained relatively constant, whereas during movement, muscle length is of course changing.

At the outset, Merton (54) conceived of the efferent command as being mediated entirely by gamma innervation of the muscle spindle. Because this rather indirect route appeared inadequate for implementing rapid motor commands, an additional direct route from supraspinal paths to alpha motoneurons was hypothesized (52). This general approach has been termed "follow-up length" servo because of the requirement that gamma modulation mediate length changes via changes in spindle afferent discharge. While the length-servo hypothesis is now felt to be inadequate, it was certainly highly original, and it motivated a great deal of important research. It is therefore useful for didactic reasons to reevaluate it on the strength of the evidence available both at that time and now.

First, with regard to the hypothesis of length regulation, no direct supporting evidence was presented at the time the hypothesis was first introduced, or has since been forthcoming. The reported finding, which was of twitch-induced electromyographic (EMG) silencing, simply indicated that muscle spindles are highly sensitive to length change, and that this sensitivity was reflected in the motor output. More direct evidence of length regulation, such as a finding that muscle length was actually held constant by reflex action or that muscle stiffness was greatly enhanced, was not provided (see next section). A finding of powerful EMG increases following limb perturbation was reported by Hammond (53), who interpreted the response as a manifestation of servo action; however, it now appears the large amplitude changes were induced by short latency reaction time movements.

Second, no clear evidence supporting this gamma-based control of muscle length was presented. All that was shown was that modulation of gamma motoneurons by descending pathways was possible, a necessary but insufficient condition for length-servo control.

3. Evaluation of Hypotheses of Reflex Action

In order to critically evaluate the length-servo hypothesis (or any other hypothesis of reflex action) it is worth diverging briefly to decide what criteria should be satisfied in order for such an hypothesis to be acceptable.

A classic length-servo device compares information from a position transducer against some central "reference" signal, and issues a corrective command or "error signal" to an actuator, if transducer reading and reference values are different. (Referring to Figure 4, the length-servo component would be that loop which includes the muscle in the forward path, and the length receptor in the feedback path—the summing junction is shown as the motoneuron, which is clearly an oversimplification.) A useful way of evaluating the performance of such a servo is to compare the behavior of the system recorded without such

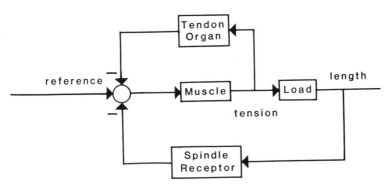

Figure 4 Block diagram of feedback loops acting to regulate muscle contraction. Increasing length evokes motoneuronal excitation which would act to shorten muscle, closing a length-negative feedback loop. Increasing tension evokes motoneuronal inhibition via tendon organ projections, closing a force-negative feedback loop.

positional feedback with that observed when the position feedback loop is operational. This approach is useful, since an effective length servo should achieve the commanded position with much greater reliability and precision when position information is available, as compared with the situation when position information is not. Expressed somewhat differently, this analysis contrasts the closed-loop performance of the system with that of the open loop.

A critical parameter for such an evaluation is the *positional stiffness* of the system, since this provides a direct measure of the accuracy with which a position can be held (or reached) in the face of an external load. Even the most rigid positional servo will show some measurable deflection during load imposition, and will therefore demonstrate a measurable stiffness (since stiffness is simply the ratio of force and length change). For the case of the muscle length (or positional) servo, an important comparison is the positional stiffness of the muscle with reflex loop intact versus the positional stiffness with loop opened. (The reflex loop can be opened by dorsal root section.)

As described in an earlier section, the classic length-tension properties of active muscle actually reflect springlike behavior. A measure of the validity of the position-servo hypothesis can therefore be provided by asking whether the stiffness of muscle with reflexes intact exceeds the stiffness of muscle recorded without any reflex regulation. One convenient way to examine the positional stiffness of the neuromuscular system is to use perturbations in position, applied via a length- (or position-) controlled muscle stretcher. This type of stretcher is able to impose the required position change, regardless of the resisting force being generated by the muscle. Since the load applied by the position-controlled stretcher is effectively infinite, the tension evoked by the stretch reflex is therefore a direct measure of the available output of the system. This tension output is, in turn, determined by the "open loop gain," which is simply the degree to which a signal injected at one point in a loop will be amplified after propagation around the loop. If the positional stiffness of the reflex is not substantially greater than that of muscle alone, then the hypothesis of length regulation is unlikely to be valid.

4. Comparison of Open-Loop with Closed-Loop Muscle Stiffness

The open-loop or "mechanical" stiffness of active muscle is a complex quantity, whose magnitude depends upon a number of parameters (14), including the level of muscular recruitment, the rate of motor unit activation, the initial muscle length, and the motor unit type (i.e., fast or slow twitch). Stiffness also varies greatly between dynamic and static conditions (8,14), and is quite different for stretch and release of muscle. For all of these reasons, comparison of reflex and mechanical stiffness has to be made under carefully specified initial conditions. While it is difficult to establish the state of recruitment and rate modulation for all of the motor units contained within a typical skeletal muscle, a range of stiffness measurements can be made for various, realistic values of important parameters, and a corresponding estimate of the range of possible stiffnesses achieved.

This comparison was made for the soleus muscle of the cat by Nichols and Houk (14). They verified that the "mechanical" stiffness of the muscle had several significant nonlinearities comparable to those described in earlier studies (8). As shown in Figure 2a, during the initial phase of muscle stretch muscle tension rises sharply for a fraction of a millimeter (the short-range stiffness) and this is followed by a sharp decline in muscular stiffness (the "yield" phase). Subsequently, restoration of appropriate tension levels takes place gradually, depending upon the level of muscle activation, and the rate of imposed stretch. If the muscle is forcibly shortened, over an amplitude and at a velocity comparable to those imposed during stretch, the initial decline in tension is rapid but then becomes more gradual, showing some overshoot before the final static level is achieved. There are no features of the tension response resembling muscle yield recorded under these conditions. An important outcome of this comparison is that muscular stiffness shows marked differences during stretch versus release, resulting in strongly asymmetric force records.

If we now compare the mechanical muscle responses with the stretch responses of muscle under reflex control (Fig. 2b), it is apparent that the stiffness of muscle is rather more constant (as shown by the relatively smooth tension change that accompanies muscle stretch or release), and it is significantly larger than the mechanical stiffness of muscle, especially during the dynamic phase of stretch. This type of analysis would appear, at least initially, to support a position-servo hypothesis, since the stiffness of the muscle under reflex control is much greater than that of the muscle alone. More detailed comparisons, however, do not sustain this impression.

For example, the mechanical muscular contribution to the total tension output increases in proportion to the level of initial force, while the reflex output does not (14). This means that under some conditions, such as at high initial forces, reflex force output is broadly comparable to that of muscle alone (14). This is not simply an outcome of saturation of motor output, since the relative mechanical and reflex contributions grade continuously from low to high initial force levels. Comparisons made during muscle shortening are even less supportive of the position-servo hypothesis, since the mechanical and reflex force profiles are then frequently similar (Fig. 2a,b).

When stretch reflex responses are examined over a broad range of conditions, such as at different initial forces, during stretch of different amplitudes, applied at different velocities, and for stretch versus release, reflex stiffness is not consistently enhanced above that of muscle alone. It follows that the length-servo model is unlikely to be appropriate.

5. Recent Modifications: Long-Loop Hypotheses

Because segmental reflex connections were thought to have insufficient potency to allow effective length regulation, a number of investigators, beginning with Phillips (55), have argued that "long-loop connections" could be used to augment muscle force in response to external perturbations. The afferent path of this long loop was thought to be composed of the cortical projections of muscle spindle afferents (56). It is also known that corticospinal neurons displaying direct projections to segmental motoneurons of forelimb muscles receive afferent input from the same muscles, thereby completing a loop (57). While the existence of such a loop appears firmly established, it remains to be shown that this loop is used to perform continuous feedback regulation. An alternative, equally feasible hypothesis is that this circuit is used for programmed movements, which are capable of being released by sensory cues, including those arising from muscle afferents. This type of sensorimotor processing would exhibit no fixed relationship between stimulus and motor response, and would not be expected to show responses consistent with either a simple position-servo or "long-loop" position-servo model.

In view of the existence of short-latency connections from muscle afferents to cortical neurons, it was reasonable to examine the limb reflex responses to transient loading, searching for evidence of reflex components occurring at latencies appropriate for such long-loop actions. A number of investigators have, in fact, observed that stretch-evoked EMG responses show bursting patterns consistent with the existence of several loops of different conduction time (46). These include a short-latency, spinal segmental input, and longer-latency supraspinal loop(s), traversing motor cortex or cerebellum (58-63). While some circumstantial support for supraspinal loops emerges from detailed analyses of the time-course of EMG responses in proximal and distal limb muscles (62), few studies have taken full account of the effects of continuing afferent excitation during a typical perturbation, and of the effects of polysynaptic processing through parallel spinal pathways. Thus, it is not altogether surprising that stretch of muscles in spinalized cat preparations was reported to evoke EMG responses to muscle stretch that are quite similar to those recorded in the intact preparation (64). While such experiments cannot exclude a long-loop contribution, they indicate that the use of EMG bursting patterns to infer connectivity of reflex pathways is fraught with difficulty, and they argue against any overly simplistic analyses of EMG response patterns.

To this point, I have argued that the responses evoked in response to muscle length change reflex responses do not promote a reliable increase in reflex stiffness, consistent with the demands of a useful position-servo device. As stated in the introductory section, regulation of muscle contraction must depend upon the information provided by muscle receptors. Since length regulation is apparently not present, it is conceivable that other variables recorded by muscle receptors (such as velocity or muscle tension) are regulated during muscle contraction. These variables could be used either directly or following some form of preliminary spinal processing which might include summation of information from different muscle sensory receptor types onto one interneuron or class of interneurons.

6. Regulated Variables

At present, there is no direct information available supporting the existence of regulatory states in which movement velocity or force is regulated directly (but note 65). In addition, no muscle receptors exist that relay muscle velocity information in any simple form. As described in Chapter 12 (this volume), for amplitudes of stretch exceeding 0.5% of the range of physiologic length change, the response of primary spindle afferents is only weakly dependent on velocity, and the response also varies as a function of absolute muscle length in a rather complex, nonlinear manner. While such complexities certainly do not eliminate the possible existence of a central neuronal transformation, reestablishing simple velocity dependence of spinal neural mechanisms, no evidence is available motivating such a supposition. Moreover, examination of reflex EMG and force dependence on stretch velocity (14) do not support the existence of a velocity-regulating process.

In similar fashion, no observations have been reported in which muscle tension is maintained at a constant value during reflex responses, or during voluntary movement (although it must be acknowledged that rather few measurements exist). At the present time, the most appealing possibility is that tendon organ and muscle spindle afferent information are combined in some manner to regulate muscle contraction.

7. Stiffness Regulation

An important current hypothesis, originating from Nichols and Houk (14), is that stretch reflex action compensates for a number of the major, nonlinear properties of muscle, giving rise to essentially springlike performance of the intact muscle. The evidence in support of this proposition is largely indirect in form but quite substantial in scope, as shown by the following observations.

First, for the intact reflex system, springlike behavior of muscle is quite common (66–68), and this stiffness is maintained under conditions in which areflexive muscle shows marked deviations from simple springlike behavior (14). These deviations include muscle yield and the marked asymmetry of muscle tension responses in stretch and release, described in earlier sections, and illustrated in Figure 2a. For the best-studied case, that of the soleus muscle in the decerebrate cat, the reflex tension evoked by muscle stretch increases roughly in proportion to stretch amplitude, for both stretch and release.

Although the stiffness of the reflex response is greater for small stretch amplitudes than for large, and the stiffness is also somewhat greater in release than stretch, nonetheless, the consistency and smoothness of the relation between length and tension is greatly enhanced in the intact system (by comparison with the responses of electrically activated muscle).

Second, for the case of the soleus again, the EMG responses to stretch and release, which are a measure of neurally mediated reflex action, are appropriate in magnitude, timing, and symmetry to exactly offset the differences in muscle mechanical responses described in the previous paragraph. As shown diagrammatically in Figure 2b, EMG increase is substantial during stretch, when muscle yielding is prominent, while EMG reduction is often minimal during shortening, when mechanical properties of muscle are essentially springlike in character. There is presumably little need for neural modification of the muscle tension response to shortening, in order to preserve springlike characteristics, since muscle displays such characteristics spontaneously. While the most detailed EMG observations have been made in the cat preparation, it is reassuring that comparable EMG asymmetry is apparent during stretch and release of elbow flexor muscles in intact, conscious human subjects (68).

Third, it can be shown theoretically (14,69,70) that a system in which both length and tension are incorporated in the feedback configuration will regulate some derived system property, such as stiffness. In a system composed of springlike elements it is theoretically impossible to regulate both force and length independently.

A number of other secondary lines of evidence have been introduced in support of a stiffness-regulation model. For example, measurements of reflex stiffness have been made during variations of initial force, in both the cat and human models (71,72). In an ideally regulated system, stiffness would remain totally constant (and therefore independent of initial force). In a totally unregulated system, stiffness would rise more or less simply in proportion to initial force magnitude. (This model presumes that force is generated by the addition of parallel force-generating elements, each with specified stiffness.) Under realistic experimental conditions, stiffness increases much less than initial force, suggesting that some regulation may have taken place. For example, a tenfold increase in initial force is typically accompanied by a two- to threefold increase in stiffness (14,71). If this evaluation is correct, then reflex action is not especially effective in maintaining precise constancy of stiffness.

A further example supporting stiffness regulation arises from careful analysis of EMG responses to symmetric stretch and release of the cat and human (14,68). As described earlier, the EMG changes are broadly appropriate to compensate for the inherent mechanical characteristics of muscle. It is often found, especially in the human experiments, that rectified EMG may actually increase during shortening (a pattern that appears to promote increased positional error).

Such EMG increases presumably act to modify muscle mechanical state, promoting the symmetry of the tension response to symmetric stretch and release.

8. Summary and Evaluation

The evidence reviewed to this point has shown that in the presence of an intact reflex loop, muscle displays behavior much closer to that of a simple spring than is shown by the same muscle under open-loop conditions (i.e., with reflex loop opened). This evidence is consistent with a stiffness-regulation hypothesis, but is not entirely conclusive, primarily because it is circumstantial, or correlative in form. Moreover, while a role for spindle receptors and tendon organs seems plausible, no direct evaluation of their role has been provided in the literature, and no test of feedback regulation (versus other forms of regulation) has yet been described.

F. Force-Feedback Regulation: Role of Tendon Organ Projections

1. Role of Tendon Organs

In most animal experiments directed toward evaluation of stretch reflex mechanisms, the test muscle is stretched with a length-servo device, and the measured variable is then muscle tension. Under these conditions, muscle spindle receptor discharge is essentially invariant (although some force-related variations might be anticipated). If a simple feedback system of stiffness regulation is operational, then the important feedback in this experimental setting would appear to arise from tendon organs. For these reasons, the role of tendon organs and their central projections has special prominence in reflex regulation of muscle stiffness.

In an earlier section, it was pointed out that tendon organ afferents evoke autogenetic inhibition via a disynaptic or trisynaptic linkage, and that inhibitory postsynaptic potentials can be recorded from motoneurons innervating muscles acting at remote joints. Inhibition of an extensor muscle is accompanied by excitation of the antagonist, giving rise to the term "inverse" myotatic reflex, in which tension increases of the agonist give rise to inhibition of the antagonist muscles. Because of these findings of autogenetic inhibition in electrophysiologic experiments it is useful to ask whether tension-mediated increases in tendon organ discharge evoke appropriate reductions in motor output in reflexively activated muscles. That is, do tendon organs and their central projections provide effective force-feedback regulation?

2. Use of Internal Disturbances to Estimate Force Feedback

The first direct attempt to quantify the efficacy of this tendon organ pathway was reported by Houk et al. (73). These authors argued that in the presence of tendon organ–mediated force feedback, the force increases generated by electrical stimulation of small ventral root fascicles would be offset by reductions in motor output to other motor units in the same muscle. The preparation used for these experiments was the decerebrate cat, and the muscle examined was the soleus. The experiment compared the increment in tension evoked by stimulating a number of motor units in a passive soleus muscle with that evoked by stimulating the same set of motor units in the presence of reflex action. This comparison revealed that the force increments evoked in the presence of motor activity (and therefore reflex action) were significantly smaller than those observed in passive muscle, suggesting that some form of force-feedback loop was operational.

A finding of force-related reductions in motor output does not automatically indicate that tendon organ pathways were responsible. Because of the existence of series-compliant elements in the muscle, and especially in the tendon, a reduction in spindle-mediated excitatory drive to spinal motoneurons could also come from the spindle shortening that parallels force-related extension of these compliant elements. Some changes in tension can also be attributed directly to this shortening of extrafusal muscle fibers, since these fibers would now be operating at a different point on their length-tension curves. In the Houk study (73), the observed decline in tension in reflexively activated muscle was apportioned into various components (i.e., spindle receptor unloading and length-tension contributions), leaving a relatively small fraction attributable to tendon organ-mediated force feedback. Expressed in terms of a dimensionless gain measurement, the loop gain of this force-feedback pathway was estimated to lie in the range of 0.2-0.5. While this loop gain is small by most standards, the authors calculated that the gain was sufficient to reduce the effects of fatigue (or other types of contractile failure) by about one-third.

Although the force-feedback experiments described were highly innovative, some uncertainties arose regarding the estimates of spindle receptor rate reductions, or "unloading" evoked during ventral root stimulation. This uncertainty arises because the contraction induced by stimulation of a small ventral root fascicle may be unevenly dispersed within the muscle, so that the magnitude of spindle afferent rate reduction, or "unloading," when assessed over the full complement of spindle receptors in the muscle may not be easily estimated from the change in net muscle tension recorded at the tendon.

In an attempt to overcome the uncertainties associated with these estimates of spindle afferent unloading, Jack and colleagues (74) repeated the Houk protocol (in which the tension evoked by stimulation of small ventral root fascicles was examined both in the presence and in the absence of reflex action) (73), but also superimposed longitudinal tendon vibration during the tension increase. This vibration acted to "clamp" the Ia afferent discharge at the vibration frequency, thereby minimizing the spindle afferent unloading effects of tension increases. Under these conditions, the effects of tension increases were significantly reduced, and the resultant gain estimates of the tendon organ pathway were even smaller, falling in the range of 0.0-0.2.

Two other approaches toward estimation of tendon organ–related force feedback have been attempted. Rymer and Hasan (75) used dantrolene sodium to impair soleus muscle contractility in the decerebrated cat preparation, and recorded soleus EMG response to muscle stretch as a measure of neural compensatory responses. They found that EMG response to stretch did not increase significantly, even in preparations where dantrolene had reduced reflex muscle stiffness by as much as 50-70%. Their estimates of force-feedback gain were indistinguishable from zero.

A different approach, reported by Hoffer and Andreassen (76), depended upon parametric estimation of length and force-feedback contributions to muscle stiffness changes. These stiffness changes were measured during ramp and hold stretches, initiated at a number of different initial forces. Their estimates of tendon organ-mediated gain were again indistinguishable from zero.

3. Summary and Evaluation

It appears that a number of estimates of tendon organ–mediated force-feedback gain have provided very small gain values, typically near zero. It is important to note, however, that all of the aforementioned estimates of force-feedback gain were based on experiments performed in hindlimb extensor muscles of the decerebrate cat preparation. It could be argued, with some justice, that the decerebrate preparation is not ideal for these studies because the responses of many segmental reflex pathways are heavily modified, as evidenced by the observation that Ib-mediated ipsilateral postsynaptic potentials (IPSPs) in homonymous motoneurons are largely suppressed, by comparison with the spinalized or even the anesthetized state. Nonetheless, *it is this same decerebrate preparation which shows strong evidence of stiffness regulation.* If this analysis is correct, then the stiffness regulation is being accomplished through means other than tendon organ feedback.

G. Predictive Compensation: A Special Role for the Primary Ending

The absence of significant effects of tendon organ projections onto the autogenetic muscle is especially difficult to reconcile with simple feedback models for stiffness regulation because, as was pointed out earlier, when muscle is stretched by a position-controlled device tendon organs become the only receptors capable of detecting inappropriate force levels (and therefore erroneus stiffness values). This is because spindle receptor discharge is largely uninfluenced by tension change during stretch. On this basis, tendon organ projections would appear to occupy a pivotal role in regulating stiffness, yet in the decerebrate animal, stiffness is apparently regulated without the help of tendon organ projections. Some alternative approach would appear to be necessary.

1. Model-Reference Control

One such approach assigns a special role to the spindle primary ending in directly regulating muscle tension, a role which is of course more readily assigned to a muscle "length" receptor. This tension regulatory role can be understood if the muscle spindle is considered to operate as a form of extrafusal muscle model. In this form of regulation, which is described as "model-reference" (77), changes in muscle length are considered to be imposed as a simultaneous input to extrafusal fibers and intrafusal fibers. The intrafusal fiber pole contains muscle broadly comparable in its mechanical characteristics to extrafusal muscle, allowing this polar region to act as the model of extrafusal muscle. The changes in tension of the polar region are then transduced by primary endings located at the equatorial region of the fiber, giving rise to a neural signal that closely reflects the mechanical changes at the pole. If the characteristics of this transduced signal are appropriate, and afferent propagation and spinal processing rapid, then the efferent spinal command to muscle might be suitable for predicting and minimizing muscle yield during stretch. To achieve this yielding compensation, the signal would be expected to arrive at an appropriate early time, to show the correct asymmetry, and to have a demonstrable role in preventing muscle yield. It appears that primary ending-mediated responses satisfy all of these requirements, thereby generating a rather strong, if somewhat circumstantial case for the "model-reference" approach toward regulation of muscle contraction.

The evidence in support of a special role for primary endings is threefold. First, the latency of EMG response to abrupt muscle stretch is appropriate for yielding compensation (78). For the case of the soleus muscle of the cat, the EMG response to abrupt muscle stretch begins approximately 10 msec after stretch onset, a latency which is composed of the following elements: receptor activation time (1-2 msec), propagation from primary endings via dorsal roots (2-3 msec), central spinal monosynaptic projection or oligosynaptic projection (1 msec), motor efferent propagation to muscle (2-3 msec), neuromuscular transmission (1 msec). While the time of yielding onset varies according to stretch velocity, and to the rate of muscle activation, yielding does not usually commence until 25 msec after stretch onset, and is usually much later. (The earliest onset recorded was 18 msec.) It appears that the onset of EMG activity is appropriate to initiate force generation within 25-30 msec of stretch onset, allowing yield prevention to occur.

A second line of evidence regarding the yield-compensating role of the primary ending is provided by close comparisons of spindle primary afferent response to symmetric muscle stretch and release with the reflex EMG and tension response of muscle recorded under similar stimulus conditions (78). As was described earlier, in the presence of significant simultaneous dynamic and static fusimotor bias, primary spindle receptor dynamic response to stretch is much larger than the response to symmetric muscle shortening. This asymmetry is precisely opposite to that shown by the tension response of areflexive muscle, but is very close to that shown in the EMG responses (see Fig. 2b). The form of the EMG response indicates that the spindle primary ending input is transmitted substantially unmodified. It appears, then, that the appropriate compensatory signal arises immediately at the periphery, as soon as muscle stretch induces a response from the primary ending. The signal is initiated rapidly, is swiftly propagated, and also has the required asymmetry to compensate for the asymmetry of muscle.

The third line of evidence concerns the effect of modulating primary spindle afferent discharge on muscle yielding, and it depends upon recordings of muscle tension made during combined stretch and vibration of the soleus muscle in the decerebrate cat preparation (78). If a reflex muscular contraction of the soleus is established by high-frequency longitudinal tendon vibration, the muscle force response evoked by superimposed large amplitude stretch is quite different from that recorded in a typical stretch reflex response. Specifically, there is a sharp decline in stiffness after vibrated muscle has been stretched for approximately 0.5 mm, a length sufficient to induce muscle yielding in areflexive muscle. It appears that longitudinal tendon vibration, which "clamps" Ia afferent discharge at the vibration frequency (79) has prevented any stretch-induced increase in spindle afferent discharge, and effectively eliminated the initial phase of yielding compensation, allowing a yieldlike reduction in muscle force to be manifested.

Although the cited observations are perhaps individually inconclusive, taken en masse they appear to support an important role for the primary ending in yielding compensation and in stiffness regulation. They also appear to vindicate the model reference framework used to motivate this approach. Since the outcome of this type of regulation is to elicit a compensatory response for muscle yielding before yielding of extrafusal muscle actually occurs, alternative and useful descriptive terms are "predictive" compensation or "anticipatory" compensation.

2. Regulation of Motor Output: Recruitment Versus Rate Modulation

Predictive compensation of muscle yield appears to depend upon abrupt increases in motor output, arising shortly after stretch onset. Increases in motor output (which appear as increases in rectified EMG activity) are generated by recruitment of new motor units, and/or rate modulation of previously active motor units. It is conceivable that motor unit recruitment and rate modulation have different roles in yielding compensation.

The roles of recruitment and rate modulation in yielding compensation were examined by Cordo and Rymer (49), who determined the patterns of recruitment and rate modulation exhibited by soleus and medial gastrocnemius motor units during muscle stretch, and then evaluated the yield compensatory effects of stimulating motor axons with these same patterns of motor output (varying both recruitment and rate modulation [80]. These studies showed clearly that motor unit recruitment was a highly effective method for minimizing overall muscle yielding because newly recruited units showed almost no tendency to yield. This yielding prevention arises presumably because newly activated muscle fibers are generating actomyosin bonds at a high rate, thereby over-riding the effects of stretch-induced bond disruption, the presumptive mechanism of muscle yielding.

On the other hand, rate modulation of previously active muscle proved to be a relatively ineffective way of minimizing muscle yielding (80). The net force increases induced by rate modulation during stretch were quite modest (especially when naturally occurring rates were used) and the increases were relatively slow to develop, so that little yielding compensation resulted. Even doublets, which are closely spaced pairs of motor unit impulses recorded typically when muscle is freshly recruited, did not appear to enhance the resistance of the muscle to yielding. This is in contrast to the observation that doublets act to greatly enhance tension in isometric muscle. Apparently, stretch disrupts the processes responsible for development of the catch.

3. Summary and Evaluation

It appears that newly recruited muscle fibers are relatively resistant to yield, indicating that recruitment may be very important in the initial phase of yield compensation. Parenthetically, it does not appear to be important that recruitment begin at exactly monosynaptic latency. Any step increase in recruitment occurring at, slightly after, or even before stretch onset appeared to be sufficient to protect against yielding.

H. Yielding Compensation at Different Muscle Tensions

One potential difficulty with the predictive compensation model is that the magnitude of stretch-induced muscle yielding varies markedly at different initial force levels (14). Specifically, at very low initial forces, the mechanical muscle contribution is quite modest, meaning that recorded reflex tension is largely generated by recruitment of fresh motor units, and by some associated rate modulation. As the initial force increases, the mechanical contribution of the muscle to the total recorded tension also increases in direct proportion to the increase in force, and this change is accompanied by a relative reduction in the size of the reflex contribution. At very high initial forces, the mechanical muscle contribution may be almost entirely responsible for the early portion of the tension record.

At first sight, it seems difficult to understand how such an arrangement could be implemented using spindle receptors, whose discharge is largely independent of muscle force. It now appears likely that the force-matching characteristics of this predictive system are embedded in the properties of the motor output, rather than in the characteristics of the afferent input. A sharp depolarization of the motoneuron pool (such as would be generated in response to rapid stretch of the homonymous muscle) induces many motor units to be recruited when the pool is largely quiescent, and much smaller numbers of units to be recruited when the motoneuronal pool is substantially activated. (This sequence is in accordance with the size principle, in that the motor units recruited initially generate little tension.) Preferential recruitment at low initial forces is exactly the response pattern required for maximizing yielding compensation, since yielding is greatest at low initial forces, where recruitment is the predominant mode of tension regulation. At higher initial forces, muscle yielding is much less prominent, so that the relatively poor yielding compensation provided by rate modulation is less telling in its consequences. In sum, the largest need for recruitment appears to arise when the rate of recruitment is greatest, a fortunate "coincidence."

I. Yielding Compensation: The Role of Fusimotor Input

On a more speculative note, it is of some interest to consider the potential role(s) of efferent spindle input in the "model-reference" hypothesis. If the polar regions of the muscle spindle serve as models of extrafusal muscle, then one possible role for gamma (and beta) efferent input to the spindle is to optimize intrafusal muscle mechanical behavior during muscle length change, over a wide range of motor output states. In this context, increasing fusimotor discharge (beta or gamma) could serve to augment stiffness of intrafusal fibers, in parallel with increasing stiffness of extrafusal fibers. One possible advantage of increasing fusimotor input at high muscle tensions is that spindle afferent discharge rate will be maintained in the face of compliance-related internal shortening of muscle.

It is also likely that simultaneous input from static and dynamic gamma (and beta) fibers increases the asymmetry of spindle afferent response to symmetric muscle stretch and release. This is because gamma (and beta) dynamic activation increases primary ending response to muscle stretch, whereas static efferent activation diminishes the muscle spindle response to muscle shortening. The net effect of this efferent input is to generate response asymmetries precisely opposite to those of muscle, and therefore potentially appropriate to compensate for the asymmetric mechanical properties of muscle.

III. ABNORMALITIES OF STRETCH REFLEX FUNCTION: THE CLASP-KNIFE REFLEX

Stretch of muscles in either the decerebrate cat or in normal humans evokes a progressive tension increase that is broadly proportional to the amplitude of stretch, and is therefore springlike in character. If the dorsolateral quadrants of the spinal cord are then sectioned, interrupting major reticulospinal pathways, a comparable stretch may now induce a profound inhibition, especially when the muscle is stretched to near maximum length (39,81). The inhibition is augmented when the stretched muscle is generating substantial force. Similar inhibition can also be evoked in an isometric muscle by stretch of a synergist. The inhibition is apparently mediated by receptors responding to increases in length and/or increases in tension (39).

It is conceivable that clasp-knife inhibition could be generated by the convergent effects of tension organs and muscle spindle afferents, acting on interneurons or motoneurons; however, there is now strong evidence supporting a special role for mechanoreceptors with free nerve ending structure (39). These free nerve endings, whose afferents may be group II, III, or IV fibers, are activated by muscle stretch and contraction, with a time-course broadly appropriate to mediate the clasp-knife response.

The evidence supporting a special role for these mechanoreceptors in mediating clasp-knife inhibition is partly exclusionary in nature and partly direct. The exclusionary evidence is that the responses of the major muscle receptors, including primary and secondary endings and Golgi tendon organs, are inappropriate in their response thresholds or in the form of their length-rate relations to mediate clasp-knife inhibition (39). For example, recordings of primary ending discharge during the clasp-knife reflex show no evidence of a decline in rate preceding the onset of inhibition, indicating that gamma inhibition (and consequent afferent rate reduction) is not a likely mechanism. Moreover, neither the length threshold nor the time-course of discharge of secondary spindle afferents corresponds to the clasp-knife response. In regard to a possible tendon organ contribution, since tendon organ discharge is strongly dependent upon active muscle tension, the development of a profound inhibition sufficient to totally suppress motoneuronal output for many seconds is hard to reconcile simply with tendon organ activity (a point made clearly by Burke et al. [80]). This is because the loss of active tension would be followed, inevitably, by a reduction of tendon organ discharge. Some additional mechanism for prolonging the central inhibitory effects of tendon organ discharge is required for such an hypothesis to be made acceptable.

The direct evidence supporting an important role for muscle free nerve endings is partly that they have appropriate responsiveness to muscle stretch and contraction (39), but also that a subpopulation of these endings is acutely sensitive to gentle mechanical stimulation of the tendon and muscle aponeuroses, a type of stimulus which is also extremely potent in inhibiting motor activity in the stimulated muscle of the spinal-lesioned cat. (This type of stimulus, while not entirely specific for free nerve endings, is disproportionately powerful in its effects on these receptors, as compared with other types of muscle receptors.) The effect of this spinal lesion appears to be mediated by releasing the activity of powerful segmental inhibitory interneurons, which are strongly excited by free nerve ending mechanoreceptors, and that project to regional motoneurons.

In sum, the clasp-knife reflex is an autogenetic inhibitory reflex, originating in the discharge of free nerve ending mechanoreceptors, and mediated via powerful inhibitory interneuronal projections that diverge to inhibit many extensor muscles in the limb and to simultaneously activate many flexor muscles. The net outcome is that activation of intramuscular receptors gives rise to a disseminated inhibition of extensors and excitation of flexors throughout the limb. The action of such a reflex appears to unload extensor muscles, but it is unclear at present whether this is an important role under normal conditions. In fact, the functional contributions of this system in the nonlesioned state remain uncertain. There is no clear description of clasp-knife type inhibition in neurologically intact subjects, although the collapse in quadriceps muscle force associated with knee cartilage injury has features reminiscent of the clasp-knife responses.

IV. MUSCLE SYNERGIES

The emphasis to this point has been on input-output properties of spinal reflexes, with particular emphasis on the autogenetic reflex mechanisms associated with stretch reflex and clasp-knife responses. Under normal conditions even such simple reflexes are not confined to single muscles. For the case of stretch reflexes elicited at a typical joint, such as the elbow, extension of the elbow would stretch and activate many or all of the muscles that cross the joint. The resultant reflex response of these muscles is partly autogenetically based (in that stretch of spindles in a particular muscle will excite homonymous motoneurons, it results partly from divergence of Ia (and perhaps group II) afferents to synergist motoneurons, and finally it probably also results from divergence of activated interneurons to motoneurons lying within different motoneuron pools. It follows that the operational unit of motor output is rarely (if ever) the single muscle. Muscles are almost always activated in some combination, which is often identified as a "synergic" pattern. In the case of reflex responses, such as those resulting from elbow extension, the pattern of motor output elicited is also dependent upon the characteristics of the sensory input, such as stimulus location, stimulus intensity, and type and rate of change of the stimulus intensity.

For voluntary or automatic behaviors that are not reflexive in nature, the source of the synergic relations is less obvious (than in reflex responses). Such synergic motor patterns may often be similar to those seen in reflexive movements, suggesting that similar neural pathways are used, however, the neuronal substrates for these patterns are largely unexplored and may not necessarily be the same. Thus, while a painful stimulus to skin will typically elicit a flexion withdrawal response in which many flexors within the limb are activated in a precise pattern, the neuronal elements responsible for generating this pattern may conceivably be different from those employed in a voluntary flexion pattern. The use of fundamentally different neuronal elements to execute closely similar movements would seem to be an inefficient "design" choice, however no evidence is presently available allowing exclusion of this alternative. A different source of synergic relations arises when we consider the relation between muscles with opposing actions.

A. Reciprocal Inhibition

Activation of Ia afferents to a particular muscle will give rise to inhibition of motoneurons in "opposing," or antagonist muscles. This pattern is termed "reciprocal inhibition," and it is the presumptive mechanism for antagonist relaxation when a group of agonist muscles with similar actions are stretched.

It has now become evident that the Ia reciprocal inhibition is mediated via a set of interneurons located in deeper regions of the intermediate spinal gray matter (82,83). These interneurons are activated monosynaptically by Ia afferents, and project directly to opposing motoneurons with inhibitory projections. These interneurons receive inhibitory projections from regional interneurons (such as Renshaw neurons), input from regional cutaneous and joint nerves, and from descending pathways (such as the corticospinal and reticulospinal projections). The degree of convergence of these different inputs onto the Ia neuron would seem to indicate that the Ia inhibitory pathway is misnamed, and that the interneuron acts as a nodal inhibitory connection in many circuits (see 83). Little direct information is available about patterns of Ia interneuronal discharge in realistic circumstances, with the exception of observations made during "fictive" locomotion. Recordings from Ia interneurons during L-DOPA-induced activation of spinal locomotion pattern generators show in-phase activation (84), even in the absence of peripheral motor activity, indicating that locomotion pattern generators also project to the Ia inhibitory interneurons.

V. SIGNAL PROCESSING IN THE SPINAL CORD: ROLE OF INTERNEURONS

Anatomic studies reveal that most of the synaptic contacts lying on spinal motoneurons originate in regional interneurons, rather than in afferent monosynaptic projections. The role of most spinal interneurons is quite unclear, and remains largely untested. Relatively few attempts have been made to record from interneurons in unanesthetized spinal cords in reduced or intact preparations. Existing classification schemes are based largely on the pattern of synaptic connections.

A. Established Interneuron Systems

There are two well-established interneuron systems, for which structural and synaptic studies appear to be relatively complete. The first, already addressed in an earlier section, is the Ia interneuron, and the second is the Renshaw neuron.

The Ia interneuron is identified on the basis of the existence of a monosynaptic Ia connection, and by Renshaw-mediated inhibition (elicited by synchronous antidromic stimulation of the ventral root). The interneuron also has a characteristic location, lying medially in the ventral gray matter. The second well-characterized interneuron is the Renshaw neuron. This neuron was first identified by Renshaw in 1946 (85). He showed that the interneuron was inhibitory, and that it was activated monosynaptically by motoneuron axon collaterals. The Renshaw neuron is therefore activated by cholinergic mechanisms. Both muscarinic and nicotinic antagonists appear to reduce neuronal discharge, indicating that each type of cholinergic receptor is present on the neuron surface, although muscarinic receptors appear to be most important. Renshaw neurons inhibit Ia interneurons and other Renshaw neurons.

In spite of the simplicity of the Renshaw circuit the functional roles remain uncertain. Use of nicotinic blocking agents (such as DHBE) during random (Poisson) stimulation of the Ia input showed moderate increases in discharge of motoneurons over certain stimulus frequencies, suggesting that some Renshaw-mediated inhibition had been eliminated, but that Renshaw action was not prominent. The effects of Renshaw discharge may have been more readily visualized if muscarinic blocking agents were used (since the muscarinic cholinergic receptor appears to be most important in modulating sustained Renshaw neuronal discharge).

There are two broadly different types of hypotheses that have been advanced regarding the functional role of Renshaw neurons. The first deals with feedback effects of Renshaw neurons onto the exciting motoneurons. Here, Renshaw neurons are regarded as stabilizing the motor unit discharge rate at some appropriate value (or range of values) (86). This hypothesis is advanced largely because the circuit is readily described as a negative feedback loop, in which rate is the regulated variable. The advantage of such rate stabilization has not been clarified, and no test of such an hypothesis has been advanced.

The second class of hypothesis argues that Renshaw neurons impose important spatial constraints on the discharge of the motoneuron pool (87), acting to limit synchrony of motoneurons, and thus promoting a smooth muscle contraction. Such an outcome can be predicted on the basis of simple simulations of motoneuron network characteristics, since the probability of discharge of a given motoneuron is diminished if other motoneurons within the region have discharged within a time period sufficient to allow Renshaw neuronal activation and subsequent motoneuronal inhibition. It follows that Renshaw neurons would tend to desynchronize discharge of neighboring motoneurons, and therefore discharge of motor units within the muscle. At present, it is unclear whether the magnitude of this desynchronizing effect is sufficient to induce noticeable changes in muscle tension. This issue is, however, under active investigation.

B. Presumptive Interneuron Types

A number of other interneuron types have been described, but they are even less extensively examined than the interneurons listed previously, and appropriate functional roles have not been proposed in most instances. It is likely that excitatory interneurons exist in the intermediate gray which receive input from Ia afferents and perhaps from group II spindle afferents as well. These interneurons are perhaps responsible for the prolonged discharge of motoneurons following longitudinal vibration, a powerful Ia afferent stimulus. Other classes of interneurons include the Ib interneuron (described earlier) and a related class of inhibitory interneurons, the Ia-Ib convergent interneuron, which are distinguished by the fact that they receive convergent Ia-Ib input from the same muscle (88,89). These Ia-Ib interneurons receive widespread convergence from cutaneous and joint afferents, they receive input from other muscles, and from corticospinal, reticulospinal, and other descending pathways. Ia-Ib interneurons also inhibit each other, and appear to inhibit neurons of Clarke's column, an unexpected projection.

The definition of the Ia-Ib neuron has relied on intracellular recording techniques, which do not readily permit an assessment of the functional potency of Ia versus Ib inputs to this series of interneurons. Nonetheless, the Ia afferent input appears to be less powerful than the Ib input. Under these conditions, the neuron could perhaps function as a variable gain element mediating force feedback. Since Ia afferent input is greatest during the dynamic phase of muscle stretch, the effects of the interneuron would be enhanced under these conditions.

REFERENCES

1. Houk, J. C., and Rymer, W. Z. (1981). Neural control of muscle length and tension. In *Handbook of Physiology: The Nervous System*, vol. 2, *Motor Control*, V. B. Brooks (Ed.), American Physiological Society, Bethesda, Maryland, pp. 257–323.
2. Rymer, W. Z. (1983). Muscle afferent contributions to the regulation of muscle length and tension. In *The Clinical Neurosciences*, vol. 5, *Neurobiology*, W. Willis (Ed.), pp. 435–470.
3. Gordon, A. M., Huxley, A. F., and Julian, F. J. (1966). The variation in isometric tension with sarcomere length in vertebrate muscle fibres. *J. Physiol. (Lond.) 184*:170–192.
4. Huxley, A. F. (1974). Muscular contraction. *J. Physiol. (Lond.) 243*:1–43.

5. Rack, P. M. H., and Westbury, D. R. (1969). The effects of length and stimulus rate on tension in the isometric cat soleus muscle. *J. Physiol. (Lond.) 204*:443–460.

6. Grillner, S., and Udo, M. (1971). Motor unit activity and stiffness of the contracting muscle fibres in the tonic stretch reflex. *Acta Physiol. Scand. 87*:420–424.

7. Hill, A. V. (1938). The heat of shortening and the dynamic constants of muscle. *Proc. R. Soc. Lond. (Biol.) 126*:136–195.

8. Rack, P. M. H., and Westbury, D. R. (1974). The short range stiffness of active mammalian muscle and its effect on mechanical properties. *J. Physiol. (Lond.) 240*:331–350.

9. Mannard, A., and Stein, R. B. (1973). Determination of the frequency response of isometric soleus muscle in the cat using random nerve stimulation. *J. Physiol. (Lond.) 229*:275–296.

10. Bawa, P., and Stein, R. B. (1976). Frequency response of human soleus muscle. *J. Neurophysiol. 39*:788–793.

11. Rack, P. M. H. (1970). The significance of mechanical properties of muscle in the reflex control of posture. In *Excitatory Synaptic Mechanisms*, Jansen and Anderson (Eds.), pp. 317–321.

12. Oguztereli, M. N., and Stein, R. B. (1977). A kinetic study of muscular contractions. *J. Math. Biol. 5*:1–31.

13. Joyce, G. C., Rack, P. M. H., and Westbury, D. R. (1969). The mechanical properties of cat soleus muscle during controlled lengthening and shortening movements. *J. Physiol. (Lond.) 204*:461–474.

14. Nichols, T. R., and Houk, J. C. (1976). The improvement in linearity and the regulation of stiffness that results from the actions of the stretch reflex. *J. Neurophysiol. 39*:119–142.

15. Partridge, L. D., and Benton, L. A. (1981). Muscle, the motor. In *Handbook of Physiology: The Nervous System*, vol. 2, *Motor Control*, V. B. Brooks (Ed.), American Physiological Society, Bethesda, Maryland, pp. 43–106.

16. Gurfinkel, V. S., and Levick, Y. S. (1974). Effects of a doublet or omission and their connection with the dynamics of the active state of human muscles. *Biofizika 19*:925–931.

17. Burke, R. E., Rudomin, P., and Zajac, F. E. (1970). Catch property in single mammalian motor units. *Science 168*:122–124.

18. Hulliger, M., Matthews, P. B. C., and Noth, J. (1977). Static and dynamic fusimotor action on the response of Ia fibres to low frequency sinusoidal stretching of widely ranging amplitude. *J. Physiol. (Lond.) 267*:811–838.

19. Crago, P. E., Houk, J. C., and Rymer, W. A. (1982). Sampling of total muscle force by tendon organs. *J. Neurophysiol. 47*:1069-1083.

20. Houk, J. C., Crago, P. E., and Rymer, W. Z. (1980). Functional properties of Golgi tendon organs. In *Segmental Motor Control in Man*, J. E. Desmedt (Ed.), Progress in Clinical Neurophysiology, Karger, Basel.

21. Paintal, A. S. (1960). Functional analysis of group III afferent fibres of mammalian muscles. *J. Physiol. (Lond.) 152*:250–270.

22. Paintal, A. S. (1961). Participation by pressure-pain receptors of mammalian muscles in the flexion reflex. *J. Physiol. (Lond.) 156*:498–514.

23. Stacey, J. J. Free nerve endings in skeletal muscle of the cat. *J. Anat. (Lond.) 105*:231–254.

24. Kniffki, K.-D., Mense, S., and Schmidt, R. F. (1976). Chemo- and mechano-sensitivity of possible metabo- and nociceptors in skeletal muscle. *Pflugers Arch. 362*:R32.

25. Kniffki, J.-D., Mense, S., and Schmidt, R. F. (1976). Mechanisms of muscle pain: A comparison with cutaneous nociception. In *Sensory Functions of the Skin in Primates*, Y. Zotterman (Ed.), Wenner-Gren Center International Symposium Series, vol. 27, Pergamon Press, New York, pp. 463–473.

26. Kniffki, J.-D., Mense, S., and Schmidt, R. F. (1978). Responses of group IV afferent units from skeletal muscle to stretch, contraction and chemical stimulation. *Exp. Br. Res. 31*:511–522.

27. Alvord, E. C., and Fuortes, M. G. F. (1953). Reflex activity of extensor motor units following muscular excitation. *J. Physiol. (Lond.) 122*:302–321.

28. Tsukahara, N., and Ohye, C. (1964). Polysynaptic activation of extensor motoneurons from group Ia afferents in the cat spinal cord. *Experientia 20*:628–629.

29. Pacheco, P., and Guzman-Flores, C. (1969). Intracellular recording in extensor motoneurones of spastic cats. *Exp. Neurol. 25*:472–481.

30. Schomburg, E. E., and Behrends, H. B. (1978). The possibility of phase-dependent monosynaptic and polysynaptic Ia excitation to homonymous motoneurones during fictive locomotion. *Brain Res. 143*:533–537.

31. Hultborn, H., Wigstrom, and H., Wangberg, B. (1975). Prolonged activation of soleus motoneurones following a conditioning train in soleus Ia afferents—A case for a reverberating loop? *Neurosci. Lett. 1*:147–152.

32 Hultborn, H., Wigstrom, H., and Wangberg, B. (1976). Prolonged excitation in motoneurones triggered by activity in Ia afferents. *Acta. Physiol. Scand. (Suppl.) 440*:62.

33. Hultborn, H., and Wigstrom, H. (1980). Motor response with long latency and maintained duration evoked by activity in Ia afferents. In *Spinal and Supraspinal Mechanisms of Voluntary Motor Control and Locomotion*, J. E. Desmedt, (Ed.), vol. 8, Progress in Clinical Neurophysiology, Karger, Basel, pp. 99–116.

34. Kanda, K. (1972). Contribution of polysynaptic pathways to the tonic vibration reflex. *Jpn. J. Physiol. 22*:367–377.

35. Eccles, J. C., Eccles, R. M., and Lundberg, A. (1957). Synaptic actions on motoneurones caused by impulses in Golgi tendon organ afferents. *J. Physiol. (Lond.) 138*:227–252.

36. Fetz, E. E., Jankowska, E., Johanisson, T., and Lipski, J. (1979). Autogenetic inhibition of motoneurones by impulses in group Ia muscle spindle afferents. *J. Physiol. (Lond.) 293*:73–195.

37. Lundberg, A., Malmgren, K., and Schomburg, E. D. (1975). Convergence from Ib, cutaneous and joint afferents in reflex pathways to motoneurones. *Brain Res. 87*:81–84.

38. Lucas, M., and Willis, W. (1979). Identification of muscle afferents which activate interneurons in the intermediate nucleus. *J. Neurophysiol. 37*: 282–293.

39. Rymer, W. A., Houk, J. C., and Crago, P. E. (1979). Mechanisms of the clasp knife reflex studied in an animal model. *Exp. Brain Res. 37*:98–113.

40. Kirkwood, P. A., and Sears, T. A. (1974). Monosynaptic excitation of motoneurones from muscle spindle. *Nature 252*:243–244.

41. Kirkwood, P. A., and Sears, T. A. (1975). Monosynaptic excitation of motoneurones from muscle spindle secondary endings of intercostal and triceps surae muscles in the cat. *J. Physiol. (Lond.) 245*:64–66P.

42. Stauffer, E. K., Watt, D. G. D., Taylor, A., Reinking, R. M., and Stuart, D. B. (1976). Analysis of muscle receptor connections by spike-triggered averaging. 2. Spindle II afferents. *J. Neurophysiol. 39*:1393–1402.

43. Munson, J. B., Sypert, G. N., and Zengel, J. G. (1982). Monosynaptic projections of individual group II afferents to type identified medial gastrocnemius motoneurons in the cat. *J. Neurophysiol. 48*:1164.

44. Brown, A. G. (1981). Organization in the spinal cord. *The Anatomy and Physiology of Identified Neurons*. Springer-Verlag, Berlin, New York.

45. Milner-Brown, H. S., Stein, R. B., and Yeman, R. G. (1973). The orderly recruitment of human motor units during isometric voluntary contraction. *J. Physiol. (Lond.) 236*:359–370.

46. Monster, W. A., and Chan, H. (1977). Isometric force production by motor units of extensor digitorum communis muscle in man. *J. Neurophysiol. 40*: 1432-1443.

47. Henneman, E., Somjen, G., and Carpenter, D. O. (1965). Functional significance of cell size in spinal motoneurons. *J. Neurophysiol. 28*:560.

48. Milner-Brown, H. S., Stein, R. B., and Yemm, R. (1973). Changes in firing rate of human motor units during linearly changing voluntary contractions. *J. Physiol. (Lond.) 230*:371–390.

49. Cordo, P. J., and Rymer, W. Z. (1982). Motor unit activation patterns in lenfthening and isometric contractions of hindlimb extensors in the decerebrate cat. *J. Neurophysiol. 47*:287–302.

50. Fulton, J. F., and Pisuner, J. (1947). A note concerning the probable function of various afferent end-organs in skeletal muscle. *Am. J. Physiol. 83*: 554–562.

51. Merton, P. A. (1951). The silent period in a muscle of the human hand. *J. Physiol. (Lond.) 114*:183–198.

52. Merton, P. A. (1953). Speculations on the servo-control of movement. In *The Spinal Cord*, Little, Brown, Boston, pp. 183–198.

53. Hammond, P. H. (1960). An experimental study of servo action in human muscular control. In *Proceedings III International Congress Medical Electronics*, London, Institution of Electrical Engineers, pp. 190-199.

54. Eldred, E., Granit, R., and Merton, P. A. (1953). Supraspinal control of the muscle spindle and its significance. *J. Physiol. (Lond.) 122*:498–523.

55. Phillips, C. G. (1969). Motor apparatus of the baboon's hand. *Proc. R. Soc. Lond. (Biol.) 173*:141–174.

56. Phillips, C. G., Powell, T. P. S., and Weisendanger, M. (1971). Projection from low-threshold muscle afferents of hand and forearm to area 3a of baboon's cortex. *J. Physiol. (Lond.) 217*:419–446.

57. Fetz, E. (1983). *Proceedings of IUPS*. Sydney, Australia.

58. Lee, R. G., and Tatton, W. G. (1975). Motor responses to sudden limb displacements in primates with specific CNS lesions and in human patients with motor system disorders. *Can. J. Neurol. Sci. 2*:285–293.

59. Marsden, C. D., Merton, P. A., and Morton, H. B. (1972). Servo action in human voluntary movement. *Nature 238*:140–143.

60. Marsden, C. D., Merton, P. A., and Morton, H. B. (1973). Is the human stretch reflex cortical rather than spinal? *Lancet 1*:759–761.

61. Marsden, C. D., Merton, P. A., and Morton, H. B. (1976). Servo action in the human thumb. *J. Physiol. (Lond.) 257*:1–44.

62. Marsden, C. D., Merton, P. A., and Morton, H. B. (1976). Stretch reflexes and servo actions in a variety of human muscles. *J. Physiol. (Lond.) 259*:531–560.

63. Marsden, C. D., Merton, P. A. Morton, H. B., Adam, J. E. R., and Hallett, M. (1978). Automatic and voluntary responses to muscle stretch in man. In *Cerebral Motor Control in Man: Long Loop Mechanisms*. Progress in Clinical Neurophysiology, vol. 4, J. D. Desmedt (Ed)., Karger, Basel, pp. 167–177.

64. Ghez, C., and Shinoda, Y. (1978). Spinal mechanisms of the functional stretch reflex. *Brain Res. 32*:55–68.

65. Tardieu, C., Tabary, J. C., and Lardien, G. (1968). Etude mechanique et electromyographique de reponses a differentes perturbation en maintien postural. *J. Physiol. (Paris) 60*:243–259.

66. Matthews, P. B. C. (1959). The dependence of tension upon extension in the stretch reflex of the soleus muscle of the decerebrate cat. *J. Physiol. (Lond.) 147*:521–546.

67. Matthews, P. B. C. (1959). A study of certain factors influencing the stretch reflex of the decerebrate cat. *J. Physiol. (Lond.) 147*:547–564.

68. Crago, P. E., Houk, J. C., and Hasan, Z. (1976). Regulatory actions of the human stretch reflex. *J. Neurophysiol. 39*:925–935.

69. Houk, J. C. (1972). The phylogeny of muscular control configurations. In *Biocybernetics*, vol. 4, H. Drischel and P. Dettmar (Eds.), Fischer, Jena, Germany, pp. 125–155.

70. Houk, J. C. (1979). Regulation of stiffness by skeletomotor reflexes. *Ann. Rev. Physiol. 41*:99–114.

71. Brown, T. I. H., Rack, P. M. H., and Ross, H. F. (1977). The thumb stretch reflex. *J. Physiol. (Lond.) 209*:30–31.

72. Hoffer, J. A., and Andreassen, S. (1981). Regulation of soleus muscle stiffness in premammillary cats: Mechanical and reflex components. *J. Neurophysiol. (Lond.) 45*:267–285.

73. Houk, J. C., Singer, J. J., and Goldman, M. R. (1970). An evaluation of length and force feedback to soleus muscles of decerebrate cats. *J. Neurophysiol. 33*:784–811.

74. Jack, J. J. B. (1978). Some methods for selective activation of muscle afferent fibers. In *Studies in Neurophysiology*, R. Porter (Ed.), Cambridge Univ. Press, Cambridge, England, pp. 155-176.

75. Rymer, W. Z., and Hasan, Z. (1980). Absence of force-feedback in soleus muscle of the decerebrate cat. *Brain Res. 184*:203-209.

76. Hoffer, J. A., and Andreassen, S.(1981). Limitations in the servo-regulations of soleus muscle stiffness in premammillary cats. In *Muscle Receptors and Movement*, A. Taylor and A. Prochazka (Eds.), Macmillan, New York, pp 311 -324.

77. Truxal, J. G. (1961). Control systems—Some unusual design problems. In *Adaptive Control Systems*, E. Michkin and L. Braun (Eds.), McGraw-Hill, New York, Chapter 4.

78. Houk, J. C., Crago, P. E., and Rymer, W. Z. (1981). Function of spindle dynamic response in stiffness regulation—A predictive mechanism provided by nonlinear feedback. In *Muscle Receptors and Movement*, A. Taylor and A. Prochazka (Eds.), MacMillan, New York, pp. 299-310.

79. Brown, M. C., Engberg, I., and Matthews, P. B. C. (1967). The relative sensitivity to vibration of muscle receptors in the cat. *J. Physiol. (Lond.) 192*: 773-800.

80. Cordo, P. J., and Rymer, W. Z.(1982). Contributions of motor unit recruitment and rate modulation to compensation for muscle yielding. *J. Neurophysiol. 47*:797-809.

81. Burke, D., Knowles, L., Andrews, C., and Ashby, P. (1972). Spasticity, decerebrate rigidity and the clasp-knife phenomenon: An experimental study in the cat. *Brain 95*:31-48.

82. Baldissera, F., Hultborn, and H. Illert, M. (1981). Integration in spinal neuronal systems. In *Handbook of Physiology: The Nervous System*, vol. 2, *Motor Control*, V. E. Brooks (Ed.), American Physiological Society, Bethesda, Maryland.

83. Hultborn, H. (1972). Convergence on interneurones in the reciprocal Ia inhibitory pathway to motoneurons. *Acta Physiol. Scand. 85*:1-42.

84. Feldman, A. G., and Orlorsky, G. N. (1975). Activity of interneurons mediating reciprocal Ia inhibition during locomotion. *Brain Res. 84*:181-194.

85. Renshaw, B. (1946). Central effects of centripetal impulses in axons of spinal ventral roots. *J. Neurophysiol. 9*:191-204.

86. Hultborn, H. S., Lindstrom, S., and Wigstrom, H. (1971). On the function of recurrent inhibition in the spinal cord. *J. Physiol. (Lond.) 215*:637-664.

87. Adam, D., Windhorst, U., and Inbar, G. F. (1978). The effects of recurrent inhibition on the cross correlated firing patterns of motoneurones. *Biol. Cybern. 29*:229-235.

88. Jankowska, E., McCrea, D., and Mackel, R. (1981). Oligosynaptic excitation of motoneurones by impulses in group Ia muscle spindle afferents in the cat. *J. Physiol. (Lond.) 316*:411-425.

89. Jankowska, E., McCrea, D., and Mackel, R. (1981). Pattern of 'non-reciprocal' inhibition of motoneurones by impulses in group Ia muscle spindle afferents in the cat. *J. Physiol. (Lond.) 316*:393-409.

14
CENTRAL PATTERN GENERATORS IN THE SPINAL CORD

Paul S. G. Stein *Washington University, St. Louis, Missouri*

I. INTRODUCTION

The spinal cord contains neuronal circuitry that can generate complex motor behaviors (1-8). After the cord has been completely transected, the segments caudal to the cut can produce motor patterns responsible for swimming, stepping, and scratching. This chapter will discuss neuronal mechanisms used by the spinal cord to produce coordinated motor output. Since our understanding of spinal motor mechanisms is far from complete, this will be a progress report of current knowledge, a statement of current experimental techniques, and a guide for strategies of future experimental work.

The experiments reported will be on vertebrates that range in complexity from the lamprey to the cat. The unifying principle emerging from this work is that the spinal cord has the necessary complexity to (1) coordinate motor units within a muscle, (2) coordinate close muscular synergies, (3) control the timing relationships between agonists and antagonists acting at a single joint, (4) coordinate the muscles acting at a joint with those acting at other joints, and (5) control the movements of one limb with that of other limbs and the trunk (1-10). These motor outputs can be produced by the spinal cord in the absence of sensory feedback (1-8,11).

A. Motor Programs: Myography

The term "motor program" is a useful concept for the experimental analyses of spinal motor control. A motor program is defined as the activation pattern of motor neuron pools and/or muscles during a behavior. Motor programs are usually monitored by recording muscle action potentials, that is, electromyographic (EMG) recordings. A given pattern of electromyographic recordings can be correlated with a specific movement sequence. Since electromyographic recordings provide a sensitive measure of neural output, electromyography is useful when a motor behavior in a spinal animal is compared to that of an intact animal. The electromyographic pattern is useful in determining what stimulus condition, for example, electrical pulses, chemical stimulation, and tactile stimulation, will elicit a movement in the spinal animal that is an excellent replica of the movement produced by an organism with an intact central nervous system.

B. Fictive Motor Programs: Neurography

An alternative method for monitoring the motor program is that of electroneurographic (ENG) recordings from the peripheral nerves that lead to individual muscles. The technique of electroneurographic recordings is especially powerful when utilized in a spinal preparation that is immobilized with a neuromuscular blocking agent such as curare or gallamine triethiodide (Flaxedil). In such a spinal immobilized preparation, appropriate stimulation can elicit an electroneurographic motor program that replicates the electromyographic program observed prior to neuromuscular blockade. Since the electroneurographic motor program of the immobilized preparation is produced in the absence of a "real" movement, it has been termed a "fictive" motor program.

When a fictive motor program is elicited, there is no movement; therefore, no phasic sensory input is available to trigger any portion of the fictive motor program. The term "centrally programmed" is utilized to designate a motor program produced in the absence of timing cues derived from phasic sensory feedback. If a motor program is centrally programmed, it follows that a set of central nervous system neurons must be responsible for the generation of the motor program. The term "central pattern generator" (CPG) is defined to be the neurons responsible for the generation of the motor pattern. If a fictive motor program is generated by a spinal preparation, then a major portion of the central pattern generator for that behavior is located within the spinal cord. The term central pattern generator serves as a convenient operational definition for studies of spinal motor mechanisms. Current techniques allow measurements of spinal central pattern generator motor output. From these data, hypotheses can be constructed concerning the neurons that belong to the spinal central pattern generators. Recordings have been obtained from candidate spinal central pattern generator neurons. Further work is needed to determine with certainty that these candidate neurons belong to a spinal central pattern generator for a motor behavior.

C. Spinal Programs: Swimming, Stepping, and Scratching

Swimming, stepping, and scratching are rhythmic motor programs that can be produced by the spinal cord after all neural connections with supraspinal structures have been severed. Swimming and stepping are rhythmic behaviors in which the organism exerts force against an external substrate; scratching is a rhythmic behavior in which the organism exerts force against itself.

For each motor program it is possible to find an agonist-antagonist pair of muscles whose activities rhythmically alternate during the movement cycle. During fish swimming left trunk muscles alternate with right trunk muscles at a given segmental level. During tetrapod scratching or stepping hip flexors alternate with hip extensors. If every other muscle active during the motor program had an activity pattern that began and ended in strict coincidence with one member of the reference agonist-antagonist pair, then the motor program would have a strictly bipartite organization. Such a strict bipartite program is rare; the most usual occurrence is that many agonist-antagonist pairs of muscles are active during a movement. Each agonist-antagonist pair can control the movements of a single degree of freedom of a joint, for example, flexion-extension of the knee, lateral bending between two adjacent vertebrae, or abduction-adduction of the hip. In any one type of motor program, a phase lag is present between those muscles controlling one degree of freedom and those controlling another. This phase lag is a characteristic of that type of program. Since the spinal cord can produce many types of motor programs, the spinal motor circuitry must have the flexibility to change the relative phasing among muscles that control different degrees of freedom. In some situations, for example, a change from forward locomotion to backward locomotion or a change from rostral scratching to caudal scratching, relative phasing can change by as much as 0.5 of a cycle! The neuronal mechanisms underlying this flexibility are not yet understood; the best working hypotheses will be discussed in the concluding remarks.

D. Strategies for Central Pattern Generator Study

The major theses of this chapter are: (1) there has been much recent progress in studies of central pattern generator function, and (2) no one organism can reveal all the properties of spinal central pattern generator mechanisms. Each organism presented in this chapter offers specific opportunities for study; the analyses of the entire spectrum of vertebrates (12-151) will provide the most comprehensive picture of spinal motor function.

II. LAMPREY

The lamprey is a primitive vertebrate that belongs to the cyclostome class of jawless fishes. Its spinal cord offers many technical advantages for studies of the spinal control of swimming (12-16). The lamprey's spinal cord is flat and lacks myelin, so that cell bodies can be visualized directly. Intense study of the lamprey in several laboratories over the past few years has produced important insights concerning the neuronal mechanisms responsible for the control of movement during locomotion (12-28).

The lamprey swims by passing rhythmic undulations of lateral bending from head to tail. The muscles in a body hemisegment display a phase lead of 0.01 of a cycle when compared with the neighboring ipsilateral caudal hemisegment (27). At a given segmental level, muscles on one side of the body are out of phase (0.5 phase difference) with muscles on the contralateral side. These phase relationships can be observed in a lamprey with a complete spinal transection whose spinal cord is bathed in a Ringer's solution containing a low concentration of an excitatory amino acid such as D-glutamic acid or N-methyl-D-aspartic acid (17,19,21). While some experiments have utilized myography to record motor output (19), most recent reports (17,18,20-28) have utilized electroneurographic recordings from a spinal cord dissected free of musculature and isolated in vitro. A preparation consisting of a few segments of the spinal cord can produce a properly phased motor output in vitro. This result does not depend upon the rostrocaudal location of the segments; as few as four spinal segments can produce the program.

The in vitro lamprey spinal cord has become an outstanding preparation for pharmacologic manipulation of the spinal circuitry responsible for motor rhythm production. Two main directions have been pursued utilizing bath application of pharmacologic agents. First, the responses to excitatory amino acids have been explored (21). Blockers of N-methyl-D-aspartic acid receptors diminish the spinal cord response to applied excitatory amino acids. It is an attractive hypothesis that the lamprey might utilize these receptors during the natural activation of swimming. Second, the responses to inhibitory amino acids have also been examined (18). Strychnine, a blocker of glycine inhibition in the spinal cord, will disturb the production of the swimming motor pattern. The blockers of γ-aminobutyric acid (GABA) inhibition do not affect the swim pattern. It therefore seems likely that glycine inhibition is utilized within the lamprey swim central pattern generator.

Although the swim motor pattern can be produced by the in vitro spinal cord in the absence of movement, an undulation of the spinal cord can excite mechanosensitive neurons that respond to spinal cord movement (25). The mechanosensitive dendrites of these neurons are located in the spinal cord, most likely next to the meninges. A movement of the spinal cord that can excite the mechanosensitive neurons can alter the timing of the swim central pattern generator so that the swim motor program is entrained to the timing of the imposed mechanical movement (20). A response of a central program generator to sensory input is seen throughout the animal kingdom (7,11) and is an important mechanism for modifying motor output to make it adapt to the mechanical properties of the organism.

The lamprey spinal cord is particularly amenable to intracellular recordings from both motor neurons and interneurons (12–16). Intracellular recordings from motor neurons (24,26,28) have revealed that each motor neuron is excited via depolarizing potentials that occur in phase with action potentials recorded in the nearest ipsilateral ventral root. Each motor neuron also receives chloride-sensitive inhibitory synaptic potentials that alternate with the excitatory potentials.

Intracellular recordings have been obtained from interneurons in the spinal cord (22–24,26) whose activity is phase-locked with the fictive swim motor program. These interneurons might either belong to the swim central program generator or be driven by the swim central program generator. The best studied class of interneurons has been the CC interneurons whose axons run caudally in the spinal cord contralateral to their cell bodies (23,24,26). Some of these interneurons have depolarizing potentials that are either in-phase or have a slight phase lead with the nearby ventral root discharge ipsilateral to their cell body. Some CC interneurons inhibit contralateral motor neurons via their contralateral axons. These cells may, therefore, assist in the proper phasing of the alternation between the left and the right sides of the body. In addition, some CC neurons receive chloride-sensitive inhibition in between their depolarizing phases. Another type of interneuron has axons that remain confined to the hemisegment of their cell body (12,22). The phasic undulations in membrane potential of some of these interneurons remain after all action potentials of the spinal cord have been blocked with tetrodotoxin. This suggests that the rhythmic membrane potentials might originate within each spinal segment and need not depend upon action potentials from neurons many segments away. This is consistent with the observation that only four spinal segments are needed to produce the fictive motor program (17). These short axon cells are excellent candidates to be part of the swim central program generator.

The experimental results on the lamprey spinal cord have been extremely encouraging. It is likely that the future work on this preparation will reveal important principles of the neuronal mechanisms utilized to produce spinal motor output.

III. ELASMOBRANCHS

A. Dogfish

The spinal dogfish can produce spontaneous swimming movements after high spinal transection (29–31). Analyses of electromyographic recordings from trunk muscles at low frequencies of swimming reveal that only red muscle fibers are activated by the spinal cord; at higher frequencies of swimming both red and white muscles are activated (31). The spinal dogfish usually displays the intersegmental coordination characteristic of forward swimming. A backward swimming motor program can also be induced by tactile stimulation of the rostroventral surface of the preparation. A preparation consisting of several adjacent segments of the spinal cord can produce a forward swimming motor program; as few as eight segments are sufficient. This implies that the central program generator for swimming is distributed throughout the spinal cord.

A spinal dogfish immobilized with curare will produce a fictive swim motor program (32). The rhythm of the fictive swim can be modified by such sensory manipulations as the experimenter rhythmically moving the tail from one lateral position to another (13,32-34). The modified motor rhythm will match the imposed movement under a wide range of stimulus conditions. Sensory receptors sufficient to produce this effect are located within the vertebral column and spinal cord, since removal of skin and muscle does not disturb the effect (34).

A second type of sensory modification, a phase-dependent reflex reversal, has also been observed in immobilized preparations (13,33). A single stimulus to the tail can have different motor effects depending upon the phase of the fictive cycle in which the stimulus is delivered.

B. Stingray

The stingray has been recently introduced as a model for the neurophysiologic study of locomotion by Leonard, Droge, and their coworkers (35-40). The stingray swims with a laterally placed pair of pectoral fins. The fins are elevated by dorsal fin musculature and depressed by ventral fin musculature. Rhythmic caudally directed waves of muscle contractions pass down the pectoral fin during swimming. Decerebrate stingrays will display spontaneous swimming; spinal stingrays can be induced to swim with L-DOPA. Decerebrate stingrays under neuromuscular blockade will display a fictive swimming program.

The motor nuclei to the dorsal fin muscles are located in a lateral position in the ventral horn; the nuclei to the ventral fin muscles are located in a medial position in the ventral horn (40). The developing limb bud of vertebrates with more complex limb structure initially contains a dorsal muscle mass and a ventral muscle mass; motor nuclei in the spinal cord of muscles formed by the dorsal muscle mass are located lateral to the motor nuclei of muscles formed by the ventral muscle mass (87,89). Studies of the stingray pectoral fin may, therefore, reveal important properties of a primitive state of spinal cord control of a limb.

IV. BONY FISH

The bony fish have not been utilized extensively in modern studies of the control of spinal motor rhythms. The classic work of von Holst (41) with movement analyses of fin rhythms of fish with medullary sections revealed the central coupling among spinal central program generators controlling the fins. This led to the development of important notions concerning the rules governing different types of limb coordination patterns that are of great interest in studies of interlimb coordination (2,5). Grillner and Kashin (42) have reviewed studies of movement analyses and electromyographic recordings during swimming in bony fish. Electrical stimulation of the midbrain can evoke swimming in a fish (43). This midbrain location is similar to that used in cats to evoke stepping (3,7,114).

An important component of swimming behavior in fish is the initial startle response to a strong stimulus. This behavior is mediated by a pair of large identifiable reticulospinal neurons, termed Mauthner cells (44–52). Mauthner cells have been well studied from anatomic, physiologic, and behavioral points of view. Direct electrical stimulation of a single Mauthner cell will lead to a bending of the contralateral trunk musculature. Such a C-shaped bending is also observed during a naturally occurring startle response. Direct recording from a Mauthner cell during the naturally occurring startle response shows that the cell is active just prior to the activation of the trunk musculature. This activation of the Mauthner cell is an important component of the startle response; the cell may serve as a "command neuron" for the startle behavior (44–52). Other reticulospinal neurons can also serve in this role, since fish with Mauthner cells ablated can still display startle responses (49).

V. AMPHIBIANS

A. Frog Wiping Reflex

The wiping reflex of the frog is a classic spinal preparation. A frog with a complete transection of the spinal cord responds to tactile stimulation of the body surface by rubbing a nearby limb against the stimulated site (8,53–58). This was described in 1846 by Paton (53) and was extensively studied in the late nineteenth century (reviewed by Baglioni in ref. 54). The behavior is termed a "wiping" reflex, since the limb wipes away the stimulus of paper soaked in a weak acid; its characteristics are identical to the scratch reflex observed in other vertebrates (8).

Recently, the elegant experiments of Fukson, Berkinblit, and Feldman (58) have revealed an important complexity present in the spinal cord. A stimulus applied to the elbow of a high spinal frog will elicit a wiping reflex by the ipsilateral hindlimb in which the hindlimb will reach up and wipe the stimulus away from the elbow. The hindlimb can display the necessary wipe trajectory when the elbow is positioned in very different locations in space, for example, the elbow can be either rostral or caudal to the shoulder. This demonstrates that the spinal cord contains a spatial map that calculates the location of the surface of a limb that can move in space. Proprioceptive and cutaneous input from the forelimb must be integrated in the formation of this map. Physiologic recordings during the wiping reflex are extremely limited. Simpson (57) reports that an intracellular recording from a hindlimb motor neuron during cutaneous stimulation will show distinct patterns of synaptic activation.

B. Swimming

Frog tadpoles swim like fish. They have a pair of Mauthner cells that degenerate after the tadpole develops into an adult frog. These cells in the tadpole show functional characteristics that are similar to those in fish (59,60). The swimming rhythm produced by trunk motor neurons in the tadpole larvae can be produced by an in vitro preparation of the tadpole central nervous system (61). In addition, electroneurographic recordings from the axons of motor neurons to the developing limb of the tadpole will display a complex swimlike limb motor program when recorded in the in vitro central nervous system preparation (62).

The embryonic origins of the tadpole swimming rhythm have been examined extensively by Roberts and his coworkers (63–69). The Stage 38 frog embryo, when dissected out of the egg case, will display swimming behavior. The preparation under curare will display a fictive motor program in which a trunk muscle motor neuron will fire once per cycle in antiphase with a contralateral motor neuron at the same segmental level. During a swim episode each motor neuron receives a tonic depolarization. In addition, during each cycle it receives a phasic excitatory potential that alternates with a phasic inhibitory potential. The inhibitory potential is directly related to the expression of the motor rhythm in the contralateral portion of the spinal cord. Intracellular recordings from interneurons that have a cell body contralateral to their axon display membrane potential changes similar to motor neurons.

C. Stepping

Stepping has been examined in newts and salamanders (70–73). This was one of the first reports of electromyographic recordings during stepping that demonstrated that a multipartite motor program would retain its structure after deafferentation. The preparation is also amenable to the surgical manipulations of transplanting limb buds to produce supernumerary limbs that can be innervated by the spinal cord itself or by explants of the spinal cord.

VI. REPTILES

A. Turtle Scratch Reflex

The spinal turtle can produce a scratch reflex in response to mechanical stimulation of the shell and skin (8,74–80). There are three different "forms" of the scratch reflex: the rostral scratch, the pocket scratch, and the caudal scratch

(77,78). Each form uses a distinct portion of the limb to achieve the rub, has its own receptive field, and has a distinct motor program. The program measured with electromyographic recordings in a preparation with movement (77) can also be observed with electroneurographic recordings in the fictive preparation (78). An in vitro preparation of shell, spinal cord, and peripheral nerve can also produce a fictive scratch program (80). Intracellular recordings from motor neurons during the fictive scratch reveal that each motor neuron is depolarized during its active phase and hyperpolarized during at least a portion of its quiescent phase (78,79).

Motor programs and limb movements during scratch reflex display: (1) rhythmic alternation between hip protractors and hip retractors, and (2) knee extension at a characteristic phase within the hip cycle (8,75-79). The rub against the stimulated site on the body surface takes place during knee extension. A site rostral to the limb is rubbed in a rostral scratch by the dorsum of the foot; in this form of scratch the knee extends while the hip is protracted. A site caudal to the limb is rubbed in a caudal scratch by the heel or the side of the foot; in this form the knee extends while the hip is retracted. The foot is not able to touch a site near the hip in the pocket region; sites in this region are rubbed with the side of the knee. During this pocket scratch, the knee extends while the hip is retracting. Thus, the phase of knee extension activity in the hip cycle is specified according to the form of scratch that is produced. The phase specified for a given form is observed with both joint angle analysis and electromyographic program analysis in turtles with movement and with electroneurographic program analysis in turtles with neuromuscular blockade.

The mechanical constraints imposed by the geometries of the limb and shell are important in determining what form of the scratch is expressed (8,77). Stimulus sites in the rostral scratch receptive field can only be reached by the dorsum of the foot. The dorsum of the foot is unable to reach sites in the pocket scratch receptive field, but the side of the knee can. The narrow boundary between the rostral scratch and the pocket scratch receptive fields, termed a transition zone, is the region of the body that can be reached by either the dorsum of the foot or the side of the knee. The spinal cord will produce either a pure rostral scratch, a pure pocket scratch, a switching behavior between rostral scratches and pocket scratches, or a hybrid of both rostral and pocket scratches in response to stimulation of the rostral-pocket transition zone. The fact that there are smooth blends and transitions between motor programs indicates that, even though the central program generator for the rostral scratch must differ at least in part from the central program generator for the pocket scratch, there must be considerable overlap or interaction between central program generators for different forms of the scratch. The "unit generator hypothesis" of Grillner (7), when modified for turtle scratching, offers an explanation of how the spinal cord can produce the different forms of scratch motor programs.

B. Turtle Swimming

The spinal turtle will not spontaneously produce swimming behavior, but it can be induced to swim via electrical pulses delivered focally to spinal cord sites within the dorsal portion of the lateral funiculus (81,82). The frequency of the swim program can be altered by alterations in the frequency of the applied electrical pulses. The correct interlimb phasing of forelimb and hindlimb is displayed by the high spinal preparation (82).

Electrical stimulation of specific sites in the midbrain of a mesencephalic turtle can elicit swimming movements of the limbs (83). The site in the turtle is similar to that utilized in fish swimming (43) and cat stepping (3,114).

VII. BIRDS

The chick embryo has provided a great deal of experimental information concerning the development of the spinal cord control of a limb (84–96). Electromyographic recordings from the chick hindlimb reveal that at very early stages of limb development there is coordination of motor units within a muscle, coactivation of synergist muscles, and alternation of activity between antagonist muscles (84,85,90,95). These characteristics are present in the 7-day embryo, a stage prior to the development of hindlimb responses to cutaneous stimulation (84,85). These can also be observed in an in vitro spinal cord and hindlimb preparation (90,95). The in vitro preparation has a transection of the spinal cord; therefore, at early stages of development the spinal cord does not depend upon supraspinal structures for generating a coordinated motor pattern. The spinal in vitro embryo, when deafferented via dorsal rhizotomies of the hindlimb enlargement, will also display a proper coordination between muscles (95). Spinal programs for intramuscular coordination present at very early stages, therefore, do not depend upon sensory inputs from dorsal roots.

Experimental manipulations of the limb bud can produce a hindlimb whose muscles are innervated by foreign motor neuron pools (94,96). In such preparations, a given muscle can either display a normal motor pattern, a completely incorrect motor pattern, or a slightly modified motor program. Therefore, in some cases, the spinal motor pools receive patterned interneuronal information that may not be modified if the motor axon innervates an incorrect muscle.

The development of motor coordination in the chick is critical to the survival of the embryo, since a very complex stereotyped motor output must be produced when the chick hatches (85,86,91). This output is normally only produced once in the life of the chicken. An already hatched chick, when placed in an appropriately sized plastic egg, will again initiate hatching (91). A bending of the neck in a hatched chick is sufficient stimulus to turn off stepping behavior and initiate hatching.

The motor program in hatched chicks during stepping has been extensively analyzed at behavioral and myographic levels in intact chicks (92). This work demonstrates that the stepping program is a tripartite program and does not simply consist of alternation between flexors and extensors. This tripartite program can also be observed in spinal chicks in response to electrical stimulation of specific loci in the lateral funiculus of the spinal cord (93). Spinal immobilized chicks when stimulated in a similar fashion will also produce a proper fictive stepping program (93).

VIII. MAMMALS

A. Scratching

The scratch reflex (8) in the dog (97,98) and the cat (99–111) has provided much excellent information about the organization of mammalian central program generators. The cat scratch has been particularly well studied with movement analysis (100), electromyographic recordings (100), electroneurographic recordings (100,102–111), extracellular unit recordings (101–104,106, 109,110), and intracellular recordings (105). The initial response of the cat hindlimb to a tactile stimulus in the scratch receptive field is a postural or tonic response; the thorax bends toward the stimulus and the hindlimb flexes in preparation to scratch. After several seconds of the postural response, the rhythmic motor program begins. It is quite regular and can readily be elicited in spinal preparations in which the limb can move. The fictive scratch program is also easily elicited after neuromuscular blockade. In contrast to the frog (54–57) and turtle (77,78), in which several forms of the scratch reflex are present, only one form has been described in the cat: a rostral scratch reflex in which the receptive field includes only the pinna and the neck.

When the electromyographic program for the cat scratch was first reported (100), a bipartite classification scheme of muscle activities was attempted in which muscles active during the long phase of the cycle were termed L-type muscles and muscles active during the short phase of the cycle were termed S-type muscles. Later reports with electroneurographic analyses (111) and intracellular recordings from motor neurons (105) demonstrate a more complex organization. Some S-type motor units turn on while L-type motor units are still active; other S-type motor units do not turn on until other S-type motor units have already turned off; and some L-type motor units turn on prior to the activation of other L-type motor units. Further studies are necessary to reveal an appropriate multipartite classification scheme.

Extracellular recordings from interneurons in the lumbosacral enlargement during a fictive scratch demonstrate that many neurons are physically active during the scratch cycle (102–104,106,109,110). The first report of interneuronal recordings sampled a large number of units in the gray matter (103,104). A set of characteristics concerning each unit was reported; no attempt was made to identify the unit according to traditional classification schemes (152,153). Berkinblit et al. (103,104) constructed a tripartite model of the scratch central program based upon the timing properties of the interneurons. The model is in need of further experimental testing with intracellular recordings from these neurons.

Further recordings from interneurons in the enlargement during the fictive scratch were obtained after identifying the units according to traditional criteria (152,153). Renshaw cells (110), Ia inhibitory interneurons (106), and ventral spinocerebellar tract neurons (102) are phasically active during the fictive scratch cycle. At least some of the input to Renshaw cells during the scratch comes from motor neuron collaterals; however, some Renshaw cells are active during a longer portion of the cycle than the motor neurons that excite them. This raises the possibility that scratch central program generator interneurons directly modulate Renshaw cells. Both Ia inhibitory interneurons and ventral spinocerebellar tract neurons are known to have powerful excitatory input from primary sensory afferents of the limb (152,153). In the preparation producing a fictive scratch, the limb is immobile and primary afferents only provide tonic input to spinal cord neurons. Thus, both Ia inhibitory and ventral spinocerebellar tract neurons must receive powerful phasic synaptic drive from scratch central program generator neurons. Of particular interest is the firing pattern of Ia inhibitory interneurons monosynaptically activated by vastus muscle spindle afferents when compared with the firing pattern of Ia inhibitory interneurons monosynaptically activated by posterior biceps and semitendinosus muscle spindle afferents. During the fictive scratch (106) these interneurons are nearly coactive. The vastus Ia inhibitory interneurons have a reciprocal inhibitory relationship with posterior biceps and semitendinosus Ia inhibitory interneurons in a preparation that is not producing a scratch motor rhythm (152-154). Thus, certain connections between these interneurons must be turned off or overridden in some motor behaviors.

The fictive motor program can also be influenced by sensory inputs coming from the limb (100,104). In particular, if the hip is extended so that the immobilized limb does not display the proper scratch posture, then the scratch stimulus will elicit only the tonic postural response. If the hip is flexed, the scratch stimulus will elicit the tonic postural response followed by many cycles of the fictive scratch rhythm.

The work with the fictive scratch in the cat represents a major breakthrough in studies of mammalian central program generators. The published work describes many important features of the scratch central program generator; future work with this system has the potential to provide the experimental data that will reveal the cellular mechanisms underlying mammalian spinal central program generators.

B. Stepping

Stepping has been extensively analyzed in the cat (1-5,7,112-143). Many of the current generalizations about the spinal control of stepping come from these studies; the rabbit (144-147) and the rat (148-151) have also been used in studies of limb motor rhythms in mammals.

The classic work of Sherrington (112) and Brown (113) established that the stepping rhythm could be produced in a spinal, deafferented cat. Both Sherrington and Brown emphasized a bipartite classification scheme in which flexor muscles were phasically alternating with extensor muscles. Brown suggested that a neuronal network consisting of paired half centers with reciprocal inhibition between the half centers might be responsible for the generation of the cat stepping rhythm. Modern evidence in favor of the half center hypothesis has been presented by Lündberg and his collaborators (115,139). These data, obtained with L-DOPA stimulation in the spinal immobilized cat, demonstrate that there are reciprocal inhibitory relationships among lumbosacral interneurons active during a fictive stepping program. The half center hypothesis is based upon the Sherrington assertion that all the flexors of the limb are active during a "flexor" phase of the cycle and that all the extensors of the limb are active during an "extensor" phase of the cycle. Lundberg (116) has presented electromyographic data showing that a more complex multipartite motor output is produced during the cat step cycle. More support for this observation has been obtained with other electromyographic recordings (7,132), electroneurographic recordings (7,135), extracellular interneuronal recordings (119), and intracellular motoneuron recordings (135). Grillner has suggested a more complex version of the half-center hypothesis that has the generality to predict a multipartite motor output and still incorporates the important observation that reciprocal inhibitory relationships are an important component of the stepping central program generator (7). In his "unit generator" hypothesis Grillner suggests that there is a strong reciprocal inhibitory relationship between interneurons controlling flexion at a joint and interneurons controlling extension at the same joint. Grillner postulates a complex synaptic relationship between those interneurons controlling movement at a given joint and those interneurons controlling movement at an adjacent joint. This complex linkage is responsible for the ability of the Grillner model to generate a multipartite stepping rhythm. The Grillner model also offers a plausible explanation of how the central program generator for forward stepping can be modified to become a central program generator for backward stepping. Further work with recordings from cat central program generator interneurons is required to test fully the Grillner model.

A wide variety of preparations have been utilized to study stepping in the cat. In three preparations stepping is produced without the need of electrical or chemical stimulation. Investigators have utilized intact cats (116,129,130, 140,142), thalamic or premammillary preparations (118,121,131,135), and chronic spinal kittens (124,127,132,133) that can step properly on a treadmill. The most popular preparation that utilizes electrical stimulation has been the mesencephalic cat with electrical stimulation of the mesencephalic locomotor region (MLR: 114,117–120,122,134,136,137,143). The most utilized preparation that utilizes chemical stimulation has been the acute spinal cat treated with L-DOPA, usually preceded by nialamide injection (115,122,123,125,126, 128,138,139). The spinal L-DOPA preparation is usually utilized in combination with neuromuscular blockade; mesencephalic locomotor region stimulation in the mesencephalic cat and spontaneous activity in the thalamic cat have also been utilized with neuromuscular blockade.

Recordings from single cells during the production of the stepping program have utilized mainly extracellular recording techniques. In addition, intracellular recordings from motoneurons have been obtained (122,135,136). The action potentials of muscle spindle afferents have been recorded in intact cats (129, 140) and in spinal cats with L-DOPA stimulation (123). Strong evidence for gamma motoneuron activation of spindle afferents during alpha motoneuron activation of the parent muscle exists in the L-DOPA preparation. In intact cats, alpha-gamma motoneuron coactivation occurs under some conditions; under other conditions, very little gamma motor drive of spindle afferents is observed. Recordings from unidentified interneurons in the lumbosacral enlargement during stepping reveal that these cells display a wide variety of activation patterns during the step cycle (104,119,122). Many interneurons appear tightly linked to the activation pattern of a given muscle; much more data from interneurons are needed to understand the full range of interneuronal activation patterns. Recordings from interneurons identified by classic techniques (152, 153) reveal that ventral spinocerebellar tract interneurons (118), Ia inhibitory interneurons (120), and Renshaw cells (134) are phasicly active during the production of the fictive step cycle.

The stepping motor program can be strongly influenced by sensory inputs. Movement of the hip joint can modify the step cycle (126,127,138). Cutaneous stimulation applied to the dorsum of the foot can produce a reflex whose characteristics will vary according to the phase of the cycle in which the stimulus is presented (124,125). When the foot is off the ground and the limb is swinging forward, the stimulation elicits an enhanced flexion that allows the foot to avoid the obstacle. When the foot is on the ground and bearing weight, the stimulation elicits an enhanced extension that helps maintain the position of the foot on the ground. A phase-dependent effect can also be observed with direct electrical stimulation of peripheral nerves (121,130). A stretch applied to ankle extensor muscles can inhibit the production of the step rhythm (131).

There is a large amount of information available on cat stepping. It is clear that further data need to be obtained before we will have a complete picture of the spinal control of stepping in the cat. An example of a complexity that has only recently been revealed is the observation that the synergist flexor digitorum longus and flexor hallucis longus muscles are activated during different times of the step cycle (142). How many other complexities of this type exist can only be revealed by further work.

IX. CONCLUSIONS

There are two major generalizations that emerge from studies of spinal cord pattern generation. First, there are many complex, highly coordinated motor programs that the spinal cord can produce in the absence of phasic sensory feedback and descending modulation from supraspinal structures. Thus, neural networks, termed central program generators, reside within the spinal cord. Second, sensory feedback can cause major adaptive changes in the amplitude and timing of central program generator output. This implies that central program generators are sensitive to feedback modification. These generalizations are at the level of neuronal systems. We need to understand the cellular mechanisms underlying these systemic properties. Do central program generator neurons have specialized membrane properties such as the capacity to produce endogenous bursting activity (155) or plateau potentials (156)? Is synaptic transmission in the absence of action potentials important (157)? Are there multiaction synapses that can produce either excitation or inhibition depending upon the history of synaptic activity (158)? It may well be that the simpler lamprey and tadpole preparations will reveal these cellular properties.

There is an important organizational level intermediate between the single cell level and the whole system level that requires further understanding. This intermediate level is that of the functional organization of the central program generator. We need to understand what subsets of interneurons function within each central program generator. For the control of trunk musculature during swimming it may be that each hemisegment acts as a "unit generator" (7,42). For the control of a multijointed limb during stepping or scratching it may be that each direction of each degree of freedom has a "unit generator" whose activity modifies the activities of all the muscles involved in that degree of freedom (7). If this unit generator hypothesis is correct, then the problem of understanding the control of movement breaks down into separable questions. First, what is the internal organization of each unit generator? Second, what synaptic linkages are possible between unit generators controlling opposite movements in the same degree of freedom? For example, during forward stepping the hip flexion generator may have a reciprocal inhibitory relationship with the hip extension generator and the hip abduction generator may have a reciprocal excitatory relationship with the hip adduction generator. Third, what synaptic linkages are possible between generators controlling different degrees of freedom? Fourth, how might these linkages change when the spinal cord changes its output from one form of a behavior to an alternative form of the same behavior; for example, when it changes from forward stepping to backward stepping or from rostral scratching to caudal scratching? Fifth, how might these linkages change when the spinal cord changes its output from one behavior to another behavior? The important feature of approaching the spinal cord with questions about this intermediate level of organization is that the question can be addressed in many or perhaps all of the preparations discussed in this chapter. A result obtained in one preparation can be utilized to produce a working hypothesis for another preparation. Since the spinal motor apparatus is conservative throughout the vertebrates, this strategy can be very efficient.

This chapter has emphasized the aspects of spinal motor generation observed in a series of organisms from the lamprey to the cat. To what extent do the generalizations observed in these animals apply to the human? The spinal cord of the human shares many organizational features with the spinal cord of other vertebrates. What features are shared at the level of spinal motor generation? Spinal humans display certain reflexes that require complex motor organization such as the flexion reflex. I am not aware of any report in which a spinal human can display either a stepping or a scratching motor program. The lack of such a report might mean that the generators for these programs are not located in the human spinal cord. An alternative possibility is that the generators for stepping and scratching are located in the human spinal cord and that we have yet to discover a technique that reveals their existence. More work is needed so that we can understand the full motor capacity of the spinal cord in animals and humans.

ACKNOWLEDGMENTS

Research in the author's laboratory has been supported by NIH Grant NS-15049. I thank Gail Robertson and Lawrence Mortin for many helpful discussions and editorial assistance.

REFERENCES

1. Grillner, S. (1975). Locomotion in vertebrates: Central mechanisms and reflex interaction. *Physiol. Rev.* 55:247–304.
2. Herman, R. M., Grillner, S., Stein, P. S. G., and Stuart, D. G. (1976). *Neural Control of Locomotion*, Plenum, New York.
3. Shik, M. L., and Orlovsky, G. N. (1976). Neurophysiology of locomotor automatism. *Physiol. Rev.* 56:465–501.
4. Wetzel, M. C., and Stuart, D. G. (1976). Ensemble characteristics of cat locomotion and its neural control. *Prog. Neurobiol.* 7:1–98.
5. Stein, P. S. G. (1978). Motor systems, with specific reference to the control of locomotion. *Annu. Rev. Neurosci.* 1:61–81.

6. Delcomyn, F. (1980). Neural basis of rhythmic behavior in animals. *Science 210*:492–498.
7. Grillner, S. (1981). Control of locomotion in bipeds, tetrapods, and fish. In *Handbook of Physiology*, Sect. 1, *The Nervous System*, Volume 2, *Motor Control*, V. B. Brooks (Ed.), American Physiological Society, Bethesda, Maryland, pp. 1179–1236.
8. Stein, P. S. G. (1983). The vertebrate scratch reflex. *Symp. Soc. Exp. Biol. 37*:383–403.
9. Weiss, P. (1941). Self-differentiation of the basic patterns of coordination. *Comp. Psychol. Monographs 17*(4):1–96.
10. Bernstein, N. (1967). *The Co-ordination and Regulation of Movements*, Pergamon Press, Oxford.
11. Wilson, D. M. (1972). Genetic and sensory mechanisms for locomotion and orientation in animals. *Am. Sci. 60*:358–365.
12. Grillner, S., McClellan, A., Sigvardt, K., Wallen, P., and Williams, T. (1982). On the neural generation of "fictive locomotion" in a lower vertebrate nervous system, in vitro. In *Brain Stem Control of Spinal Mechanisms*, B. Sjolund and A. Bjorklund (Eds.), Elsevier Biomedical Press, New York, pp. 273–295.
13. Wallen, P. (1982). Spinal mechanisms controlling locomotion in dogfish and lamprey. *Acta Physiol. Scand. (Suppl.) 503*:1–45.
14. Grillner, S., Wallen, P., McClellan, A., Sigvardt, K., Williams, T., and Feldman, J. (1983). The neural generation of locomotion in the lamprey— An incomplete account. *Symp. Soc. Exp. Biol. 37*:285–304.
15. Rovainen, C. M. (1983). Identified neurons in the lamprey spinal cord and their roles in fictive swimming. *Symp. Soc. Exp. Biol. 37*:305–330.
16. Rovainen, C. M. (1983). Neurophysiology. In *The Biology of Lampreys*, vol. 4, I. C. Potter and M. W. Hardisty (Eds.), Academic Press, London, pp. 1–136.
17. Cohen, A. H., and Wallen, P. (1980). The neuronal correlate of locomotion in fish. "Fictive swimming" induced in an in vitro preparation of the lamprey spinal cord. *Exp. Brain Res. 41*:11–18.
18. Grillner, S., and Wallen, P. (1980). Does the central pattern generation for locomotion in lamprey depend on glycine inhibition? *Acta Physiol. Scand. 110*:103–105.
19. Poon, M. L. T. (1980). Induction of swimming in lamprey by L-DOPA and amino acids. *J. Comp. Physiol. 136*:337–344.
20. Grillner, S., McClellan, A., and Perret, C. (1981). Entrainment of the spinal pattern generators for swimming by mechanosensitive elements in the lamprey spinal cord in vitro. *Brain Res. 217*:380–386.
21. Grillner, S., McClellan, A., Sigvardt, K., Wallen, P., and Wilen, M. (1981). Activation of NMDA-receptors elicits "fictive locomotion" in lamprey spinal cord in vitro. *Acta Physiol. Scand. 113*:549–551.
22. Sigvardt, K. A., and Grillner, S. (1981). Spinal neuronal activity during fictive locomotion in the lamprey. *Soc. Neurosci. Abstr. 7*:362.

23. Buchanan, J. T. (1982). Identification of interneurons with contralateral, caudal axons in the lamprey spinal cord: Synaptic interactions and morphology. *J. Neurophysiol. 47*:961–975.

24. Buchanan, J. T., and Cohen, A. H. (1982). Activities of identified interneurons, motoneurons, and muscle fibers during fictive swimming in the lamprey and effects of reticulospinal and dorsal cell stimulation. *J. Neurophysiol. 47*:948–960.

25. Grillner, S., McClellan, A., and Sigvardt, K. (1982). Mechanosensitive neurons in the spinal cord of the lamprey. *Brain Res. 235*:169–173.

26. Kahn, J. A. (1982). Patterns of synaptic inhibition in motoneurons and interneurons during fictive swimming in the lamprey, as revealed by Cl⁻ injections. *J. Comp. Physiol. 147*:189–194.

27. Wallen, P., and Williams, T. L. (1982). Intersegmental coordination in the isolated spinal cord of the lamprey during "fictive locomotion" as compared with swimming in the intact and spinal lamprey. *J. Physiol. (Lond.) 325*:30P–31P.

28. Russell, D. F., and Wallen, P. (1983). On the control of myotomal motoneurones during "fictive swimming" in the lamprey spinal cord in vitro. *Acta Physiol. Scand. 117*:161–170.

29. Roberts, B. L., and Williamson, R. M. (1983). Motor pattern formation in the dogfish spinal cord. *Symp. Soc. Exp. Biol. 37*:331–350.

30. Gray, J., and Sand, A. (1936). The locomotory rhythm of the dogfish *(Scyllium canicula). J. Exp. Biol. 13*:200–209.

31. Grillner, S. (1974). On the generation of locomotion in the spinal dogfish. *Exp. Brain Res. 20*:459–470.

32. Grillner, S., Perret, C., and Zanger, P. (1976). Central generation of locomotion in the spinal dogfish. *Brain Res. 109*:255–269.

33. Wallen, P. (1980). On the mechanisms of a phase-dependent reflex occurring during locomotion in dogfish. *Exp. Brain Res. 39*:193–202.

34. Grillner, S., and Wallen, P. (1982). On peripheral control mechanisms acting on the central pattern generators for swimming in the dogfish. *J. Exp. Biol. 98*:1–22.

35. Livingston, C. A., Williams, B. J., and Leonard, R. B. (1981). Locomotor activity elicited by spinal cord stimulation in the stingray, *Dasyatis sabina. Soc. Neurosci. Abstr. 7*:363.

36. Williams, B. J., Droge, M. H., Hester, K., and Leonard, R. B. (1981). Induction of swimming in the high spinal stingray by L-DOPA. *Brain Res. 220*:208–213.

37. Williams, B. J., Livingston, C. A., and Leonard, R. B. (1982). The effect of subtotal spinal cord lesions on locomotion in the stingray, *Dasyatis sabina. Soc. Neurosci. Abstr. 8*:876.

38. Droge, M. H., and Leonard, R. B. (1983). The swimming pattern in intact and decerebrated stingrays. *J. Neurophysiol. 50*:162–177.

39. Droge, M. H., and Leonard, R. B. (1983). Swimming rhythm in paralyzed, decerebrated stingrays: Normal and abnormal coupling. *J. Neurophysiol. 50*:178–191.

40. Droge, M. H., and Leonard, R. B. (1983). Organization of spinal motor nuclei in the stingray, *Dasyatis sabina. Brain Res. 276*:201–211.

41. von Holst, E. (1973). *The Behavioral Physiology of Animals and Man*, vol. 1, translated by Robert Martin. University of Miami Press, Coral Gables, Florida.

42. Grillner, S., and Kashin, S. (1976). On the generation and performance of swimming in fish. In *Neural Control of Locomotion*, R. M. Herman, S. Grillner, P. S. G. Stein, and D. G. Stuart (Eds.), Plenum, New York, pp. 181–201.

43. Kashin, S. M., Feldman, A. G., and Orlovsky, G. N. (1974). Locomotion of fish evoked by electrical stimulation of the brain. *Brain Res. 82*:41–47.

44. Faber, D. S., and Korn, H. (Eds.) (1978). *Neurobiology of the Mauthner Cell*, Raven, New York.

45. Zottoli, S. J. (1977). Correlation of the startle reflex and Mauthner cell auditory responses in unrestrained goldfish. *J. Exp. Biol. 66*:243–254.

46. Eaton, R. C., and Kimmel, C. B. (1980). Directional sensitivity of the Mauthner cell system to vibrational stimulation in zebrafish larvae. *J. Comp. Physiol. 140*:337–342.

47. Kimmel, C. B., Eaton, R. C., and Powell, S. L. (1980). Decreased fast-start performance of zebrafish larvae lacking Mauthner neurons. *J. Comp. Physiol. 140*:343–350.

48. Eaton, R. C., Lavender, W. A., and Wieland, C. M. (1981). Identification of Mauthner-initiated response patterns in goldfish: Evidence from simultaneous cinematography and electrophysiology. *J. Comp. Physiol. 144*: 521–531.

49. Eaton, R. C., Lavender, W. A., and Wieland, C. M. (1982). Alternative neural pathways initiate fast-start responses following lesions of the Mauthner neuron in goldfish. *J. Comp. Physiol. 145*:485–496.

50. Hackett, J. T., and Faber, D. S. (1983). Mauthner axon networks mediating supraspinal components of the startle response in the goldfish. *Neuroscience 8*:317–331.

51. Eaton, R. C. (1983). Is the Mauthner cell a vertebrate command neuron? A neuroethological perspective on an evolving concept. In *Advances in Vertebrate Neuroethology*, J. P. Ewert, R. R. Capranica, and D. J. Ingle (Eds.), Plenum, New York, pp. 629–636.

52. Eaton, R. C., and Hackett, J. T. (1984). The role of the Mauthner cell in fast-starts involving escape in teleost fishes. In *Neural Mechanisms of Startle Behavior*, R. C. Eaton (ed.), Plenum, New York, pp. 213–266.

53. Paton, G. (1846). On the perceptive power of the spinal cord, as manifested by cold-blooded animals. *Edinburgh Med. Surg. J. 65*:251–269.

54. Baglioni, S. (1913). Die hautreflexe der amphibien (frosch und krote). *Ergeb. Physiol. 13*:454–546.

55. Baglioni, S. (1913). Sur riflessi cutanei degli anfibi e sui fattori che li condizionano. *Zeit. fur Alleg. Physiol. 14*:161–234.

56. Franzisket, L. (1963). Characteristics of instinctive behavior and learning in reflex activity of the frog. *Anim. Behav. 11*:318–324.

57. Simpson, J. I. (1976). Functional synaptology of the spinal cord. In *Frog Neurobiology*, R. Llinás and W. Precht (Eds.), Springer-Verlag, Berlin, pp. 728–749.

58. Fukson, O. I., Berkinblit, M. B., and Feldman, A. G. (1980). The spinal frog takes into account the scheme of its body during the wiping reflex. *Science 209*:1261–1263.

59. Rock, M. K. (1980). Functional properties of Mauthner cell in the tadpole *Rana catesbeiana. J. Neurophysiol. 44*:135–150.

60. Rock, M. K., Hackett, J. T., and Brown, D. L. (1981). Does the Mauthner cell conform to the criteria of the command neuron concept? *Brain Res. 204*:21–27.

61. Stehouwer, D. J., and Farel, P. B. (1980). Central and peripheral controls of swimming in anuran larvae. *Brain Res. 195*:323–335.

62. Stehouwer, D. J., and Farel, P. B. (1983). Development of hindlimb locomotor activity in the bullfrog (*Rana catesbeiana*) studied in vitro. *Science 219*:516–518.

63. Kahn, J. A., and Roberts, A. (1982). The central nervous origin of the swimming motor pattern in embryos of *Xenopus laevis. J. Exp. Biol. 99*: 185–196.

64. Kahn, J. A., and Roberts, A. (1982). Experiments on the central pattern generator for swimming in amphibian embryos. *Philos. Trans. R. Soc. Lond. (Biol.) 296*:229–243.

65. Kahn, J. A., Roberts, A., and Kashin, S. M. (1982). The neuromuscular basis of swimming movements in embryos of the amphibian *Xenopus laevis. J. Exp. Biol. 99*:175–184.

66. Roberts, A., and Kahn, J. A. (1982). Intracellular recordings from spinal neurons during "swimming" in paralyzed amphibian embryos. *Philos. Trans. R. Soc. Lond. (Biol.) 296*:213–228.

67. Soffe, S. R., and Roberts, A. (1982). Activity of myotomal motoneurons during fictive swimming in frog embryos. *J. Neurophysiol. 48*:1274–1278.

68. Soffe, S. R., and Roberts, A. (1982). Tonic and phasic synaptic input to spinal cord motoneurons during fictive locomotion in frog embryos. *J. Neurophysiol. 48*:1279–1288.

69. Clarke, J. D. W., Roberts, A., and Soffe, S. R. (1983). Candidate reciprocal inhibitory interneurons in the spinal cord of *Xenopus* embryos. *J. Physiol. (Lond.) 336*:61P–62P.

70. Szekely, G., and Czeh, G. (1976). Organization of locomotion. In *Frog Neurobiology*, R. Llinás and W. Precht (Eds.), Springer-Verlag, Berlin, pp. 765–792.

71. Szekely, G., Czeh, G., and Voros, G. (1969). The activity pattern of limb muscles in freely moving and deafferented newts. *Exp. Brain Res. 9*:53–62.

72. Czeh, G., and Szekely, G. (1971). Muscle activities recorded simultaneously from normal and supernumerary forelimbs in ambystoma. *Acta Physiol. Acad. Sci. Hung. 40*:287–301.

73. Szekely, G., and Czeh, G. (1971). Activity of spinal cord fragments and limbs deplanted in the dorsal fin of urodele larvae. *Acta. Physiol. Acad. Sci. Hung. 40*:303–312.

74. Valk-Fai, T., and Crowe, A. (1978). Analyses of reflex movements in the hind limbs of the terrapin *Pseudemys scripta elegans. J. Comp. Physiol. 125*:351–357.

75. Stein, P. S. G., and Grossman, M. L. (1980). Central program for scratch reflex in turtle. *J. Comp. Physiol. 140*:287–294.

76. Bakker, J. G. M., and Crowe, A. (1982). Multicyclic scratch reflex movements in the terrapin *Pseudemys scripta elegans. J. Comp. Physiol. 145*: 477–484.

77. Mortin, K. I., Keifer, J., and Stein, P. S. G. (1982). Three forms of the turtle scratch reflex. *Soc. Neurosci. Abstr. 8*:159.

78. Robertson, G. A., Keifer, J., and Stein, P. S. G. (1982). Central programs for three forms of the turtle scratch reflex. *Soc. Neurosci. Abstr. 8*:159.

79. Stein, P. S. G., Robertson, G. A., Keifer, J., Grossman, M. L., Berenbeim, J. A., and Lennard, P. R. (1982). Motor neuron synaptic potentials during fictive scratch reflex in turtle. *J. Comp. Physiol. 146*:401–409.

80. Keifer, J., and Stein, P. S. G. (1983). In vitro motor program for the rostral scratch reflex generated by the turtle spinal cord. *Brain Res. 266*:148–151.

81. Lennard, P. R., and Stein, P. S. G. (1977). Swimming movements elicited by electrical stimulation of turtle spinal cord. I. Low-spinal and intact preparations. *J. Neurophysiol. 40*:768–778.

82. Stein, P. S. G. (1978). Swimming movements elicited by electrical stimulation of the turtle spinal cord: The high spinal preparation. *J. Comp. Physiol. 124*:203–210.

83. Kazennikov, O. V., Selionov, V. A., Shik, M. L., and Yakovleva, G. V. (1980). The rhombencephalic "locomotor region" in turtles. *Neurophysiology (Kiev) 12*:251–257.

84. Bekoff, A., Stein, P. S. G., and Hamburger, V. (1975). Coordinated motor output in the hindlimb of the 7-day chick embryo. *Proc. Natl. Acad. Sci. USA 72*:1245–1248.

85. Bekoff, A. (1976). Ontogeny of leg motor output in the chick embryo: A neural analysis. *Brain Res. 106*:271–291.

86. Hamburger, V. (1977). The developmental history of the motor neuron. *Neurosci. Res. Program Bull. Suppl. 15*:1–37.

87. Landmesser, L. (1978). The distribution of motoneurones supplying chick hindlimb muscles. *J. Physiol. (Lond.) 284*:371–389.

88. Landmesser, L. (1978). The development of motor projection patterns in the chick hindlimb. *J. Physiol. (Lond.) 284*:391–414.

89. Hollyday, M. (1980). Organization of motor pools in the chick lumbar lateral motor column. *J. Comp. Neurol. 194*:143–170.

90. O'Donovan, M. J., Cooper, M. W., and Landmesser, L. T. (1981). Electromyographic activity patterns of embryonic chick hindlimb muscles. *Soc. Neurosci. Abstr. 7*:688.

91. Bekoff, A., and Kauer, J. A. (1982). Neural control of hatching: Role of neck position in turning on hatching leg movements in post-hatching chicks. *J. Comp. Physiol. 145*:497–504.

92. Jacobson, R. D., and Hollyday, M. (1982). A behavioral and electromyographic study of walking in the chick. *J. Neurophysiol. 48*:238–256.

93. Jacobson, R. D., and Hollyday, M. (1982). Electrically evoked walking and fictive locomotion in the chick. *J. Neurophysiol. 48*:257–270.

94. O'Donovan, M. J., and Landmesser, L. T. (1982). Activity patterns of chick hindlimb muscles with inappropriate innervation. *Soc. Neurosci. Abstr. 8*:708.

95. Landmesser, L. T., and O'Donovan, M. J. (1984). Activation patterns of embryonic chick hindlimb muscles recorded *in ovo* and in an isolated spinal cord preparation. *J. Physiol. (Lond.) 347*:189–204.

96. Landmesser, L. T., and O'Donovan, M. J. (1984). The activation patterns of embryonic chick motoneurons projecting to inappropriate muscles. *J. Physiol. (Lond.) 347*:205–224.

97. Sherrington, C. S. (1906). *The Integrative Action of the Nervous System*, Yale University Press, New Haven, Connecticut.

98. Sherrington, C. S. (1906). Observations on the scratch-reflex in the spinal dog. *J. Physiol. (Lond.) 34*:1–50.

99. Sherrington, C. S. (1910). Notes on the scratch-reflex of the cat. *Q. J. Exp. Physiol. 3*:213–220.

100. Deliagina, T. G., Feldman, A. G., Gelfand, I. M., and Orlovsky, G. N. (1975). On the role of central program and afferent inflow in the control of scratching movements in the cat. *Brain Res. 100*:297–313.

101. Feldman, A. G., Orlovsky, G. N., and Perret, C. (1977). Activity of muscle spindle afferents during scratching in the cat. *Brain Res. 129*:192–196.

102. Arshavsky, Y. I., Gelfand, I. M., Orlovsky, G. N., and Pavlova, G. A. (1978). Messages conveyed by spinocerebellar pathways during scratching in the cat. II. Activity of neurons in the ventral spinocerebellar tract. *Brain Res. 151*:493–506.

103. Berkinblit, M. B., Deliagina, T. G., Feldman, A. G., Gelfand, I. M., and Orlovsky, G. N. (1978). Generation of scratching. I. Activity of spinal interneurons during scratching. *J. Neurophysiol. 41*:1040–1057.

104. Berkinblit, M. B., Deliagina, T. G., Feldman, A. G., Gelfand, I. M., and Orlovsky, G. N. (1978). Generation of scratching. II. Nonregular regimes of generation. *J. Neurophysiol. 41*:1058–1069.

105. Berkinblit, M. B., Deliagina, T. G., Orlovsky, G. N., and Feldman, A. G. (1980). Activity of motoneurons during fictitious scratch reflex in the cat. *Brain Res. 193*:427–438.

106. Deliagina, T. G., and Orlovsky, G. N. (1980). Activity of Ia inhibitory interneurons during fictitious scratch reflex in the cat. *Brain Res. 193*:439–447.

107. Baev, K. V., and Kostyuk, P. G. (1981). Primary afferent depolarization evoked by the activity of spinal scratching generator. *Neuroscience 6*:205–215.

108. Baev, K. V. (1981). The central program of activation of hind-limb muscles during scratching in cats. *Neurophysiology (Kiev) 13*:38–44.

109. Baev, K. V., Degtyarenko, A. M., Zavadskaya, T. V., and Kostyuk, P. G. (1981). Activity of lumbosacral interneurons during fictitious scratching. *Neurophysiology (Kiev) 13*:45–52.

110. Deliagina, T. G., and Feldman, A. G. (1981). Activity of Renshaw cells during fictive scratch reflex in cat. *Exp. Brain Res. 42*:108–115.

111. Deliagina, T. G., Orlovsky, G. N., and Perret, C. (1981). Efferent activity during fictitious scratch reflex in the cat. *J. Neurophysiol. 45*:595–604.

112. Sherrington, C. S. (1910). Flexion-reflex of the limb, crossed extension reflex, and reflex stepping and standing. *J. Physiol. (Lond.) 40*: 28–121.

113. Brown, T. G. (1911). The intrinsic factors in the act of progression in the mammal. *Proc. R. Soc. Lond. (Biol.) 84*:308–319.

114. Shik, M. L., Severin, F. V., and Orlovsky, G. N. (1966). Control of walking and running by means of electrical stimulation of the midbrain. *Biophysics 11*:756–765.

115. Jankowska, E., Jukes, M. G. M., Lund, S. and Lundberg, A. (1967). The effect of DOPA on the spinal cord. 5. Reciprocal organization of pathways transmitting excitatory action to alpha motoneurones of flexors and extensors. *Acta Physiol. Scand. 70*:369–388.

116. Engberg, I. and Lundberg, A. (1969). An electromyographic analysis of muscular activity in the hindlimb of the cat during unrestrained locomotion. *Acta Physiol. Scand. 75*:614–630.

117. Kulagin, A. S., and Shik, M. L. (1970). Interaction of symmetrical limbs during controlled locomotion. *Biophysics 15*:171–178.

118. Arshavsky, Y. I., Berkinblit, M. B., Fukson, O. I., Gelfand, I. M., and Orlovsky, G. N. (1972). Origin of modulation in neurones of the ventral spinocerebellar tract during locomotion. *Brain Res. 43*:276–279.

119. Orlovsky, G. N., and Feldman, A. G. (1972). Classification of lumbosacral neurons according to their discharge patterns during evoked locomotion. *Neurophysiology (Kiev) 4*:311–317.

120. Feldman, A. G., and Orlovsky, G. N. (1975). Activity of interneurons mediating reciprocal Ia inhibition during locomotion. *Brain Res. 84*:181–194.

121. Duysens, J., and Pearson, K. G. (1976). The role of cutaneous afferents from the distal hindlimb in the regulation of the step cycle of thalamic cats. *Exp. Brain Res. 24*:245–255.

122. Edgerton, V. R., Grillner, S., Sjostrom, A. and Zangger, P. (1976). Central generation of locomotion in vertebrates. In *Neural Control of Locomotion*, R. M. Herman, S. Grillner, P. S. G. Stein, and D. G. Stuart (Eds.), Plenum, New York, pp. 439–464.

123. Sjostrom, A., and Zangger, P. (1976). Muscle spindle control during locomotor movements generated by the deafferented spinal cord. *Acta Physiol. Scand. 97*:281–291.

124. Forssberg, H., Grillner, S., and Rossignol, S. (1977). Phasic gain control of reflexes from the dorsum of the paw during spinal locomotion. *Brain Res. 132*:121–139.

125. Andersson, O., Forssberg, H., Grillner, S., and Lindquist, M. (1978). Phasic gain control of the transmission in cutaneous reflex pathways to motoneurones during "fictive" locomotion. *Brain Res. 149*:503–507.

126. Andersson, O., Grillner, S., Lindquist, M., and Zomlefer, M. (1978). Peripheral control of the spinal pattern generators for locomotion in the cat. *Brain Res. 150*:625–630.

127. Grillner, S., and Rossignol, S. (1978). On the initiation of the swing phase of locomotion in chronic spinal cats. *Brain Res. 146*:269–277.

128. Grillner, S., and Zangger, P. (1979). On the central generation of locomotion in the low spinal cat. *Exp. Brain Res. 34*:241–261.

129. Loeb, G. E., and Duysens, J. (1979). Activity patterns in individual hindlimb primary and secondary muscle spindle afferents during normal movements in unrestrained cats. *J. Neurophysiol. 42*:420–440.

130. Duysens, J., and Loeb, G. E. (1980). Modulation of ipsi- and contralateral reflex responses in unrestrained walking cats. *J. Neurophysiol. 44*:1024–1037.

131. Duysens, J., and Pearson, K. G. (1980). Inhibition of flexor burst generation by loading ankle extensor muscles in walking cats. *Brain Res. 187*: 321–332.

132. Forssberg, H., Grillner, S., and Halbertsma, J. (1980). The locomotion of the low spinal cat. I. Coordination within a hindlimb. *Acta Physiol. Scand. 108*:269–281.

133. Forssberg, H., Grillner, S., Halbertsma, J., and Rossignol, S. (1980). The locomotion of the low spinal cat. II. Interlimb coordination. *Acta Physiol. Scand. 108*:283–295.

134. McCrea, D. A., Pratt, C. A., and Jordan, L. M. (1980). Renshaw cell activity and recurrent effects on motoneurons during fictive locomotion. *J. Neurophysiol. 44*:475–488.

135. Perret, C., and Cabelguen, J. M. (1980). Main characteristics of the hindlimb locomotor cycle in the decorticate cat with special reference to bifunctional muscles. *Brain Res. 187*:333–352.

136. Pratt, C. A., and Jordan, L. M. (1980). Recurrent inhibition of motoneurons in decerebrate cats during controlled treadmill locomotion. *J. Neurophysiol. 44*:489–500.

137. Steeves, J. D., Schmidt, B. J., Skovgaard, B. J., and Jordan, L. M. (1980). Effect of noradrenaline and 5-hydroxytryptamine depletion on locomotion in the cat. *Brain Res. 185*:349–362.

138. Andersson, O., and Grillner, S. (1981). Peripheral control of the cat's step cycle. I. Phase dependent effects of ramp-movements of the hip during "fictive locomotion." *Acta Physiol. Scand. 113*:89–101.

139. Lundberg, A. (1981). Half-centers revisited. *Adv. Physiol. Sci. 1*:155–167.

140. Prochazka, A. (1981). Muscle spindle function during normal movement. *Int. Rev. Physiol. 25*:47–90.

141. Bayev, K. V., and Kostyuk, P. G. (1982). Polarization of primary afferent terminals of lumbosacral cord elicited by the activity of spinal locomotor generator. *Neuroscience 7*:1401–1409.

142. O'Donovan, M. J., Pinter, M. J., Dum, R. P., and Burke, R. E. (1982). Actions of FDL and FHL muscles in intact cats: Functional dissociation between anatomical synergists. *J. Neurophysiol. 47*:1126–1143.

143. Shik, M. L. (1983). Action of the brain stem locomotor region on spinal stepping generators via propriospinal pathways. In *Spinal Cord Reconstruction*, C. C. Kao, R. P. Bunge, and P. J. Reier (Eds.). Raven, New York, pp. 421–434.

144. Viala, D., and Buser, P. (1971). Modalités d'obtention de rythmes locomoteurs chez le lapin spinal par traitements pharmacologiques (DOPA, 5-HTP, D-Amphetamine). *Brain Res. 35*:151–165.

145. Viala, D., and Vidal, C. (1978). Evidence for distinct spinal locomotion generators supplying respectively fore- and hindlimbs in the rabbit. *Brain Res. 155*:182–186.

146. Vidal, C., Viala, D., and Buser, P. (1979). Central locomotor programming in the rabbit. *Brain Res. 168*:57–73.

147. Viala, D., and Freton, E. (1983). Evidence for respiratory and locomotor pattern generators in the rabbit cervico-thoracic cord and for their interactions. *Exp. Brain Res. 49*:247–256.

148. Cohen, A. H., and Gans, C. (1975). Muscle activity in rat locomotion: Movement analysis and electromyography of the flexors and extensors of the elbow. *J. Morphol. 146*:177–196.

149. Bekoff, A., and Trainer, W. (1979). The development of interlimb coordination during swimming in postnatal rats. *J. Exp. Biol. 83*:1–11.

150. Gruner, J. A., and Altman, J. (1980). Swimming in the rat: Analysis of locomotor performance in comparison to stepping. *Exp. Brain Res. 40*: 374–382.

151. Gruner, J. A., Altman, J., and Spivack, N. (1980). Effects of arrested cerebellar development on locomotion in the rat: Cinematographic and electromyographic analysis. *Exp. Brain Res. 40*:361–373.

152. Burke, R. E., and Rudomín, P. (1977). Spinal neurons and synapses. In *Handbook of Physiology*, Sect. 1, *The Nervous System*, Vol. 1, *Cellular Biology of Neurons*, E. R. Kandel (Ed.), American Physiological Society, Bethesda, Maryland, pp. 877–944.

153. Baldissera, F., Hultborn, H., and Illert, M. (1981). Integration in spinal neuronal systems. In *Handbook of Physiology*, Sect. 1, *The Nervous System*, Vol. 2, *Motor Control*. V. B. Brooks (Ed.), American Physiological Society, Bethesda, Maryland, pp. 509–595.

154. Hultborn, H., Illert, M., and Santini, M. (1976). Convergence on interneurones mediating reciprocal Ia inhibition of motoneurons. I. Disynaptic Ia inhibition of Ia inhibitory interneurons. *Acta Physiol. Scand. 96*:193–201.

155. Miller, J. P., and Selverston, A. I. (1982). Mechanisms underlying pattern generation in lobster stomatogastric ganglion as determined by selective inactivation of identified neurons. II. Oscillatory properties of pyloric neurons. *J. Neurophysiol. 48*:1378–1391.

156. Russell, D. F., and Hartline, D. K. (1978). Bursting neural networks: A re-examination. *Science 200*:453–456.

157. Pearson, K. G. (1976). Nerve cells without action potentials. In *Simpler Networks and Behavior*, J. C. Fentress (Ed.), Sinauer, Sunderland, Massachusetts, pp. 99–110.

158. Getting, P. A. (1981). Mechanisms of pattern generation underlying swimming in *Tritonia*. I. Neuronal network formed by monosynaptic connections. *J. Neurophysiol. 46*:65–79.

15

THE SPINAL LEMNISCAL PATHWAYS

Charles J. Vierck, Jr. *University of Florida College of Medicine,*
Gainesville, Florida

I. INTRODUCTION

In order to deal experimentally and conceptually with as diverse a sensory modality as somesthesis, we are compelled to divide the afferent input into categories that appear to us as elemental channels of information. We are aided by categorical divisions of receptor populations that transduce selective stimulus configurations, respond with characteristic patterns, and project to restricted portions of the central nervous system (1,2). Simplifying the receptor categories that have received considerable attention, there are four varieties of superficial cutaneous receptors: quickly adapting (QA), slowing adapting (SA), Pacinian, and hair receptors. Within each of these classes, there are variations. For example, the slowly adapting touch-pressure receptors can be divided in some animals and some areas of skin into a type I (associated with distinctive domes in the hairy skin of cats) and a stretch-sensitive type II. Similarly, hair receptors have different properties, depending upon the animal, the type of hair, and its location. Three of the four "major" categories of tactile receptors can be associated with distinctive sensations: vibration (Pacinian corpuscles), pressure (slowly adapting receptors), and hair bending. The onset of sensation of touch is determined in large part by quickly adapting receptors, but they seldom operate in isolation. At high velocities of skin deformation, both the quickly adapting and Pacinian receptors are stimulated, and the sensitivities of quickly and slowly adapting receptors overlap at low velocities. In fact, few if any somatosensations result from activity in one class of cutaneous receptor, and receptors deep to the skin must be considered as well. It is clear that vibration excites superficial and deep Pacinian corpuscles and muscle receptors and some joint receptors. Similarly, the sensation of flutter has been attributed to quickly adapting receptors that are entrained by 10–40 Hz tactile stimulation (3), but slowly adapting and Pacinian receptors also can be active in this range of oscillation (4).

The dilemma of unique but interactive input channels has fostered a number of arguments concerning the importance of receptor specificity for different sensations and has challenged our ability to define the elemental building blocks of the somatosensory systems. Because the interactions between receptor categories and their pathways of projection increase as we ascend the central nervous system, we are faced with the necessity of describing the sorting and resorting of information at each level of the neuraxis. To the extent that the functional significance(s) of each new combination of input categories can be established, we should understand the coding operations of the systems. To this end, investigation of the functional relevance of information sorting at the spinal level should establish principles that are embellished at supraspinal levels. Furthermore, the anatomic segregation of well-defined, ascending pathways in the spinal white matter is of practical importance, permitting selective stimulation, interruption, or isolation.

In addition to the problem, shared by vision and audition, of responding to an enormous range of stimulus intensities and frequencies, the spatial demands on somatosensory coding are unique. The distance senses represent the external world on a spatially limited but orderly and densely packed sheet of receptors of a few distinct categories. In contrast, the somatosensory receptors are distributed widely (in three dimensions) throughout the domain that is sensed. Because of the variety of tissues comprising the somatosensory domain, covering the territory requires integration of many receptor categories, rather than adding more of a given receptor type (e.g., stimulating more rods to cover a wider visual angle). Thus, variations in intensity of a stimulus impinging on the skin will progressively recruit superficial tactile receptors, muscle, tendon, ligament, and joint receptors and nociceptors in the skin, muscles, fascia, and viscera. Depending on such factors as the temperature, sharpness, force, and velocity of the stimulus, the sensory experience will differ and will be derived from activity in different proportions of certain receptor categories.

Classically, a functional distinction has been made between large peripheral afferent fibers that ascend the dorsal spinal columns (DC), without synapse in the dorsal spinal gray matter, and the ascending spinal pathways that originate from the dorsal horn. Based upon clinical cases involving selective disruption of large afferents (e.g., tabes dorsalis) or accidental severance of the ipsilateral white matter, the dorsal columns (fasciculi gracilis and cuneatus) have been credited with all of the epicritic somesthetic sensations (5,6). That is, fine discriminations of the relative intensity, quality, or location of light tactile and proprioceptive sensations were thought to depend critically upon integrity of the ipsilateral dorsal columns. The epicritic sensations were contrasted with protopathic sensations that have been attributed to the contralateral spinothalamic (ST) tracts. Protopathic messages were thought to provide few bits of information, but to signal the presence of tactile, thermal, or painful stimuli and to alert the organism. Spatial, temporal, and intensive resolution were described as rudimentary when supported solely by the contralateral spinothalamic pathways (7). Conversely, detection of minimal stimulation (e.g., drawing a wisp of cotton across the skin surface) was described as intact following ipsilateral lesions of the spinal cord. Because anterolateral cordotomy also does not reliably impair detection of light tactile stimuli (see, however, 8), "gross" touch was ascribed to a presumed ventral spinothalamic tract (9).

There is little reason to think that a neural system that can support subtle distinctions between the qualities, locations, and intensities of tactile experiences (the dorsal column–lemniscal system) could not provide cues sufficient to recognize the mere occurrence of tactile events. Although the spinothalamic system contributes substantial input to the reticular formation (10), lending credence to a unique role in alerting and arousing the organism, it is more likely to regulate motoric and emotional reactions to aversive stimulation than to mediate orienting and detecting reactions to light tactile stimuli. Both the spinothalamic and the lemniscal pathways share access to brain systems implicated in orientation to and conscious recognition of minimal stimuli (10-14), and touch detection survives complete section of the ipsilateral or the contralateral long ascending spinal pathways in primates (8,15).

Redundancy of simple tactile recognition is a functional expression of an interdigitation of projection fields from the different spinal pathways onto common targets in the brain stem and thalamus (16). Thus, many of the somatosensory functions that we can define by convenient tests will not be mediated exclusively by a single pathway. More realistically, each pathway can be expected to transmit some messages uniquely and to share other functions with different tracts. In the latter case, touch detection is normal (or nearly so) following interruption of any of the major ascending spinal pathways (in other words, each tract is not necessary for touch detection).

II. ORIGINS OF THE ASCENDING SPINAL PATHWAYS

Consistent with the classic separation of inputs critically concerned with conduction of pain and temperature information versus discriminative touch and proprioception, an early distinction between medial and lateral divisions of the

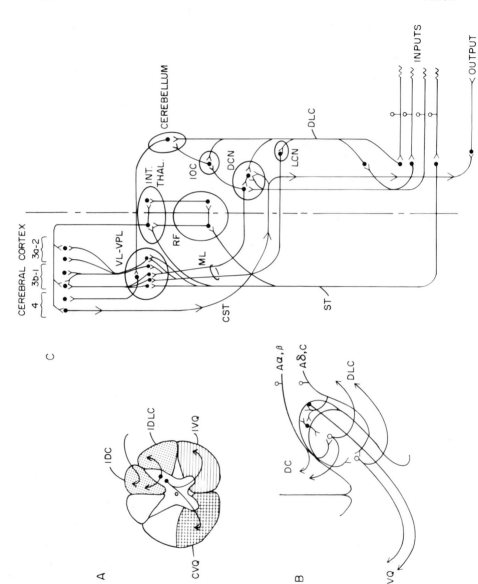

Figure 1 Highly schematic representations of the distribution of somesthetic inputs to the spinal gray matter and from the spinal white matter to the brain and back to motoneurons of the ventral horn. The connections shown do not approximate the complexity of available pathways and synaptic interactions, but the main thoroughfares emphasized in this review are shown. A, The spinal lemniscal pathways in the ipsilateral dorsal columns (IDC) and dorsolateral columns (IDLC) are speckled and are shown to receive primary axons (IDC only) and secondary axons from the dorsal horn. The ventral white matter contains the spinothalamic tract in the contralateral ventral quadrant (CVQ) and bilateral spinoreticular pathways (CVQ and IVQ). B, The major sources of input to the lemniscal and spinothalamic pathways are diagrammed. Large peripheral afferents (Aα and β fibers) project rostrally within the dorsal columns and synapse on dorsal horn cells that send axons into the ipsilateral dorsal and dorsolateral columns (DC and DLC) and the spinothalamic tract in the CVQ. Small myelinated (Aδ) and unmyelinated (C) peripheral afferents form a lateral division of the dorsal roots and synapse superficially and deep within the dorsal horn onto cells of origin of the spinothalamic tract. The small cells in the substantia gelatinosa distribute input from small-diameter afferents to multireceptive cells in the dorsal horn that project into the long ascending pathways. C, The projections of the lemniscal pathways from spinal cord to thalamus to the cerebral cortex are depicted, along with associated projections via the cerebellum and the spinothalamic pathway. The corticospinal projection to the medulla and spinal cord is included. LCN = lateral cervical nucleus; DCN = dorsal column nuclei (gracilis and cuneatus); IOC = inferior olivary complex; ML = medial lemniscus; RF = brain stem reticular formation; INT. THAL. = intralaminar thalamic nuclei; VL–VPL = nuclei ventralis lateralis and ventralis posterolateralis of the thalamus; CST = corticospinal tract; ST = spinothalamic tract.

dorsal roots (17) has been confirmed with modern techniques that reveal differential distributions of large (primary non-nociceptive) and small (primarily nociceptive and thermal) afferents onto cytoarchitectural laminae of the dorsal horn (18) (Fig. 1). Small myelinated (Aδ) and unmyelinated (C) fibers enter via the lateral division of the dorsal root and distribute primarily to laminae I and II (the marginal zone and substantia gelatinosa) and to laminae V and VI. Cells of origin of the spinothalamic tract are located primarily in laminae I, V, and VI (19). Lamina II processes small-fiber input and projects onto dorsal horn neurons and to the propriospinal system (via Lissauer's tract) for modulation of transmission through the spinal gray matter (20). Large myelinated afferents (Aα and β) enter the medial division of the dorsal roots and ascend the dorsal columns directly or synapse in laminae III-VI of the dorsal horn. Dorsal horn cells in lamina III-V give rise to axons that ascend ipsilaterally and contribute to the lemniscal system (21). Thus, large and small primary afferents have exclusive and shared projection fields within the dorsal horn, and the spinothalamic and lemniscal neurons have separate and shared locations in the dorsal horn (as do the dendrites of these cells).

Tactile and proprioceptive input to the dorsal horn from a given locus on or in the body is distributed over a number of cord segments by direct input at the level of entry, from collaterals of dorsal column afferents, and from terminals of afferents that exit the dorsal columns. Despite this rostrocaudal spread of input, the body is mapped coherently in the dorsal horn (22). It is important to recognize the presence of spatial order in the dorsal horn because it provides the substrate for spatial coding outside the dorsal columns. The contribution of dorsal horn pathways to spatial resolution often has not been considered seriously because a somatotopic order of projections from the dorsal horn has been difficult to demonstrate at rostral targets (23). Nevertheless, behavioral data demonstrating excellent spatial discrimination on certain tasks after dorsal column section force us to regard the dorsal horn projection system as spatially precise in its rostral projections.

The pathways of projection are numerous for dorsal horn neurons receiving tactile or proprioceptive inputs (24). A few of the major output channels are: (1) the postsynaptic dorsal column tract (PSDC), (2) the dorsal column–dorsolateral column–dorsal column (DC-DLC-DC) projection, via the dorsolateral columns to the dorsal column nuclei, (3) the spinocervicothalamic tract (SCT), (4) the spinothalamic tract (ST), (5) the spinoreticular tract, and (6) the spinocerebellar tracts (Fig. 1). Faced with a plethora of routes by which dorsal horn cells could influence or mediate discriminative somesthetic capacities, a useful opening approach to functional characterization is to determine the information conveyed by three independently dissectable cord sectors: (1) the ipsilateral dorsal columns (IDC), containing primary afferent and secondary (dorsal horn) projections to the dorsal column nuclei and then the medial lemniscus; (2) the ipsilateral lateral column (ILC), including secondary axons projecting to the medial lemniscus via the dorsal column nuclei and the lateral cervical nucleus; and (3) the contralateral ventral quadrant (CVQ), containing the spinothalamic tracts. The discussion to follow will concentrate on these tracts from the spinal cord to the thalamus, because evidence supports the contention that conscious somatosensation depends upon the lemniscal and spinothalamic projection systems (25-27). The potential contribution of spinocerebellocortical pathways to somatic sensibility has been negated (28-30), but it has not been ruled out, and the possibility that lesions of either lateral column have an effect by virtue of spinocerebellar tract interruption must be kept in mind. Independent lesions of pure lemniscal and cerebellar pathways are feasible, but they have been utilized rarely (29,30,30a).

III. THE MEDIAL LEMNISCUS

The medial lemniscus receives more complex inputs from the spinal cord than those provided by primary afferent fibers in the dorsal columns (Fig. 1). The primary dorsal column axons send collaterals to the spinal dorsal horn, providing touch and proprioceptive input onto cells in laminae III-VI. Cells in laminae IV (nucleus proprius) project in both the dorsal and dorsolateral columns to lemniscal projection cells at upper cervical and lower bulbar levels (21,31-33). Thus, inputs to the medullary dorsal column nuclei are: (1) from primary dorsal column afferents, (2) from relayed dorsal column afferents, and (3) from relayed dorsolateral column afferents. In addition, dorsolateral column axons synapse in the lateral cervical nucleus (a small, lateral extension of the dorsal horn from C1-C3) (1,34,35). Cells in the lateral cervical nucleus send axons across the midline, at the levels of the nucleus, to form the spinocervicothalamic tract, in the contralateral lateral columns of C1-C3 (36,37). In the medulla, the spino-cervicothalamic tract axons join fibers from the contralateral dorsal column nuclei. In anatomic terms, since the medial lemniscus (ML) originates in the dorsal column and lateral cervical nuclei, the spinal lemniscal pathways include axons in the dorsal and the dorsolateral columns.

Behavioral data from a variety of tasks give functional meaning to a definition of the lemniscal system as extending beyond the dorsal columns to include the dorsolateral columns (38). This view is not at variance with early clinical observations that focused attention on the dorsal column component of the spinal lemniscal pathways. For example, descriptions of dorsal column degeneration in tabes dorsalis patients were taken to mean that only the dorsal columns were affected, but the syphilis spirochete attacks large afferents that project into the dorsal horn as well. Tabes should affect: (1) dorsal column primary afferents, (2) the predominant input to dorsal horn cells projecting in the dorsal and dorsolateral columns, and (3) convergent inputs (e.g., with high-threshold afferents) onto secondary cells of the ventral spinal pathways. Hence, tabes represents a global loss of touch and proprioceptive input to all of the spinal pathways.

Until recently, data from patients sustaining accidental, focal interruption of the lemniscal pathways did not have the benefit of surgical or histological determination of the lesion extent. Typically, patients with spinal lesions producing ipsilateral loss of fine touch and proprioception also have ipsilateral pyramidal tract signs and contralateral attenuation of pain and temperature sensibility (the Brown-Séquard syndrome [7]). Clearly, these lesions involve most of the white matter on one side of the spinal cord. For analysis of the relative importance of the dorsal column and dorsolateral column components of the lemniscal system, it is necessary to obtain behavioral observations with histologic verification of restricted and combined dorsal column and dorsolateral column sections.

A. The Dorsal Columns

Primary afferent inputs to the dorsal columns enter in bands that are stacked laterally as the cord is ascended. Each band represents input from one dermatome, and the areas innervated by adjacent dorsal roots overlap extensively. Because orderly spatial relationships are maintained within the dorsal column projection from each root, a structured map of some of the body surface is formed by the dorsal column axons in cross section at each rostrocaudal level. At lower spinal levels, the map contains disjunctive shifts; that is, adjacent cells do not always have overlapping or adjacent receptive fields (RFs). However, at cervical levels, the dorsal column axons have become arranged so that a continuous trajectory along the surface of the body is traced by consecutive receptive fields encountered by a penetrating microelectrode (39). The rearrangement of dorsal column afferents to form a coherent map of the body surface confirms classic descriptions of an orderly spatial representation within the dorsal column-lemniscal system.

Experiments that have compared the composition of the dorsal columns at cervical versus thoracolumbar levels have shown that the dorsal columns differ substantially from the classic view as being: (1) the exclusive channel of input to the medial lemniscus from large peripheral afferents, and (2) comprised exclusively of primary dorsal root afferents. Most of the studies have involved carnivores, but the available information on primates is confirmatory for the overall pattern of lemniscal sorting that occurs in carnivores (39,40). Of the total population of primary afferents that enter the dorsal columns from the hindlimbs, only 23% extend to the gracile nucleus to form a monosynaptic connection from the periphery to projection cells of the medial lemniscus (41), but only 15% of the cervical fasciculus gracilis consists of secondary axons (i.e., from cells in the dorsal horn) (33). Thus, primary afferents make up the bulk of the long dorsal column projection, but a substantial proportion of large afferents from the dorsal root synapse within the dorsal horn.

The modality composition of the long and short primary dorsal column axons differs in a number of respects. The long primary axons are, in general, quickly adapting, but there are differences among experiments (and possibly species and fasciculi gracilis vs. cuneatus) in the proportion of axons of a given modality category that project to the dorsal column nuclei relative to the number that exit the dorsal columns. For example, all slowly adapting primaries may exit the dorsal columns (39), or the slowly adapting I axons exit, but the slowly adapting II afferents stay (42), or more slowly adapting I than slowly adapting II afferents project directly to the medulla (43), or vice verse (44). If we favor positive evidence, assuming that negative findings can result easily from sampling errors, few categories of large afferents are excluded from the group of long primaries, but the representation of slowly adapting afferents in the long dorsal column projection is low (45). It is clear that the monosynaptic projection to the nucleus gracilis is dominated by axons that mark the onset (and offset) of tactile or proprioceptive stimulation (46). Most of the primary afferents are quickly adapting, and, therefore, movement rather than position of the skin or joints is conveyed monosynaptically to the dorsal column nuclei. For the skin, which has been studied more thoroughly than proprioceptors, velocities of indentation in the midrange are detected amply by the primary quickly adapting afferents, and fast or slow rates of indentation are underrepresented by the paucity of Pacinian or slowly adapting afferents, respectively. In fact, within categories of skin afferents, the more quickly adapting subclasses tend to be more substantially represented as long dorsal column primaries (42). Not only are the primary dorsal column afferents tuned selectively to phasic stimuli, but the skin-to-nucleus conduction time appears to be adjusted for conduction distance such that simultaneous stimulation of proximal versus distal loci produces near simultaneous activity in the appropriate portions of the dorsal column nucleus (47). Thus, the primary dorsal column afferents convey with exquisite precision the location *and* timing of movement onto (or movement of) different portions of the body—particularly the distal extremities.

Secondary dorsal column afferents are typical of long-tract projection neurons of the dorsal horn, in that submodality convergence is common. Up to 75% of the relayed dorsal column afferents are classified as multireceptive on the basis of responsivity to stimulation of hairs, skin touch, stretch of muscles, and noxious mechanical and thermal stimulation (32,33,48,49). The remainder are quickly adapting touch or nociceptor-specific units. The secondary dorsal column axons make up a minor portion of the long dorsal column projection from the lumbosacral plexus to the nucleus gracilis, but the secondary dorsal column afferents are more plentiful in monkeys than in cats (21). Interpretation of the physiologic basis of deficits from dorsal column section must take the postsynaptic system into account. This becomes apparent when the receptive characteristics of lemniscal projection neurons in the dorsal column nuclei are compared with the sensitivities of long primary afferents. A substantial number of cells within the medial lemniscus are multireceptive or respond to input categories that are meagerly represented or absent in the population of long primary dorsal column afferents (50).

It is likely that the secondary dorsal column projection contributes directly to the doral column-lemniscal ouput. Therefore, the consequences of dorsal column section cannot be attributed exclusively to a loss of quickly adapting touch and proprioception. This follows from involvement of secondary axons by dorsal column lesions and from the fact that quickly adapting input is not restricted to the long dorsal column system. A small percentage of quickly adapting primaries exit the dorsal columns to terminate in the dorsal horn (42), and collaterals of long dorsal column axons are distributed to the spinal gray matter (1). Input from quickly adapting afferents to dorsal horn cells is likely to be underestimated because of masking by convergent interactions from other receptor categories. For example, slowly adapting tactile afferents respond to movement of the skin with an onset transient response that could be enhanced by convergent interactions with quickly adapting afferents, but the postsynaptic response would be classified as slowly adapting because of a sensitivity to maintained indentation. Tactile input to spinal cells of projection to the dorsal, dorsolateral, and anterolateral columns clearly includes quickly adapting afferents, as shown by responses to stimulation of hairs (51,52). The dorsal column-lemniscal pathway is unique in preserving a large population of modality-specific velocity detectors, but it is not the exclusive ascending pathway for quickly adapting somesthetic receptors. Accordingly, a dorsal column lesioned animal can appear to detect stimulation of quickly adapting afferents (53) (see Fig. 2).

Issues of considerable interest and importance for understanding principles of somatosensory coding at supraspinal levels are presented by organization of the dorsal column nuclei into: (1) a core of relatively modality-specific projection neurons with characteristics similar to dorsal column primaries, and (2) associated, reticular regions that contain neurons with a high degree of submodality convergence, reminiscent of dorsal horn cells (21,54,55). In cats and monkeys, long primary dorsal column afferents project to a core region of the nucleus gracilis that contains lemniscal projection neurons. Dorsal horn cells send axons in the dorsal and dorsolateral columns to synapse within rostral and ventral portions of the dorsal column nuclei that contain few, if any, lemniscal projection neurons. These convergent reticular zones also receive substantial descending input from the somatosensorimotor cerebral cortex (56). Observations that cortical influences are excitatory to cells of the convergent zones but are predominantly inhibitory on the dorsal column-lemniscal

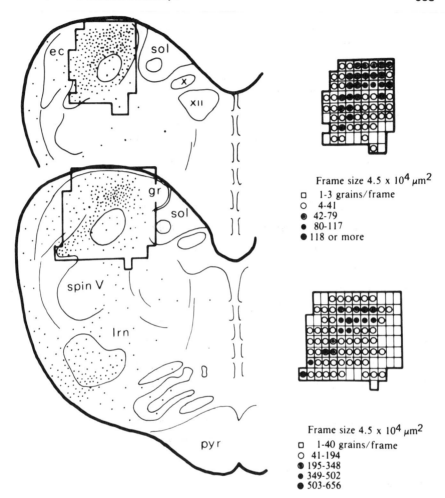

Figure 2 Following injection of tritiated amino acid into the brachial dorsal horn of a monkey, autoradiographic silver grains are numerous within the cuneate nucleus, except for the encircled core region. Automated grain counts within the cuneate nucleus are shown to the right of each section. (From Ref. 21.)

projection neurons (57) suggest that inhibitory modulations of lemniscal projection cells are produced by interneurones from the reticular zones. It is likely that the inhibition can be generated by ascending or descending inputs to these interneurones (58). Furthermore, excitatory driving or modulation of lemniscal projection neurons could result from convergent interactions between cortical and dorsal horn projections to the reticular regions of the dorsal column nuclei.

Table 1 Summary of the Anatomic and Physiologic Characteristics of the Core and Convergent Regions of the Dorsal Column Nuclei (DCN)

Core DCN system	Convergent DCN system
20 μ Round cells, bushy dendrites	12 μ Irregular cells, long, sparse dendrites
Primary afferent input from DC	Input from dorsal horn (DC and DLC), somatosensori-motor cortex, and reticular formation
Projection to VPL	Projection to VPL, PO, ZI, tectum, pretectum, cerebellum, and dorsal accessory olive
Thalamic projection in dense clusters	Scattered thalamic projection
Small projection from SM cortex	Substantial projection from SM cortex
Inhibited by SI stimulation	Facilitated by SI stimulation
Distal representation exceeds proximal	Proximal representation exceeds distal
Precise somatotopy	Less obvious somatotopy
Small RFs, little overlap, contralateral	Larger range of RFs, more overlap, ipsilateral and contralateral
Precise afferent inhibition	Afferent facilitation
Sharp RF boundaries	Large subliminal fringe
Receptor specificity	Submodality convergence
Low thresholds for activation	Broader range of thresholds
Narrow dynamic range	Wider dynamic range
Short latency	Greater range of latencies
Fast adapting	Fast and slow adapting
High frequency following	Lower frequency following
Anesthesia resistant	Anesthesia sensitive

It is worth emphasizing again that the lemniscal cells respond to afferent input categories that are not present among the long dorsal column primaries (Table 1).

The dorsal column–lemniscal system is unique among the ascending spinal pathways with regard to the spatial precision of inhibitory influences. Early descriptions of inhibitory receptive fields characterized them as surrounding the excitatory fields (59), and only a small percentage of somatosensory neurons could be shown to have spatially limited center-surround receptive field patterns. Modern utilization of the condition-test paradigm has shown that a large portion of lemniscal neurons have overlapping excitatory and inhibitory receptive fields

(60), and it can be inferred that inhibitory surrounds occur in a subpopulation with larger inhibitory than excitatory fields. Consistent with the overlap of receptive fields for excitation and inhibition, evidence favors a degree of sub-modality autoinhibition, with quickly adapting input providing most of the excitation and the inhibition (61,62). These findings reiterate the spatial precision of inhibitory influences on a system of high spatial excitatory resolution, but they also force consideration of the temporal order of excitatory and inhibitory influences.

A discrete tactile stimulus to a quiet subject will elicit: (1) A brief discharge within the primary dorsal column–lemniscal system that is unsculptured by afferent inhibition. If the stimulus moves across the skin, the location and timing of impingement upon a sequence of receptive fields will be signaled accurately in space and time by a succession of quickly adapting responses across the somato-topic map of the dorsal column–lemniscal system. (2) If the stimulus remains within a given receptive area, the threshold for excitation will be elevated by afferent inhibition, and the frequency of discharge to suprathreshold stimuli will be decreased, phasically (for up to 200 msec).

It is presumed that spatial resolution will be enhanced by inhibition that could reduce receptive field areas and increase the signal-to-noise ratio (63), but these effects might be counterbalanced by a reduction in the size and magnitude of the population response (64-66). In either case, reception of a tactile stimulus presents at least two types of message over the dorsal column–lemniscal system: (1) An early response to fast-conducting, highly secure transmission via primary afferents. Primary afferent endings in the dorsal nuclei are specialized (67-69), and projection neurons typically respond with a doublet of action potentials (70,71). (2) Later transmission is not restricted to primary afferents, but includes input from dorsal horn cells, and the dorsal horn nuclear output is shaped by inhibition. The modulating influences appear to arise from inter-actions in regions of the dorsal column nuclei that receive input from the dorsal horn and from the cerebral cortex. The latter input probably is elicited in part by primary afferent projection to the medial lemniscus and on to the highly ordered postcentral gyrus.

Passive reception of a novel tactile stimulus can be expected to elicit several reactions that could depend critically upon the lemniscal system. The first, the orienting response would require fast, secure conduction, moderately accurate localization, and access to motor systems for directing the head, eyes, and extremities with respect to the stimulus (depending upon its perceived significance). Projections of the dorsal column–lemniscal system to the somatosensory and motor cortex, cerebellum, tectum, pretectum, reticular formation, red nucleus, and subthalamus (11-14) meet these needs. Subsequent tactile evaluation of the stimulus could benefit from improved spatial resolution, permitting examination of the form and/or texture of the stimulus object. Secondary appreciation of stimulus features would be aided, presumably, from convergence of a variety of receptor categories—particularly the slowly adapting afferents that most effectively resolve textural patterns (72). The combination of primary and secondary projections to the dorsal column nuclei appears to meet these requirements.

In the real world of behaving organisms, significant tactile stimuli are most often encountered and explored by the process of active touch, involving the distal extremities that are richly supplied by the dorsal column–lemniscal system. Although superior tactile resolution for active palpation versus passive reception has not been demonstrated beyond doubt (73), interactions between motor activity and somatosensory sensitivity have been shown. In particular, rostral somatosensory conduction is reduced during gross movement of digits (74) or of limbs in the process of ambulation or during ballistic projection (75,76), but tactile and proprioceptive information is permitted access to the motor cortex during fine, adjustive movements of the distal extremities (77). Similarly, detailed examination of somatosensory input to the cortex during different phases of ambulation reveals units in the somatosensory cortex that respond during footfall but are otherwise suppressed (78). Taken together, results from rats, cats, and monkeys suggest that inhibition of somatosensory conduction is selective in time relative to motor as well as to sensory events. The channel is open when there is a need to evaluate with the distal extremities the consequences of a motor act, but information is excluded during gross movements, when a response to the stimuls would interfere with completion of the programmed movement. For example, a brachiating monkey must complete each reaching movement, ignoring incidental cutaneous stimulation during limb projection, and then the timing, exact placement, and resistance encountered by the hands must be evaluated quickly and accurately when the targets are contacted.

Additional studies of sensory-motor processing are required to determine: (1) whether motor-related sensory modulation affects sensory acuity in a more subtle manner than switching conduction on or off, (2) whether different submodalities are selectively affected during different phases of motor acts (e.g., proximal proprioceptive and distal tactile inputs should be sampled at different times) (79), and (3) the degree of dependence of accurate motor programming on somatosensory input and gating. The latter question is of considerable interest with respect to the dorsal column–lemniscal system because the dorsal columns constitute the spinal pathway for tactile and proprioceptive input to the precentral motor cortex (80). Characteristics of the dorsal column--lemniscal system that would be important for rapid and accurate motor programming by the corticospinal system are: (1) precise somatotopic mapping of the distal extremities by both systems in register in the motor cortex (81), providing match-mismatch comparisons of output and input (82,83), (2) a constant and rapid conduction time from different loci on the body (47), and (3) precise marking of the onset of movement (by proprioceptors) and the termination of the motor act (by touch). Thus, it is clear that the lemniscal system must be evaluated in relation to sensorimotor coordination in addition to its role in structuring conscious sensations of touch and proprioception.

Discussion of the anatomy and physiology of the dorsal column–lemniscal system to this point has concentrated on the fasciculus gracilis because it has been studied more thoroughly than its forelimb equivalent, the fasciculus cuneatus. However, given the specialized use of the hands in active touch by many species (especially primates), it is imperative that the organization of the forelimb lemniscal pathways be elucidated in detail. Although the sorting of primary and secondary afferents within the fasciculus cuneatus has not been fully explicated, similarities between the fasciculi gracilis and cuneatus have been suggested. Primary afferents that enter the fasciculus cuneatus may not exit in significant proportions before synapsing in the nucleus cuneatus, but there is a preferential selection for quickly adapting afferents (45). Secondary afferents are present in the fasciculus cuneatus and have physiologic properties and anatomic projection patterns similar to the postsynaptic axons in the fasciculus gracilis (21). The major differences between the dorsal column fasciculi are as follow: (1) recordings from the medial lemniscus indicate that the preponderance of lemniscal axons supply the forelimb (50), and (2) the fasciculus cuneatus contains a significant number of primary afferents supplying slowly adapting proprioceptors, including muscle receptors (84). Some of the axons in the fasciculus cuneatus terminate outside the nucleus cuneatus (e.g., in the cuneate nucleus; 85), which projects both to the cerebellum and to the thalamus (85a). Overall, the lemniscal projection of "deep" somatosensory receptor categories is more substantial for the forelimbs than the hindlimbs. Based upon recent demonstrations that muscle, joint, and tactile receptors each contribute to sensations of movement and position of the fingers and hand (86), the increased representation of proprioceptor categories within the fasciculus cuneatus is consistent with a requirement for feedback regulation of manual dexterity. The pyramidal motor system has been strongly implicated in the control of digital fractionation and of force output by the hand (87–89), and dorsal column–lemniscal input to the primary sensorimotor cortex is ideally suited for guidance and regulation of these functions.

B. The Dorsolateral Lemniscal Pathways

The ipsilateral dorsolateral spinal column contains at least two distinct pathways that contribute input to the medial lemniscus. The cells of origin of these tracts are located predominantly in laminae IV of the dorsal horn and project to the dorsal column nuclei or to the lateral cervical nucleus (1,21,35,90). Dorsolateral axons to the dorsal column nuclei have not been characterized thoroughly, but they appear to be quite similar in physiologic properties to secondary axons in the dorsal columns (91). The dorsolateral–dorsal column axons are fewer in number than the secondary dorsal column fibers (21), suggesting that they provide a minor contribution to lemniscal coding, but this has not been determined and may depend upon submodality. For example, dorsal horn cells with input from muscle afferents supplying the hindlimb project to nucleus z, at the rostral tip of the nucleus gracilis (35,92,93). Although some cells in nucleus z project into the medial lemniscus (94), there is dispute on this point (95), and there is some difficulty in deciding whether nucleus z should be considered as being separate from the reticular (convergent) zones of the nucleus gracilis (93). Thus, nucleus z could project directly to the lemniscus and indirectly via interneurons to dorsal column-lemniscal projection cells. In either case, it is important to note that sensory information from muscles and joints of the hindlimb project via the dorsolateral funiculus to the medial lemniscus and then the thalamo-cortical projection system.

The spinocervicothalamic tract reflects the convergent properties of lamina IV neurons. The predominant input to cells in the lateral cervical nucleus is from hair receptors, with a variety of additional contributions from touch, pressure, noxious thermal, and noxious mechanical receptors in the skin (1,90,95). There is a small representation from high-threshold joint and muscle receptors, but little or no input from proprioceptors. The spinocervicothalamic tract contribution to the medial lemniscus complements in several respects the distal representation of the dorsal columns by providing fast, synaptically secure conduction from proximal body parts. The spinocervicothalamic tract differs from the dorsal columns in the relatively high proportion of convergent neurons in the spinocervical tract. However, the spinocervicothalamic tract displays an unusual capacity for submodality filtering by descending projections to the dorsal horn cells of origin. When under the influence of descending inhibition from the brain stem, spinocervicothalamic tract cells respond primarily to stimulation of hairs (51) and, therefore, accurately time the onset of stimuli to the surface of the proximal limbs and trunk by presenting a quickly adapting barrage of impulses. The receptive fields of neurons in the lateral cervical nucleus can be quite small, but they are more variable than dorsal column-lemniscal projection cells. This is not surprising, since receptive fields in all somesthetic pathways increase in size with more proximal locations, and spatial resolution becomes less precise in a distal to proximal progression (96).

IV. COMPARISON OF THE SPINOTHALAMIC AND LEMNISCAL PATHWAYS

The spinothalamic projection can be divided into at least two systems (97,98): (1) a long tract providing direct input to the lateral thalamus (the neospino-thalamic system), and (2) direct and relayed connections to the medial thalamus (the paleospinothalamic and spinoreticulothalamic systems). Neospinothalamic and paleospinothalamic fibers course in the anterolateral and ventral columns. Hence, it is necessary to interrupt an entire ventral quadrant of spinal white matter in order to completely interrupt the crossed spinothalamic systems. When this is accomplished, pain and thermal sensitivity are substantially reduced, but not eliminated, for months following surgery in primates (5,8,9, 100,100a). A special role in the coding of pain and temperature sensations by the spinothalamic tract is indicated by these findings. Although the lemniscal pathways receive some input from thermal and nociceptive afferents (1,22,32, 90,95), and pain reactions can be modulated by dorsal spinal pathways (101), evidence is lacking for a critical role in coding of thermal or pain sensations by the lemniscal system (102). Hence, these somesthetic submodalities will not be considered further in this review.

Because the spinothalamic tract contains cells receiving input from tactile and proprioceptive afferents (103), the contralateral ventral quadrant must be considered as a potential factor in coding of fine somesthetic sensations that have been attributed to the lemniscal system. Dorsal horn cells of projection to the contralateral thalamus share some similarities with spinal cord cells projecting to the dorsal column and lateral cervical nuclei: (1) Physiologically, a substantial proportion of spinothalamic cells exhibit convergence of non-noxious and nociceptive, cutaneous afferents (103–105). The cell bodies of these multireceptive neurons are located primarily in laminae IV-VI, and they respond to hair, touch, or pressure stimulation, usually in combination with different nociceptive inputs from the skin, muscles, or viscera (106). (2) Although the dominant input source to the spinothalamic tract involves slowly conducting peripheral afferents, spinothalamic transmission from the dorsal horn to the thalamus is fast (mean: 36 m/sec) (107), and therefore the conduction time from periphery to cortex for stimuli involving large peripheral afferents is not slowed appreciably when transmission is limited to the spinothalamic tract. (3) The thalamic terminations of the spinothalamic tract overlap extensively with the projection from the medial lemniscus to the nucleus ventralis posterolateralis (VPL) (16). Although it has not been demonstrated that spinothalamic and lemniscal axons synapse on the same thalamic cells of projection to the cerebral cortex, it is reasonable to presume that the two projection systems terminate in register and that each contributes to somatotopic order in the nucleus ventralis posterolateralis. Axons of the spinothalamic tract are ordered somatotopically (108), but the receptive fields for touch and pressure stimulation are large relative to high-threshold spinothalamic neurons or to lemniscal axons (104). This result suggests that the spinothalamic tract subserves localization of noxious stimuli but is not a significant factor in spatial coding of light tactile stimuli. (4) The contribution of proprioceptive afferents to the dorsal column, spinocervicothalamic, and spinothalamic pathways is small in each case and often involves convergence with different receptor categories. Part of the difficulty in defining the physiologic substrates of proprioceptive sensations arises from selective inattention of experimenters to deep receptor categories because of the difficulty in defining the location and the classification of the receptors. The conscious perception of limb positions appears to depend upon a variety of sensory cues (109) that are conveyed primarily by the lemniscal system, after spinal conduction via the dorsal columns or the spinocerebellar tract (109a).

V. SENSORY FUNCTIONS OF THE DORSAL COLUMNS

A. Spatiotactile Discrimination

The dorsal column-lemniscal system is highly specialized for conduction of tactile information from the distal extremities to the cerebral cortex, and this pathway is most developed in mammals with excellent manual and pedal dexterity (110). The most distinctive feature of the fasciculi gracilis and cuneatus is the high degree of somatotopic organization, and dorsal column lesions produce a profound deafferentation of the distal extremity core of the high-resolution primary somatosensory "map" in awake primates (111). It is understandable, therefore, that textbooks of neurology have for years advocated simple tests of spatiotactile resolution for detection of damage to the dorsal column-lemniscal pathway. These tests ordinarily involve the ability of patients to localize or resolve punctate stimuli delivered to the skin in a manner closely resembling the procedures that have been utilized to characterize receptive fields and spatial organization in physiologic experiments that have revealed the highest spatial resolution in the dorsal columns. Thus, it has been disorienting to learn that spatial discriminations involving punctate stimulation can be little affected by complete interruption of the dorsal columns (38).

A fundamental assumption concerning the presence of topographic maps within sensory systems is that the location of an adequate stimulus is "read off" the map(s) by some scanning process that detects the spatial locations of evoked neural activity (112). If this is the case, then a dorsal column lesion should disrupt the capacity to localize punctate stimulation of the distal extremities because the spatial representation of highest resolution has been removed. However, tests of absolute localization on the hindlimbs of monkeys (113) or human patients (114; see Fig. 3) with complete transection of the dorsal columns have demonstrated no significant deficit. Whenever a discrepancy of this sort arises, we are left unsure as to whether the neural system or the functional test has been indicted, but in the case of absolute localization, the latter is most likely. Errors of localization are common among normal subjects (115)—even with stimulation of the fingers or toes, where receptive fields are small, innervation density is high, spatial discrimination on other tests is excellent, and confusion between digits is clearly unexpected. The test of absolute localization appears not to require the fine spatial resolution of the dorsal column–lemniscal system, which is consistent with theoretical predictions that localization can be mediated by systems with large or small receptive fields, given a minimal innervation density (66). The high degree of spatial order in the dorsal column–lemniscal projection system is especially adapted to discrimination of certain relationships between moving or multiple punctate stimuli (116,117), but not for revealing the absolute localization of individual points.

Considering the circumstances in which sensory stimuli are normally received, it is understandable that localization by tactile cues could be imprecise. The need for perceptual localization by touch pertains almost exclusively to novel stimuli; and the distance senses are enlisted in the early stages of identification of most stimulus objects by mammals. Once localization is accomplished, then attention shifts to examination of features other than the object's position relative to the body surface. Thus, a crudely directed orienting reaction to a tactile stimulus puts the object under visual control and permits a more precise, secondary evaluation. However, when the need for directed motoric reactions to tactile stimuli is taken into account, it seems that fast and accurate somato-sensorimotor localization would be a necessity. Quick, adjustive reactions occur during orienting reactions, requiring spatially detailed and comprehensive motor programs, in order to attend toward and act upon the object while maintaining balance. Fast transmission of onset information to somatotopically ordered motor systems by the dorsal column–lemniscal pathway could underlie these adjustive reactions, and the presence of a directed motor act could be necessary to reveal localization deficits following dorsal column lesions.

In the study of absolute tactile localization by monkeys (113), the task was structured as follows: (1) The animal pressed a lever and held it down until onset of a 10-Hz stimulus to either foot, after a variable period. (2) Release of the lever after stimulus onset (the detection latency) permitted pressing one of six small buttons on a front panel. The buttons were located on figurine drawings of a monkey's feet, at locations corresponding to points that could be stimulated on the glabrous skin surface. (3) Pressing a button terminated the trial and produced reinforcement if the correct button was pressed (i.e., corresponding to the location of the activated stimulator). The time from bar release to button press was termed the transit time. Disruptions of spatiomotor programming could have shown up as changes in detection latencies or transit times (or both) and were separable from direct effects on coordination (since afferents from the responding arm enter above the thoracic dorsal column lesion) or on perceptual localization (since the lesions did not affect the percentage of correct responses). Neither detection latencies nor transit times were lengthened by the dorsal column lesions, indicating that localization of punctate, tactile stimuli is not served uniquely by the dorsal columns, even when the response measure requires fast and accurate motor programming. Dorsal column lesions do produce a specific pattern of motoric deficits in the affected limb (see following discussion), but these effects are not to be explained by disruptions of the body image or impaired localization of stimuli on the body surface. These results indicate that the functional significance of the earliest dorsal column–lemniscal response relates primarily to direct reactions of the stimulated limb.

In contrast to the normal imprecision of tactile localization on the distal extremities and its susceptibility to manipulations of visual attention (115), the classic two-point threshold for spatial resolution is tightly correlated with receptive field size (112,118), and therefore appears to be determined by the spatial resolving power of the somatosensory system. The abundant use of the two-point or compass test has been dictated by convenience for clinical testing of patients and by assumptions that the threshold for resolution of two points reflects the capacity to identify more complex patterns. Furthermore, it once was assumed that pattern recognition represents an adequate test for integrity of the spatially precise core projection systems to the primary somatosensory or visual cortices. Investigators of both sensory systems have been quite surprised at the results of direct tests of these long-standing hypotheses. Ablation of the striate visual cortex in cats produces only subtle deficits of pattern recognition (119), and section of the dorsal columns does not elevate two-point thresholds on the hands or feet of monkeys (120) or humans (114,121). Taken together, these results pose fundamental questions about the roles of serial and parallel processing of spatial codes by component pathways within sensory systems.

It is important to recognize that the two-point threshold is not an appropriate clinical test for interruption of the dorsal columns. However, it is inappropriate to conclude from this test that the dorsal columns are not critical for any aspect of spatiotactile resolution. Other tests must be evaluated, and one approach to the problem is to assume that tests that generate the lowest spatial thresholds will most sensitively reflect integrity of the most precise somatotopic system. Comparing methods of spatial threshold testing with punctate stimuli, variations of the point-localization test yield thresholds well below those obtained with the compass test (96,122). In the point-localization procedure, the punctate stimuli are applied sequentially to the skin, and the subject identifies whether the same or different loci were touched. Improved temporal resolution of individual skin contacts has also been shown by asking subjects to resolve rapidly sequenced taps to different (rather than the same) spots on the skin (123). Thus, spatial resolution is improved by temporal disparity, and temporal resolution is facilitated by spatial disparity (124). An implication of this type of result is that the overlap of inhibitory with excitatory receptive fields within the dorsal column–lemniscal system (60) works against resolution of simultaneous stimuli but for resolution of a succession of stimuli across the skin surface. This possibility has been tested with several approaches.

In an experiment with monkeys, two punctate stimulations were delivered a second apart to the lateral calf, and discrimination of the spatial sequence (proximal then distal or vice versa) was required (117). The location of the first stimulus varied from trial to trial, so that the task could not be solved on the basis of absolute location, and the deliberate pace of the stimulus sequence put no demands upon the system for temporal resolution. Interruption of the dorsal columns elevated thresholds from 10 mm to 36 mm, but isolation of the dorsal columns produced no deficit. The adequacy of the isolated dorsal column was tested by interrupting the ipsilateral lateral column and the contralateral ventral quadrant. This experiment demonstrates a predominant role for the dorsal columns in coding the relative location of stimuli; the pathway appeared to be necessary and sufficient for spatial sequence recognition, even though the stimuli were not presented to a distal extremity. Comparison of this finding with the absolute localization and two-point tests (113,120) verifies physiologic studies indicating that the relative location of receptive fields is the spatial feature most faithfully preserved within the distorted map of the body surface in the postcentral gyrus (116).

With extended training over months following a dorsal column lesion, thresholds for tactile sequence recognition returned to normal values. Interpretations of this recovery process and the "responsible" pathways will follow later; for the present, it is important to note that no spatial test involving purely vertical indentations of the skin (as opposed to movement across the skin surface) has revealed *permanent* deficits from a dorsal column lesion. Thus, while it can be shown that the dorsal columns are normally involved in coding of spatial patterns applied orthogonally to the skin, as revealed by dorsal column isolations and by temporary dorsal column deficits on some tasks, conduction via the lateral and ventral columns can suffice when the animals are retrained on the discrimination following removal of the dorsal column input.

B. Spatiotemporal Discriminations of Tactile Stimulation

Comparisons of pattern recognition by the visual and somatosensory systems are available in an extensive literature that has evaluated reading of Braille characters or other patterns of punctate, vibratory stimulation (125). These studies have shown clearly that touch is inferior to vision with respect to usable spatial bandwidth, effective field of "view," and memory capacity. The spatially limited attention for touch and the low pass characteristics of skin force a sequential scanning strategy involving movement of a limited area of the receptor surface (e.g., a fingertip) over the stimulus (or the stimulus over the skin). With the expectation that the movement sensitivity of the dorsal column–lemniscal system is appropriate for this preferred sampling strategy, several investigations have demonstrated substantial deficits of spatial discrimination in monkeys or humans following dorsal column lesions. The tests involved identification of the direction of movement of a stimulus across the skin (126) or discrimination of geometric forms that are drawn on the skin (114). In the former case, involving monkeys, the lesions were confined to the dorsal columns, and recovery did not occur over a year of testing on the hindlimbs. Therefore, the clinical test of graphesthesia is appropriate for detecting interruption of the dorsal spinal columns. Furthermore, and most important for understanding the contributions of the dorsal column–lemniscal system to somesthetic sensations, these results indicate that *spatiotemporal sequences* are coded uniquely and critically by the dorsal columns. This conclusion is entirely consistent with the characteristic spatial *and* temporal precision of excitatory and inhibitory influences on dorsal column–lemniscal projection cells.

C. Discrimination of Textures

Compared with point-localization thresholds of several millimeters on the finger-tips of human subjects (96,122), the ability to distinguish spatial patterns by drawing a finger over surfaces of different spatial frequencies is hyperacuitive by several orders of magnitude (considering the distance between the point or edge contours) (128). This comparison stresses again the improved spatial acuity for stimulation that progresses across the skin in an uninterrupted trajectory. Although the reduplication of contours (and gaps) in a geometric pattern could improve resolution over the pair of stimuli in the point-localization test, this appears not to be a major factor. Discrimination between reduplicated patterns of punctate indentation by fixed stimulators with different average spacings can be poor even when the points are widely spaced on the hands (129). There is some advantage to a cascaded ("times square") activation of orthogonal stimulators (130), but a marked increase in acuity appears to result from tangential movement across the ridges of glabrous skin (131).

Given the deficits of direction sensitivity and graphesthesia that occur with dorsal column lesions (114,117,126,127), it is to be expected that discrimination of the spatiotemporal patterns that are presented by palpation of surfaces differing in roughness would be impaired by dorsal column lesions. Cortical lesions restricted within the core, dorsal column projection region of SI (in cytoarchitectonic area 1) do produce deficits of roughness discrimination (26,27). As it has been tested in previous investigations, however, this is not the case following dorsal column section. Ambulation over sandpaper surfaces (cats) or palpation of sandpaper cylinders (monkeys) reveals slight and temporary or no deficits following dorsal column lesions (132–134). These studies have involved both the hands and the feet, whereas the graphesthesia and direction deficits were demonstrated on the lower extremities.

Early conjecture concerning the peripheral afferents providing the most useful information for texture discrimination focused on Pacinian afferents (135), but recent and direct investigations of pattern recognition have offered convincing arguments and evidence for a maximal contribution by slowly adapting afferents, relatively degraded but supportive input from quickly adapting afferents, and little resolution of different spacings by Pacinian afferents (72,136). If Pacinian afferent input were critical for roughness discrimination, the lack of a dorsal column deficit would be understandable on the basis of a minimal projection in the dorsal columns and a lack of change in vibratory detection following dorsal column lesions (1,53), although discrimination of suprathreshold frequencies is more germane to this question. Similarly, the minor representation of slowly adapting afferents in the dorsal columns could explain the lack of roughness deficits following a dorsal column lesion. It would seem, however, that a substantial deafferentation of the distal extremities, loss of some slowly adapting conduction via the postsynaptic dorsal column path, removal of most of the supportive quickly adapting input, and disruption of the lemniscal somatotopy would impair roughness discrimination significantly—at least in the early postoperative period. An important factor for interpretation of the available data may be the use of sandpaper surfaces as textured stimuli in the lesion studies but utilization of dot patterns for the investigation of peripheral afferent responses. With the latter methodology, spatiotemporal resolution is assessed relatively purely (although wider spacings of dots will produce deeper, local indentations). Different grades of sandpaper employ different grit materials, sizes, spacings, and elevations from the layer of glue, producing qualitative changes in sharpness, penetration, and friction. These special characteristics of sandpaper could present sensory cues quite distinct from spatial pattern. For example, the distinction between sharp and dull has been attributed to the spinothalamic tract (114,137).

The exquisite sensitivity that has been demonstrated for discrimination of textural patterns questions a fundamental assumption that has permeated the majority of physiologic studies of somatosensory coding—that the receptive fields of individual units constitute the irreducible building blocks and the limiting parameter for spatial resolution. That is, tactile receptive fields are generally considered as being indiscriminate for different qualities or locations of stimulation within the boundaries of an arbitrarily defined skin area, giving the impression that the parent cell necessarily "confuses" different patterns of stimulation within its receptive field. This argument has seemed particularly compelling for units displaying uniform, rather than spotty, receptive fields (e.g., quickly adapting afferents). However, it has recently been shown that the discharge of single peripheral afferents, including quickly acting units, can differentiate the locations or the number of multiple points with a receptive field (138,138a,138b). In the simplest case, the unit can distinguish direct deformation at the receptive field center from stimulation elsewhere in the field, but other patterns of selective sensitivity and/or spatial summation have been described. For example, the discharge of a peripheral slowly adapting afferent to small probes can be equal to the summed discharge of spike frequencies produced by each probe singly (138). These results provide potential explanations for hyperacuitive tactile sensitivity, and they point to a need for descriptions of the microsensitivities of dorsal horn and dorsal column nuclear cells. It seems that orderly patterns of punctate sensitivity within receptive field borders would be most likely within the dorsal column nuclei, where convergence is limited to one or a few receptor categories. In contrast, the multireceptive dorsal horn cells appear to combine spatial summation with intensity sensitivity (159), which is an understandable consequence of convergence from many receptor categories from different tissue depths and with different receptive field patterns.

D. Stereognosis

Another test of active touch that involves movement of skin across the stimulus object and has been linked traditionally to the dorsal columns is stereognosis or object recognition by haptic palpation (139). Of particular interest is the combination of proprioceptive and tactile cues to form an holistic impression of the size and shape of the object, its hardness or softness and texture, and the relative orientation and extent of any edge contours. A deficit of stereognosis from a dorsal column lesion could mean that any one or more of these component discriminations is deteriorated and essential or that the combination of cues to form an overall Gestalt is particularly dependent upon the dorsal column-lemniscal system. A lack of deficit could indicate that none of the component cues is deteriorated by the lesion, or some unaffected signals could compensate for the disruption of others. The latter explanation may be appropriate to explain little or no deficit in discriminating geometric forms (e.g., cubes from hexahedrons) (134). These findings stand in contrast to the following dorsal column deficits: (1) elevated thresholds for discriminating the relative size of discs impressed on the skin (140), (2) raised thresholds for discriminating different pressures applied to the skin (15), (3) impaired ability to regulate motoric force within a narrow range (141), (4) diminished facility with fractionated movements of the digits (142), (5) decreased sensitivity to relative hardness (134), and (6) an inability to discriminate directions of movement over the skin (126) or identify shapes that are cut in relief and traced (without visual cues) by scanning the fingers along edge contours (127). How can a monkey discriminate, by palpation, between three-dimensional forms when there is difficulty: timing movements of the fingers, regulating the pressure exerted during grasp, sensing resistance of the object to palpation or grasp, knowing the direction in which the object moves over the skin, and appreciating the presence, orientation, and relative locations of edge contours? Most of the deficits on tests of component capacities for stereognosis were subtotal and temporary, and it is not known whether transient stereognostic deficits would have been observed at threshold levels of difference in object shapes. Criterion performance on the stereognostic task required some retraining with discriminanda clearly supra-threshold for differences in shapes with edge contours, and a round-oval discrimination required more trials to relearn than were needed preoperatively (134). Thus, it is concluded that dorsal column lesions do not produce an enduring astereognosis, but component sensory and sensory-motor capacities are disrupted to the extent that at least temporary impairment of fine, haptic distinctions of three-dimensional objects should be observed. The multiplicity of available cues for stereognostic discriminations makes it an undesirable test, unless certain features can be varied to the exclusion of others; and thresholds should be measured (143).

An important question posed by tests of stereognosis concerns the relative contributions of proprioceptors versus cutaneous receptors for object discrimination. The dorsal column deficit in recognition of patterns cut in relief (127) could depend upon a loss of spatiotemporal, tactile cues (126) presented as a finger follows an edge contour and changes occur in the direction and location of cutaneous stimulation (e.g., at a corner). Also, sequential "readings" of proprioceptive input and/or motor output could form an image of the finger's path in space. The severe deficit of contour recognition by tracing that occurs following a dorsal lesion suggests critical involvement of the dorsal columns in spatiotemporal sequences of proprioceptive input because proprioceptive cues did not compensate for the expected tactile deficit. A concordance of tactile and proprioceptive effects would be consistent with the preponderance in the dorsal columns of quickly adapting movement detectors from both superficial and deep receptors. In contrast, the lack of deficits on tests of stereognosis involving grasp of objects could mean that position sense is intact for the hands following dorsal column interruption. That is, the preferred strategy for judging the size and shape of three-dimensional discriminanda may be to grasp and hold the objects and monitor the relative positions of the fingers as signaled by slowly adapting position detectors. Slowly adapting proprioceptors are underrepresented in the fasciculus gracilis (144), and static position sense (at the knee) is unaffected by dorsal column lesions (145). More information is needed on the effects of dorsal column lesions on senses of movement and position of joints at the distal extremities, particularly the hand.

E. Summary

There have been few experiments that have demonstrated enduring sensory deficits following complete dorsal column lesions. An enduring or "permanent" impairment is defined here as a significant decrease of sensitivity that is maintained through more than 2 months of postoperative training on the relevant sensory test. Discriminations of the speed (114) or direction (126) of stimulus movement over the skin are lost irrevocably and appear to underlie enduring deficits on tests of graphesthesia. There are disruptions of some motor functions of the distal extremities (see later), and these may or may not be accompanied by losses of "conscious" proprioception. The evidence is incomplete on whether vibratory sensitivity is affected, since it is necessary to distinguish between detection thresholds and capacities for frequency discrimination within the ranges of quickly acting and Pacinian afferents. Negative findings are to be expected on tasks requiring simple detection of a stimulus because none of the receptor categories is exclusively represented in the dorsal columns. Tests of spatiotactile resolution can reveal deficits from dorsal column lesions (117,140), but recovery has been observed with retraining on all purely spatial discriminations. Only spatiotemporal coding of tangential cutaneous stimulation and spatiotemporal programming of certain motor sequences are disturbed irrevocably by interruption of the dorsal columns (54,126,134,141,146,147). This leaves a variety of presumed lemniscal functions that are dependent upon non-dorsal column conduction or are coded by combined inputs from the dorsal columns and another pathway or other pathways.

The few experiments that have lesioned and isolated the dorsal columns and tested for tactile or proprioceptive capacities have demonstrated a functional redundancy of the dorsal columns with other pathways for touch detection (148,149), sequence recognition for punctate touch (117), and static position sense at the knee joint (145). Performance on these tests can be normal with lesion or isolation of the dorsal columns. Similarly, although sufficiency of the dorsal columns has not been assessed by dorsal column isolation on the following tasks, recovery of touch intensity (15), geometric form (134,140), and roughness (132,133), discriminations after dorsal column lesions demonstrates that some other pathway(s) can compensate for the absence of dorsal column conduction. Selective interruption of the ipsilateral lateral column or contralateral ventral quadrant, in combination with dorsal column lesions, has indicated that some, but not all, of these functions depend upon dorsal or dorsolateral input to the medial lemniscus.

VI. CONTRIBUTIONS TO CUTANEOUS AND PROPRIOCEPTIVE SENSATIONS BY PATHWAYS IN THE LATERAL AND VENTRAL SPINAL COLUMNS

Lesions of the ipsilateral dorsal quadrant should produce total deafferentation of the spinal inputs to the medial lemniscus (24). Dorsal quadrant sections in carnivores have produced deficits of touch thresholds (delivered by air puffs to hairy skin) (150) and induced a loss of reactivity to slowly adapting tactile input (151).

In contrast, touch detection thresholds are unaffected by ipsilateral dorsal quadrant lesions in primates (15), and difference thresholds for touch intensity are elevated only transiently. The disparity between carnivores and monkeys with respect to touch detection thresholds could be related to procedural variations or to organizational features of the pathways. The studies of carnivores involved stimulation of proximal hairy skin, but the primates were stimulated on glabrous skin of the feet. The stimuli received by cats and dogs were selective for proximally located hair afferents (150) or slowly adapting receptors (151) that project primarily to the dorsal horn, but the application of von Frey hairs to the glabrous skin of monkeys would activate quickly adapting and pacinian receptors at threshold intensities (152). Also, the capacity for recovery with extensive training was not assessed for the carnivores. Thus, we are still in doubt as to whether the "protopathic" detection of light cutaneous contact is primarily lemniscal, spinothalamic, or both. In contrast, primates with dorsal quadrant lesions exhibit "permanently" elevated thresholds for spatiotactile discriminations of point separation (the two point test), relative locations of points (spatial sequence recognition), or the distance between edge contours (117,120,140).

A. Spatiotactile Discrimination

Spatiotactile discriminations of simplistic punctate patterns or geometric forms are: (1) deteriorated temporarily (or not at all) by a dorsal column lesion (117, 120,134,140), (2) not affected by lesions of the lateral columns (either the ipsilateral dorsolateral column or the contralateral ventral quadrant, or both) (117,120); and (c) significantly and "permanently" disrupted by interruption of the spinal lemniscal tracts (the primary and secondary dorsal column systems, the dorsal column-dorsolateral column-dorsal column projection, and the spinocervicothalamic tract) (114,117,120,140). These findings are of historical interest because they revive the conclusion that the medial lemniscus is the critical channel for high spatiotactile resolution. More specifically, the somatotopic map of the lemniscal system is necessary for spatial resolution, but a high level of spatial discrimination can be maintained by *either* dorsal or lateral column inputs to the mapping system(s). It can be presumed that the dorsal and the dorsolateral funiculi support spatial discrimination by providing different but complementary forms of spatial information.

When human subjects judge the size of an object impressed on the skin (e.g., a disc, presenting a flat surface bounded by a continuous edge contour), discriminations can be made on the basis of distances between edge contours and/or by comparing the surface areas of the stimuli (153). Sensations related to the edge are more salient than those of the interior surface, and therefore discrimation of size should be disrupted, at least temporarily, by loss of inputs that contribute to the clarity of the sensation elicited by an edge contour. Physiologic evidence for such an effect of dorsal column lesions is provided by observations that responsive ventrobasal units in lesioned animals often exhibit poorly defined receptive field boundaries (154), which contrast with the sharp receptive field limits observed in intact animals. Possibly, the transient impairment of tactile size discrimination following a dorsal column lesion (140) can be attributed to less sharply defined spatial configurations of the evoked neural activity. The recovery of size discrimination could then be based on relearning to interpret the new spatial profiles of neural activity. For example, calculations of convergence factors for spinocervical tract neurons has revealed a constancy that would permit derivation of stimulus area by "counting" the number of active spinocervicothalamic units (1). Detailed information is needed on the aggregate neural responses to spatially defined stimuli following lesions of the lemniscal pathways, permitting correlation of available spatial codes with sensory capacity.

It has seened reasonable to assume that the clarity of edge contours is provided by afferent inhibitory interactions within the central nervous system (112, 155). If this were the case, then dorsal column lesions should permanently impair discriminations requiring edge detection because of the unusual precision of inhibitory and excitatory receptive field sizes and locations within the dorsal column projection (60). However, it has been shown that both quickly and slowly adapting peripheral afferents are selectively sensitive to contours, producing high rates of discharge to points or edges as compared with compression by surfaces (156-158). Thus, the profile of activity in dorsal horn cells of projection to the lateral columns should reflect to some extent the locations of contours. In addition, the discharge of the secondary cells is gradated in proportion to the area of a stimulus within the confines of the receptive fields (159), and area provides a relevant cue for derivation of stimulus size by human subjects (153).

B. Anatomic and Physiologic Correlates of Recovery of Spatial Discriminations Following Dorsal Column Lesions

Afferents in the dorsal and the dorsolateral columns converge onto the dorsal column nuclei and collaborate in determining the output of medial lemniscus projection cells (21), and dorsal column-lemniscal and spinocervicothalamic tract-lemniscal projection cells converge onto a common zone of thalamic cells (16). The lemniscal system contains both a core of exclusive projections by the dorsal columns and a fringe of convergent systems with flexible capacities to accept inputs from different channels and to survive loss of one channel. Following *acute* transection of the fasciculus gracilis in cats, responsive units can be found in the cell nest region of the nucleus gracilis (the dorsal column core) (160), but they are few in number, and their response properties are quite different from normal. Receptive fields can be quite large, somatotopy is no longer evident, responses are weak, and habituation to repeated stimulation is frequently seen. A maximum of 50% of the few drivable cells in the core region are responsive to light tactile stimulation. Many cells give only weak responses and have high thresholds, which presumes input from deep receptors (e.g., muscle and joint receptors) or nociceptors. Numerous cells exhibit spontaneous activity (not seen in normal nuclei) but are not activated by peripheral stimulation; this should produce a high level of noise in rostral relays of the lemniscal system.

Within 7-14 days following dorsal column section, the number of synaptic boutons decreases within the cell nest region of the gracile nucleus, and cell somata sizes are reduced in the same region (161). When recordings are made within the dorsal column nuclei (162) or the somatosensory cortex (111) following a *chronic* dorsal column lesion, there appears to be little filling in of the core projection system. Cells with small receptive fields for light tactile stimulation within the dorsal column–deafferented area are absent or rare, with response patterns different from normal (e.g., rapid habituation). There can be a filling in of the fringes of the core region, with expansion of the distribution of cells with receptive fields in afferented skin regions, but the core representation of the distal extremity does not recover from dorsal column lesion. "New" receptive fields within the zone of deafferentation have been reported not to have orderly somatotopic relationships. Possibly, an important feature of chronically reduced input to the dorsal column nuclei (relative to acute lesions) is a reduced proportion of cells with spontaneous activity but no sensory-related discharge (162).

Following deafferentation of the core system, the noncore, convergent lemniscal projection system is presumed to subserve rudimentary spatial discrimination in the acute stages of dorsal column deafferentation; absolute localization, two-point discrimination, and stereognosis are intact in the early postoperative period (113,120,134). Furthermore, and quite important, the convergent projection system appears to be capable of anatomic and physiologic reorganization and functional recovery; thresholds for relative localization of points and edges on the skin return to normal levels with retraining after dorsal column section (117,140).

Following a dorsal column lesion, the core dorsal column–lemniscal system is severely deafferented from the peripheral receptor sheet; noise levels are high, somatotopy is lost, and anatomic reorganization is minimal, if present. In contrast, by sparing sources of spatially organized input to the fringe lemniscal system (from the contralateral ventral quadrant and the ipsilateral lateral column) an organizational fabric of spatial referents is maintained within the somatotopic thalamocortical projections to SI and SII. Spared ascending and intrahemispheric and interhemispheric projections to these maps are in spatial register within the convergent system, and therefore sprouting over short distances by these intact systems should increase the population of central cells with appropriately ordered receptive fields. That is, a reafferented central cell is likely to have a recovered receptive field similar to the original field. Numerous frustrated attempts to define differences in dorsal column-lesioned animals in the gross structure of noncore, somatosensory maps within the cerebral cortex make apparent a high degree of somatotopic precision within the convergent system (163-166). Furthermore, anatomic reorganization in the central nervous system by axonal sprouting has been shown to be optimal and qualitatively distinct in regions of convergent projection following partial deafferentation (167).

A great deal more information is needed on the relationships between the core and convergent regions at different levels of the neuraxis (dorsal column nuclei, nucleus ventralis posterolateralis, and SI cortex) in order to understand the mechanisms of functional recovery from dorsal column lesions, but certain patterns are emerging. For example, the area of the nucleus ventralis posterolateralis in the cat that receives the most dense convergence from the dorsal column and spinocervicothalamic lemniscal paths (the fringes of VPL_1 and VPL_m) (168) is also a divergent pathway that distributes information widely to the somatosensory and motor cortices. The core dorsal column–lemniscal system is connected to cytoarchitectural areas 3B and 1 of the postcentral gyrus (170); the fringe lemniscal system of projections from the dorsal and lateral columns sends thalamocortical afferents to the motor, SI, and SII cortical areas (169). The distribution of lemniscal information to each of the cortical somatotopic maps fits expectations that the medial lemniscus would serve as the principal resource of highly ordered input for spatial somatosensory-motor functions.

The acute deficits of spatial resolution that have been observed following a dorsal column lesion are to be expected on the basis of severe deafferentation of the core lemniscal system and a substantial, but subtotal, loss of ascending inputs to the fringe lemniscal system. However, if the animals are retrained on the affected discriminations, a consistent pattern of recovery is observed. Following several weeks to several months of testing, thresholds begin to drop from levels in excess of four times preoperative values, and discrimination gradually improves to normal over 2-3 months of testing (171). The onset of recovery is consistent with the expected time course of axonal sprouting within the fringe lemniscal system (172). This can be shown most clearly following a second dorsal column lesion in animals that have learned previously to discriminate the sensory signals that have been altered by a primary lesion of the other dorsal column (171). An animal that has recovered completely from the first dorsal column lesion should be able to respond to the relevant new cues on the side of the second lesion, as soon as these signals are present. The onset of recovery is earlier, on the average, following the second dorsal column lesion, but it does not appear earlier than 2 weeks postoperatively. Furthermore, the time-course of recovery, from onset of improvement to achievement of normal discrimination, is the same following primary and secondary dorsal column lesions. These observations indicate that anatomic reorganization makes functional recovery possible with retraining, but the occurrence of grossly observable sprouting does not, by itself, provide functional restitution following dorsal column lesions. It is not yet clear whether the anatomic reorganization depends upon retraining (173) or whether the retraining is required to adapt to the altered information provided by a process of sprouting that occurs independent of training (or whether a combination of these possibilities is operative). It is apparent that there is little transfer of recovery from one dorsal column lesion to another in the same animal; and the process of functional restoration is quite gradual and dependent upon task-specific practice. The same conclusion has resulted from systematic study of recovery from deficits in tactile discrimination of spatial frequency following cortical lesions (174).

Primary lesions of the dorsolateral column leave the core projection intact and only partially deafferent the fringe areas of lemniscal termination (111,170, 175). The absence of spatiotactile deficits following ipsilateral dorsolateral column lesions (or even after isolation of the dorsal column lemniscal pathway) (117) indicates that an intact core projection compensates for partial deafferentation of the fringe lemniscal zones. Thus, the results of a dorsal column or ipsilateral dorsolateral column lesion suggest that the core and fringe lemniscal systems can independently or cooperatively mediate spatiotactile resolution. It should be recognized that complete deafferentation of the lemniscal fringe is not produced by either dorsal column or ipsilateral dorsolateral column lesions. In fact, combined section of the dorsal and dorsolateral columns does not remove all ascending input to the thalamic fringe zones of lemniscal projection, since spinothalamic convergence within these areas is now apparent (16). These recent anatomic findings may explain the fact that ipsilateral dorsal quadrant lesions do not obliterate all discriminative tactile or proprioceptive functions in primates.

Although the two-point tactile test is not affected by ipsilateral dorsal column or dorsolateral column lesions, thresholds are elevated greater than fourfold by ipsilateral dorsal quadrant section (M. Levitt, C. Vierck, and R. Schwartzman, unpublished observations). Combination of ipsilateral dorsal column and spinothalamic section does not disrupt two-point discrimination on the feet, and therefore the test is specific for integrity of the lemniscal spinal pathways as a whole (both the dorsal and dorsolateral columns must be lesioned to produce a deficit). Because of absent to minimal two-point deficits following dorsal column section but substantial impairments after dorsal quadrant lesion, the two-point test can serve as an accurate and convenient indicant of complete lemniscal interruption.

A   Lesion common to both patients - bilateral interruption of dorsal
    columns. Bilateral deficits:

SPEED OF MOVEMENT OVER SKIN   SPEED OF MOVEMENT OVER SKIN

GRAPHESTHESIA   GRAPHESTHESIA

DIRECTION OF MOVEMENT   DIRECTION OF MOVEMENT OVER
    OVER SKIN   SKIN

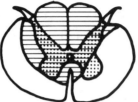

B   Additional deficits from R. side of patient #1; lesion of the
    ipsilateral dorsal column and portions of the dorsolateral-lemniscal
    and spinothalamic tracts:

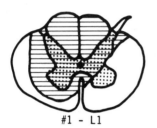

TWO-POINT DISCRIMINATION

TACTILE LOCALIZATION

SHARP-DULL DISCRIMINATION

THERMOSENSITIVITY

#1 - L1

C   Additional deficits from both sides of patient #2; complete lesion
    of the dorsal and dorsolateral lemniscal pathways:

TWO-POINT DISCRIMINATION   TWO-POINT DISCRIMINATION

TACTILE LOCALIZATION   TACTILE LOCALIZATION

VIBRATION DETECTION   VIBRATION DETECTION

PRESSURE DETECTION   PRESSURE DETECTION

DETECTION OF MOVEMENT OVER   DETECTION OF MOVEMENT OVER
    SKIN   SKIN

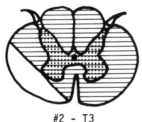

#2 - T3

D   Unilateral <u>sparing</u> in patient #2 from isolation of the ipsilateral
    or contralateral anterolateral column:

JOINT MOVEMENT DETECTION   SHARP-DULL DISCRIMINATION

DISCRIMINATION OF JOINT   THERMOSENSITIVITY
    MOVEMENT DIRECTION

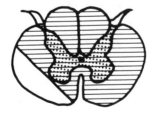

In some respects, the test of spatial sequence recognition serves also as an indicant of lemniscal integrity, since normal discrimination recovers after dorsal column section, is unaffected by an ipsilateral dorsolateral column lesion, and is permanently impaired by interruption of the ipsilateral dorsal quadrant (117; Fig. 4B). However, enduring deficits are produced similarly by combining dorsal column with spinothalamic tract lesions. For this discrimination of the relative position of points on the body surface, loss of either the dorsolateral or spinothalamic contributions to the topographic thalamocortical projection system disrupts discrimination (in the absence of the dorsal columns). Thus, an absolute separation of lemniscal and spinothalamic functions may be artificial, albeit useful. It is clear that the spinothalamic tract is not solely responsible for discriminative tactile or proprioceptive functions (i.e., primary contralateral ventral quadrant lesions produce no deficit), but afferents to the topographic thalamocortical projection system can be reduced such that inputs from both the dorsolateral and the spinothalamic systems are required for spatial resolution. This dependency on spinothalamic tract input occurs when the contralateral ventral quadrant lesion is primary or secondary in relation to interruption of the dorsal columns. Therefore, the effect cannot be ascribed to removal of an abnormally strong contribution from the spinothalamic tract by sprouting in response to a primary dorsal column lesion. Furthermore, evidence from human patients with partial transections of the spinal cord confirms dependency of spatiotactile resolution on both lateral columns in the absence of the dorsal columns (114). Dorsal column lesions did not produce impairments of absolute localization or two-point discrimination (Fig. 3A), whereas dorsal column plus contralateral ventral quadrant involvement (Fig. 3B) or isolation of the spinothalamic tract (Fig. 3C) produced substantial deficits on both tasks.

C. Proprioception

Monkeys have been trained to discriminate movement at the knee joint to different end positions of the calf (145; M. Levitt, C. Vierck, and J. Ovelman-Levitt,

Figure 3 The results of sensory evaluation of two human patients after traumatic, subtotal interruption of the spinal white matter at L1 (patient no. 1) or T3 (patient no. 2) are summarized as. A, Bilateral deficits common to both patients and attributable primarily to interruption of the dorsal columns. B, Additional deficits from one side of patient no. 1, attributable to complete interruption of the dorsal columns and partial involvement of the IDC and CVQ. C, Bilateral deficits in patient no. 2 (but not patient no. 1) attributable to complete interruption of the dorsal and dorsolateral columns bilaterally. D, Functions that are *spared* in patient no. 2 and are therefore conveyed by the IVQ (left side) or the CVQ (right side). (Adapted from Ref. 114.)

unpublished observations), and thoracic spinal lesions affected thresholds as follows (Fig. 4A): (1) no change following DC lesions, (2) no impairment as the result of severing the ipsilateral dorsoal column and the dorsal half of the ipsilateral dorsolateral column, (3) a doubling of thresholds following ipsilateral hemisection, (4) no ipsilateral or contralateral deficit consequent to section of one ventral quadrant, (5) normal thresholds following isolation of either the ipsilateral dorsal column or lateral column, and (6) severe deficits after lesions of the ipsilateral dorsal quadrant and the contralateral ventral quadrant. These results demonstrate sufficiency for the ipsilateral dorsal column or the ipsilateral lateral column (item 5 in previous list) but not for the spinothalamic tract (item 3; although some residual information concerning limb position is available following ipsilateral hemisection). All deficits resulted from damage to *both* the dorsal and the lateral columns *ipsilaterally*, and the amount of damage to the lateral column(s) appeared to be an important determinant of the extent to which thresholds were elevated (item 2 vs. 3 or 6). These conclusions are supported by studies of human patients showing that: (1) isolation of one dorsal column by section of the ipsilateral lateral column and the contralateral ventral quadrant produced no detectable impairment of limb position sense (176); and (2) lesions of the ipsilateral dorsal column, produced no obvious deficit (Fig. 3A); but (3) interruption of the ipsilateral dorsal column and the ipsilateral lateral column produced impairments in discrimination of the direction of joint movement (Fig. 3D, right side). An important contribution by axons in the midportion of the ipsilateral lateral column is indicated by comparison of the left and right sides of panel D in Figure 3. This finding is supported by a recent physiologic study showing slowly adapting proprioceptive input to cells with axons distributed in the midportion of the ipsilateral lateral column (177).

Apparently, accurate determination of the endpoint of a passive limb movement can be accomplished either on the basis of quickly adapting afferents in the dorsal columns or by the dorsal horn projections to the lateral columns by multireceptive neurons receiving slowly adapting input. In contrast to the classic notion that position sense depends critically upon the dorsal columns, current knowledge of slowly adapting afferent sorting from the fasciculus gracilis leaves us surprised that the isolated dorsal column preparation can sense limb position. In order for the dorsal columns to provide the sole source of afferent information for derivation of limb position, it would appear that an integration of velocity would have to be performed, if dorsal column–lemniscal projection cells do not have restricted receptive fields for joint angle (144). The velocity of movement to the discriminated end positions was randomized for monkeys, and they responded quickly (within 500 msec) following termination of the passive limb movement. Hence, simple velocity was not a relevant cue. In order for the animals to derive the end positions from the discharge of afferents that respond to movement through most of the physiologic range, it would be necessary to monitor the rate and duration of discharge (determined by velocity and distance). This "strategy" applies both to quickly and slowly adapting afferents, since the animals discriminated end positions during the velocity-dependent onset discharge of slowly adapting joint afferents (178).

What is the afferent pathway in the ipsilateral lateral column that carries information sufficient to support limb position sense for the hindlimbs? An apparent lack of sensitivity to combined dorsal column and superficial dorso-lateral column interruption (Fig. 4A), coupled with substantial deficits follow-ing lesions involving the dorsal column and most of the ipsilateral dorsal column, indicates that the dorsolateral lemniscal pathways may not be the responsible channels. In contrast, on tests of spatiotactile resolution even slight involvement of the ipsilateral dorsolateral column adds significantly to the consequences of a dorsal column lesion (117,140). Furthermore, recordings from the core region of the nucleus gracilis suggest that slowly adapting information from joints and muscles is not relayed to the thalamus from this major source of lemniscal pro-jection neurons (144). These observations indicate that the lemniscal projection of slowly adapting hindlimb proprioceptors emanates from a separate region of the dorsal column nuclear complex (e.g., nucleus z [92]). This explanation would depend upon a segregation of tactile and proprioceptive afferents in the ipsilateral lateral column, with the deep afferents projecting in the midlateral column to nucleus z and the cutaneous pathway traversing the dorsolateral column to nucleus gracilis and the spinocervicothalamic tract. Afferents to nucleus z appear to course both in the dorsolateral column (35,92) and via collaterals of the dorsal spinocerebellar tract (179). The midlateral location of the proprioceptive pathway suggests revival of the possibility that the spino-cerebellar tracts supply critical information for conscious proprioception (178a). This could be accomplished by collaterals to the dorsal column nuclear complex or by projection via the cerebellum (179,179a). The evidence does not favor dependence of the hindlimb lemniscal system upon conduction to and from the cerebellum (30,91,180).

D. Population Coding of Touch Intensity by the Convergent Spinal Projection Systems

In order to understand the composition of the lemniscal pathways it has been necessary to characterize single units, but to appreciate the functional capacities of the system it is important to reconstruct the total profiles of neural activity that are offered by the component pathways in response to tactile stimuli. It is obvious that spatial coding must be accomplished by interpretation of activity in populations of cells, but evidence is beginning to suggest that other somato-sensory discrimintions that might be derived from the rate of activity in properly tuned single cells rely additionally on the number of cells (or the particular set

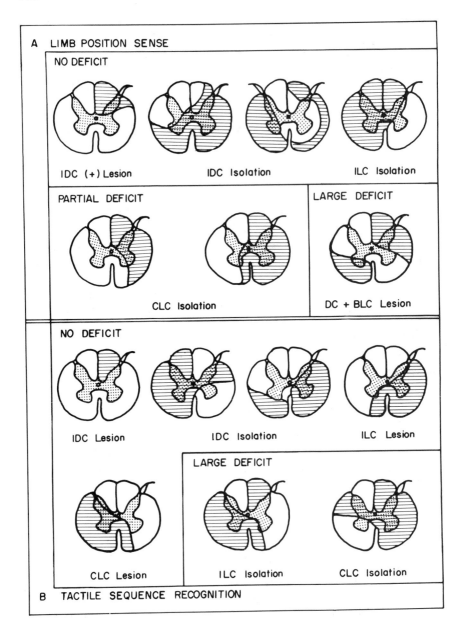

A LIMB POSITION SENSE

NO DEFICIT

IDC (+) Lesion   IDC Isolation   ILC Isolation

PARTIAL DEFICIT   LARGE DEFICIT

CLC Isolation   DC + BLC Lesion

NO DEFICIT

IDC Lesion   IDC Isolation   ILC Lesion

LARGE DEFICIT

CLC Lesion   ILC Isolation   CLC Isolation

B TACTILE SEQUENCE RECOGNITION

of cells) activated by each stimulus. An example is provided by sensations of touch-pressure.

Activity in one or a few peripheral afferents can permit detection of a tactile stimulus (181), and terminals from all classes of low-threshold afferents are distributed both to the dorsal column nuclei and to the dorsal horn. The rostral projections of slowly adapting afferents have not been determined with certainty, but they terminate extensively in dorsal horn laminae III-V (1), gaining access to multireceptive cells with secondary projections in the ipsilateral dorsal column ipsilateral lateral column, and contralateral ventral quadrant. Therefore, it is not surprising that touch detection thresholds are little changed by interruption of each major cord sector (15,114,151). Also, it is possible that the rate of discharge by one or a few slowly adapting tactile afferents could support discrimination of the relative intensities of different stimuli to the same receptive field, since correlations have been good between slowly adapting discharge and magnitude estimations of skin indentation (182). If the assumptions of a widely distributed projection and a capacity to discriminate levels of activity in one or a few slowly adapting cells are correct, then difference thresholds for light pressure should survive section of individual pathways. Surprisingly, significant deficits of pressure discrimination: (1) result from dorsal column section, (2) recover with retraining, (3) return following secondary interruption of the ipsilateral dorsolateral column, and (4) recover again with extensive testing (15).

Even a temporary deficit of pressure discrimination following a dorsal column lesion is surprising because of emphasis that has been placed on the dominance of quickly adapting afferents within the dorsal column and their lack of sensitivity to amount of skin indentation (2,39). However, the threshold sensitivity at the receptive field center for different quickly adapting afferents

---

Figure 4 Idealized drawings of spinal cord lesions administered to monkeys trained to produce psychophysical thresholds for limb position sense at the knee (A; upper panels) or discrimination of the order in which two points were touched on the lateral calf (B; lower panels). The presence of a dorsal root indicates the laterality of threshold tests referred to in each panel. A, Limb position sense was unimpaired by lesion or isolation of either the IDC or the ILC. Interruption of both the IDC and the ILC produced an elevation of thresholds from an average of 5.9–13.4° of rotation (four animals). Interruption of the IDC, ILC, and CVQ produced an inability to discriminate 34° of rotation (one animal). B, Tactile sequence recognition was unimpaired or recovered from partial deficits after interruption or isolation of the IDC, but combined lesions of the IDC with either the ILC or the CVQ produce substantial threshold elevations, from an average of 10.4 mm to >40 mm. (A from M. Levitt, C. J. Vierck, and J. Ovelman-Levitt, unpublished observations; B from Ref. 117.)

varies over a substantial range that may be expanded at higher levels of the central nervous system (183). Also, the sensitivity of peripheral and especially of central quickly adapting units falls off toward the periphery of the receptive field (138a,138b). These features provide the basis for a population code for pressure by units that do not individually differentiate between a substantial range of forces applied to the skin. That is, the number of quickly adapting cells responding to a stimulus could reflect the force of its application to the skin, and if so, dorsal column lesions would disrupt pressure discrimination. Alternatively, the projection of slowly adapting afferents to the postsynaptic dorsal column system could account for a contribution to pressure discrimination by the dorsal columns. Either way, the succession of deficits and recovery following dorsal and dorsolateral lesions argues for population coding of pressure discrimination.

The saturation of dorsal column output with activity in a proportion (approximately 50%) of its input from a peripheral nerve (184) indicates that the dorsal columns present useful information only for light stimuli. That is, tactile receptors supplying the dorsal columns are located superficially and give saturated responses to relatively light pressures, and dorsal column afferents converge onto lemniscal projection cells such that maximum output is achieved with activity in 50% of the incoming afferents. Possibly, the fringe projection to the lemniscal system from the dorsal horn codes intensity by total neural activity, which would depend primarily on the number of active cells at intensities near threshold and the total number of impulses at higher values. Discrimination of the intensity of skin vibration also has been ascribed to population codes derived from the number of active cells or the number of impulses (185). These considerations dictate that psychophysical measurements evaluate discriminability throughout a stimulus continuum in order to characterize coding operations involved in representation of a sensory quality. That is, measurement of detection thresholds can be insensitive to actual involvement of a neural system in coding of suprathreshold discriminations along a sensory continuum (100).

VII. MOTOR FUNCTIONS OF THE DORSAL COLUMNS

A. Dorsal Column Inputs to Motor Systems

Feedback regulation of motor activities is accomplished by input from receptors in the skin, joint capsules, ligaments, tendons, and muscles, and these afferent categories distribute in various proportions to a plethora of motor systems that converge ultimately onto spinal motoneurones. The dorsal column-lemniscal system projects to the cerebellum directly (179) and via the dorsal accessory portion of the inferior olivary complex (14), to the brain stem reticular formation (e.g., medullary nucleus gigantocellularis) (12) and the inferior central raphe nucleus (179a), to the intercollicular nucleus and the red nucleus within the midbrain (11,14), to diencephalic portions of circuitry relating the basal ganglia with motor areas of the cerebral cortex (e.g., zona incerta; 186), and via the ventrobasal thalamus (16,186) to the pericruciate motor-sensory cortex (MsI; cytoarchitectural area 4 [187]) and the sensory-motor cortex (SmI and SmII; cytoarchitectural areas 3, 1, 2, and the parietal operculum [170]). It would be restrictive to label these structures as motor, but each is implicated in motor control. Since most subroutines of motor programming can utilize fast, spatially discrete feedback concerning the progress and consequences of somatic activity, it is not surprising that the dorsal columns project to most of the major motor systems.

As obvious as the preceding statement seems, there are numerous examples of adaptive motoric capacities recovering in human patients or laboratory animals with lesions of the dorsal spinal roots (142,188,189), thalamic motor relays (190), or the corticospinal tract (87,191,192). For example, animals deafferented by dorsal rhizotomy can ambulate or reach and grasp accurately in space, with or without visual guidance. Apparently, the specific functions performed by afferent input to the motor systems listed previously (plus the recipients of further efferent projections) are expressed as refinements to more general programs for moving about in proper orientation to objects in three-dimensional space. As an example, consider the intercollicular projection from the dorsal column-lemniscal system, contributing to sensory-motor programs that integrate directed attention via orienting reactions involving the different sensory modalities. For each of the sensory projections to the tectum from the visual, auditory, and somatosensory systems the input cells are topographically ordered and preferentially responsive to transient stimulus movement (193). The lemniscal system provides these characteristics (194), and some behavioral deficits following dorsal column lesions could be attributed to a loss of tectal functions. When attempting to perform complex sequential acts to capture a moving target (simulating prey-catching behavior) dorsal column-lesioned cats frequently become disoriented if the target is missed and displaced (147). Although normal or lesioned cats can perform integrated sequences of muscular contractions that result in projection of the body and one limb to meet the moving target, certain fine details or components of the motor act are disrupted by a dorsal column lesion. One of these is the ability to adjust to rapid changes in trajectory of the target at the point of contact. Other sensorimotor impairments can be identified by focusing in on different aspects of movement control in controlled testing situations (discussed later).

B. Initiation of Motor Acts

Initiation of "conscious" motor acts may well involve complex interactions between the frontal and parietal cortices (195-198), the cerebellum (199), the basal ganglia (200), and the thalamus (201). Convergence of lemniscal inputs with these systems in thalamic nuclei ventralis posterolateralis and ventralis lateralis (170,187,202), and distribution of lemniscal information from SI to the frontal and posterior parietal cortex (197,203) suggests that some aspects of intentional movement should be disrupted by dorsal column lesions. For example, the spatial program for a directed ballistic projection of a limb could be voided or disrupted by an absent or distorted somatosensory estimate of limb position. In addition, accurate moment-to-moment information concerning limb position and movement and the timing and location of contact with the environment constitute critical links in the match-mismatch functions attributed to the motor cortex (MsI) (204).

Standing on the dorsum of the foot, which can be observed for weeks following a dorsal column lesion (205-207), constitutes striking evidence that proprioceptive input concerning the distal limbs is insufficiently utilized by the animals to initiate adaptive behavior. Other dorsal column deficits in the early postoperative period (of several weeks to several months) are indicative of inadequate tactile and proprioceptive feedback for motor programming. Observations of reduced "spontaneous" motor activity, reluctance to use a limb affected by a unilateral dorsal column lesion, and catatonic postures in blindfolded monkeys (206) suggest a strong lemniscal contribution to the initiation of purposive motor acts. However, these gross abnormalities of posture and motoric initiative recover with time and experience. Also, to be sure that the programming of limb movements is affected by lemniscal lesions, it is necessary to eliminate the possibility that the animals simply are not motivated to use the affected limb. That is, the deficits could be related to coordination rather than to initiation, and the monkeys could "give up" on a limb that is suddenly awkward. To circumvent this problem, it is necessary to train animals to emit certain motor actions for reinforcement, when the normally innervated control limb is restrained from participation in the task.

Surprisingly few studies have measured reaction times in situations that permit control of the eliciting stimuli, but there is a suggestion that initiation of jumping responses (in cats) by visual cues is delayed slightly (147). These results contrast with the previously discussed finding of normal reaction times for a spatially directed projection of a normal limb, cued by spatially discrete stimulation of a dorsal column–deafferented limb (113). Thus, direct feedback from the limb to be moved is important for response initiation and is supplied in part by the dorsal columns, but a more general specification of the body image is not dependent upon integrity of the dorsal columns. Many of the functions served exclusively by the dorsal column–lemniscal system involve "unconscious" feedback regulation of motor actions.

Involvement of the dorsal column–lemniscal system in the initiation of automatic motor functions is indicated by deficits in reflexive placing reactions that have been observed following dorsal column interruption (205-207). Exacerbation of these effects is produced by interruption of the dorsolateral column with the dorsal columns (205,207) or by dorsal column lesions near the entry levels of the relevant afferents (i.e., just rostral to the brachial or lumbosacral plexus) (207). For example, both tactile and proprioceptive placing of a limb following touch of hairs or bending the digits against a surface (with vision occluded) are diminished in frequency by combined dorsal column and dorsolateral column lesions, but only tactile placing is noticeably affected by lesions confined to the dorsal columns (207), and recovery is observed over weeks (205,209).

C. Guidance of Ballistic Limb Movements

When the demands for precision of the terminal motor activities of the distal extremity are varied systematically, and the animals are forced to rely upon somatosensory feedback, the factors influencing ballistic limb projection can be made apparent. Most of the paradigms that have been used to investigate the motor capacities of animals with partial or total somatosensory deafferentation have relied upon visual cues to define the goal location, and visualization of the limbs is often permitted as the animals perform the task. Under these optimal conditions, rats and cats grossly misplace the distal extremities on elevated beams following dorsal column lesions or dorsal rhizotomy (205,210,217), but substantial recovery is observed (205,208,210,217). When monkeys are required to project a limb to targets in extrapersonal space, distal extremity placement is most revealing of limb deafferentation. For example, when the start point of a well-trained motor act is constant from trial to trial and the target points are varied along a single plane of movement, rhizotomized or dorsal column-lesioned monkeys can quickly and accurately direct a forelimb to the goal location (189,211), but dextrous manipulation of the goal objects, at the endpoint of the ballistic limb placement, is severely impaired (142). It should be stated that the ballistic movements are not identical to normal trajectories of the same limb before surgery; subtle differences are clear to an observer (188) or with detailed analyses (212-214).

Elimination of visual following of the movement sequences leaves ballistic projection intact and exacerbates the deficits of distal extremity orientation. When monkeys are trained to project the hand into different compartments behind an opaque barrier, a partially deafferented hand or foot (following dorsal column section) is not oriented for entry into small compartments (142,146). Rather than straighten, elevate, and partially supinate the hand or foot to fit the rectangular compartment (oriented vertically), the lesioned monkeys bang against or crudely grasp the walls of the correct compartment. However, with frequent practice, gross orientation of the distal extremities (with or without visual guidance) recovers to functional levels closely approximating normal performance on stereotyped, well-learned tests (142,146).

One of the difficulties inherent in highly quantified studies of thoroughly practiced movements is that the trajectories are generally simple, progressing from a constant start position to various points along a single plane of movement. The need for proprioceptive and tactile guidance of motoric actions should increase when the start and endpoints vary randomly in three dimensions, as is the case for a primate in its natural environment. Some response measurement opportunities are lost by permitting movement in three dimensions, but latencies to the completed motor act are reliably indicative of motoric efficiency. For example, dorsal column–lesioned and limb-deafferented monkeys have been compared on a task in which: (1) the goal locations were varied from trial to trial within the area of a frontal plane accessible to the responding arm, requiring projections within a coordinate system to points at different distances along each of the three spatial dimensions; (2) the targets were observed in bright illumination, and then the room was completely dark for a variable foreperiod (5-15 sec) before trial onset; (3) the responding arm was moved passively by the experimenter during the foreperiod, and trial onset was defined by release of the arm; and (4) food reinforcement was produced and the lights were turned on when the animal contacted the peg (171,188). The animals could not predict the startpoint of movement, were forced to rely upon memory of the goal location, and could not see the limb movements. Normal response times were 275 msec for the hands, a value quite close to choice reaction times on tasks requiring simple responses (215).

Monkeys deafferented by dorsal rhizotomy (from C3-T3) could not direct the affected limb to the target within several seconds with testing over nearly 2 months, and although considerable recovery occurred (188), response times averaged 700 msec or more (2.6 times control values) following a year of postoperative training. Similarly, following complete interruption of the dorsal columns, monkeys were slowed substantially in accurate projection of the forelimbs (4.4 times control times to location of the goal object) and the hindlimbs (2.6 times control values). However, complete recovery, as judged by movement time, occurred with practice over 8 months (forelimbs) or 2 months (hindlimbs). Thus, input from the dorsal column–lemniscal system is utilized normally for somatosensory programming and evaluation of ballistic limb movements, when the start- and endpoints vary from trial to trial. Other pathways can provide compensatory inputs with retraining.

In summary, initiation of ballistic limb projections can occur with training following somatosensory deafferentation. In addition, execution of programs for ballistic movement appears not to rely upon a moment-to-moment evaluation of the movement trajectory. Possibly, the motor systems can be programmed to set the amount of contraction in antagonistic muscle groups, which specifies end position with minimal or no reliance on proprioceptive feedback during movement (189). This method of generating different end positions could depend upon monitoring the outputs of the motor systems directly, without interposition of proprioceptors in the circuit (216). When the beginning and endpoints of the limb projection are constant from trial to trial, sensory cues are not required to establish or execute appropriate motor programs. However, when the start and endpoints are not predictable, sensory cues are necessary for directing limb projections. Visual or somatosensory signals will suffice. Following exclusion of visual cues, the usefulness of somatosensory cues can be demonstrated by deafferentation or dorsal column lesions, but accurate spatial programming can be reestablished in the absence of the dorsal column–lemniscal system. Complete recovery from dorsal column interruption would not be expected with added demands for rapid sequencing of different movements and precise orientations of the hand.

D. Coordinating Movement Sequences

It seems likely that coordination of two to four limbs in a precisely timed sequence of integrated movements would require feedback concerning the timing of events (e.g., footfalls when running) and the relative positions of different limbs. Observation of cats with extensive rhizotomies has revealed expected deficits of interlimb coordination when the animals run on a platform or treadmill in the early postoperative period, but considerable recovery is seen (217,218). Dorsal column lesions produce a deficit of interlimb coordination only following caudal lesions (T12) that would interrupt proprioceptive afferents to the dorsal horn (46) and would involve relevant propriospinal connections between the forelimbs and hindlimbs (219). The principal conclusion of these studies is that gross coordination of well-learned and natural movement sequences, such as running or climbing, is not permanently lost following dorsal column–lemniscal lesions or dorsal rhizotomy. Certainly, there are deficits, and these are graded in severity according to the extent of deafferentation and for more difficult motor sequences, but the timing of events for different limbs is not disrupted severely and permanently when the demands on the distal extremity for precision and dexterity are minimized.

Following restriction of somesthetic feedback by lesions of the dorsal columns or dorsal roots, some deficits of movement control are maintained despite daily practice for months on a given motor task. Compensation for perturbations of a programmed motor sequence cannot occur with normal efficiency when the perturbation cues a new program for a corrective motor act (188,189). Accelerating, slowing, or even stopping a movement can be accommodated by adjusting muscular tensions until the programmed endstate is achieved (189), but rapidly changing motor programs to circumvent an unexpected obstacle or to follow a newly significant somatosensory cue obviously is dependent upon the spatial and temporal resolution of the signals from the periphery. It is for this reason, in part, that the dorsal column–lemniscal system is thought to be especially involved with control of the distal extremities. Because the purpose of most motor actions is to engage some object with the hand or foot, it is the distal portion of the extremity that must make the major compensation for errors, given an approximately accurate trajectory of the whole limb. And the distal extremity is maximally adapted to perform rapid sequences of movements. Hence, dorsal column lesions appear to disrupt sequences of individual movements (220) when the program for each component of the sequence depends on quickly sensing the consequences of the preceding component. If the dorsal column–lemniscal system is a critical source of input for altering the course of movement sequences, then it should be in the periods of transition from one movement to another that dorsal column–lemniscal input is important for adjustive reprogramming.

The capacity for emitting repetitive sequences of movements of the distal extremity can be tested by training a monkey to press a lever on a fixed-ratio operant schedule. When different ratios of responses per reinforcement are utilized (fixed ratios of five to 50 responses/reinforcement), in order to establish rates of responding that vary from two to four responses/sec, high cervical interruption of the fasciculi gracilis and cuneatus produces severe early deficits for the hand, but minimal to no slowing of the foot (146). Interruption of the spinocerebellar tracts produces deficits of repetitive motor sequencing (e.g., the test for adiadokokineses), and interruption of dorsal column–cerebellar connections could account for slowing of fixed ratio responding by the hand (221, 221a). This interpretation is supported by the minor deficit and rapid and complete recovery of motoric sequencing by the feet, because hindlimb dorsal column–cerebellar axons exit the dorsal columns well below the cervical lesions.

The ability to emit repetitive cycles of manual flexion and extension recovers to or near control frequencies for dorsal column–lesioned animals after months of practice on the fixed ratio task. Recovery of the capacity for rapid execution of simple, well-learned flexion-extension sequences following dorsal column–lemniscal lesions leaves other aspects of response evaluation and programming to be investigated in more detail. For example, the bar response does not require a refined specification of muscular exertion or of the spatial extent of each movement because the response is halted by an external stop. The repetitive response is executed by all the fingers acting in concert, and the movement occurs almost entirely at the wrist. The effects of dorsal column lesions should be evaluated for patterns of movement that require adaptation by inserting new motor programs that are directed by peripheral feedback.

E. Force Feedback

The cues available for judging (and controlling) muscular force can be provided by: (1) motor reafference, the "sense of effort" (216), (2) comparisons of motor output with muscle spindle and tendon organ input (109), (3) comparisons of motor output with movement distance (e.g., from joint afferents), or (4) superficial cutaneous and subcutaneous pressure receptors. It is difficult to isolate these cues for independent experimental analysis, but some useful information has been provided by investigations of the effects of spinal tract section on the capacity to discriminate between objects of different weights but identical sizes and shapes. Weight discrimination has been reported not to be deteriorated by a dorsal column lesion, even when section of the inferior cerebellar peduncle is added in a separate surgical procedure (29), or the entire medial lemniscus is sectioned (30a). In these important studies, monkeys or apes pulled objects of equal size and shape toward them by grasping attached ropes. For some dorsal column-lesioned animals, the objects were placed behind a screen and were not viewed until pulled to a stop, where the selected object was investigated for presence or absence of the reward. Thus, the necessary strategy involved testing the resistance of both objects with short pulls, followed by a long pull of the selected container, without visual monitoring of the distance moved.

The weight discrimination task that has been utilized, involving movement of objects that offer resistance in proportion to the friction produced by differing weights, represents another example of a sensory test that is not sensitive to dorsal column-lemniscal interruption because of a multiplicity of available cues. For example, the rate of movement of the object can be determined crudely from auditory cues by an experienced subject, and the movement distance can be derived from auditory cues and experience (the distance remains constant from trial to trial). Weight discrimination could be accomplished by monitoring pressure sensations, and if this were the only exterosensory cue available, elevations of thresholds for weight discrimination would be expected because pressure discrimination is deteriorated following dorsal column-lemniscal lesions (15). Also, dorsal column-lesioned monkeys cannot actively generate a constant force against an oscillating manipulandum (141)—a result that would follow from distorted or insufficient feedback concerning the pressure exerted against an object. However, discrimination of cutaneous pressures recovers to normal levels following dorsal column lesions (15), and the slowly adapting cutaneous and proprioceptive input to the lemniscal pathways in the lateral column could explain sparing of weight discrimination following interruption of the dorsal columns. The conclusion that brain stem lesions of the medial lemniscus do not impair weight discrimination is more difficult to understand. Even slight sparing of the medial lemniscus could spare discriminatory somatosensations, and the lemniscal boundaries are less obvious in the brain stem than in the spinal cord.

Since most of the interactions of animals with the environment involve forcible displacement of objects (e.g., throwing or pushing) or movement of the body relative to a surface or structure, force feedback constitutes a critical source of information concerning operations performed by the distal extremities. In fact, for many motor functions of the distal extremities, knowledge of the relative positions of the digits is less important than accurate information concerning the position and resistance of an object (or surface) at certain critical points in time. For example, imagine the demands of a task requiring that subjects throw objects differing in size, shape, and weight a given distance. The configuration of the grasp would differ considerably from trial to trial, and it would matter little which fingers contacted the object. The exact form of the grasp would determine motor efficiency (e.g., restricting the grasp to the thumb and little finger would impair power and accuracy), but it would not be a critical determinant of sensory feedback. The sensed resistance of the object just before the point of release would be a crucial determinant of the different amounts of muscular power required to project the dissimilar objects the same distance.

Cutaneous pressure receptors can be important contributors to the sensations of resistance, and muscle and tendon receptors are clearly important. Recent evidence implicates cutaneous, joint, and muscle receptors in the mediation of sensations of pressure, movement, and position for the hand (86, 222,223). Reductions of motor output (e.g., by partial paralysis) cause an overestimation of sensed resistance (possibly because of an increased sense of effort; 224), but some afferent activity is required for sensations of movement (109, 225). That is, sensations of movement and resistance appear to depend upon a correlation of a sense of effort with afferent feedback. The dorsal column-lemniscal system is likely to be the critical source of this input to the corticospinal system for control of fine movement at precise points in time (discussed later), but the purely sensory appreciation of force is not provided exclusively by the dorsal columns (15,29).

F. Relationships Between Dorsal Column–Lemniscal Input and Corticospinal Output

Both the lemniscal and the pyramidal systems especially innervate the distal limbs (and the mouth) (226). For the corticospinal motor system, the preferential innervation of the distal extremities is not only a quantitative matter, involving a more dense projection to cord levels supplying the brachial and lumbosacral plexuses. Direct corticospinal projections to motoneurons are observed to occur uniquely at segments supplying the distal limbs (227). In addition, afferent innervation of corticospinal neurons is supplied exclusively by the dorsal column component of the lemniscal system (80), and only the portions of SI cortex that supply the distal extremities are severely deafferented by dorsal column lesions (111). Thus, the dorsal columns exclusively supply corticospinal neurons that uniquely couple the cerebral cortex with motoneurons, and the preferential targets of this long loop are the distal extremities, which are most skilled for environmental manipulation. These relationships suggest functions for the dorsal column--pyramidal linkage that will not be duplicated by other sensorimotor systems.

The dorsal column and corticospinal pathways are qualitatively distinct in primates versus other mammals (110,228), in simian versus prosimian primates (229), and for New versus Old World monkeys (230). In addition, the sizes of the dorsal column-lemniscal and pyramidal systems increase disproportionately in man (231,232). The capacity for fractionation of the movements of individual digits increases in pace with the neural projection patterns and with peripheral alterations of structure that are most pronounced for the hand (233). Special requirements for coordination of the digits are imposed on the hands during manipulation of environmental objects, and the dorsal column-lemniscal and pyramidal systems preferentially innervate the upper extremities (particularly the fingers; 50,55,111,234). The latter point is worth emphasizing because the more profound effects of dorsal column section on motoric functions of the hand relative to the feet have been ascribed to the presence of spinocerebellar afferents in the fasciculus cuneatus (206,221). However, the more obvious and enduring deficits of manual (as compared with pedal) dexterity following a dorsal column lesion are likely to result in part from interruption of dorsal column-lemniscal projections that are adapted to the more complex and delicate functions of the more sophisticated peripheral structure.

The dorsal column-lemniscal and pyramidal systems are reciprocally connected to an extent that justifies use of the term dorsal column-pyramidal system. A large proportion of corticospinal projection neurons that have been sampled by microelectrodes receive inputs from joint, muscle, and/or cutaneous receptors, and the responses are characteristic of dorsal column-lemniscal cells (e.g., short latency, quickly adapting, submodality specific, and topographically precise; 81,235). Interruption of the dorsal columns eliminates somatosensory responsivity for these motor cortical cells (80). The projection of the dorsal column-lemniscal system to corticospinal neurons provides for parallel cortical processing via direct pathways to the SI and MI areas (80,170) and by reciprocal connections between the precentral and postcentral gyri (203,236). A large proportion of the dorsal column-lemniscal projection cells are influenced by a projection of cortical pyramidal cells to the gracile and cuneate nuclei (directly or via the brain stem reticular formation) (56,57,237,238) and to the ventro-basal complex (239). The dorsal column-pyramidal interactions at each level (brain stem, thalamus, and cortex) are in register spatially, interrelating the refined somatotopy of the descending and ascending pathways. Conduction speed is high in both directions, suggesting precise temporal interactions (237) that are consistent with the unique spatiotemporal functions ascribed to the dorsal column-lemniscal and pyramidal tracts (126,240), but it should be recognized that both portions of the dorsal column–pyramidal system contain slowly conducting elements that have not been characterized fully (241,242).

The outflow of pyramidal activity that precedes and accompanies a limb projection filters the feedback that is obtained by the corticospinal system during the movement (243,244). Proprioceptive inputs can be allowed through as conduction of tactile information is gated out (239). Also, proprioceptive stimulation is effective in driving pyramidal neurons during the execution of precise distal extremity movements, but limb perturbation during ballistic movements does not excite the pyramidal neurons (77). Thus, the pyramidal-dorsal column system determines its accessibility to peripheral feedback according to the afferent submodality, the type of movement, and time relative to certain movements (corrected for conduction times) (237). Proprioceptive inputs contribute to the programming and execution of fine, adjustive or manipulative activities, and tactile and proprioceptive information is utilized to determine the consequences of the component movements in a manipulative sequence. The gating of pyramidal input in relation to motor actions involves the lemniscal system substantially, and other afferent sources are modulated as well. Dorsal horn neurons projecting to the spinothalamic tract are affected by the corticospinal outflow (246), and peripheral afferent influences on moto-neuron discharge are inhibited presynaptically by pyramidal activity (247).

Following pyramidotomy or section of the fasciculus cuneatus above the brachial plexus, some forms of movement control are affected only transiently. Monkeys with chronic dorsal column–pyramidal lesions can initiate a ballistic limb projection or flex (or extend) the wrist or a finger at normal latencies (87,88,142,248), and the limbs can be directed accurately during running or climbing (38,88). However, even though the trajectories of replicated ballistic movements closely approximate those of intact limbs, observers readily note a reduction of the grace and fluidity of movement following pyramidotomy or dorsal column section (146,249). The subtle and yet obvious deterioration of coordination results partly from faulty orientation and adjustment of the hand at the endpoint of the movement sequences, but other effects are likely to con-tribute to the less than facile performance. For example, corticospinal cells are active well in advance of response onset (198), "priming" alpha and gamma motoneurons that are dependent upon spatial and temporal summation of inputs, and contributing to the distribution of reciprocal inhibition of antag-onists (250). Loss or disrupted timing of the smooth crescendo of alpha-gamma coactivation by the corticospinal system is expected to predispose toward abrupt movement transitions and to reduce feedback from unloaded muscle spindles in agonist muscles, altering the balance of spindle discharge from muscles acting on the relevant joints. The resulting deficits should be expressed primarily by the hands but also in the fixation of proximal joints, since corticospinal influ-ences are not exclusive of proximal motoneurones.

Interruption of the corticospinal tract, ordinarily by section of the bulbar pyramid, produces profound, flaccid paralysis in the immediate postoperative interval, but dramatic recovery occurs within the first 2 postoperative weeks. When pyramidotomized animals have been observed for several months or more, and when they have been retested or retrained repeatedly in structured situations (providing reliable data and ensuring motivation to perform), the following chronic deficits have been described: (1) flexor hypotonicity (191,240,251), (2) reduction of strength (252,254), (3) loss of placing reactions (240,251,255), (4) reduction of flexor reflex strength (191,251,256), (5) inability to release manual grasp (88,240,249), (6) elevation of choice reaction times (87,252,257), (7) impairment of digital dexterity and prehension of objects (192,240,249,255, 257), (8) loss of precision grip (i.e., thumb, forefinger opposition) (88,240), (9) inability to fractionate digital movements (88,240), (10) reduction of the speed of movements (248,253,254), and (11) impairment in adjusting to displacement of a limb (191). Some of these deficits appear to result from direct deafferentation of motoneurons and are not present (or are transient) following lesions of the dorsal columns or the medial lemniscus. Disruptions of tone and of the speed or strength of reflexive or conscious movement are minimal or absent following lemniscal interruption (208,258). However, dextrous actions of the distal extremities (3 and 7-9 in previous list) are impaired similarly by dorsal column and by pyramidal lesions (54,142,146,206,207).

Somatosensory responsivity and premotor discharges of pyramidal neurons have been observed in detail as monkeys manipulate the position of a manipulandum (primarily involving wrist pronation and supination) and respond to perturbations of the manipulandum (259). Variations of the behavioral paradigm permit comparisons of ballistic versus slow or fine adjustive or braking movements, and active versus passive pronation or supination. Variation of the recording locations has identified different categories of pyramidal neurons in the rostral and caudal motor cortex (81,82) and areas 3, 3b, and 1 of the primary somatosensory cortex and areas 2 and 5 of the parietal cortex. Clearly, somatosensory input modulates pyramidal output, producing prominant peaks of activity in pyramidal tract cells following perturbation (260). Related peaks of electromyographic activity occur in agonist muscles in association with reflexive and voluntary actions. The earliest electromyographic response (M1) is dependent primarily upon segmental inputs, but it is affected by corticospinal activity (261). Pyramidal and segmental interactions determine the magnitude of the early reflexive response to perturbation, but the occurrence of the M1 response is not dependent upon integrity of the lemniscal or pyramidal systems (262-264). The second peak (M2) may be dependent upon the lemniscal-pyramidal linkage (262,263), but it has not been determined whether or not the dorsal columns are the critical lemniscal pathway for preservation of the second pyramidal or M2 responses. That is, patients with clinical signs indicating complete interruption of the spinal lemniscal pathways do not produce the M2 response (264), but selective interruption of the dorsal columns has not been employed in companion investigations of laboratory animals. Evocation of the transcortical responses is relevant to adaptive movements and promotes rapid somatosensorimotor reaction times (as compared with reactions to visual or auditory stimulation) (265).

The M2 response to perturbation can be related to corticospinal activity and has been termed a transcortical reflex. Although the M2 response occurs at short latency and is determined by a paucisynaptic linkage (a minimum of four synapses), the M2 is accompanied by pyramidal discharge that is influenced by a variety of factors associated with voluntary reactions. For example, the pattern of discharge by individual pyramidal tract neurons, or specific populations of corticospinal neurons that commence discharging at 30 msec or more following a perturbation, can distinguish: (1) active from passive movement (83), (2) prior instructions to assist or oppose a perturbation (263), (3) different load conditions (259), (4) ballistic versus pursuit or fine adjustive reactions (83), (5) large versus small and fast versus slow reactions (83), (6) the force or speed of the motor act (89,266), (7) the direction of movement (259), (8) active versus passive braking or termination of the response (259), and (9) the degree of training on the task (267). The variety of activity patterns across the population and the complexity of the gating operations that differentially affect the categories of corticospinal neurons makes it apparent that the dorsal column–pyramidal system is pivotal to the exquisite flexibility of distal extremity movements that is necessitated by interactions with the environment. The particular influences of dorsal column–lemniscal versus cerebellar and other sources of input remain to be determined (268), but the absence of peripheral driving of pyramidal neurons in the motor cortex following dorsal column section (80), and the characteristics of somatosensory responses (spatially discrete, quickly adapting, and submodality specific) (81,235) indicate a primary or even an obligatory contribution from the dorsal columns. Accordingly, dorsal column or pyramidal tract lesions produce similar deficits of movement that are especially apparent on tasks requiring fine adjustive reactions of the hands that are dictated by instructions or training and are directed by the spatiotemporal sequence of somatosensory stimulation.

G. Recovery of Motor Performance Following Dorsal Column–Lemniscal Lesions

Because the dorsal columns may supply all peripheral somatosensory input to a pyramidal system that especially serves skilled responses established and directed by training and experience, it is possible that only stereotyped motor responses would survive dorsal column or pyramidal lesions. That is, the capacity for new motoric learning could be compromised severely by dorsal column–pyramidal system damage. Certainly, this is not the case in a global sense, as evidenced by substantial recovery of a variety of motor capacities following dorsal column or pyramidal system lesions. As expected, movements produced by proximal musculature and ballistic (open loop) projections of the limbs reveal the earliest and most complete recovery (87,88,171), but considerable improvement of object manipulations by the hand has been reported also (134,171,191,254,256).

Tests of motor performance provide reliable indicants of neural plasticity following injury, because the error feedback can be immediate and precise and the object of the task remains obvious, in contrast to purely sensory tests, where altered sensory cues may not be attended to by the subject (171). The onset of motoric recovery following a dorsal column lesion occurs typically at 2 weeks postsurgically (171), and the initial improvement in performance can be abrupt and substantial, suggesting the occurrence of anatomic reorganization (e.g., sprouting) at that point in time. Further sharpening of performance is observed consistently with extended practice. This secondary, slow form of improvement is dependent upon task-specific practice, showing little transfer from training the same limb in other contexts or from testing the contralateral limb on the same task (171). For example, a dorsal column- or pyramidal-lesioned monkey can regain a great deal of facility for reaching and grasping during climbing and in social interactions in a large, communal enclosure, and yet performance in a formal testing situation remains impaired. Improvement with formal testing beyond the first month after dorsal column section is not related to time per se but progresses at comparable rates in animals that begin the retraining regimen early or as long as 5 months after surgery (188). Consistent with the process of motor learning that is experienced by normal individuals during development or in the learning of a new sport, retraining the dorsal column–deafferented motor systems is laborious, requiring many repetitions that can be distributed over months. There are cumulative effects of practice that can be stored over days in "registers" that apply specifically to a given task and limb. Thus, it is apparent that motoric learning is not dependent strictly upon the dorsal columns or the pyramidal system.

What deficits remain from DC *or* pyramidal lesions after time and retraining; or, what motor capacities are dependent critically upon the dorsal column–pyramidal system? Tone is reduced "permanently" in monkeys following pyramidotomy (191), but it appears to be reduced only transiently following dorsal column lesions in monkeys (207,209). Reduction of tone following pyramidotomy is likely to be related to loss of the majority of pyramidal axons that are small (241). This large population of small pyramidal cells has not been sampled thoroughly, and therefore the relevance of dorsal column inputs has not been determined. It is possible that these cells contribute substantially to modulation within the dorsal column nuclei and to priming the gamma efferents (269).

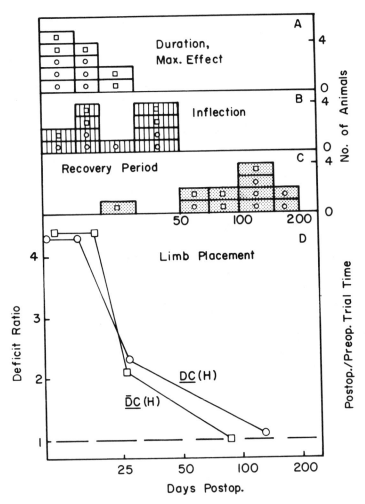

Figure 5 D, Recovery of hindlimb projection terminating in accurate placement of the foot in a vertical, 32-mm-wide, 80-mm-long compartment (two monkeys) or requiring accurate grasp of food pellets resting on a 25-mm-square column (two monkeys) or on a slick surface (two monkeys). All monkeys received complete unilateral DC lesions at the first surgery [DC(H)] and five monkeys received complete DC lesions on the other side at the second surgery [D̄C(H)]. The histograms give the timing, for individual animals, of the onset of recovery (A), the transition from rapid to slow recovery (B), and the endpoint of recovery (C). The slow phase of recovery was considerably shorter on those tasks requiring crude grasp or foot placement than on tasks requiring precision grip. The fast phase is most apparent on tasks that depend critically upon proximal musculature. (From Ref. 171.)

Some distal extremity facility is lost irrevocably following dorsal column or pyramidal lesions, but the details of the impairments have not been worked out. Prehension is lost, even under visual control, which stands in contrast with the successful visual guidance of ballistic limb projections (88,142,240) and of manipulative search strategies (134,254). The interpretation that the animals cannot fractionate movements of individual digits seems compelling. However, it has been claimed that prehension can occur when the dorsal column nuclei are ablated, even when the lemniscal lesion is added to dorsal rhizotomy (270), and the permanent loss of precision grip by pyramidotomized monkeys has been challenged (191,254). Thus, following dorsal column or pyramidal lesions, the hand can be formed into different configurations for scraping, pushing, squeezing, and grasping with different combinations of finger movements that adapt to the sizes and shapes of objects. The motoric deficits resulting from dorsal column section or dorsal column nuclear lesions appear to involve disruption of the spatiotemporal precision of movements more than an inability to form the hand in different spatial configurations.

VIII. OVERVIEW

Claims that the dorsal columns provide critical input for conscious somatosensations or are utilized for direct motor feedback have made several cycles through the somatosensory literature (for example, 6,126,140,271). Clearly, the answer is that both claims are correct, and the anatomicophysiologic basis for distributing information from the dorsal columns to both sensory and motor systems is sound. The dorsal columns project directly, and with high spatial resolution and order, to frontal and parietal cortical areas that are implicated in the planning, initiating, programming, monitoring, and evaluation of active motoric exploration of the environment. Accordingly, the dorsal column-lemniscal system is essential for certain sensory and sensorimotor capacities that are integral to the process of active touch (38). However, other spinal pathways can substitute for dorsal column feedback in the mediation or relearning of many sensory discriminations or motor skills, and therefore it is necessary to control and manipulate a variety of inputs and to observe animals over long periods of training in order to define the obligatory contributions of the dorsal column-lemniscal system. As expected, the sensory and motor functions served uniquely by the dorsal column-lemniscal system rely upon high spatial *and* temporal resolution (126). The conscious sensory functions dependent upon the temporal resolution of the dorsal column-lemniscal system have not been investigated as vigorously as has spatial resolution.

It seems likely that some motor processes are guided by dorsal column input that is "insulated" from conscious sensation. For example, the intermediate latency (30-60 msec) motoric adjustments to perturbations of a manipulandum

(259,262,264) appear to depend upon dorsal column input, but they probably occur without full conscious recognition of the force and direction of the brief, precisely timed and spatially appropriate motor responses. It is not adaptive to focus attention on the continuous flow of precise adjustments required to maintain balance and interact with an environment containing numerous irregularities (e.g., when running on uneven terrain). However, if the motor task requires a sequence of volitional actions involving evaluation of each component movement and choice of the successive movement, a degree of conscious discrimination of relevant sensations is a natural outcome. For example, during active palpation of objects the skin is moved over the surfaces, and appreciation of the direction and path of movement of each contour is important for planning each active movement and for building up a perception of form. Sensations of direction and form for stimuli moving across the skin surface are lost following dorsal column interruption. These deficits are not dependent upon active exploration (126), but they occur with active touch and involve disruption of sensations that ordinarily occur during active manipulation. Other sensory consequences of active palpation of objects for stereognistic recognition can be undisturbed by interruption of the dorsal column–lemniscal system (134); these sensations appear to result from static cues of position. For example, input from slowly adapting tactile receptors does not project substantially within the dorsal columns (40).

Propulsion of objects or the body in space requires precise regulation of muscular force, expressed at the distal extremities and sensed by receptors in the distal skin, joints, muscles, tendons, and ligaments. Consistent with regulation of muscular force by the pyramidal system (89,266), demonstrable deficits of cutaneous pressure discrimination following dorsal column lesions (15), and intimate interconnections within the dorsal column–pyramidal system (56,80), doral column–lesioned monkeys or cats cannot regulate force output to match changing environmental contingencies (141,147). These deficits in motion contrast with a lack of impairments on tasks permitting discrimination of static cues of position or location on the basis of proprioception or touch (113,120, 121,145,271). The lack of impairments or transient deficits on a variety of tests that provide static cues and put no constraints on response speed is understandable in view of the nearly exclusive representation of velocity or acceleration detectors in the dorsal column lemniscal system (1,39,42,46). Exquisite sensitivity of dorsal column afferents to movement of the limbs or of the skin relative to objects, combined with fast conduction, secure transmission, and fast adaptation, provide temporal resolution that is necessary for precise timing of adaptive motor responses. The dorsal column–lemniscal system combines information from superficial and deep receptors to inform the organism of *changes* in the relationships between body parts and the environment; and direct connections to the pyramidal and other motor systems regulate adjustments requiring phasic, voluntary reactions. Adjustive motoric reactions can be directed spatially by dorsal column conduction that is allowed to pass the selective filter of pyramidal inhibition (83). The dorsal column–lemniscal system provides input that is crucial for motoric plasticity, in the sense of improvising movements that are directed relative to a dynamic environment, but motoric learning is not dependent upon the dorsal column–lemniscal system.

The somatotopic maps within the central nervous system can subserve a variety of spatial sensory discriminations in the absence of: the dorsal columns (Table 2.A,B), the dorsolateral columns (Table 2.E), the spinothalamic tract (Table 2.G), or the dorsolateral and spinothalamic tracts (Table 2.C). The dorsal column–lemniscal pathway is the most effective contributor to spatial resolution (117), but projections from the dorsal horn via the lateral and ventral columns can support a variety of spatiotactile capacities. On most tests of discriminative somesthesis that have been used to evaluate different lesion combinations, complete lemniscal lesions (of the dorsal and dorsolateral columns) produce more profound deficits than dorsal column and spinothalamic interruption (Table 2.D vs. 2.F), confirming the Brown-Séquard pattern of deficits in humans (7) and suggesting a preeminence of dorsolateral over spinothalamic contributions to discriminative somesthetic sensations. For some discriminations, however, addition of either dorsolateral *or* spinothalamic section to a dorsal column lesion produces profound and enduring deficits (117). Thus, it is likely that spatial discriminations depend upon a minimal innervation density provided to the somatosensory maps by convergent projections from each of the major ascending pathways (16,117). The dorsal columns provide an exclusive core representation of the distal extremities that is not convergent with or exactly duplicated by the lateral and ventral pathways (111,170), but other portions of the somatotopic mapping systems receive input from the dorsal, lateral, and ventral spinal pathways (16,23,37). These convergent mapping systems (e.g., in the "fringes" of SI and in SII) are optimal sites for anatomic reorganization following partial deafferentation by selective spinal lesions (167), which could provide a foundation for the impressive relearning of sensory and sensory-motor capacities that can occur after subtotal spinal injury (171).

Multidisciplinary investigations of the sorting of information among the spinal pathways to the thalamus and cortex have revealed subsystems that repeatedly interact to expand the number of functional categories (e.g., the types of submodality convergence onto single cells) and the adaptability of the overall somatosensory representation to loss of some portion of its input. Gone is the notion that each of the apparently fundamental somatosensory capacities is subserved by a single, relatively isolated pathway of rostral conduction. This applies to functions that can be related to a given receptor (e.g., vibration and the Pacinian corpuscle) and to processes that depend upon specific requirements for a population code (e.g., spatial acuity, with specifications for receptive field

Table 2 Effects of Spinal Lesions Restricted to the Ipsilateral Dorsal Columns (IDC), the Ipsilateral Lateral Column (ILC), the Contralateral Lateral Column (CLC), or Combinations of These Cord Sectors[a]

Deficit	Recovery or no deficit
A. IDC lesion—sensory tests:	
Graphesthesia*	------------------------------
Ph: 114	
Tactile direction disc.*	------------------------------
Ph: 114, 126, 274	
Tactile velocity disc.*	------------------------------
Ph: 114	
Hypalgesia	------------------------------
Ph: 101	
Tactile size disc.	Tactile size disc.
Ph: 140	Ph: 140
Tactile sequence disc.	Tactile sequence disc.
Ph: 117	Ph: 117
Texture disc.*	Texture disc.*
Cf,h: 132, 133	Cf,h: 132, 133; Pf: 134
Stereognosis*	Stereognosis*
Pf: 134, 273	Pf: 54, 134
Hardness disc.	Hardness disc.
Pf: 134	Pf: 134
Weight disc.	Weight disc.
Pf: 29	Pf: 29
Tactile pressure disc.	Tactile pressure disc.
Pf: 15	Ph: 15
Electrical stim. detect.	Electrical stim. detect.
Pf: 134	Pf: 134
------------------------------	Tactile pressure detect.
Ph, Ch: 15, 114, 151	
------------------------------	Tactile movement detect.*
Ph: 114, 126	
------------------------------	Hair movement detect.*
Ch: 150	
------------------------------	Vibration detection
Pf,h: 53, 114	
------------------------------	Tactile localization
Ph: 113	Pf,h: 114, 273; Cf,h: 205
------------------------------	Two-point disc.
Pf,h: 114, 120, 121	
------------------------------	Limb position sense
Ph: 145	

Table 2 *(Continued)*

Deficit	Recovery or no deficit

B. IDC lesion—sensorimotor tests:

Force regulation   ------------------------
    Pf; Ch: 141, 147
Body projection   ------------------------
    Ph; Ch: 147, 275, 276
Distal limb dexterity   ------------------------
    Pf,h: 54, 134, 142, 146, 206, 207
Grasp reflex   ------------------------
    Pf,h: 207
Reaction time   Reaction time
    Pf; Ch: 147, 258   Pf: 258
Ballistic movement   Ballistic movement
    Pf,h; Cf: 142, 146, 147, 258   Pf,h: 142, 146, 258
Balance   Balance
    Ph; Ch: 132, 205, 275, 277   Ph; Ch: 132, 205, 275, 277
Placing reaction   Placing reaction
    Ph; Ch: 132, 205, 207, 273   Ph; Ch: 205, 273
Hypotonicity   Muscular tone
    Pf,h: 208   Pf,h: 208
------------------------   Stepping, interlimb coordination
    Cf,h: 219

C. IDC isolation (ILC + CLC lesion)—sensory tests:

------------------------   Tactile stimulus detect.
    Ch: 148, 149
------------------------   Tactile sequence disc.
    Ph: 117
------------------------   Limb position sense
    Ph: 145

D. Lemniscal lesion (IDC + ILC)—sensory tests:

Graphesthesia   ------------------------
    Ph: 114
Tactile direction disc.*   ------------------------
    Ph: 114
Tactile velocity disc.*   ------------------------
    Ph: 114
Hyperalgesia   ------------------------
    Ph: 101
Tactile size disc.   ------------------------
    Ph: 140

Table 2 *(Continued)*

Deficit	Recovery or no deficit
D. (continued)	
Tactile sequence disc.	-------------------------
Ph: 117	
Texture disc.*	-------------------------
Cf,h: 132, 133	
Vibration detection	-------------------------
Ph: 114	
Tactile localization	-------------------------
Ph; Ch: 114, 105	
Two-point disc.	-------------------------
Ph: 114, 120	
Limb position sense	-------------------------
Ph: 145	
Hair movement detect.	-------------------------
Ch: 150	
Tactile pressure disc.	Tactile pressure disc.
Ph: 15	Ph: 15
Tactile pressure detect.	Tactile pressure detect.
Ph; Ch: 114, 151	Ph: 15
Tactile movement detect.*	Tactile movement detect.*
Ph: 114, 126	Ph: 126
-------------------------	Limb movement detect.
Ph: 114	
-------------------------	Limb movement direction sense
Ph: 114	
E. ILC lesion—sensory tests:	
Texture disc.*	-------------------------
Cf,h: 133	
Hyperalgesia	-------------------------
Ph: 126	
-------------------------	Tactile sequence disc.
Ph: 117	
-------------------------	Limb position sense
Ph: 145	
Tactile pressure detect.	Tactile pressure detect.
Ch: 151	Ph: 15
Hair movement detect.	Hair movement detect.
Ch: 150	Ch: 150

Table 2 *(Continued)*

Deficit	Recovery or no deficit
F. ILC isolation (IDC + CLC lesion)—sensory tests:	
Tactile sequence disc.	-------------------------
Ph: 117	
-------------------------	Two-point disc.
Pf,h: 120	
-------------------------	Limb position sense
Ph: 145	
-------------------------	Limb movement direction sense
Ph: 114	
G. CLC lesion—sensory tests:	
-------------------------	Tactile sequence disc.
Ph: 117	
-------------------------	Limb position sense
Ph: 145	
Two-point disc.	Two-point disc.
Ph: 278	Ph: 120
Tactile pressure detect.	Tactile pressure detect.
Ph: 8, 279	Ph: 279
Pain threshold and magnitude	Pain threshold and magnitude
Pf,h: 100, 102, 137	Pf,h: 102, 137
Thermal sensitivity	Thermal sensitivity
Pf,h: 137	Pf,h: 137

[a]Tests involving movement of stimuli across the skin surface are indicated by *. The subjects and limbs tested and the references are listed below each dependent variable (Ph: 114 indicates testing of primates on the hindlimbs by reference 114; Cf: refers to evaluation of carnivore forelimbs). Listing a test in the left and right columns indicates that a deficit was obtained, but performance returned to normal levels. Entries on the left and dashes on the right refer to deficits that did not recover. Entries on the right and dashes on the left indicate that no deficit occurred (references on the left) or that recovery occurred (references on the right). Only those tests are listed with each lesion category that have been studied; an impairment that occurs with an IDC lesion can be presumed to occur with IDC and ILC interruption but is not listed in the latter category unless tested. Absence of a reference in the right column can mean that recovery was not tested.

configuration and order). Nevertheless, each pathway has evolved with the acquisition of particular skills (110,232), and therefore, there are distinguishing functions that have been demonstrated for at least two of the major ascending spinal pathways. The spinothalamic tract clearly is most important for perception of pain (8,137), and the dorsal columns are: (1) sufficient for mediation of spatiotactile resolution and limb position sense that are present following isolation of the dorsal column-lemniscal projection (Fig. 4) (117), and (2) necessary for sensory discriminations and motoric skills that require spatial resolution *and* precise timing of somatosensory feedback (126).

Specific functions for the dorsolateral pathways have not been identified beyond contributions to spatial and intensive discriminations that are conveyed redundantly by the dorsal columns (Table 2). It is now apparent that the lemniscal system extends beyond the dorsal columns to include dorsolateral spinal pathways that contribute input to lemniscal projection cells in the dorsal column nuclei or the lateral cervical nucleus. The dorsolateral lemniscal pathways modulate and are modulated by a dorsal column-lemniscal tract (91,272) that contains some axons descending to synapse in the dorsal horn (272a), implying a functional interdependence between primary and relayed lemniscal afferents that has not been demonstrated behaviorally. That is, isolated lesions of the dorsal column or dorsolateral column frequently produce little or no deficit, but unilateral lesion of an entire dorsal quadrant of spinal white matter can produce profound, obvious, and enduring disruptions of spatial somesthetic discrimination on the same tasks. The classic clinical tests of two-point resolution or point-localization define a lesion that interrupts the spinal lemniscal pathways for touch (including both the ipsilateral dorsolateral and dorsal columns).

The distribution of touch input to the dorsal and dorsolateral columns appears to be similar for the forelimbs and hindlimbs. In contrast, the fasciculus cuneatus conveys proprioceptive afferents directly to the cuneate nuclear complex, but slowly adapting muscle and joint afferents from the hindlimb exit the fasciculus gracilis to synapse in the dorsal horn for relay via the lateral column to the gracile nuclear complex (46,84). High cervical lesions of the dorsal columns produce more substantial and enduring impairments of motoric coordination for the forelimbs than the hindlimbs, and the deficits are observed in the programming and evaluation of movements involving adjustive interactions with the environment (146,206,221). Sensations of limb movement, direction, and position have not been tested adequately for the forelimbs after dorsal column-lemniscal interruption. Position sense at the knee is conveyed by the dorsal columns and by axons located midlaterally (Fig. 4A) (presumably by spinocerebellar collaterals to the gracile nuclear complex).

This review has emphasized information obtained from investigation of primate species, but it has included comparisons with carnivores because of the wealth of data available from cats. The distal extremities of primates and carnivores are adapted for functions that differ between the species and are likely to be subserved by specialized lemniscal characteristics that have yet to be identified. The dorsolateral pathways may be more "important" in cats than in monkeys, but in general, the principles of organization of the lemniscal pathways appear to be quite similar in cats, monkeys, and man. The major differences in organization of the ascending spinal pathways pertain to a relatively more developed spinothalamic system of primates, which contributes to touch and proprioception as well as to pain and temperature sensations. The spinothalamic tract of primates provides inputs that can supplement and enhance the capacities of the lemniscal pathways, but epicritic functions depend critically upon different portions of the ipsilateral spinal pathways. Hence, the following lesions can be distinguished on the basis of neurologic evaluation of somatosensory capacities for the hindlimbs of primates: (1) dorsal columns (e.g., graphesthesia), (2) dorsal and dorsolateral columns (e.g., two-point discrimination), (3) dorsal and lateral columns (e.g., limb position sense), and (4) anterolateral and ventral columns (e.g., pain and temperature sensations).

REFERENCES

1. Brown, A. G. (1981). *Organization in the Spinal Cord*. Springer-Verlag, New York.
2. Burgess, P. R., and Perl, E. R. (1981). Cutaneous mechanoreceptors and nociceptors. In *Handbook of Sensory Physiology*, vol. 2, A. Iggo (Ed.), Springer-Verlag, Berlin, pp. 29–78.
3. Lamotte, R. H., and Mountcastle, V. B. (1975). Capacities of humans and monkeys to discriminate between vibratory stimuli of different frequency and amplitude. *J. Neurophysiol. 38*:539–559.
4. Tapper, D. N., Galera-Garcia, C., and Brown, P. B. (1972). Sinusoidal mechanical stimulation of the tactile pad receptor: Tuning curves. *Brain Res. 36*:223–227.
5. Head, H. (1920). *Studies in Neurology*, Oxford, London.
6. Mountcastle, V. B. (1961). Some functional properties of the somatic afferent system. In *Sensory Communications*, W. A. Rosenblith (Ed.), Massachusetts Institute of Technology, Cambridge, pp. 403–436.
7. Brown-Séquard, C.-E. (1855). *Experimental and Clinical Resarches on the Physiology and Pathology of the Spinal Cord*. Colin and Nowlan, Richmond.
8. Walker, A. E. (1940). The spinothalamic tract in man. *Arch. Neurol. Psychiat. 43*:284–298.
9. May, W. P. (1906). Reviews: The afferent path. *Brain 29*:742–803.
10. Mehler, W. R., Feferman, M. E., and Nauta, W. J. H. (1960). Ascending axon degeneration following anterolateral cordotomy: An experimental study in the monkey. *Brain 83*:718–750.
11. Robards, M. J. (1979). Somatic neurons in the brainstem and neocortex projecting to the external nucleus of the inferior colliculus: An anatomical study in the opossum. *J. Comp. Neurol. 184*:547–566.
12. Salibi, N. S., Saade, N. E., Banna, N. R., and Jabbur, S. J. (1980). Dorsal column input into the reticular formation. *Nature 288*:481–483.

13. Blomquist, A., Flink, R., Bowsher, D., Griph, S., and Westman, J. (1978). Tectal and thalamic projections of dorsal column and lateral cervical nuclei: A quantitative study in the cat. *Brain Res. 141*:335–341.

14. Berkley, K. J., and Hand, P. J. (1978). Efferent projections of the gracile nucleus in the cat. *Brain Res. 153*:263–283.

15. Vierck, C. J. (1977). Absolute and differential sensitivities to touch stimuli after spinal cord lesions in monkeys. *Brain Res. 134*:529–539.

16. Berkley, K. J. (1980). Spatial relationships between the terminations of somatic sensory and motor pathways in the rostral brainstem of cats and monkeys. I. Ascending somatic sensory inputs to lateral diencephalon. *J. Comp. Neurol. 193*:283–317.

17. Ranson, S. W. (1913). The course within the spinal cord of the non-medullated fibers of the dorsal roots: A study of Lissauer's tract in the cat. *J. Comp. Neurol. 23*:259–282.

18. Light, A. R., and Perl, E. R. (1977). Differential termination of large-diameter and small-diameter primary afferent fibers in the spinal dorsal gray matter as indicated by labeling with horseradish peroxidase. *Neurosci. Lett. 6*:59–63.

19. Trevino, D. L., and Carstons, E. (1976). Confirmation of the location of spinothalamic neurons in the cat and monkey by the retrograde transport of horseradish peroxidase. *Brain Res. 98*:177–182.

20. Denny-Brown, D., Kirk, E. J., and Yanagisawa, N. (1973). The tract of Lissauer in relation to sensory transmission in the dorsal horn of spinal cord in the macaque monkey. *J. Comp. Neurol. 151*:175–200.

21. Rustioni, A., Hayes, N. L., and O'Neill, S. (1979). Dorsal column nuclei and ascending spinal afferents in macaques. *Brain 102*:95–125.

22. Brown, P. B., and Culberson, J. L. (1981). Somatotopic organization of hindlimb cutaneous dorsal root projections to cat dorsal horn. *J. Neurophysiol. 45*:137–143.

23. Boivie, J. (1979). Anatomical reinvestigation of the termination of the spinothalamic tract in the monkey. *J. Comp. Neurol. 186*:343–370.

24. Willis, W. D., and Coggeshall, R. E. (1978). In *Sensory Mechansims of the Spinal Cord*, Plenum, New York.

25. Lamotte, R. H., and Mountcastle, V. B. (1979). Disorders in somesthesis following lesions of parietal lobe. *J. Neurophysiol. 42*:400–419.

26. Carlson, M. (1981). Characteristics of sensory deficits following lesions of Brodmann's areas 1 and 2 in the postcentral gyrus of Macaca mulatta. *Brain Res. 204*:424–430.

27. Semmes, J., Porter, L., and Randolph, M. C. (1974). Further studies of anterior postcentral lesions in monkeys. *Cortex 10*:55–68.

28. Holmes, G. (1922). Cronnian lectures on the clinical symptoms of cerebellar disease. *Lecture IV, Lancet 2*:111–115.

29. Devito, J. L., Ruch, T. C., and Patton, H. D. (1964). Analysis of residual weight discriminatory ability and evoked potentials following section of dorsal columns in monkeys. *Indian J. Physiol. Pharmacol. 8*:117–126.

→ 30.   Liebman, R. S., and Levitt, M. (1973). Position sense after combined spinal tractotomies and cerebellectomies in macaques. *Exp. Neurol. 40*: 170-182.

→ 30a. Sjoquist, D., and Weinstein, E. A. (1942). The effect of section of the medial lemniscus on proprioceptive functions in chimpanzees and monkeys. *J. Neurophysiol. 5*:69-74.

31.   Dart, A. M., and Gordon, G. (1973). Some properties of spinal connections of the cat's dorsal column nuclei which do not involve the dorsal columns. *Brain Res. 58*:61-68.

→ 32.   Uddenberg, N. (1968). Functional organization of long, second order afferents in the dorsal funiculus. *Exp. Brain Res. 4*:377-382.

33.   Angaut-Petit, D. (1975). The dorsal column system: I. Existence of long ascending postsynaptic fibres in the cat's fasciculus gracilis. *Exp. Brain Res. 22*:457-470.

34.   Morin, F. (1955). A new spinal pathway for cutaneous impulses. *Am. J. Physiol. 183*-252.

35.   Nijensohn, D. E., and Kerr, F. W. L. (1975). The ascending projections of the dorsolateral funiculus of the spinal cord in the primate. *J. Comp. Neurol. 161*:459-470.

36.   Ha, H. (1971). Cervicothalamic tract in the rhesus monkey. *Exp. Neurol. 33*:205-212.

37.   Boivie, J. (1980). Thalamic projections from lateral cervical nucleus in monkey. A degeneration study. *Brain Res. 198*:13-26.

38.   Vierck, C. J., Jr. (1978). The mechanism of recognition of objects by manipulation: a multidisciplinary approach. In *Active Touch*, G. Gordon (Ed.), Pergamon Press, Oxford, pp. 139-159.

39.   Whitsel, B. L., Petrucelli, L. M., Ha, H., and Dreyer, D. A. (1972). The resorting of spinal afferents as antecedent to the body representation in the post central gyrus. *Brain Behav. Evol. 5*:303-341.

40.   Whitsel, B. L., Petrucelli, L. M., and Sapiro, G. (1969). Modality representation in the lumbar and cervical fasciculus gracilis of squirrel monkey. *Brain Res. 15*:67-78.

41.   Glees, P., and Soler, J. (1951). Fibre content of the posterior column and synaptic connections of nucleus gracilis. *Z. Zellforsch. 36*:381-400.

42.   Horch, K. W., Burgess, P. R., and Whitehorn, D. (1976). Ascending collaterals of cutaneous neurons in the fasciculus gracilis of the cat. *Brain Res. 117*:1-17.

43.   Brown, A. G. (1968). Cutaneous afferent fiber collaterals in the dorsal column of the cat. *Exp. Brain Res. 5*:293-305.

44.   Bromberg, M. B., and Whitehorn, D. (1974). Myelinated fiber types in the superficial radial nerve of the cat and their central projections. *Brain Res. 78*:157-163.

45.   Pubols, L. M., and Pubols, B. H. (1973). Modality composition and functional characteristics of dorsal column mechanoreceptive afferent fibers innervating the raccoon's forepaw. *J. Neurophysiol. 36*:1023-1035.

46. Burgess, P. R., and Clark, F. J. (1969). Characteristics of knee joint receptors in the cat. *J. Physiol. 203*:301–317.

47. Whitehorn, D., Bromberg, M. B., Howe, J. F., Putnam, J. E., and Burgess, P. R. (1972). Activation of gracile nucleus: Time distribution of activity in presynaptic and postsynaptic elements. *Exp. Neurol. 37*:312–321.

48. Jankowska, E., Rastad, J., and Zarzecki, P. (1979). Segmental and supraspinal input to cells of origin of non-primary fibres in the feline dorsal columns. *J. Physiol. (Lond.) 290*:185–200.

49. Brown, A. G., and Fyffe, R. E. W. (1981). Form and function of dorsal horn neurones with axons ascending the dorsal columns in cat. *J. Physiol. (Lond.) 321*:31–47.

50. Brown, A. G. (1974). A study of single axons in the cat's medial lemniscus. *J. Physiol. 236*:225–246.

51. Brown, A. G. (1973). Ascending and long spinal pathways: Dorsal columns, spinocervical tract and spinothalamic tract. In *Handbook of Sensory Physiology*, vol. 2, A. Iggo (Ed.), Springer-Verlag, Berlin, pp. 315–338.

52. Willis, W. D., Trevino, D. L., Coulter, J. D., and Maunz, R. A. (1974). Responses of primate spinothalamic tract neurons to natural stimulation of hindlimb. *J. Neurophysiol. 37*:358–372.

53. Schwartzman, R. J., and Bogdonoff, M. D. (1969). Proprioception and vibration sensibility discrimination in the absence of the posterior columns. *Arch. Neurol. 20*:349–353.

54. Beck, C. M. (1976). Dual dorsal columns: A review. *Can. J. Neurol. Sci. 3*:1–7.

55. Keller, J. H., and Hand, P. J. (1970). Dorsal root projections to nucleus cuneatus of the cat. *Brain Res. 20*:1–17.

56. Kuypers, H. G. J. M., and Tuerk, J. D. (1964). The distribution of the cortical fibres within the nuclei cuneatus and gracilis of the cat. *J. Anat. 98*:143–162.

57. Gordon, G., and Jukes, M. G. M. (1964). Descending influences on the exteroceptive organizations of the cat's gracile nucleus. *J. Physiol. (Lond.) 173*:291–319.

58. Bromberg, M. B., Blum, P., and Whitehorn, D. (1975). Quantitative characteristics of inhibition in the cuneate nucleus of the cat. *Exp. Neurol. 48*:37–56.

59. Mountcastle, V. B., and Powell, T. P. S. (1959). Neural mechanisms subserving cutaneous sensibility with special reference to the role of afferent inhibition in sensory perception and discrimination. *Bull. Johns Hopkins Hosp. 105*:201–232.

60. Laskin, S. E., and Spencer, W. A. (1979). Cutaneous masking. II. Geometry of excitatory and inhibitory receptive fields of single units in somatosensory cortex of the cat. *J. Neurophysiol. 42*:1061–1082.

61. Aoki, M. (1981). Afferent inhibition on various types of cats cuneate neurons induced by dynamic and steady tactile stimuli. *Brain Res. 221*:257–269.

62. Bystrzycka, E., Nail, B. S., and Rowe, M. (1977). Inhibition of cuneate neurons: its afferent source and influence on dynamically sensitive 'tactile' neurones. *J. Physiol. (Lond.) 268*:251-270.

63. Mountcastle, V. B. (1978). *Medical Physiology*, Mosby, St. Louis.

64. Vierck, C. J., Jr., and Jones, M. B. (1970). Influences of low and high frequency oscillation upon spatio-tactile resolution. *Physiol. Behav. 5*:1431-1435.

65. Mountcastle, V. B., Talbot, W. H., Sakata, H., and Hyvarinen, J. (1966). In *Touch, Heat and Pain*, A. V. S. de Reuck and J. Knight (Eds.), Little, Brown, Boston, pp. 325-351.

66. Erickson, R. P. (1968). Stimulus coding in topographic and non-topographic modalities: On the significance of the activity of individual sensory neurons. *Physiol. Rev. 75*:447-465.

67. Rustioni, A., and Sotelo, C. (1974). Synaptic organization of the nucleus gracilis of the cat. Experimental identification of dorsal root fibers and cortical afferents. *J. Comp. Anat. 4*:441-468.

68. Rustioni, A., and Ellis, L. C. (1978). Ultrastructural identification of non-primary afferent terminals in the nucleus gracilis of cats. *Brain Res. 146*: 358-365.

69. Blomquist, A., and Westman, J. (1976). Interneurons and initial axon collaterals in the feline gracile nucleus demonstrated with the rapid Golgi technique. *Brain Res. 111*:407-410.

70. Galindo, A., Krnjević, K., and Schwartz, S. (1968). Patterns of firing in cuneate neurones and some effects of Flaxedil. *Exp. Brain Res. 5*:87-101.

71. Calvin, W. H., and Loeser, J. D. (1975). Doublet and burst firing patterns within the dorsal column nuclei of cat and man. *Exp. Neurol. 48*:406-426.

72. Darian-Smith, I., Davidson, I., and Johnson, K. O. (1980). Peripheral neural representation of spatial dimensions of a textured surface moving across the monkey finger pad. *J. Physiol. (Lond.) 309*:135-146.

73. Gordon, G. (1978). Introduction. In *Active Touch*, G. Gordon (Ed.), Pergamon Press, Oxford, pp. XIII-XXII.

74. Coquery, J.-M. (1978). Role of active movement in control of afferent input from skin in cat and man. In *Active Touch*, G. Gordon (Ed.), Pergamon Press, Oxford, pp. 161-170.

75. Ghez, C., and Pisa, M. (1972). Inhibition of afferent transmission in cuneate nucleus during voluntary movement in the cat. *Brain Res. 40*: 145-151.

76. Coulter, J. D. (1974). Sensory transmission through lemniscal pathway during voluntary movement in the cat. *J. Neurophysiol. 37*:831-845.

77. Fromm, C., and Evarts, E. V. (1978). Motor cortex responses to kinesthetic inputs during postural stability, precise fine movement and ballistic movement in the conscious monkey. In *Active Touch*, G. Gordon (Ed.), Pergamon Press, Oxford, pp. 105-118.

78. Chapin, J. K., and Woodward, D. J. (1982). Somatic sensory transmission to the cortex during movement: Gating of single cell responses to touch. *Exp. Neurol. 78*:654-669.

79. Tsumoto, T., Nakamura, S., and Iwama, I. (1975). Pyramidal tract control over cutaneous and kinesthetic sensory transmission in the cat thalamus. *Exp. Brain Res.* 22:281.

80. Brinkman, J., Bush, B. M., and Porter, R. (1978). Deficient influences of peripheral stimuli on precentral neurons in monkeys with dorsal column lesions. *J. Physiol. (Lond.)* 276:27–48.

81. Strick, P. L., and Preston, J. B. (1982). Two representations of the hand in area 4 of a primate. II. Somatosensory input organization. *J. Neurophysiol.* 48:150–159.

82. Strick, P. L., and Preston, J. B. (1982). Two representations of the hand in area 4 of a primate. I. Motor output organization. *J. Neurophysiol.* 48: 139–149.

83. Evarts, E. V., and Fromm, C. (1978). The pyramidal tract neuron as summing point in a closed-loop control system in the monkey. In *Cerebral Motor Control in Man: Long Loop Mechanisms*, J. E. Desmedt (Ed.), *Progr. Clin. Neurophysiol.* 4:56–69.

84. Rosen, I. (1969). Afferent connections to group I activated cells in the main cuneate nucleus of the cat. *J. Physiol. (Lond.)* 205:209–236.

85. Shriver, J. E., Stein, B. M., and Carpenter, M. B. (1968). Central projections of spinal dorsal roots in the monkey. I. Cervical and upper thoracic dorsal roots. *Am. J. Anat.* 123:27–74.

85a. Boivie, J., Grant, G., Albe-Fessard, D., and Levante, A. (1975). *Neurosci. Lett.* 1:3.

86. Gandevia, S. C., and McCloskey, D. I. (1976). Joint sense, muscle sense, and their combination as position sense, measured at the distal interphalangeal joint of the middle finger. *J. Physiol. (Lond.)* 206:387–407.

87. Lawrence, D. G., and Kuypers, H. G. J. M. (1968). The functional organization of the motor system in the monkey. 1. The effects of bilateral pyramidal lesions. *Brain* 91:1–14.

88. Beck, C. H., and Chambers, W. W. (1970). Speed, accuracy and strength of forelimb movement after unilateral pyramidotomy in rhesus monkeys. *J. Comp. Physiol. Psychol.* 70:1–22.

89. Evarts, E. V. (1968). Relation of pyramidal tract activity to force exerted during voluntary movement. *J. Neurophysiol.* 31:14.

90. Bryan, R. N., Trevino, D. L., Coulter, J. D., and Willis, W. D. (1973). Location and somatotopic organization of cells of origin of the spinocervical tract. *Exp. Brain Res.* 17:177–189.

91. Dart, A. M., and Gordon, G. (1973). Some properties of spinal connections of the cat's dorsal column nuclei which do not involve the dorsal columns. *Brain Res.* 58:61–68.

92. Landgren, S., and Silfvenius, H. (1971). Nucleus Z, the medullary relay in the projection path to the cerebral cortex of group I muscle afferents from the cat's hind limb. *J. Physiol. (Lond.)* 218:551–571.

93. Johansson, H., and Silfvenius, H. (1977). Input from ipsilateral proprio- and exteroceptive hind limb afferents to nucleus Z of the cat medullar oblongata. *J. Physiol. (Lond.)* 265:371–393.

94. Grant, G., Boivie, J., and Silfvenius, H. (1973). Course and termination of fibres from the nucleus Z of the medulla oblongata. An experimental light microscopical study in the cat. *Brain Res. 55*:55–70.

95. Cervero, F., Iggo, A., and Molony, V. (1977). Responses of spinocervical tract neurones to noxious stimulation of the skin. *J. Physiol. (Lond.) 267*: 537–558.

96. Weinstein, S. (1968). Intensive and extensive aspects of tactile sensitivity as a function of body part, sex and laterality. In *The Skin Senses*, D. Kenshalo (Ed.), Charles C Thomas, Springfield, Illinois, pp. 195–222.

97. Melzack, R., and Casey, K. L. (1968). Sensory, motivational and central control determinants of pain. In *The Skin Senses*, D. Kanshalo (Ed.), Charles C Thomas, Springfield, Illinois, pp. 423–444.

98. Kerr, F. W. L., and Lippman, H. H. (1974). The primate spinothalamic tract as demonstrated by anterolateral cordotomy and commissural myelotomy. In *Advances in Neurology*, vol. 4, J. J. Bonica (Ed.), Raven, New York, pp. 147–156.

99. Kerr, F. W. L. (1975). The ventral spinothalamic tract and other ascending systems of the ventral funiculus of the spinal cord. *J. Comp. Neurol. 159*: 335–356.

100. Vierck, C. J., Jr., Cooper, B. Y., Franzén, O., Ritz, L. A., and Greenspan, J. D. (1983). Behavioral analysis of CNS pathways and transmitter systems involved in conduction and inhibition of pain sensations and reactions in primates. In *Progress in Psychobiology and Physiological Psychology*, J. Sprague and A. Epstein (Eds.), Academic Press, New York, pp. 113–165.

100a. King, R. B. (1957). Postchordotomy studies of pain threshold. *Neurology 7*:610–669.

101. Vierck, C. J., Jr., Hamilton, D. M., and Thornby, J. I. (1974). Pain reactivity of monkeys after lesions to the dorsal and lateral columns of the spinal cord. *Exp. Brain Res. 13*:140–158.

102. Vierck, C. J., Jr., and Luck, M. M. (1979). Loss and recovery of reactivity to noxious stimuli in monkeys with primary spinothalamic cordotomies, followed by secondary and tertiary lesions of other sectors. *Brain 102*: 233–248.

103. Willis, W. D., Trevino, D. L. Coulter, J. D., and Maunz, R. A. (1974). Responses of primate spinothalamic tract neurons to natural stimulation of hindlimb. *J. Neurophysiol. 37*:358–372.

104. Applebaum, A. E., Beall, J. E., Foreman, R. D., and Willis, W. D. (1975). Organization and receptive fields of primate spinothalamic tract neurons. *J. Neurophysiol. 38*:572–586.

105. Price, D. D., and Mayer, D. J. (1975). Neurophysiological characterization of the anterolateral quadrant neurons subserving pain in Macaca mulatta. *Pain 1*:59–72.

106. Foreman, R. D., Schmidt, R. F., and Willis, W. D. (1977). Convergence of muscle and cutaneous input onto primate spinothalamic tract neurons. *Brain Res. 124*:555–560.

107. Giesler, G. J., Jr., Yezierski, R. P., Gerhard, K. D., and Willis, W. D. (1981). Spinothalamic tract neurons that project to medial and/or lateral thalamic nuclei: Evidence for a physiologically novel population of spinal cord neurons. *J. Neurophysiol. 46*:1285-1308.

108. Weaver, T. A., and Walker, A. E. (1941). Topical arrangement within spinothalamic tract of monkey. *Arch. Neurol. Psychiat. 46*:877-883.

109. Matthews, P. B. C. (1977). Muscle afferents and kinaesthesia. *Br. Med. Bull. 33*:137-142.

109a. Tracey, D. J. (1982). Pathways for proprioception. In *Proprioception, Posture and Emotion*, D. Garlick (Ed.), University of New South Wales, Kensington, pp. 23-55.

110. Schroeder, D. M., and Jane, J. A. (1971). Projection of dorsal column nuclei and spinal cord to brainstem and thalamus in the tree shrew, Tupaia glis. *J. Comp. Neurol. 142*:309-350.

111. Dreyer, D. A., Schneider, R. J., Metz, C. B., and Whitsel, B. L. (1974). Differential contributions of spinal pathways to both representation in postcentral gyrus of Macaca mulatta. *J. Neurophysiol. 37*:119-145.

112. von Bekesy, G. (1967). In *Sensory Inhibition*, Princeton University, Princeton.

113. Vierck, C. J., Jr., and Rand, R. (1979). Localization of touch on glabrous skin following dorsal column lesion in a primate. *Neurosci. Abst. 5*:715.

114. Wall, P. D., and Noordenbos, W. (1977). Sensory functions which remain in man after complete transection of dorsal columns. *Brain 100*:641-653.

115. Halnan, C. R. E., and Wright, G. H. (1960). Tactile localization. *Brain 83*: 677-699.

116. Werner, G., and Whitsel, B. L. (1968). Topology of the body representation in somatosensory area 1 of primates. *J. Neurophysiol. 311*:856-869.

117. Vierck, C. J., Jr., Cohen, R. H., and Cooper, B. Y. (1983). Effects of spinal tractotomy on spatial sequence recognition in macaques. *J. Neurosci. 2*: 280-290.

118. Vallbo, A. B., and Johansson, R. S. (1978). The tactile sensory innervation of the glabrous skin of the human hand. In *Active Touch*, G. Gordon (Ed.), Pergamon Press, Oxford, pp. 29-54.

119. Berkley, M. A. (1982). The geniculo cortical system and visual perception. In *Changing Concepts of the Nervous System*, A. R. Morrison and P. L. Strick (Eds.), Academic Press, New York, pp. 295-320.

120. Levitt, M., and Schwartzman, R. J. (1966). Spinal sensory tracts and two-point tactile sensitivity. *Anat. Rec. 154*:377.

121. Cook, A. W., and Browder, E. J. (1965). Function of posterior columns in man. *Arch. Neurol. Psychiat. 12*:72-79.

122. Zigler, M. J. (1935). The experimental relation of the two-point limen to the error of location. *J. Gen. Psychol. 13*:316-332.

123. Rosner, B. S. (1961). Neural factors limiting cutaneous spatiotemporal discriminations. In *Sensory Communications*, W. A. Roseblith (Ed.), Massachusetts Institute of Technology, Cambridge, pp. 725-738.

124. Hirsh, I. J., and Sherrick, C. E., Jr. (1961). Perceived order in different sense modalities. *J. Exp. Psychol. 62*:423-432.

125. Loomis, J. M. (1981). Tactile pattern perception. *Perception 10*:5–27.
126. Vierck, C. J., Jr. (1974). Tactile movement detection and discriminating following dorsal column lesions in monkeys. *Exp. Brain Res. 20*: 331–346.
127. Azulay, A., and Schwartz, A. S. (1975). The role of the dorsal funiculus of the primate in tactual discriminations. *Exp. Neurol. 46*:315–332.
128. Taylor, M. M., and Lederman, S. J. (1975). Tactile roughness of grooved surfaces: A model and the effect of friction. *Percept. Psychophys. 17*: 28–36.
129. Hill, J. W., and Bliss, J. D. (1968). Modeling a tactile sensory register. *Percept. Psychophys. 4*:91–101.
130. Beauchamp, K. L., Matheson, D. W., and Scadden, L. A. (1971). Effect of stimulus-change method on tactile-image recognition. *Percept. Mot. Skills 33*:1067–1070.
131. Grunewald, A. P. (1978). On braille and braille machines. *Sensory World 3*:4.
132. Dobry, P. K. J., and Casey, K. L. (1972). Roughness discrimination in cats with dorsal column lesions. *Brain 44*:385–397.
133. Kitai, S. T., and Weinberg, J. (1968). Tactile discrimination study of the dorsal column-medial lemniscal system and spino-cervico-thalamic tract in cat. *Exp. Brain Res. 6*:234–246.
134. Schwartz, A. S., Eidelberg, E., Marchok, P., and Azulay, A. (1972). Tactile discrimination in the monkey after section of the dorsal funiculus and lateral lemniscus. *Exp. Neurol. 37*:582–596.
135. Kreuger, L. E. (1970). David Katz's "Der Aufbau der Tastwelt (The World of Touch): A Synopsis. *Percept. Psychophys. 7*:337–341.
136. Lederman, S. J., Loomis, J. M., and Williams, D. A. (1982). The role of vibration in the tactual perception of roughness. *Percept. Psychophys. 32*:109–116.
137. White, J. C., and Sweet, W. H. (1969). *Pain and the Neurosurgeon*, Charles C Thomas, Springfield, Illinois.
138. Phillips, J. R., and Johnson, K. O. (1981). Tactile spatial resolution. III. A continuum mechanics model of skin predicting mechanoreceptor responses to bars, edges, and gratings. *J. Neurophysiol. 46*:1204–1225.
138a. Gardner, E. P., and Spencer, W. A. (1972). Sensory funneling. I. Psychophysical observations of human subjects and responses of cutaneous mechanoreceptive afferents in the cat to patterned skin stimuli. *J. Neurophysiol. 35*:925–953.
138b. Goodwin, A. W., Youl, B. D., and Zimmerman, N. P. (1981). Single quickly adapting mechanoreceptive afferents innervating monkey glabrous skin: Responses to two vibrating probes. *J. Neurophysiol. 45*:227–242.
139. Critchley, M. (1953). In *The Parietal Lobes*, Williams & Wilkins, Baltimore.
140. Vierck, C. J., Jr. (1973). Alterations of spatio-tactile discrimination after lesions of primate spinal cord. *Brain Res. 58*:69–79.
141. Dyhre-Poulsen, P. (1965). Impairment of tactile tracking after dorsal column lesions in monkeys. *Exp. Brain Res. (Suppl.) 23*:64.

142. Vierck, C. J., Jr. (1975). Proprioceptive deficits after dorsal column lesions in monkeys. In *The Somatosensory System*, H. H. Kornhuber (Ed.), George Thieme, Stuttgart, pp. 311–318.

143. Roland, E. (1976). Astereognosis. Tactile discrimination after localized hemispheric lesions in man. *Arch. Neurol. 33*:543–550.

144. Williams, W. J., BeMent, S. L., Yim, T. C. T., and McCall, W. D. (1973). Nucleus gracilis responses to knee joint motion; a frequency response study. *Brain Res. 64*:123–140.

145. Vierck, C. J., Jr. (1966). Spinal pathways mediating limb position sense. *Anat. Rec. 254*:437.

146. Vierck, C. J., Jr. (1978). Comparison of forelimb and hindlimb motor deficits following dorsal column section in monkeys. *Brain Res. 146*: 279–294.

147. McCormack, M., and Dubrovsky, B. (1979). Impairment in limb actions after dorsal funiculi section in cats. *Exp. Brain Res. 37*:31–40.

148. Myers, D. A., Hostetter, G., Bourassa, C. M., and Swett, J. E. (1974). Dorsal columns in sensory detection. *Brain Res. 70*:350–355.

149. Frommer, G. P., Trefz, B. R., and Casey, K. L. (1977). Somatosensory function and cortical unit activity in cats with only dorsal column fibers. *Exp. Brain Res. 27*:113–129.

150. Norrsell, U. (1966). The spinal afferent pathways of conditioned reflexes to cutaneous stimuli in the dog. *Exp. Brain Res. 2*:269–282.

151. Tapper, D. M. (1970). Behavioral evaluation of the tactile pad receptor system in hairy skin of the cat. *Exp. Neurol. 26*:447–459.

152. Johansson, R. S., and Vallbo, A. B. (1979). Detection of tactile stimuli. Thresholds of afferent units related to psychophysical thresholds in the human head. *J. Physiol. (Lond.) 297*:405–422.

153. Jones, M. B., and Vierck, C. J., Jr. (1973). Length discrimination on the skin. *Am. J. Psychol. 86*:49–60.

154. Millar, J. (1973). The topography and receptive fields of ventroposterolateral thalamic neurons excited by afferents projecting through the dorsolateral funiculus of the spinal cord. *Exp. Neurol. 41*:303–313.

155. Ratliff, F. (1965). *Mach Bands: Quantitative Studies on Neural Networks in the Retina*, Holden-Day, San Francisco.

156. Vierck, C. J., Jr. (1979). Comparison of punctate, edge and surface stimulation of peripheral, slowly-adapting, cutaneous, afferent units of cats. *Brain Res. 175*:155–159.

157. Phillips, J. R., and Johnson, K. O. (1981). Tactile spatial resolution. II. Neural representation of bars, edges and gratings in monkey primary afferents. *J. Neurophysiol. 46*:1192–1203.

158. Johansson, R. S., Landstom, U., and Lundstrom, R. (1982). Sensitivity to edges of mechanoreceptive afferents units innervating the glabrous skin of the human head. *Brain Res. 244*:27–32.

159. Brown, P. B. (1969). Response of cat dorsal horn cells to variations of intensity, location and area of cutaneous stimuli. *Exp. Neurol. 23*:249–265.

160. Dostrovsky, J. O., and Millar, J. (1977). Receptive fields of gracile neurons after transection of the dorsal columns. *Exp. Neurol. 56*:610–621.

161. Bernstein, J. J., and Ganchrow, D. (1981). Relationship of afferentation with soma size of nucleus gracilis neurons after bilateral dorsal column lesion in the rat. *Exp. Neurol. 71*:452–463.

162. Millar, J., Basbaum, A. I., and Wall, P. D. (1976). Restructuring of the somatotopic map and appearance of abnormal neuronal activity in the gracile nucleus after partial deafferentation. *Exp. Neurol. 50*:658–672.

163. Levitt, M., and Levitt, J. (1968). Sensory hind limb representation of Sm I cortex of the cat after spinal tractotomies. *Exp. Neurol. 22*:276–302.

164. Anderson, S. A. (1962). Projection of different spinal pathways to the second somatic sensory area in cat. *Acta Physiol. Scand. (Suppl. 94)*: 1–74.

165. Eidelberg, E., and Woodbury, C. M. (1972). Apparent redundancy in the somatosensory system in monkeys. *Exp. Neurol. 37*:573–581.

166. Dobry, P. J. K., and Casey, K. L. (1972). Coronal somatosensory unit responses in cats with dorsal column lesions. *Brain Res. 44*:399–416.

167. Goldberger, M. E., and Murray, M. (1978). Recovery of movement and axonal sprouting may obey some of the same laws. In *Neuronal Plasticity*, C. W. Cotman (Ed.), Raven, New York, pp. 73–96.

168. Andersen, P., Andersson, S. A., and Landgren, S. (1966). Some properties of the thalamic relay cells in the spino-cervico-lemniscal path. *Acta Physiol. Scand. 68*:72–83.

169. Spreafico, R., Hayes, N. L., and Rustioni, A. (1981). Thalamic projections to the primary and secondary somatosensory cortices in cat: Single and double retrograde tracer studies. *J. Comp. Neurol. 203*:67–90.

170. Jones, E. G., and Friedman, D. P. (1982). Projection pattern of functional components of thalamic ventrobasal complex on monkey somatosensory cortex. *J. Neurophysiol. 48*:521–544.

171. Vierck, C. J., Jr. (1982). Plasticity of somatic sensations and motor capacities following lesions of the dorsal spinal columns in monkeys. In *Changing Concepts of the Nervous System*, A. R. Morrison and P. L. Strick (Eds.), Academic Press, New York, pp. 151–170.

172. Tessler, A., Glazer, E. Artymyshyn, R., Murray, M., and Goldberger, M. E. (1980). Recovery of substance P in the cat spinal cord after unilateral lumbosacral deafferentation. *Brain Res. 191*:459–470.

173. Vrensen, G., and Nunes Cardozo, J. (1981). Changes in size and shape of synaptic connections after visual training: An ultra structural approach of synaptic plasticity. *Brain Res. 218*:79–97.

174. Finger, S., and Reyes, R. (1977). Long-term deficits after somatosensory cortical lesions in rats. *Physiol. Behav. 15*:289–293.

175. Fadiga, E., Haimann, C., Margnelli, M., and Sotgiu, M. L. (1978). Variability of peripheral representation in ventrobasal thalamic nuclei of the cat: Effects of acute reversible blockade of the dorsal column nuclei. *Exp. Neurol. 60*:484–498.

176. Nathan, P. W., and Smith, M. C. (1973). Effects of two unilateral cordotomies on the motility of the lower limbs. *Brain 96*:471–494.

177. Wei, J. Y., Simon, J., Randíc, M., and Burgess, P. R., Personal communication.

178. Skoglund, S. (1956). Anatomical and physiological studies of knee joint innervation in the cat. (1956). *Acta Physiol. Scand. (Suppl.) 36*:124.

178a. Bourassa, C. M., and Swett, J. E. (1982). Behavioral detection of subcortical stimuli: Comparison of somatosensory and motor circuits. *J. Comp. Physiol. Psychol. 96*:679–690.

179. Johansson, H., and Silfvenius, H. (1977). Axon collateral activation by dorsal spinocerebellar tract fibers of group I relay cells or nucleus Z in the cat medulla oblongata. *J. Physiol. (Lond.) 265*:341–369.

179a. Saade, N. E., Jundi, A. S., Jabbur, S. J., and Banna, N. R. (1982). Dorsal column input to inferior raphe centralis neurons. *Brain Res. 250*:345–348.

180. Grant, G., Boivie, J., and Brodal, A. (1968). The question of a cerebellar projection from the lateral cervical nucleus re-examined. *Brain Res. 9*: 95–102.

181. Torebjörk, H. E., and Ochoa, J. L. (1980). Specific sensations evoked by activity in single identified sensory units in man. *Acta Physiol. Scand. 110*: 445–447.

182. Werner, G., and Mountcastle, V. B. (1965). Neural activity in mechanoreceptive cutaneous afferents: Stimulus-response relations, Weber functions, and information transmission. *J. Neurophysiol. 28*:359–397.

183. Whitsel, B. L., Jr., Schreiner, C., and Essick, G. K. (1976). An analysis of variability in somatosensory cortical neuron discharge. *J. Neurophysiol. 40*:589–607.

184. Walsh, J. P., and Whitehorn, D. (1981). An input-output analysis of the dorsal column nuclei. *Exp. Neurol. 73*:186–198.

185. Johnson, K. O. (1974). Reconstruction of population response to vibratory stimulus in quickly adapting mechanoreceptive afferent fiber population innervating glabrous skin of the monkey. *J. Neurophysiol. 37*:48–72.

186. Boivie, J. (1978). Anatomical observations on the dorsal column nuclei, their thalamic projection and the cytoarchitecture of some somatosensory thalamic nuclei in the monkey. *J. Comp. Neurol. 178*:17–48.

187. Tracey, D. J., Asanuma, C., Jones, E. G., and Porter, R. (1980). Thalamic relay to motor cortex: Afferent pathways from brain stem, cerebellum and spinal cord in monkeys. *J. Neurophysiol. 44*:532–554.

188. Vierck, C. J., Jr. (1982). Comparison of the effects of dorsal rhizotomy or dorsal column transection on motor performance of monkeys. *Exp. Neurol. 75*:566–575.

189. Polit, A., and Bizzi, E. (1979). Characteristics of motor programs underlying arm movements in monkeys. *J. Neurophysiol. 42*:183–194.

190. Smith, M. C. (1967). Stereotactic operations for Parkinson's disease; anatomical observations. In *Modern Trends in Neurology*, D. Williams (Ed.), Butterworths, London, pp. 21–52.

191. Chapman, C. E., and Wiesendanger, M. (1982). Recovery of function following unilateral lesions in the bulbar pyramid in the monkey. *Electroenceph. Clin. Neurophysiol.* *53*:374–387.
192. Bucy, P. C., Keplinger, J. E., and Siqueria, E. B. (1954). Destruction of the pyramidal tract in man. *J. Neurosurg.* *21*:295–298.
193. Stein, B. E., Magalhaes-Castro, B., and Kruger, L. (1976). Relationship between visual and tactile representations in cat superior colliculus. *J. Neurophysiol.* *39*:401–419.
194. Bitar, M., Saade, N. E., Banna, N. R., and Jabbur, S. J. (1981). Interactions of inputs from dorsal columns and ventral tracts with visual inputs on single neurons of cat superior colliculus. *Brain Res.* *220*:356–361.
195. Mountcastle, V. B., Lynch, J. C., Georgopoulos, A. Sakata, H., and Acuna, C. (1975). Posterior parietal association cortex of the monkey: Command functions for operations within extrapersonal space. *J. Neurophysiol.* *38*: 871–908.
196. Delacour, J., Libouban, S., and McNeil, M. (1972). Premotor cortex and instrumental behavior in monkeys. *Physiol. Behav.* *8*:299–305.
197. Pandya, D. N., and Kuypers, H. G. J. M. (1969). Cortico-cortical connections in the Rhesus monkey. *Brain Res.* *13*:13–36.
198. Evarts, E. V. (1966). Pyramidal tract activity associated with a conditioned hand movement in the monkey. *J. Neurophysiol.* *29*:1011–1027.
199. Thach, W. T. (1978). Correlation of neural discharge with pattern and force of muscular activity, joint position, and direction of intended next movement in motor cortex and cerebellum. *J. Neurophysiol.* *41*:654–676.
200. DeLong, M. R., and Strick, P. L. (1974). Relation of basal ganglia, cerebellum, and motor cortex units to ramp and ballistic limb movements. *Brain Res.* *71*:327–335.
201. Strick, P. L. (1976). Activity of ventrolateral thalamic neurons during arm movement. *J. Neurophysiol.* *39*:1032–1044.
202. Asanuma, C., Thach, W. T., and Jones, E. G. (1983). Distribution of cerebellar terminations and their relation to other afferent terminations in the ventral lateral thalamic region of the monkey. *Brain Res. Rev.* *5*:237–265.
203. Jones, E. G., Coulter, J. D., and Hendry, S. H. C. (1978). Intracortical connectivity of architectonic fields in the somatic sensory, motor and parietal cortex of monkeys. *J. Comp. Neurol.* *181*:291–348.
204. Phillips, C. G. (1969). The Ferrier lecture, 1968. Motor apparatus of the baboon's hand. *Proc. R. Soc. Lond. (Biol.)* *173*:141–174.
205. Liu, C. N., Yu, J., Chambers, W. W., and Ha, H. (1975). The role for the medial lemniscal and spinocervicothalamic pathways on tactile reactions in cats. *Acta Neurobiol. Exp.* *35*:149–157.
206. Gilman, S., and Denny-Brown, D. (1966). Disorders of movement and behavior following dorsal column lesions. *Brain* *89*:397–418.
207. Schneider, R. J., Kulics, A. T., and Ducker, T. B. (1977). Proprioceptive pathways of the spinal cord. *J. Neurol. Neurosurg. Psychiat.* *40*:417–433.

208. Heckman, T., and Bourassa, S. M. (1981). Lesions of the dorsal column nuclei or medial lemniscus of the cat: Effect on motor performance. *Brain Res. 244*:405–411.
209. Christiansen, J. (1966). Neurological observations of macaques with spinal cord lesions. *Anat. Rec. 154*:330.
210. Ganchrow, D., Margolin, J., Perez, L., and Bernstein, J. J. (1980). Component analysis of hind limb behavioral alterations after damage to the rat dorsal funiculus. *Exp. Neurol. 70*:339–355.
211. Bossom, J., and Omaya, A. K. (1968). Visuomotor adaption (to prismatic transformation of the retinal image) in monkeys with bilateral dorsal rhizotomy. *Brain 91*:161–172.
212. Gilman, S., Carr, D., and Hollenberg, J. (1976). Kinematic effects of deafferentation and cerebellar oblation. *Brain 99*:311–330.
213. Taub, E., Goldberg, I. A., and Taub, P. (1975). Deafferentation in monkeys: Pointing at a target without visual feedback. *Exp. Neurol. 46*:178–186.
214. Terzuolo, C. A., Soechting, J. F., and Ranish, N. A. (1974). Studies on the control of some simple motor tasks. V. Changes in motor output following dorsal root section in squirrel monkey. *Brain Res. 70*:521–526.
215. Leonard, J. A. (1959). Tactual choice reactions: I. *Q. J. Exp. Psychol. 11*: 76–82.
216. Sperry, R. W. (1950). Neural basis of spontaneous optokinetic response produced by visual inversion. *J. Comp. Physiol. Psychol. 43*:482–489.
217. Goldberger, M. E. (1977). Locomotor recovery after unilateral hindlimb deafferentation in cats. *Brain Res. 123*:59–74.
218. Wetzel, M. C., Atwater, A. E., Wait, J. V., and Stuart, C. G. (1976). Kinematics of locomotion by cats with a single hindlimb deafferented. *J. Neurophysiol. 39*:667–678.
219. English, A. W. (1980). Interlimb coordination during stepping in the cat: Effects of dorsal column section. *J. Neurophysiol. 44*:270–279.
220. Dubrovskyu, B., Davelaar, F., and Garcia-Rill, E. (1971). The role of dorsal columns in serial order acts. *Exp. Neurol. 33*:93–102.
221. Ferraro, A., and Barrera, S. E. (1934). Effects of experimental lesions of the posterior columns in macacus Rhesus monkeys. *Brain 57*:307–332.
221a. Beaubaton, D., and Trouche, E. (1982). Participation of the cerebellar dentate nucleus in the control of a goal-directed movement in monkeys. Effects of reversible or permanent dentate lesion on the duration and accuracy of a pointing response. *Exp. Brain Res. 46*:127–138.
222. Roland, P. E., and Ladegaard-Pedersen, H. (1977). A quantitative analysis of sensations of tension and of kinaesthesia in man. *Brain 100*:671–692.
223. Marsden, C. D., Rothwell, J. C., and Traub, M. M. (1979). Effect of thumb anesthesia on weight perception, muscle activity and the stretch reflex in man. *J. Physiol. 294*:303–315.
224. Gandevia, S. C., and McCloskey, D. I. (1977). Sensations of heaviness. *Brain 100*:345–354.
225. McCloskey, D. I., and Torda, T. A. G. (1975). Corollary motor discharges and kinaesthesia. *Brain Res. 100*:467–470.

226. Kuypers, H. G. J. M. (1964). The descending pathways to the spinal cord, their anatomy and function. *Prog. Brain Res.* *11*:178–200.

227. Liu, C. N., and Chambers, W. W. (1964). An experimental study of the cortico-spinal system in the monkey (Macaca mulatta): The spinal pathways and preterminal distribution of degenerating fibers following discrete lesions of the pre- and postcentral gyri and bulbar pyramid. *J. Comp. Neurol.* *123*:257–284.

228. Schoen, J. H. R. (1964). Comparative aspects of the descending fibre systems in the spinal cord. *Prog. Brain Res.* *11*:203–222.

229. Campbell, C. B., Yashon, D., and Jane, J. A. (1966). The origin, course and termination of corticospinal fibers in the slow loris, Nycticebus coucang (boddaert). *J. Comp. Neurol.* *127*:101–112.

230. Petras, J. M. (1968). Corticospinal fibers in New World and Old World simians. *Brain Res.* *8*:206–208.

231. Sherrington, C. S. (1900). The spinal cord. In *Textbook of Physiology*, E. A. Schafer (Ed.), vol. 2, Pentland, Edinburgh, pp. 783–883.

232. Heffner, R., and Masterton, B. (1975). Variation in form of the pyramidal tract and its relationship to digital dexterity. *Brain Behav. Evol.* *12*:161–200.

233. Bishop, A. (1964). Use of the hand in lower primates. In *Evolutionary and Genetic Biology of Primates*, J. Buettner-Janusch (Eds.), vol. 2, Academic Press, New York, pp. 133–225.

234. Clough, J. F., and Sheridan, J. D. (1968). A fast pathway for cortical influence on cervical gamma moto-neurones in the baboon. *J. Physiol. (Lond.)* *195*:26P–27P.

235. Lemon, R. N., and Porter, R. (1976). Afferent input to movement–related precentral neurones in conscious monkeys. *Proc. R. Soc. Lond. (Biol.)* *194*:313–339.

236. Asanauma, H., Waters, R. S., and Yumiya, H. (1982). Physiological properties of neurons projecting from area 3a to area 4g of feline cerebral cortex. *J. Neurophysiol.* *48*:1048–1057.

237. Cole, J. D., and Gordon, G. (1976). Differences in timing of cortico-cuneate and corticogracile actions. In *Sensory Functions of the Skin*, Y. Zotterman, (Ed.), Pergamon Press, Oxford, pp. 231–240.

238. Levitt, M., Carreras, M., Liu, C. N., and Chambers, W. W. (1964). Pyramidal and extrapyramidal modulation of somatosensory activity in gracile and cuneate nuclei. *Arch. Ital. Biol.* *102*:197–229.

239. Tsumoto, T., Nakamura, S., and Iwama, K. (1975). Pyramidal tract control over cutaneous and kinesthetic sensory transmission in the cat thalamus. *Exp. Brain Res.* *22*:281–294.

240. Tower, S. S. (1940). Pyramidal lesions in the monkey. *Brain* *63*:36–90.

241. Lassek, A. M. (1948). Pyramidal tract: Basic considerations of corticospinal neurones. *Res. Publ. Ass. Nerv. Ment. Dis.* *27*:106–128.

242. Hwang, Y. C., Hinsman, E. J., and Roesel, O. F. (1975). Caliber spectra of fibers in the fasciculus gracilis of the cat cervical spinal cord: A quantitative electron microscopic study. *J. Comp. Neurol.* *162*:195–204.

243. Towe, A. L. (1973). Somatosensory cortex: Descending influences on ascending systems. In *Handbook of Sensory Physiology*, vol. 2, A. Iggo (Ed.), Springer-Verlag, Berlin, pp. 315–338.

244. Dyhre-Poulsen, P. (1978). Perception of tactile stimuli before ballistic and during tracking movements. In *Active Touch*, G. Gordon (Ed.), Pergamon Press, Oxford, pp. 171–176.

245. Andersen, P., Eccles, J. C., Schmidt, R. F., and Yokota, T. (1964). Depolarization of presynaptic fibers in the cuneate nucleus. *J. Neurophysiol.* 27:92–106.

246. Coulter, J. D., Maunz, R. A., and Willis, W. D. (1974). Effects of stimulation of sensorimotor cortex on primate spinothalamic neurons. *Brain Res.* 65:351–356.

247. Andersen, P., Eccles, J. C., and Sears, T. A. (1964). Cortically evoked depolarization of primary afferent fibers in the spinal cord. *J. Neurophysiol.* 27:63–77.

248. Hepp-Reymond, M.-C., Trouche, E., and Wiesendanger, M. (1974). Effects of unilateral and bilateral pyramidotomy on a conditioned rapid precision grip in monkeys (Macaca fasicularis). *Exp. Brain Res.* 21:519–527.

249. Hore, J., Phillips, C. G., and Porter, R. (1973). The effects of pyramidotomy on motor performance in the brush-tailed possum (Trichosurus vulpecula). *Brain Res.* 49:181–184.

250. Jankowska, E., and Tanaka, R. (1974). Neuronal mechanism of the disynaptic inhibition evoked in primate spinal motoneurones from the corticospinal tract. *Brain Res.* 75:163–166.

251. Laursen, A. M., and Wiesendanger, M. (1966). Motor deficits after transection of a bulbar pyramid in the cat. *Acta Physiol. Scand.* 68:118–126.

252. Laursen, A. M., and Wiesendanger, M. (1967). The effect of pyramidal lesions on response latency in cats. *Brain Res.* 5:207–220.

253. Hepp-Reymond, M.-C., and Wiesendanger, M. (1972). Unilateral pyramidotomy in monkeys: Effect on force and speed of a conditioned precision grip. *Brain Res.* 36:117–131.

254. Bucy, P. C., Ladpli, R., and Ehrlich, A. (1966). Destruction of the pyramidal tract in the monkey. *J. Neurosurg.* 25:1–20.

255. Phillips, E. G. T., and Phillips, C. G. (1944). Pyramidal section in the cat. *Brain* 67:1–9.

256. Schwartzman, R. J. (1978). A behavioral analysis of complete unilateral section of pyramidal tract at the medullary level in Macaca mulatta. *Ann. Neurol.* 4:234–244.

257. Castro, A. J. (1972). The effects of cortical ablations on digital usage in the rat. *Brain Res.* 37:173–185.

258. Eidelberg, E., Kreinick, C. J., and Langescheid, C. (1975). On the possible functional role of afferent pathways in skin sensation. *Exp. Neurol.* 47:419–432.

259. Evarts, E. V., and Fromm, C. (1981). Transcortical reflexes and servo control of movement. *Can. J. Physiol. Pharmacol.* 59:757–775.

260. Sakai, T., and Preston, J. B. (1978). Evidence for a transcortical reflex: Primate corticospinal tract neuron responses to ramp stretch of muscle. *Brain Res. 159*:463–467.

261. Lloyd, D. P. C. (1941). The spinal mechanism of the pyramidal system in cats. *J. Neurophysiol. 4*:525–546.

262. Lee, R. G., and Tatton, W. G. (1975). Motor responses to sudden limb displacements in primates with specific CNS lesions and in human patients with motor system disorders. *Can. J. Physiol. Pharmacol. 2*: 285–293.

263. Evarts, E. G., and Tanji, J. (1974). Gating of motor cortex reflexes by prior instruction. *Brain Res. 71*:479–494.

264. Marsden, C. D., Merton, P. A., and Morton, H. B. (1973). Is the human stretch reflex cortical rather than spinal? *Lancet 1*:759–761.

265. Evarts, E. V., and Vaughn, W. J. (1978). Intended arm movements in response to externally produced arm displacements in man. In *Cerebral Motor Control in Man: Long Loop Mechanisms. Progress in Clinical Neurophysiology* (J. E. Desmedt, Ed.), vol. 4, Karger, Basel, pp. 178–192.

266. Smith, A. M., Hepp-Reymond, M.-C., and Wyss, U. R. (1975). Relation of activity in precentral cortical neurones to force and rate of force change during isometric contractions of finger muscles. *Exp. Brain Res. 23*:315–332.

267. Evarts, E. V. (1973). Motor cortex reflexes associated with learned movements. *Science 179*:501–503.

268. Hallett, M., Shahani, B. T., and Young, R. R. (1975). EMG analysis of stereotyped voluntary movements in man. *J. Neurol. Neurosurg. 38*: 1154–1162.

269. Fidone, S. J., and Preston, J. B. (1969). Patterns of motor cortex control of flexor and extensor cat fusimotor neurones. *J. Neurophysiol. 32*:103–115.

270. Teodoru, D. E., Tran, T., and Berman, A. J. (1978). Forelimb function after dorsal column nuclei lesion or dorsal rhizotomy. *Soc. Neurosci. Abst. 4*:307.

271. Wall, P. D. (1970). The sensory and motor role of impulses traveling in the dorsal columns towards cerebral cortex. *Brain 93*:505–524.

272. Brown, A. G., Kirk, E. J., and Martin, H. F. (1973). Descending and segmental inhibition of transmission through the spinocervical tract. *J. Physiol. (Lond.) 230*:689–705.

272a. Burton, H., and Loewy, A. D. (1977). Projections to the spinal cord from medullary somatosensory relay nuclei. *J. Comp. Neurol. 173*:773–792.

273. Brinkman, J., and Porter, R. (1978). Movement performance and afferent projections to the sensorimotor cortex in monkeys with dorsal column lesions. In *Active Touch*, G. Gordon (Ed.), Pergamon Press, Oxford, pp. 119–138.

274. Schneider, R. J., and Burke, R. (1980). Detection of sensory spinal tract dysfunction with signal detection theory. *Soc. Neurosci. Abst. 6*:727.

275. Beck, C. H. M. (1973). Compensation of postural control by squirrel monkeys following dorsal column lesions. In *Control of Posture and Locomotion*, R. B. Stein, K. G. Pearson, R. S. Smith, and J. B. Redford (Eds.), Plenum Press, New York, pp. 421–424.

276. Melzack, R., and Bridges, J. A. (1971). Dorsal column contributions to motor behavior. *Exp. Neurol. 33*:53–68.

277. Reynolds, P. J., and Talbott, Z. E., and Brookhart, J. M. (1972). Control of postural reactions in the dog: The role of the dorsal column feedback pathway. *Brain Res. 40*:159–164.

278. Kruger, L., and Mosso, J. (1974). An evaluation of duality in the trigeminal afferent system. *Adv. Neurol. 4*:73–82.

279. Greenspan, J. D., Vierck, C. J., Jr., and Ritz, L. A. (Unpublished observations.)

16

DORSAL HORN MECHANISMS OF PAIN

Donald D. Price   *Medical College of Virginia, Virginia Commonwealth University, Richmond, Virginia*

I. INTRODUCTION

The dorsal gray matter of the mammalian spinal cord is the origin of ascending somatosensory pathways. Impulses from thermoreceptive, nociceptive, and mechanoreceptive afferents excite various types of second-order neurons of the dorsal horn. Radical transformations are made of these inputs such that responses to somatosensory stimuli do not simply passively reflect the responses of cutaneous receptors. These transformations have important implications for our perception of somatosensory sensations. The dorsal horn also is the central focal point for autonomic and somatomotor reflexes initiated by stimulation of body tissues. This region clearly does not function autonomously but is under the influence of several descending control mechanisms. For these reasons and others, the dorsal horn has been more extensively investigated than many other central nervous system areas.

This chapter will review much of what is currently known about dorsal horn mechanisms of pain. The first part of this review will discuss the input-output relationships of different types of dorsal horn neurons that are likely to be involved in pain mechanisms. These relationships account for some of the sensory attributes of pain, many of which cannot be explained on the basis of primary afferent physiology. The second part of the chapter will focus on the microcircuitry of the dorsal horn that helps to explain the input-output relationships of the dorsal horn. The anatomic-functional connections of this circuitry will be explained in terms of their role in the phenomena described in the first part of the chapter.

II. INPUT-OUTPUT RELATIONSHIPS OF THE DORSAL HORN

A. Classes of Spinal Cord Neurons

There are several distinct classes of spinal cord interneurons and spinothalamic tract neurons. These classes of neurons are based on the types of primary afferent neurons that excite them and upon their receptive field organization. The characteristics of nociceptive neurons will be emphasized in the following discussion.

1. Wide Dynamic Range Neurons

Wide dynamic range (WDR) neurons have been more extensively studied than any other class of nociceptive neurons (1,2). Their potential involvement in pain is a critical aspect of the gate control theory (1,3,4). This theory proposes that both large-diameter afferents and small-diameter afferents converge on central cells of this type and that the final output of these neurons (called T cells) is controlled by interactions between large- and small-fiber input and by descending pathways from the brain. Wide dynamic range neurons exist in high concentrations in lamina V of the dorsal horn and to a lesser extent in laminae I, II, IV, and VI (5-8). Many wide dynamic range neurons in laminae I and V are spinothalamic tract neurons (5-10). Wide dynamic range neurons receive excitatory effects from impulses in both large-diameter ($A\beta$) sensitive mechanoreceptive afferents and in small-diameter ($A\delta$ and C) nociceptive afferents (5-9). Receptive fields of these neurons range considerably in size, but they are usually much larger than those of primary afferents (see Fig. 1). They are often organized into central zones in which the neuron responds with increasingly higher frequencies of impulse discharge to gentle touch, firm pressure, and noxious pinching (5-8). These central zones are surrounded by less sensitive zones in which firm pressure and noxious stimuli evoke impulse discharge. Finally, these latter zones are often surrounded by even less sensitive zones in which only frankly noxious stimulation evokes impulse discharge. Recordings from wide dynamic range neurons in awake behaving monkeys have shown that these receptive field zones expand or contract depending on the attentional set of the animal (11,12). The receptive field areas from which neural responses could be evoked by noxious temperatures *expanded* during a thermal discrimination task and *contracted* during a visual discrimination task.

There is considerable evidence that wide dynamic range neurons have an important function in pain mechanisms. These neurons respond to noxious

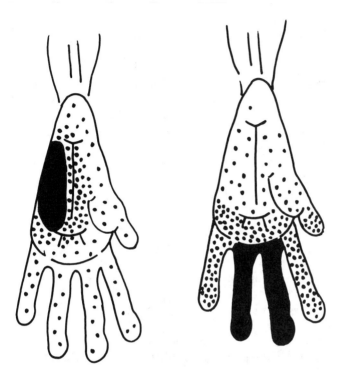

Figure 1 Drawing illustrating the gradients of responsivity recorded from two different WDR neurons (*left* and *right*) observed in an anesthetized monkey. The central portions of their receptive fields (darkly shaded) are most sensitive and respond with increasing frequency as the intensity of mechanical stimulation is increased from touch to pressure to pinch with toothed forceps. The more peripheral regions of the receptive fields are systematically less sensitive, responding differentially only to pressure and pinch (heavily stippled) or to pinch only (lightly stippled). (Redrawn from Ref. 13.)

mechanical or noxious heat stimulation with a frequency of impulse discharge that is higher than that which can be evoked by any form of innocuous stimulation (5-8). Thus, their increased response to nociceptive as compared to tactile stimulation can provide information that is sufficient to distinguish between these two levels of stimulation.

   In addition, there are several parallels between physiologic characteristics of wide dynamic range neurons and characteristics of human pain experience that strengthen the hypothesis that such neurons have a direct function in pain (1). Responses of wide dynamic range neurons to graded levels of noxious thermal stimulation increase monotonically over a 45–51°C range (5,7,11). The stimulus-response functions obtained in unanesthetized behaving monkeys (11) are similar to those obtained in anesthetized monkeys (5–8). The growth of response magnitude fits a power function with an exponent of 2.3 (temperature is computed as T_1-T_0, where 35°C is considered physiologic zero, or T_0). This power function closely parallels human psychophysical magnitude responses to this same temperature range. The latter has an exponent of 2.2 (based on data in ref. 13). Similar to pain perception, responses of wide dynamic range neurons to nociceptive skin temperatures are influenced by the psychologic set of the organism (11,12). The impulse frequency responses of these neurons to 45–49°C skin temperatures are higher when the monkey is making a thermal as compared to a visual discrimination (11). Another parallel is related to the observation that wide dynamic range neurons of the lower thoracic and upper lumbar spinal cord receive excitatory inputs from both visceral and cutaneous nociceptive afferents (14,15). Moreover, stimulation of visceral nociceptive afferents can inhibit subsequent responses of these neurons to stimulation of cutaneous nerves and vice versa (14,15). This convergence of inputs and their interactions may well provide part of the basis of referred pain (4,16) and the inhibitory interactions that are known to take place between visceral and cutaneous pain. Clearly, responses of wide dynamic range neurons to controlled noxious stimuli are not simply direct functions of receptor responses but reflect a variety of central nervous system temporal and spatial facilitatory mechanisms and inhibitory mechanisms. These mechanisms have important influences on pain perception and will be discussed later.

Many wide dynamic range neurons can be antidromically activated from the contralateral thalamus (6,9,17). These include both spinothalamic and nucleus caudalis trigeminothalamic neurons. Therefore, these neurons have central anatomic connections consistent with an involvement in pain mechanisms. These neurons appear to be most effectively antidromically activated from that portion of the ventrobasal complex that when stimulated in man produces pain (1).

2. Nociceptive-Specific Neurons

Spinal cord neurons that respond exclusively or nearly exclusively to noxious stimuli exist in high concentrations in the superficial layers of the dorsal horn (laminae I and II) and to a lesser extent in laminae IV and V. Nociceptive-specific (NS) spinothalamic tract neurons originate mainly in lamina I and to a lesser extent in laminae IV and V (5–9,18). Nociceptive-specific neurons receive exclusive excitatory effects from impulses in slowly conducting afferents. A major source of input to these neurons is from various types of primary nociceptive afferents, including high-threshold Aδ mechanosensitive afferents and C polymodal nociceptive afferents. Receptive fields of these cells are usually smaller than those of wide dynamic range neurons and sometimes show a gradient of

sensitivity similar to that of wide dynamic range neurons. There is a somatotopic organization of these cells within the marginal layer. For example, monkey
spinothalamic neurons in the 7th lumbar segment whose receptive fields are
located on the ventral surface of the foot exist in the medial part of the dorsal
horn, whereas spinothalamic cells with dorsal receptive fields are in the lateral
part of the dorsal horn (19).

Two general types of nociceptive-specific neurons have been identified.
One neuron type is unequivocally nociceptive specific, since it responds only
to a definitely noxious mechanical stimulus, such as pinching with toothed
forceps, and appears to be exclusively activated by high-threshold Aδ mechanosensitive afferents (6-18,18). The other type of nociceptive-specific cell responds
to firm nonpainful pressure of the skin (i.e., 1-10 g/mm^2), but it responds with
a higher impulse frequency to tissue-damaging stimuli (6-8,18). It is possible
that such a cell could signal intense but nonpainful information as well as nociceptive information. Some of these neurons respond to C-fiber stimulation and
to noxious thermal stimuli. These physiologic response characteristics of nociceptive-specific neurons have been found in both anesthetized (1,6-9) as well
as in unanesthetized monkeys (11,12). The potential involvement of nociceptive-
specific neurons in pain is a critical aspect of the specificity theory, which states
that the neural system involved in pain is one that responds exclusively to
nociceptive stimuli and that it is not activated by other types of somatic stimuli
(see refs. 3 and 4 for review of this concept).

Nociceptive-specific spinal cord neurons also are likely to be a part of
ascending pathways for pain. Their small receptive fields, somatotopic organizations, and modality-specificity indicates that they are well adapted to provide
information about location and type of noxious stimulus. Their responses to
graded noxious skin temperatures (44°-51°C) are monotonic functions and are,
therefore, generally consistent with human psychophysical data (13,20).
However, their stimulus-response functions are less steep than those of wide
dynamic range neurons and, therefore, show less of a parallel to human psychophysical responses (11,12). Similar to wide dynamic range neurons, responses of
nociceptive-specific neurons to 45-49°C skin temperatures are enhanced when
monkeys are making temperature discriminations as compared to visual discriminations (11,12). Many nociceptive-specific neurons can be antidromically activated from the ventrocaudal part of the ventrobasal thalamus. Thus, these cells
have anatomic connections appropriate for a role in pain.

3. Low-Threshold Mechanoreceptive Neurons

There is a third general category of central neurons in the dorsal horn that
responds to light touch, pressure, or hair movement, and appears to receive
input exclusively from sensitive mechanoreceptive afferents (1,6). Most of
these primary afferents are large myelinated Aβ afferents. *Low-threshold*

mechanoreceptive (LTM) neurons do not respond to noxious heat or exhibit higher discharge rates to noxious than to innocuous stimuli. Low-threshold mechanoreceptive neurons are concentrated in laminae III and IV (6,7,21). Very few low-threshold mechanoceptive neurons project in the spinothalamic tract (1,6,7). It is very unlikely that low-threshold mechanoceptive neurons are part of a nociceptive pathway.

B. The Function of Second-Order Nociceptive Neurons in Awake Primates

The nociceptive stimulus-response functions and other physiologic character-istics of wide dynamic range and nociceptive-specific neurons make it appear that both classes of neurons are important for pain. However, since most studies of these neurons were performed in anesthetized or spinalized animals, one might wonder whether their physiologic properties recorded in conscious animals could account for pain-related behavior. Furthermore, one might also wonder whether activation of either wide dynamic range or nociceptive-specific neurons is sufficient to evoke the experience of pain in awake primates, particu-larly humans. Two types of experiments have been carried out to answer these questions.

In the first, nucleus caudalis wide dynamic range and nociceptive-specific neurons were recorded in awake monkeys trained to make panel releases in order to escape unrewarded noxious heat trials (>43°C) or to secure reinforcement by detecting the end of an innocuous (<43°C) temperature (11,12). Simultaneous recording of escape behavior and neural responses have provided evidence that both wide dynamic range and nociceptive-specific neurons are capable of provid-ing information with which to discriminate intensities of stimulation within the noxious range. Escape latencies to 49°C heat stimuli were all <4 sec, whereas latencies on 47°C trials were all >4.0 sec. The greater increase in discharge of wide dynamic range and nociceptive-specific neurons to 49°C as compared to 47°C occurred early enough to provide signals related to the shorter escape latencies at 49°C. Such data indicate that these neurons are capable of discrim-inating different intensities of noxious stimulation. The extent to which this dis-crimination can be directly linked to sensory or affect-motivational dimensions requires further experiments.

In the second type of experiment, spinothalamic tract axons within the cervical spinal cord were electrically stimulated in awake humans and the parameters of stimulation were adjusted so as to stimulate *only* the axons of wide dynamic range neurons (22). This stimulus condition was inferred by com-paring electrical threshold and refractory period of monkey spinothalamic tract axons with similar parameters required to evoke pain in awake patients (23). The refractory periods and electrical thresholds of wide dynamic range neurons but not nociceptive-specific neurons matched the refractory periods and electrical thresholds of anterolateral quadrant (ALQ)-evoked pain. Since the electrical thresholds of nociceptive-specific axons were higher than current levels required to evoke pain in humans, then it appears that activation of wide dynamic range neurons is a sufficient condition to evoke pain. Whether selective stimulation of nociceptive-specific neurons also results in pain perception is a hypothesis yet to be tested.

C. Spatial Transformations of Primary Nociceptive Afferent Input

Radical spatial transformations take place between input from primary nociceptive afferents and output of spinothalamic tract neurons (6-8). These transformations are related to the manner in which primary afferent input is dispersed within the dorsal horn and to the propriospinal interconnections within the spinal gray matter. Such transformations are important for central summation and appear to account for such phenomena as radiation of suprathreshold painful sensations that occur under pathologic as well as normal circumstances.

At least two spatial factors are important for transmission of nociceptive information within the dorsal gray matter: somatotopic organization and receptive fields with extensive gradients of sensitivity. These factors have two important implications. The first is that the total number of dorsal horn sensory projection neurons activated is greater with a noxious than with an innocuous stimulus. Given the receptive field organization described previously (i.e., the area mapped by noxious stimuli is much larger than that mapped by touch), one could infer that a noxious stimulus would activate a larger number of nociceptive sensory projection neurons than touch applied to an equivalent area of skin. Touch would activate only the smaller, more sensitive zones within the receptive fields of these neurons. As stimulus intensities increased into the noxious range, however, more nociceptive neurons would be recruited, since a given. stimulus would also lie within the less sensitive peripheral zones of receptive fields of other neurons. For example, a gentle tactile stimulus applied to the third toe would activate the neuron whose receptive field is shown at the right in Figure 1. A mildly nociceptive stimulus (e.g., 45°C or pinch with fine-toothed forceps) would evoke a higher frequency impulse discharge in this neuron, but it would not activate the neuron whose receptive field is shown at the left (Fig. 1). If the stimulus intensity extended to even higher levels (e.g., 47°C or heavy pinch), the neuron whose receptive field is shown at the left also would be recruited. This recruitment would increase the total number of central sensory neurons activated. Both the frequency of impulse discharge and the total number of central sensory neurons activated could contribute to the overall perceived intensity of pain. A second implication of this type of receptive field organization is that painful sensations would radiate when stimulus intensities extend above pain threshold. At pain threshold, only those neurons would be activated whose most sensitive receptive field regions lie within the area of the stimulus. As stimulation intensity increased within the noxious range, more nociceptive neurons would be activated, since the stimulus would activate wide dynamic range neurons with very extensive receptive fields and whose most sensitive receptive field regions are remote from the actual stimulus. Since such neurons within the nucleus caudalis and the spinal cord dorsal horn are somatotopically organized, sensation would radiate to surrounding zones as stimulus intensities increase in the noxious range. In support of this explanation, it has been shown that suprathreshold pain evoked by heat radiates to surrounding areas whose temperatures are in fact not elevated (7). Radiation also is a salient feature of many types of pain and pathologic pain (16).

The work of Denny-Brown and coworkers (24) has shown that pain is more vulnerable to a loss of central spatial summation than is touch or temperature sense. In particular, the authors showed that interruption of the descending tract of the fifth nerve or section of dorsal roots results in zones of sensory loss that are greater for pain than for touch. These analgesic zones are not constant, but they can be contracted by subconvulsive doses of strychnine or by small lesions of the medial portion of Lissauer's tract (24). They can be expanded by picrotoxin or lesions of the lateral portion of Lissauer's tract. Thus, pain sensibility is under the control of intrinsic facilitatory and inhibitory interconnections within the spinal cord. The facilitatory connections may provide part of the basis for the widespread receptive fields with extensive gradients of sensitivity. Indeed, this idea has been partly confirmed by Yokota et al. (25) who found that subconvulsive doses of strychnine greatly expanded the nociceptive portions of wide dynamic range receptive fields and picrotoxin contracted them. Interestingly, picrotoxin expanded the tactile portion of the receptive fields (26).

Studies of pain evoked by stimulation of the cervical anterolateral quadrant in humans also support the idea that central spatial summation is important for pain (22,23). When the frequency was held constant (50 Hz), it was found that the perception of anterolateral quadrant-evoked pain invariably required larger stimulus intensities and presumably activation of a larger number of anterolateral quadrant axons than that required for perceptions of tingle, warmth, or cooling. The amount of spatial summation was critical, since stimulus intensities just sufficient to evoke tingle would *only* evoke nonpainful sensations even when stimulus frequencies extended up to 500 Hz. In contrast, when stimulus intensities were increased to activate a critical number of axons, much lower frequencies (5-25 Hz) evoked pain.

D. The Role of Propriospinal Interconnections

Propriospinal interconnections undoubtedly play a major role in central summation and facilitatory mechanisms of pain. Many of these interconnections arise from laminae IV–VI of the dorsal horn (27,28). The longest propriospinal connections, extending from cervical to lumbosacral levels, originate from lamina V, a major site of origin of primate spinothalamic tract neurons (27,28). The extent to which propriospinal interconnections originate from neurons that also project in somatosensory pathways is unknown. However, spinothalamic tract neurons are likely to be strongly influenced by intersegmental connections, since such connections and sensory relay neurons originate from the same dorsal horn layers. This influence is certainly consistent with the extensive receptive fields of some spinothalamic neurons, some of which extend across several spinal dermatomes. Some of the input to these neurons, then, are likely to originate from interneurons many spinal cord segments away.

The role of propriospinal interconnections in dorsal horn input-output relationships is illustrated schematically in Figure 2. One can discern from this diagram that interruption of spinothalamic neurons at one level (e.g., lumbar) would leave open the possibility that somatosensory information could still pass via propriospinal connections to sensory neurons at another level (i.e., cervical). The latter, in turn, could be spinothalamic neurons or interneurons. Initially, the partial interruption of this pathway would result in a zone of analgesia related to interruption of a critical pathway as well as to a decrement in the total number of sensory neurons conveying nociceptive information. The gradual return of pain would depend upon preexisting propriospinal interconnections and upon processes related to increased efficacy of synaptic transmission (e.g., denervation sensitivity). Contrary to previous explanations about the return of pain after anterolateral cordotomy, it is not necessary to postulate alternative long ascending pathways nor short axon multineuronal pathways for pain (16).

E. Temporal Transformations of Primary Nociceptive Input

Certain types of skin sensations show evidence of temporal summation and after-responses. Since responses of primary afferent neurons do not temporally summate nor long outlast the duration of stimulation, such phenomena must occur within the central nervous system. Several studies have demonstrated that the spinal cord dorsal horn is a site of origin of temporal summation and after-responses and that such phenomena show striking parallels to sensory phenomena in humans (7).

One series of studies (7,29) has utilized controlled brief heat pulses to compare human psychophysical responses to first and second pain with primary afferents and spinothalamic tract neuronal responses. Peripherally, first and second pain are a consequence of synchronous activation of $A\delta$ and C nociceptive afferents, both of which directly excite spinothalamic tract neurons. A single heat pulse (peak temp. = $51°C$) to the skin reliably evokes first and second pain in humans and early and long latency impulse discharges in monkey wide

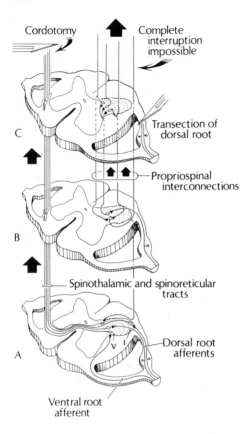

Figure 2 Schematic diagram illustrating the anatomic role of propriospinal interconnections in ascending spinal pathways subserving pain. Dorsal root nociceptive afferents as well as some ventral root afferents converge on neurons within the spinal cord gray matter. Dorsal horn neurons in lamina I and V form the origin of spinothalamic and spinoreticular pathways. Propriospinal neurons with long ascending and descending interconnections provide some input to sensory projection neurons. This input could provide an alternative means of channeling lumbosacral nociceptive input to the brain after the lumbosacral spinothalamic tract is directly interrupted by a surgical lesion.

dynamic range and nociceptive-specific spinothalamic neurons (7,29). The early neuronal response, like first pain, *decreases* in magnitude with each successive heat pulse. The late neuronal response, like second pain, *increases* in magnitude with each successive heat pulse. Summation of the late neuronal response and of second pain occur only with interstimulus intervals of 3 sec or less. Since responses of C primary nociceptive afferent neurons *do not* temporally summate with identical types of heat pulses, such summation must take place within the dorsal horn. Details of these summation mechanisms will be discussed in terms of the possible microcircuitry involved (see later).

Noxious somatic stimuli sometimes evoke sensations that persist beyond the duration of the stimulus and beyond the arrival of primary afferent impulses that evoke them (7,16,29). After-discharges lasting several hundred milliseconds can be evoked in spinothalamic neurons by single electrical shocks to Aδ and C cutaneous afferents and by brief noxious heat stimuli, described previously (1,6,8,21). Similar stimuli applied to human nerves or skin will evoke after-sensations (29,30).

Some non-noxious stimuli also evoke prolonged after-responses in spino-thalamic neurons and after-sensations (7). For example, a very gentle moving tactile stimulus applied to glabrous skin of a monkey's foot will evoke 20–60-sec after-discharges in wide dynamic range spinothalamic neurons. These after-discharges can be abruptly terminated by rubbing the stimulated region. Like-wise, a similar stimulus applied to humans evokes a long-lasting after-sensation that can be terminated by rubbing the stimulated area (7,31). Interestingly, wide dynamic range neurons are the only class of dorsal horn neurons that exhibit tactile-evoked after-responses. Second-order low-threshold mechano-receptive neurons, although activated by the same primary afferents that trigger after-sensations, do not have prolonged evoked after-responses—thus, there may be an intriguing relationship between tactile-evoked after-responses and pain mechanisms. Such a relationship may partly account for certain pathologic pain syndromes, such as tic douloureux, wherein very gentle stimulation can evoke intense paroxysmal pain (4,16).

Vaginal stimulation, which evokes behavioral after-responses in cats, also evokes prolonged after-discharges in cat dorsal horn neurons (32). Similar to tactile-evoked after-responses, wide dynamic range neurons are the only class of dorsal horn neurons that respond with after-discharges to vaginal probing.

Temporal summation and extension of somatosensory signals beyond stimulus duration may be important for certain somatic sensations, especially those that have both sensory and motivational significance. Certainly, the types of after-responses and summation described previously are most often experi-enced as unpleasant or pleasant. That spinothalamic tract neurons participate in both sensory and motivational functions is indirectly indicated by the observation that interrupting the spinoreticular and spinothalamic pathways at cervical levels results not only in a loss of pain but also of other types of pleasant and unpleasant somatosensory sensations, including sexual sensations (33). The electrophysiologic observation that spinothalamic neurons have collateral axons to medial brain stem structures (7) lends support to this idea, since medial brain stem structures have been proposed to participate in affective-motivational dimensions of pain (4).

F. Inhibition of Dorsal Horn Sensory Neurons

Response characteristics of wide dynamic range and nociceptive-specific spino-thalamic neurons also reflect a variety of inhibitory mechanisms related to noci-ception. Perhaps the most well-documented type of inhibition is one that is initiated by stimulation of low-threshold mechanoreceptive afferents (34). Most low-threshold mechanosensitive (touch) afferents have rapid conduction velocities and large-diameter axons. Their inhibitory role in pain mechanisms is one of the main features of the gate control theory (3). Repetitive stimulation of these afferents can be accomplished by electrical stimulation of the dorsal columns or by low-intensity electrical stimulation of peripheral cutaneous nerves (17,34). Both kinds of stimulation reduce the magnitude of spinothalamic neuron responses to nociceptive thermal and mechanical stimuli as well as their responses to electrical stimulation of Aδ and C afferents (17,34). This form of inhibition, which does not long outlast the stimulation period, is mediated at least partly by postsynaptic mechanisms. Dorsal column stimulation evokes brief inhibitory postsynaptic potentials (IPSPs) in spinothalamic nociceptive neurons. This inhibition is likely to be mediated by local interneuronal mechanisms because the latency to these inhibitory postsynaptic potentials follows within 1 to 2 msec after the onset of dorsal column stimulation (34). Presynaptic inhibi-tory mechanisms also may play a role in this form of inhibition, since dorsal column–evoked inhibitory periods are accompanied by increased excitability (i.e., lowered electrical thresholds) of primary afferent terminals (34). Presum-ably then, these terminals are partially depolarized and release less transmitter substance during each action potential.

The inhibition of nociceptive responses of wide dynamic range and noci-ceptive-specific spinothalamic neurons by dorsal column and peripheral nerve stimulation have their parallels in analgesia produced by dorsal column stimula-tion and by transcutaneous electrical stimulation of peripheral nerves (called TENS) in humans (33). Although the use of dorsal column stimulation has been reduced because of technical reasons, transcutaneous electrical nerve stimula-tion is becoming widely used as a conservative noninvasive form of chronic pain therapy.

Another form of inhibition can be evoked in wide dynamic range neurons by intense stimulation of specific body zones that are quite remote from the neuron's receptive field. This form of inhibition has been verified in rats (36,37), cats (1), and monkeys (1). Spontaneous impulse discharge and nociceptive responses of monkey wide dynamic range neurons, whose receptive fields in-clude the foot or part of the foot, often can be inhibited by intense mechanical stimulation of the contralateral foot, contralateral hand, ipsilateral hand, base of the tail, or zones within the trigeminal region. The optimum stimulus required for this form of inhibition is clearly noxious, although firm, but innocuous, pressure is minimally effective. The potency of this inhibition is sufficient to completely or nearly completely suppress C-fiber–evoked responses of wide dynamic range neurons (36). The early latency responses of these neurons are less effected. This phenomenon also has its parallel in human sensory experience. Intense pressure applied to the contralateral hand will nearly completely suppress second pain sensation evoked by electrical stimulation of C afferents of the hand (3).

Finally, there is now a considerable literature on endogenous pain control mechanisms whose final stage of inhibitory action exists within the dorsal horn (38–40). Both opiate- and nonopiate-related neural systems originating within such structures as the periaqueductal gray, periventricular gray, locus coeruleus, nucleus raphe alatus, and nucleus raphe magnus, descend to dorsal horn laminae I, II, and to some extent lamina V (38–41). At this level, inhibition of nociceptive responses of wide dynamic range and nociceptive-specific neurons are probably mediated partly by serotonergic and noradrenergic mechanisms as well as by enkephalinergic interneuronal mechanisms within the dorsal horn itself (42,43). Some of these powerful descending controls are triggered by intense somatosensory input, as in the case of acupuncture (34,38) or by psychologic factors that occur during stress (39,44,45). Descending pain inhibitory controls, triggered partly by somatosensory input, is a concept that is an integral part of the gate control theory (3,4). Current investigations are showing the complex interactions within the dorsal horn related to these controls.

G. Possible Dorsal Horn Coding Mechanisms of Nociception

It is evident that radical transformations take place between the inputs of primary nociceptive afferents and outputs of spinothalamic tract neurons. The information encoded by the primary nociceptive afferents is preserved in these input-output relationships but not in a one-to-one fashion. The different functional classes of spinothalamic neurons do not correspond directly to the different classes of primary afferents. Their responses to nociceptive stimuli also differ from those of primary afferents. These transformations raise questions about possible coding mechanisms of nociception. Are different qualities of painful sensations coded by separate dorsal horn neuron populations? Are different dimensions of pain experience such as affect, arousal, and sensation coded by separate dorsal horn neuron populations?

Our present level of knowledge of dorsal horn physiology indicates that one cannot easily label central neurons or pathways in terms of the presumed sensations they elicit. For example, first pricking pain can be evoked by stimulation of Aδ nociceptive afferents and second pain can be evoked by stimulation of C nociceptive afferents. However, both Aδ and C nociceptive afferents often converge on the same second-order nociceptive neurons of the dorsal horn

(1,6–8,21,23,46). Thus, it would be misleading and wrong to propose that first and second pain (or epicritic and protopathic sensibility) are represented by *different* central neural populations or pathways. A similar case can be made for the distinction between mechanically induced and thermally induced pain. The latter appears to be subserved by subsets of neurons that also respond to mechanical nociceptive stimulation (1,6–8,21,23,46). The representation of different qualities of pain sensation may depend largely on activation of different proportions or combinations of nociceptive-specific and wide dynamic range neurons by a particular stimulus and on their connectivity at higher levels of the neuraxis. Thus, penetration of the skin by a needle would activate nociceptive-specific neurons that respond exclusively to nociceptive mechanical stimuli *as well as* wide dynamic range neurons that respond to both mechanical and thermal stimuli. Activation of both types of neurons may be necessary for the unique quality of sensation that is evoked by needle penetration.

Studies of human pain evoked by anterolateral quadrant stimulation shed some light on questions about coding mechanisms of pain sensation. First, it is of considerable significance that pain evoked by stimulation of wide dynamic range axons (see refs. 22 and 23 for details) was similar to that evoked by naturally occurring stimuli. Most of the reports were of burning pain, but descriptions of dull aching pain, cramping, and sharp pain were also given. These types of pain were evoked by 50-Hz trains of regularly spaced pulses, a pattern that is not likely to be generated by natural stimuli. Therefore, it is unlikely that pain is subserved by some special temporal pattern that depends upon the exact intervals of impulses in spinal cord nociceptive neurons. However, the intensity of pain was found to be dependent on the overall frequency in anterolateral quadrant neurons over a range of 5-100 Hz. A linear relationship was found between stimulation frequency and percentage of subjects reporting pain. One hundred percent of subjects reported pain at 25 Hz and none reported pain at 5 Hz. Similarly, monkey wide dynamic range neurons responded to graded noxious heat with a frequency of 5-25 Hz over a skin temperature range of 44-45.5°C (7,23), the range over which most human heat pain threshold values are distributed (47). In contrast, the frequency of nociceptive-specific responses extend between 5-25 Hz over a skin temperature range of 46-48°C. These temperature values evoke suprathreshold pain in most human subjects. Thus, the coding of pain sensation threshold intensity appears critically related to an overall frequency range of 5-25 Hz in wide dynamic range neurons.

A second question about dorsal horn coding mechanisms of pain is whether all dimensions of pain are uniformly represented in spinothalamic and spinoreticular pathways or whether there is some functional separation within these pathways. The idea of functional separation is strongly indicated by the popular assertion that the paleospinothalamic pathway is more important for affective-motivational aspects of pain and the neospinothalamic pathway carries mainly sensory-discriminative information (4). The latter idea is based mainly on anatomic grounds (4). It suggests that the spinothalamic pathway has two components ascending in the brain stem. The medial component of this pathway (paleospinothalamic tract) gives off numerous collaterals to brain stem structures thought to be involved in arousal (e.g., reticular formation structures) or affect (central gray, tectal area). The lateral component (neospinothalamic tract) is thought to have fewer collaterals to medial brain stem structures and to project to areas that are mostly involved in sensory-discriminative functions.

There are several lines of evidence that would support a more uniform representation of function within the spinothalamic pathway. First, stimulation of spinothalamic tract axons within the cervical spinal cord has been shown to give rise to pain that has both sensory-discriminative *and* affective components (22). The pains evoked by anterolateral quadrant stimulation were clearly aversive, although certainly tolerable. Behavioral responses and reports indicating that the pain was unpleasant (i.e., "bad," "hurts") were given without provocation or suggestion. Since the currents and frequencies were adjusted so as to activate the axons of wide dynamic range neurons, these indications of aversion are significant. They lead to the inference that wide dynamic range neurons activate central mechanisms related to the affective-motivational dimension of pain as well as to the central mechanisms related to sensory discrimination.

A second line of evidence provided by Nathan and Smith (48) is that numerous lesions have been made within the human cervical spinal cord that only partially interrupt the spinothalamic tract. Such lesions produce a restricted zone of analgesia in which all of the components of pain are interrupted at once. Thus, there is no selective loss of aversive components of pain as compared to sensory components.

Finally, spinothalamic tract axons, whose terminals end within the sensory thalamic nucleus, ventralis posterolateralis (VPL), are now known to have collaterals to medial brain stem structures such as central gray (7). These collateral terminations indicate that individual spinothalamic tract neurons participate in multiple functions. These neurons, which include wide dynamic range and nociceptive-specific types, have physiologic characteristics similar to those that *do not* appear to have collaterals to the medial brain stem and to those which *only* project as far as the mesencephalon. Spinal cord afferent neurons with similar physiologic characteristics project to varying levels of the brain stem. All of these observations indicate that classic functional subdivisions of the spinothalamic pathway are oversimplified and misleading (4,16). The spinothalamic pathway appears to contain many neurons that participate in different components of pain and some neurons with more restricted outputs. There does not appear to be a sharp functional subdivision of the different components of pain within the spinothalamic pathway.

III. MICROCIRCUITRY OF THE DORSAL HORN

The foregoing discussion indicates that the dorsal gray matter is the site of origin of spinothalamic pathways and it is a site wherein temporal and spatial transformations are made of somatosensory input. It also is a site of local and intersegmental inhibitory mechanisms and is the last stage of action of descending control mechanisms. Recently, considerable advances have been made in elucidating the complex circuitry of this region, especially the uppermost layers (laminae I-III). Indeed the superficial dorsal horn has become an excellent model of local circuitry, one that rivals that of the retina, olfactory bulb, and cerebellar cortex.

To be helpful, local circuitry analysis should help explain some function such as vision, movement, or perception of pain. In this regard, the dorsal horn has several advantages. For one, the types of primary nociceptive afferents that synapse within the dorsal horn have been well characterized and the terminals of some of these afferents have been described anatomically (49-51). For another, the cells of origin of somatosensory pathways (i.e., spinothalamic, spinocervical pathways) have been identified within specific laminae. Finally, as shown previously, responses of sensory neurons within the dorsal horn have been shown to parallel psychophysical responses of human observers. Thus, the inputs and outputs of this region are known to a fair degree and responses of sensory neurons of this region have been related to human sensory experience.

The remaining discussion will focus on details of neuronal circuitry within the dorsal horn that could further account for input-output relationships of this complex region. Figure 3 should serve as a guideline in understanding the circuitry involved.

A. Distribution and Termination of Primary Afferents

It has been proposed that the dorsoventral progression of physiologic types of neurons in the dorsal horn is at least partially explicable in terms of the dorsoventral progression of the terminal arbors of the various functional categories of primary afferents (52). In general, primary nociceptive afferents have been shown to terminate in laminas I and II (49; see ref. 53 for a review). Some of these afferents have collaterals that arborize in lamina V. Although the evidence is indirect, unmyelinated polymodal nociceptive afferents are considered to terminate in laminae I and IIa and possibly also in lamina V (53). Direct evidence for termination of Aδ high-threshold mechanoreceptive afferents in laminae I and IIa comes from horseradish peroxidase (HRP) injections (from the recording microelectrode) into axons of functionally identified afferents (49). HRP filled the terminal arbors of these afferents and its reaction product was identified in laminae I and IIa with both light and electron microscopic analyses.

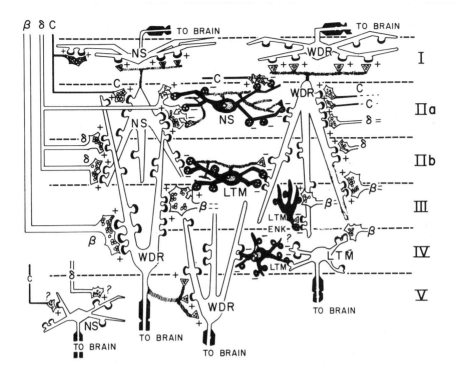

Figure 3 Schematic diagram illustrating the major morphologic-functional characteristics of neurons within dorsal horn laminae I–V. Projection neurons are indicated in laminae I, IV, and V. These include NS and WDR spinothalamic tract neurons. These neurons directly receive primary afferent excitatory input through synapses on their dendritic spines. In addition, lamina I projection neurons are likely to receive excitatory input from stalked cells in lamina IIa. Stalked cells are either NS (left neuron in lamina IIa) or WDR (right neuron in lamina IIa). NS stalked cells receive their input via axodendritic synapses on their spines in laminae IIa and IIb. WDR stalked cells receive nociceptive afferent input in laminae IIa and IIb as well as (LTM) in laminae III and IV. Lamina V projection neurons receive interneuronal excitatory input from lamina IV neurons. Several types of inhibitory interneurons also are shown and are designated in black. The lamina IIa NS islet cell receives exclusive input from nociceptive afferents and it inhibits the output of stalked cells via axoaxonic, axodendritic, dendrodendritic, and dendroaxonic synapses. The more ventral islet cell in laminae IIb and III receives input from LTM afferents and inhibits the output of stalked cells via axodendritic and dendrodendritic synapses. Other inhibitory interneurons exist in lamina III and IV. These are mostly LTM neurons. Some of these contain enkephalin.

In contrast, low-threshold mechanoreceptive primary afferents, also identified morphologically by HRP injections of their axons, terminate heavily in
laminae III and IV and sparsely in lamina IIb (50,51). This differential distribution of nociceptive and non-nociceptive afferents at least partially accounts for
the predominance of second-order nociceptive neurons in laminae I and IIa (52)
and the predominance of low-threshold mechanoreceptive interneurons in
laminae III and IV (49-52; see Fig. 3).

B. Morphologic Neuron Types Within the Dorsal Horn

Morphologically distinct types of neurons have been identified within each of
Rexed's lamina (53). Those of the uppermost three laminae have been well
characterized anatomically and physiologically within the last several years
(8,53-56).

Lamina I consists mainly of Golgi type I neurons or projection neurons
that send their axons out of the dorsal horn to various destinations within
the brain stem. Indeed, many are spinothalamic tract neurons (53). These
include spiny and smooth pyramidal neurons and some multipolar neurons
(53). The dendrites of these neurons are confined to lamina I. Some of the
same neurons that project axons into ascending pathways also have local collaterals (53,56).

Lamina II consists mainly of two types of interneurons—stalked cells and
islet cells (53-56). The cell bodies of stalked cells, so called because of their
short, stalklike branches, are found in greatest numbers in the dorsal half of
lamina II. Their cone-shaped dendritic arbors are mediolaterally compressed
and extend ventrally across lamina II and sometimes into lamina III (8,53-56).
Few stalked cells send dendrites as far as lamina IV (see Fig. 3).

Since both the terminal arborizations of primary afferents in laminae
I-III and the dendrites of stalked cells occupy mediolaterally flattened territories, this organization helps account for the mediolateral somatotopic organization described earlier (6,19).

Stalked cell axons extend dorsally into lamina I where they arborize in an
extensive umbrellalike canopy above the cell body. Thus, lamina I is the principal synaptic target of the stalked cell, although some stalked cell axonal
terminals have been seen in lamina II as well (53-56).

The other major neuron type found in lamina II is the islet cell, an interneuron that is found in small clusters or islands (53). Lamina II islet cells
generate extensive rostral and caudal dendritic arbors. The mediolateral and
dorsoventral extensions of the dendrites are much more restricted, the latter
often being confined within lamina II. Unlike the axonal arborizations of stalked
cells, those of islet cells branch repeatedly *within* the confines of the dendritic
arbors and do not extend into lamina I. Thus, the islet cell more closely resembles the classic Golgi type II interneuron found elsewhere.

Lamina III consists mainly of islet cells, a few inverted stalked cells, and a third type of interneuron (53). The latter generate sparse, dorsally directed arbors that extend only as far as lamina IIb. Most of their dendrites are confined to lamina III. Many cells of this type have been shown to contain enkephalin (42,58).

Lamina IV consists of pyramidal cells of varying sizes whose apical dendrites extend into the uppermost laminae as well as other types of neurons whose dendrites are confined to this layer. Some of the pyramidal cells are Golgi type I neurons whose axons project into ascending somatosensory pathways. These pathways include the spinocervical tract (1,21) and to a lesser extent the spinothalamic tract (58). Similar to some lamina I neurons, some lamina IV neurons have axons that ascend in sensory pathways as well as local axonal arborizations that extend into lamina V (see schematic in Fig. 3, and see ref. 59).

Lamina V contains large pyramidal neurons whose apical dendrites extend dorsally and many of these are spinothalamic tract neurons (58). They resemble the large pyramidal neurons of the cerebral cortex. Other smaller types of neurons also occupy lamina V.

C. Excitatory Interconnections Within the Dorsal Horn

The connections between types of neurons described previously would be consistent with a dorsal-ventral progression of physiologic types of neurons. Indeed, such a progression was conceptualized in terms of a cascade model several years ago (60). A major tenet of this model is that lamina IV neurons excite lamina V neurons that, in turn, converge on neurons of lamina VI. This model served to explain three important observations. The first was that within a given vertical microelectrode trajectory, the receptive field locations were similar among laminae IV-VI neurons. The second was that receptive field areas increased as microelectrode recordings progressed from laminae IV-VI (60). Receptive fields of lamina IV neurons were usually small and had sharply defined borders. Lamina V neurons were mostly wide dynamic range neurons that had larger receptive fields with gradients of sensitivity. Lamina VI wide dynamic range neuron receptive fields were even larger, often encompassing a major portion of a limb (21,60). Finally, excitatory convergence from different types of primary afferents increased as recordings progressed from laminae IV-VI (21,60). Major consequences of this type of vertical organization include somatotopic representation and functional columns of neurons wherein the dorsal neurons tend to have modality specificity and the ventral neurons have greater convergence of input. The dorsal neurons would likely provide more information about location and types of stimulation, while the ventral neurons would provide such information to a lesser degree. The ventral neurons, most of which would be wide dynamic range neurons, would provide more information about intensity.

A vertical organization within laminae I–III can now be added to this scheme, as is shown in Figure 3. Connections within these uppermost layers appear especially critical for nociceptive mechanisms and for the first time can be reviewed in some detail.

A major excitatory interconnection within laminae I and II is likely to exist between lamina II stalked cells and layer I projection neurons. The evidence for this connection, like those of the vertically directed connections in laminae IV–VI, is indirect and is based on several lines of evidence. One line of evidence is from a study wherein extracellular recordings were made of dorso-ventrally adjacent pairs of neurons in laminae I and II (8). The dorsal cell of each pair was antidromically activated from the thalamus and, thus, was almost certainly a lamina I neuron (58). The ventral cell of each pair was a histologically confirmed lamina II neuron; many of these were likely to be stalked cells (52–55). It was found that the lamina II neurons pattern of primary afferent convergence was the same or a subset of the pattern of input of the lamina I neuron above it and that both neurons had very similar receptive field locations and gradients of sensitivity. It was also found that the lamina II neurons usually had a smaller receptive field than that of the lamina I neuron above it. The lamina II neuron also had a shorter first-spike latency.

A second line of evidence that stalked cells are excitatory begins with the observation that many lamina I projection neurons are excited by activation of nociceptive afferents *and* by activation of low-threshold mechanoreceptive afferents (7,8,46). Since low-threshold mechanoreceptive afferents do not terminate directly in lamina I (53), this input must get relayed to lamina I via an interneuron. The only interneuron whose axon extensively arborizes in lamina I is the stalked cell. In direct corroboration of this hypothesis, stalked cells, stained intracellularly with HRP, have been characterized physiologically as wide dynamic range neurons (54). Interestingly, those stalked cells whose dendrites extended ventrally into layer III were wide dynamic range neurons and those whose dendrites terminated more dorsally were nociceptive-specific neurons. Thus, wide dynamic range stalked cells, whose proximal dendrites receive nociceptive afferent input and whose distal dendrites receive low-threshold mechanoceptive input in lamina III (Fig. 3), are excellent candidates for relaying excitatory effects from different types of primary afferents to lamina I projection neurons. One cannot exclude the possibility that some stalked cells have other functions and some may even be inhibitory. However, the bulk of the available evidence indicates stalked cells are excitatory.

The interconnections of stalked cells with primary afferents and with lamina I projection neurons have a critical bearing on neural mechanisms related to slow temporal summation of C-fiber–mediated responses (e.g., second pain) and sensory after-responses. Stalked cells, which directly receive primary nociceptive afferent and low-threshold mechanoceptive input, are the first central neurons to display response characteristics reflective of these neural mechanisms (8,54, 55). Electron microscopic analysis of stalked cell dendrites spines shows that they are heavily invested with primary afferent synapses and a single primary afferent terminal may synapse on several spine heads of a single stalked cell (55). Thus, the prolonged after-discharges and temporal summations evoked in stalked cells by synchronous afferent inputs may well be partly related to this type of highly secure synaptic arrangement. An additional factor in these phenomena is likely to include a long-lasting neurotransmitter or neuromodulatory substance. Substance P, which is likely to be released by C polymodal afferents and exerts prolonged and powerful excitatory effects on laminae I and II neurons, is likely to play an important role in C-fiber-mediated after-responses and temporal summation (61).

The response characteristics of laminae IV-VI nociceptive neurons are generally similar to those in laminae I-II. Proportionately more wide dynamic range neurons and fewer nociceptive-specific neurons exist in the ventral layers. Otherwise, prolonged discharges and temporal summation of C afferent-evoked responses are similar in both locations (1). There are two possible reasons for these similar response characteristics that are not mutually exclusive. First, some individual primary nociceptive afferents have been shown to send two axon collaterals into the dorsal horn, one branch arborizing in laminae I and/or II and the other arborizing in laminaes IV and V (49; see Fig. 3). Thus, it is quite possible that primary afferent nociceptive neurotransmitter mechanisms account, at least in part, for the similar responses observed in laminae I and II and IV-VI. Another possible explanation is that some lamina IV neurons have dendrites that extend dorsally into the uppermost layers (53). These laminae IV neurons would then be effected by nociceptive mechanisms that exist in laminae I and II. Such neurons might then relay these effects to more ventral neurons. Both of these explanations need to be tested in future anatomic and physiologic studies.

D. Inhibitory Interconnections Within the Dorsal Horn

Several types of inhibitory interneurons appear to exist within the dorsal horn and are represented in the schematic in Figure 3. These interneurons are likely to partially mediate the various forms of inhibition described earlier. Two major types of interneurons have been characterized anatomically and physiologically—the islet cell and the lamina III enkephalin cell (see Sec. III.B).

As mentioned in Sec. III.B, the islet cell is a Golgi type II cell comparable to inhibitory interneurons at other central nervous system areas. In addition, similarities between the ultrastructural appearance of GAD (glutamic and decarboxylase—the enzyme which synthesizes GABA[γ-aminobutyric acid])-stained profiles and those of islet cell dendritic and axonal synaptic profiles, has lead Bennett et al. (54), and Gobel et al. (55) to suspect that at least some islet cells contain GABA, a neurotransmitter whose effects are generally inhibitory. This inhibition is likely to be both pre- and postsynaptic, since dendroaxonic, dendrodendritic, axodendritic, and axoaxonal synapses are formed by islet cells (54,55). The identity of the dendrites that receive islet cells' dendrodendritic synapses has not been conclusively demonstrated, but the available evidence (54,55) strongly indicates that at least some of them belong to stalked cells (Fig. 3). Because the dendritic arbors of lamina I neurons are mostly contained in lamina I, while the dendrites and axons of islet cells are confined to lamina II, islet cell–induced inhibition is not likely to affect lamina I neurons directly. If the stalked cell is an excitatory interneuron, then the islet cell can indirectly inhibit the lamina I neuron's input via postsynaptic inhibition of the stalked cell dendrites or via presynaptic inhibition of the primary afferent terminals in lamina II.

The islet cells of lamina IIb and III are activated predominantly by low-threshold mechanoreceptive primary afferents. These islet cells are likely to mediate some of the short-duration inhibitory effects of low-threshold mecano-ceptive stimulation on nociceptive responses of sensory projection neurons. On the other hand, more superficial islet cells in lamina IIa receive nociceptive primary afferents and may be involved in inhibitory phenomena that are initiated by noxious stimuli (e.g. "hyperstimulation analgesia"; cf. ref. 4).

Islet cells and stalked cells also are likely to be involved in the effects pro-duced by activation of descending pain inhibitory pathways of brain stem origin. Layer II is known to be a major locus of termination of serotinergic and nor-adrenergic pathways (62). Ruda and Gobel (62) have shown serotonergic con-nections to lamina II dendrites.

The lamina III enkephalin cell is activated exclusively by low-threshold mechanoceptive afferents and often by a single type (57). This cell may be involved in a long-duration form of pain inhibition activated by low-threshold tactile afferents. Other enkephalin neurons are found in lamina II and less often in lamina I (42,57). Although their exact functional role in inhibition is less clear than that of other interneurons, it has been conclusively demonstrated that local enkephalinergic terminals directly contact the dendrites and cell bodies of spinothalamic tract neurons (63). Thus, it is clear that dorsal horn enkephalin-ergic mechanisms directly control the output of sensory relay nociceptive neurons.

IV. SOME CONCLUSIONS AND A PERSPECTIVE

The progress made in elucidating the complex circuitry involved in spinal cord processing of nociceptive information is encouraging and indicates that similar analysis may be applicable to other sensory, motivational, or affective systems.

It appears clear that nociceptive input-output relationships of the dorsal gray matter are anything but simple direct reflections of "pain receptor" activity. Instead, complex spatial and temporal transformations of nociceptive input take place within the dorsal horn. These transformations are reflected in the response characteristics of interneurons and sensory projection neurons within this region. Most importantly, response characteristics such as after-discharge, slow temporal summation, and receptive field gradients can partly account for some of the perplexing features of experimental pain and clinical pain. In addition, elucidation of efferent control of this region provides further insight into the nature of afferent processing, especially when this efferent control is examined in the context of a behavioral experiment (11,12).

The analysis of dorsal horn nociceptive mechanisms has recently been extended to include the complex microcircuitry and neurochemistry of this region. Thus, the physiology of the dorsal horn can now begin to be explained in concepts similar to those used in the functional analysis of the cerebellar cortex, olfactory bulb, and retina.

Ultimately, the phenomena to be explained in physiologic-anatomic studies of the dorsal horn are those that we perceive in ordinary experience—pains that radiate, summate, and last longer than the stimulus itself. We should not lose sight of these phenomena in our attempts to understand the physiology of the dorsal horn.

REFERENCES

1. Price, D. D., and Dubner, R. (1977). Neurons that subserve the sensory-discriminative aspects of pain. *Pain 3*:307–338.
2. Hayes, R. L., Price, D. D., and Dubner, R. (1979). Behavioral and physiological studies of sensory coding and modulation of trigeminal nociceptive input. In *Advances in Pain Research and Therapy*, vol. 3, J. J. Bonica, J. C. Leibeskind, and D. G. Albe-Fessard (Eds.), Raven, New York, pp. 219–243.
3. Melzack, R., and Wall, P. D. (1965). Pain mechanisms: A new theory. *Science 150*:971–979.
4. Melzack, R. (1973). *The Puzzle of Pain*, Basic Books, New York.
5. Kenshalo, D. R., Jr., Leonard, R. B., Chung, J. M., and Willis, W. D. (1979). Responses of primate spinothalamic neurons to graded and to repeated noxious heat stimuli. *Neurophysiol. 42*:1370–1389.
6. Price, D. D., Dubner, R., and Hu, J. W. (1976). Trigeminothalamic neurons in nucleus caudalis responsive to tactile, thermal, and nociceptive stimulation of monkey's face. *J. Neurophysiol. 39*:936–953.
7. Price, D. D., Hayes, R. L., Ruda, M. A., and Dubner, R. (1978). Spatial and temporal transformations of input to spinothalamic tract neurons and their relation to somatic sensation. *J. Neurophysiol. 41*:933–947.

8. Price, D. D., Hayashi, H., Dubner, R., and Ruda, M. A. (1979). Functional relationships between neurons of marginal and substantia gelatinosa layers of primate dorsal horn, *J. Neurophysiol. 42*:1590–1608.

9. Willis, W. D., Trevino, D. L., Coulter, J. D., and Maunz, R. A. (1974). Responses of primate spinothalamic tract neurons to natural stimulation of hindlimb. *J. Neurophysiol. 37*:358–372.

10. Willis, W. D., Kenshalo, D. R., Jr., and Leonard, R. B. (1979). The cells of origin of the spinothalamic tract. *J. Comp. Neurol. 188*:543–574.

11. Hayes, R. L., Dubner, R., and Hoffman, D. S. (1981). Neuronal activity in medullary dorsal horn of awake monkeys trained in a thermal discrimination task II: Behavioral modulation of responses to thermal and mechanical stimuli. *J. Neurohphysiol. 46*:428–443.

12. Hoffman, D. S., Dubner, R., Hayes, R. L., and Medlin, T. P. (1981). Neuronal activity in medullary dorsal horn of awake monkeys trained in a thermal discrimination task I: Responses to innocuous and noxious thermal stimuli. *J. Neurophysiol. 46*:409–427.

13. Price, D. D., Barrell, J. J., and Gracely, R. H. (1980). A psychophysical analysis of experiential factors that selectively influence the affective dimension of pain. *Pain 8*:137–150.

14. Blair, R. W., Weber, R. N., and Foreman, R. D. (1981). Characteristics of primate spinothalamic tract neurons receiving viscerosomatic convergent inputs in T_3-T_5 segments. *J. Neurophysiol. 46*:797–811.

15. Foreman, R. D. (1977). Viscerosomatic convergence onto spinal neurons responding to afferent fibers located in the inferior cardiac nerve. *Brain Res. 137*:164–168.

16. Noordenbos, W. (1959). *Pain*, Amsterdam: Elsevier.

17. Willis, W. D. (1979). Physiology of dorsal horn and spinal cord pathways related to pain. In *Mechanisms of Pain and Analgesia Compounds*, R. F. Beers, Jr., and E. G. Bassett (Eds.), Raven, New York, pp. 143–156.

18. Kumazawa, T., and Perl, E. R. (1978). Excitation of marginal and substantia gelatinosa neurons in the primate spinal cord: Indications of their place in dorsal horn functional organization. *J. Comp. Neurol. 177*:417–434.

19. Applebaum, A. E., Beall, J. E., and Foreman, R. D., and Willis, W. D. (1975). Organization and receptive fields of primate spinothalamic tract neurons. *J. Neurophysiol. 38*:572–586.

20. Hardy, J. D., Wolff, H. G., and Goodell, H. (1952). *Pain Sensations and Reactions*, Williams & Wilkins, Baltimore.

21. Price, D. D., and Browe, A. C. (1975). Responses of spinal cord neurons to graded noxious and non-noxious stimuli. *Exp. Neurol. 48*:201–221.

22. Mayer, D. J., Price, D. D., and Becker, D. P. (1975). Neurophysiological characterization of the anterolateral spinal cord neurons contributing to pain perception in man. *Pain 1*:51–58.

23. Price, D. D., and Mayer, D. J. (1975). Neurophysiological characterization of the anterolateral quadrant neurons subserving pain in *M. mulatta*. *Pain 1*:59–72.

24. Denny-Brown, D., Kirk, E. J., and Yanagisawa, N. (1972). The tract of Lissauer in relation to sensory transmission in the dorsal horn of the spinal cord in the macaque monkey, *J. Comp. Neurol. 151*:175–200.

25. Yokota, T., Nishikawa, N., and Nishikawa, Y. (1979). Effects of strychnine upon different classes of trigeminal subnucleus caudalis neurons. *Brain Res. 168*:430–434.

26. Yokota, T., and Nishika, Y. (1979). Action of picrotoxin upon trigeminal subnucleus caudalis in the monkey. *Brain Res. 171*:369–373.

27. Yezierski, R. P., Culberson, J. L., and Brown, P. B. (1980). Cells of origin of propriospinal connections to cat lumbosacral grey as determined with horseradish peroxidase. *Exp. Neurol. 69*:493–512.

28. Matsushita, M., Michiko, I., and Hosoya, Y. (1979). The location of spinal neurons with long descending axons in the cat: A study with the horseradish peroxidase technique. *J. Comp. Neurol. 184*:63–80.

29. Price, D. D., Hu, J. W., Dubner, R., and Gracely, R. H. (1977). Peripheral suppression of first pain and central summation of second pain evoked by noxious heat pulses. *Pain 3*:57–68.

30. Price, D. D. (1972). Characteristics of second pain and flexion reflexes indicative of prolonged central summation. *Exp. Neurol. 37*:371–391.

31. Melzack, R., and Eisenberg, H. (1968). Skin sensory afterflows. *Science 351*:445–449.

32. Price, D. D., Bushnell, M. C., and Iadarola, M. J. (1981). Responses of primary afferents and sacral spinal cord neurons to vaginal probing in the cat. *Neurosci. Lett. 26*:67–73.

33. White, A. R. and Sweet, W. C. (1971). *Pain and the Neurosurgeon: A Forty Year Experience*, Charles C Thomas, Springfield, Illinois.

34. Foreman, R. D., Applebaum, A. E., Beall, J. E., Trevino, D. E., and Willis, W. D. (1976). Responses of primate spinothalamic tract neurons to electrical stimulation of hindlimb peripheral nerves. *J. Neurophysiol. 39*:543.

35. Long, D. M., Campbell, J. N., and Gucer, G. (1979). Transcutaneous electrical stimulation for relief of chronic pain. In *Advances in Pain Research and Therapy*, vol. 3, J. J. Bonica, J. C. Leibeskind, and D. G. Albe-Fessard (Eds.), Raven, New York, p. 593.

36. LeBars, D., Dickenson, A. H., and Besson, J. M. (1979). Diffuse noxious inhibitory controls (DNIC). I. Effects on dorsal horn convergent neurons in the rat. *Pain 6*:283–304.

37. LeBars, D., Dickenson, A. H., and Besson, J. M. (1979). Diffuse noxious inhibitory controls (DNIC). II. Lack of effect on non-convergent neurons, supraspinal involvement, and theoretical implications. *Pain 6*:305–327.

38. Mayer, D. J., and Price, D. D. (1976). Central nervous system mechanisms of analgesia. *Pain 2*:379–404.

39. Mayer, D. J., and Watkins, L. R. (1981). The role of endorphins in pain control systems. In *Modern Problems of Pharmacopsychiatry: The Role of Endorphins in Neuropsychiatry*, H. M. Emrich (Ed.), Karger, Basel, p. 378.

40. Mayer, D. J. (1980). The centrifugal control of pain. In *Pain Discomfort, and Humanitarian Care*, L. Ng and J. J. Bonica (Eds.), Elsevier, Amsterdam, p. 228.

41. Basbaum, A. I., Clanton, C. H., and Fields, H. L. (1978). Three bulbospinal pathways from the rostral medulla of the cat: An autoradiographic study of pain nodulating systems. *J. Comp. Neurol. 178*:209-224.

42. Glazer, E. J., and Basbaum, A. I. (1981). Enkephalin perikarya in the marginal layer and sacral autonomic nucleus of the cat spinal cord. *J. Comp. Neurol. 146*:377-390.

43. Ruda, M. A. (1982). Enkephalinergic synapses in direct contact with spinothalamic tract neurons. *Science 215*(19):1523.

44. Hayes, R. L., Bennett, G. J., Newlon, P. G., and Mayer, D. J. (1978). Behavioral and physiological studies of non-narcotic analgesia in the rat elicited by certain environmental stimuli. *Brain Res. 155*:69-90.

45. Hayes, R. L., Price, D. D., and Bennett, G. J., Wilcox, D. L., and Mayer, D. J. (1978). Differential effects of spinal cord lesions on narcotic and non-narcotic suppression of nociceptive reflexes: Further evidence for the physiological multiplicity of pain modulation. *Brain Res. 155*:91-101.

46. Chung, J. M., Kenshalo, D. R., Jr., Gerhart, K. D., and Willis, W. D. (1979). Excitation of primate spinothalamic neurons by cutaneous C-fiber volleys. *J. Neurophysiol. 42*:1354-1369.

47. Hardy, J. D. (1953). Thresholds of pain and reflex contraction as related to noxious stimuli. *J. Appl. Physiol. 5*:725-739.

48. Nathan, P. W., and Smith, M. C. (1979). Clinico-anatomical correlation in anterolateral cordotomy. In *Advances in Pain Research and Therapy*, vol. 3, J. J. Bonica, J. C. Leibeskind, and D. G. Albe-Fessard (Eds.), Raven, New York, pp. 921-926.

49. Light, A. R., and Perl, E. R. (1979). Differential termination of large-diameter and small-diameter primary afferent fibers in the spinal dorsal grey matter as indicated by labelling with horseradish peroxidase. *J. Comp. Neurol. 186*:117-139.

50. Brown, A. G., Rose, P. K., and Snow, P. J. (1977). The morphology of hair follicle afferent fiber collaterals in the spinal cord of the cat. *J. Physiol. (Lond.) 272*:779-797.

51. Brown, A. G., Rose, P. K., and Snow, P. J. (1978). Morphology and organization of axon collaterals from afferent fibers of slowly adapting type I units in cat spinal cord. *J. Physiol. (Lond.) 277*:15-27.

52. Dubner, R., Gobel, S., and Price, D. D. (1976). Peripheral and central "pain" pathways. In *Advances in Pain Research and Therapy*, vol. 1, J. J. Bonica and D. G. Albe-Fessard (Eds.), Raven, New York, pp. 137-148.

53. Gobel, S. (1979). Neural circuitry in the substantia gelatinosa of Rolando: Anatomical insights. In *Advances in Pain Research and Therapy*, vol. 3, J. J. Bonica, J. C. Leibeskind, and D. G. Albe-Fessard (Eds.), Raven, New York, pp. 175-195.

54. Bennett, G. J., Abdelmoumene, M., Hayashi, H., and Dubner, R. (1980). Physiology and morphology of substantia gelatinosa neurons intracellularly stained with horseradish peroxidase. *J. Comp. Neurol. 194*:809-827.

55. Gobel, S., Falls, W. M., Bennett, G. J., Abdelmoumene, M., Hayashi, H., and Humphrey, E. (1980). An EM analysis of the synaptic connections of horseradish peroxidase-filled stalked cells and islet cells in the substantia gelatinosa of the adult cat spinal cord. *J. Comp. Neurol. 194*:781-807.

56. Bennett, G. J., Hayashi, H., Abdelmoumene, M., and Dubner, R. (1979). Physiological properties of stalked cells of the substantia gelatinosa intracellularly stained with horseradish peroxidase. *Brain Res. 164*:285–289.

57. Bennett, G. J., Abdelmoumene, M., Hayashi, H., Hoffert, M. J., Ruda, M. A., and Dubner, R. (1981). Physiology, morphology and immunocytology of dorsal horn layer III neurons. *Pain* (Suppl. 1):291.

58. Willis, W. D., Kenshalo, D. R., Jr., and Leonard, R. B. (1979). The cells of origin of the primate spinothalamic tract. *J. Comp. Neurol. 188*:553–574.

59. Brown, A. G., Rose, P. K., and Snow, A. J. (1977). The morphology of spinocervical tract neurons revealed by intracellular injection of horseradish peroxidase. *J. Physiol. (Lond.) 270*:747–764.

60. Wall, P. D. (1967). The physiological laminar organization of the dorsal horn. *J. Physiol. (Lond.) 188*:403–425.

61. Barber, R. P., Vaughan, J. E., Saito, K., McLaughlin, B. J., and Roberts, E. (1978). GABAergic terminals are presynaptic to primary afferent terminals in the substantia gelatinosa of the rat spinal cord. *Brain Res. 141*:35–55.

62. Ruda, M. A., and Gobel, S. (1980). Ultrastructural characteristics of axonal endings in the substantia gelatinosa which take up (3 H) sensatonin. *Brain Res. 184*:57–83.

63. Ruda, M. A. (1982). Enkephalinergic synapses in direct contact with spinothalamic tract neurons. *Science 215*(19):1523–1527.

17
THE SPINAL CORD
AND THE AUTONOMIC NERVOUS SYSTEM

Kiyomi Koizumi and Chandler McC. Brooks *Downstate Medical Center, State University of New York, Brooklyn, New York*

I. INTRODUCTION

Spinal control and involvement in the actions of the autonomic nervous system is undeniably present and constantly functioning but normally in conjunction with medullary, hypothalamic, and higher cerebral integrative "centers." Anatomically and functionally, the nervous system is a united totality. There is a cephalization, a hierarchical organization and there are obvious specializations of structure and function, but normally no parts act independently. When isolated from other structures of the central nervous system a component reveals considerable intrinsic functional activity and potential, but this does not reveal exactly what that component does and can do when retaining its normal state and interconnections.

However, in considering the spinal cord and its idiosyncratic role relative to function of the autonomic nervous system some generalizations can be made. First of all, the spinal cord is less of an integrating center than it is a transporter of incoming signals to and of outgoing signals from the hierarchy of higher control centers. It does receive all sensory signals coming in by way of dorsal roots from the viscera and tissues of the somatic system except those stimuli carried by the vagi and other cranial nerves. Under normal circumstances in the intact animal and to a lesser degree in the spinal preparation, upward-coursing signals are modified locally by intrinsic feedback. The spinal cord contains also

779

the descending efferent pathways and thus the final common pathways that carry the behavioral directives from the integrative centers to visceral and somatic effector systems: skeletal and visceral smooth muscle, blood vessels, secretory glands, and tissues. It is obvious that the efferent signals are subject to modification in passage and their ultimate effects are conditioned to a high degree by states of motoneuron pools and by local interactions in the spinal cord.

Our commission, however, is not viewed as requiring us to describe autonomic activity resulting from signals carried by cord pathways to higher centers and carried downward from higher centers to the preganglionic autonomic neurons. We shall discuss the autonomic activity that originates in and is mediated by the cord before and after interconnections with higher centers have been severed. We would like to point out, however, that higher centers by their facilitatory and inhibitory influences can and do affect what the cord generates and transmits. The cord mediates reactions but not the complex organized flow of patterned responses we term behavior.

Before proceeding with descriptions of what effect disconnection of the spinal cord from higher nervous system centers may have on its ability to control and mediate autonomic activity, a generalization can be made. Section of the cord produces the same kind of deficiencies in autonomic system function as are observed in the somatic behavioral reactions. The two systems are irrevocably linked; autonomic reactions accompany somatic reactions like shadows (1). The autonomic system innervates all body tissues, normally integrates visceral and somatic functions, is supportive of all behavior, is a modulator of reactions, and has a determinative influence on all reactions, local or general. In the spinal preparation the system performs similar type functions but in a much more simplistic and fragmented fashion than in the intact animal. It should also be said that in the absence of higher controls autonomic system behavior is different in the sense that it is not well balanced or integrated or even functionally appropriate.

II. DISCOVERY OF THE COMPONENTS OF THE AUTONOMIC SYSTEM AND THEIR ORIGIN IN THE BRAIN AND SPINAL CORD

Although the terms "involuntary nervous system," advanced by Thomas Willis in the mid 1600s, and "vegetative nervous system," proposed by J. G. Reil and M. F. X. Bichal in 1807, still have their usefulness, the nomenclature proposed by J. N. Langley in 1921 is most commonly employed. By this concept, the autonomic nervous system is an efferent complex consisting of parasympathetic and sympathetic divisions. The parasympathetic complex brackets the sympathetic, or thoracolumbar, outflow and is comprised of a cephalic outflow of cranial nerves and a sacral outflow of nerves originating from nuclei within the sacral cord. This concept of Langley, adapted by W. B. Cannon, eliminates the effort to define an autonomic afferent system. All stimuli affect the total organism; afferents that initiate reactions of the somatic system also evoke autonomic system responses, although some afferents are more effective in arousing one system than the other. One afferent system serves the two cooperating outflows, somatic and autonomic, relatively simultaneously. Thus, as in the case of the somatic system, the cord is the channel of major sensory inflow and motor neuron outflow from the central nervous system.

Attainment of our present knowledge of the autonomic nervous system and its function has required approximately 20 centuries. Galen (A.D. 130-201) was the first to identify the nerves supplying the viscera; he thought they were responsible for the sympathies. Later, in 1732, they were called sympathetic nerves by B. J. Winslow. Galen not only identified the chains of ganglia associated with segmental spinal roots but also the vagi, the splanchnics, the superior and inferior cervical, and the semilunar ganglia. He saw the rami communicantes, but he thought that the sympathetic chains, like the vagi, originated from the brain as an additional pair of cranial nerves. The early gross dissections performed and published by Vesalius in 1543 were much improved upon by Eustachius (1552), Thomas Willis (1621-1675), and B. J. Winslow (1669-1760). These anatomists, however, retained the thought that the "intercostal nerves" (lateral sympathetic chains) originated from the brain.

A retired French army neurosurgeon, François Pourfoir du Petit, however, in 1727, contested this conclusion that the lateral chains of ganglia have a cerebral origin. He showed that they actually originate from the segmental rami communicantes. Reil, in 1857, also emphasized this concept that the rami serve as connectors between the central nervous system and the "vegetative" or sympathetic system. By the mid 1800s, the early histologists Jacob Henle (1808-1885), Robert Remak (1815-1865), and C. G. Ehrenberg (1795-1876) had described the preganglionic and postganglionic fiber types and their cell bodies in the cord the ganglia (2,3).G. Meissner (1857) and L. Auerbach (1864) described the myenteric plexuses, and gradually the extent and distributions of the nerves and ganglia were determined. Probably, W. H. Gaskell (1847-1914) and J. N. Langley (1852-1925) deserve the most credit for describing the composition of the rami communicantes and the projection of the fibers of each to the peripheral ganglia and which organs were influenced by each segmental outflow (4).

Studies of the origin and differentiation of the components of the autonomic nervous system have become enormously complex in recent years as new methods have been developed. The system originates from the neural tube and/or crest during embryologic differentiation. In the development of the autonomic nervous system a regionalization of the neural crest can be recognized: The sympathetic chains derive from the entire length of the neural crest,

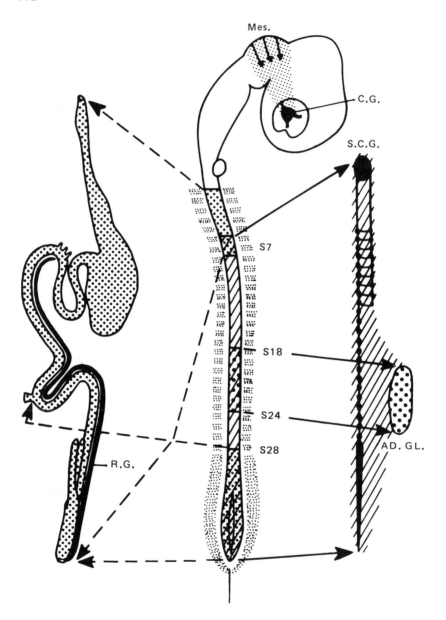

Figure 1 Diagram of the sites of origin of the sympathetic ganglia and plexuses and the enteric and ciliary ganglia in the neural crest (middle drawing). The enteric ganglion of the preumbilical gut and innervation of the postumbilical gut (left) originate from the vagal level of the neural crest (somites 1–7). The lumbosacral components of the neural crest give rise to the ganglion of Remak (R.G.)

from the level of the sixth somite caudad. Chromaffin cells that form the adrenal medulla originate from the region of somites 18-24. Most of the enteric ganglia arise from the "vagal" neural crest opposite somites 1-7. The details of the development of these various components of the somatic and autonomic nervous system are described by Le Douarin (5) and others who contributed to a recent symposium on the *Development of the Autonomic System* (6) (Fig. 1). A considerable degree of plasticity characterizes the autonomic system neurons and various factors can influence what types of fibers they become relative to production of transmitter substances. It still is not clear whether these nerves find their effector sites as a result of "guidance" or "attraction" or both. Nerve growth factor is important, but it is now necessary to consider effects of many other agents. There is also the problem of "recognition" in developing permanent association of nerves and specific effector cells. These connections are for some reason essential to the survival of the neurons. Certainly, an interplay between spinal cord and differentiating peripheral organs occurs in the development and maturation of function of the sympathetic and sacral parasympathetic complexes.

Knowledge of the complexity of the development process provides some clues as to the genesis or cause of autonomic system abnormalities. These can occur in cord development or as a result of a more peripheral failure. Aganglionosis, or Hirschsprung's disease, is one of the commoner developmental abnormalities and results in inadequate myenteric innervation and impaired function of the hindgut and defecation. Other abnormalities in reflex actions are also created by hypoganglionosis and hyperganglionosis (7), but these are peripheral rather than central abnormalities.

In addition to developmental abnormalities, there are pathologic occurrences that affect the spinal cord and its control of autonomic system function. Examples are disseminated sclerosis, amyotrophic lateral sclerosis, poliomyelitis, and tabes dorsalis. Parasympathetic and sympathetic abnormalities develop in diabetes and in infectious diseases that injure the cord and other regions of the nervous system (8). During pregnancy autonomic neurons degenerate and subsequently regenerate. In aging there is a gradual failure in autonomic reactions of central and peripheral origin. These problems are gradually coming under study (9,10). The primary objective of this present review, however, is to present our current knowledge of what autonomic system functions can occur and are sustained by the spinal cord.

---

and some ganglion cells of the postumbilical gut. The ciliary ganglia (C.G.) and cervical autonomic components arise from the mesencephalic (Mes.) crest. The sympathetic chain and plexuses originate from the neural crest caudal to the fifth somite. The adrenal medulla (suprarenal gland AD.GL.) originates from the level of the eighteenth to twenty-fourth somite (S). The sites of origin of the superior cervical ganglia (S.C.G.) and chains (right) are shown. (From Ref. 5.)

III. THE THORACOLUMBAR, SYMPATHETIC DIVISION OF THE AUTONOMIC NERVOUS SYSTEM: MORPHOLOGY AND PROPERTIES OF PREGANGLIONIC NEURONS—TONIC ACTIVITY

A. Morphology

The spinal cord contains preganglionic sympathetic neurons from which preganglionic fibers originate at each segment from the first thoracic to the third lumbar level in man, and from the first thoracic to the fourth or fifth lumbar levels in dogs and cats. Figure 2 shows a comparison of the segmental autonomic

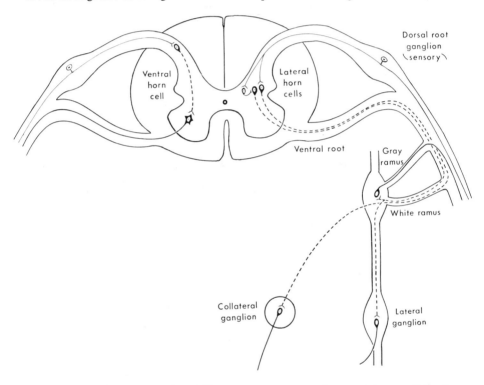

Figure 2 Diagram illustrating different arrangements of neurons in somatic and autonomic nervous systems. Single polysynaptic spinal reflex arc of somatic system is shown at left; that of sympathetic division of autonomic system is shown at right. These segmental arcs are bilateral and superimposed. At right, preganglionic neurons are represented by broken lines and postganglionic neurons by solid lines. Preganglionic fibers coming out through a white ramus make synaptic connection in more than one lateral chain ganglion and in collateral ganglia. Interneurons are also thought, as shown, to intervene between afferents and some preganglionic neurons. (Modified from Ref. 39.)

organization with that of the somatic system in the spinal cord. In simplified terms, spinal preganglionic neurons are situated in the intermediolateral horn, variously referred to as the intermediolateral cell column, superior nucleus intermediolateralis, lateral splanchnic motor cell column, superior lateral sympathetic nucleus, or thoracolumbar cell group (4). The preganglionic fibers are included in the ventral roots and accompany the somatic nerve trunks as they leave the spinal column. Shortly thereafter, these thinly myelinated fibers branch off to form the white rami. Most of these fibers make synaptic connections in the lateral ganglia, but some extend to the collateral ganglia before synapsing. Table 1 shows distribution of the sympathetic outflow in man.

The cells of the intermediolateral cell column are smaller than the ventral horn cells and measure from 12-60 μm in diameter in man and are described as bi- or multipolar cells (4). It has been suggested that the intermediolateral cell column is not restricted to the thoracolumbar levels of the cord (see 4 for ref.). Using various recently developed morphologic methods, the exact locus of origin of sympathetic preganglionic neurons has been reexamined in cats and in monkeys. They have been found to lie in the intermediolateral cell column, central autonomic gray, intercalated nucleus, and lateral funiculus. There is evidence that interneurons also exist within the intermediomedial cell column, dorsal horn, and Clarke's nucleus dorsalis to which afferent fibers connect before a synapse is made with sympathetic preganglionic neurons (11-15). There exist long intraspinal sympathetic pathways also, and impulses reaching the cord may travel several segments rostrally or caudally before exiting from a particular ventral root.

B. Properties of Sympathetic Preganglionic Neurons—Tonic Activity

Intracellular recordings from sympathetic preganglionic neurons have been carried out by a few investigators in situ (16,17,18) and in vitro (18a). Antidromically activated intracellularly recorded action potentials of sympathetic neurons show characteristic separation between IS (initial segment) and SD (somadendritic) components. Unlike those of somatic motoneurons, the potentials from preganglionic neurons have a long duration, between 4 and 15 msec, regardless of how the neurons are activated; antidromically, orthodromically, or by direct current injection (16,18). However, others have found (18a) the duration to be short, 1.8-3.5 msec. The passive electrical properties of these sympathetic preganglionic cells are more like those of autonomic ganglion cells than those of somatic motoneurons. The action potentials are followed by distinct after-hyperpolarizations lasting between 25 and 200 msec (18).

It is interesting that in studies carried out in vitro on the spinal cord slice preparations (18a), it has been found that in many preganglionic neurons the action potential has a long-lasting after-hyperpolarization of 1-7 sec., while in

Table 1 The Spinal Sympathetic Outflow to Ganglia and Body Parts in Man[a]

	Head, neck	Heart lung	Upper extremity	Upper abdominal organs	Adrenal	Kidney, ureter, testis, ovary	Pelvic organs	Lower extremity
Spinal outflow	(C-8) T1–T4 (T6)	T1–T5 (T6)	T2–T9 (T10)	T4–T9	T10–T11	T12–L2	T12–L2	T9–L2
Postganglionic synapse	Cervical sympathetic ganglia	Upper thoracic ganglia	Lower cervical Upper thoracic	Celiac Superior mesenteric ganglia	Adrenal	Celiac Renal ganglia	Celiac Inferior mesenteric ganglia	Lumbar Upper sacral ganglia
Postganglionic fibers	Vertebral neuron Internal and external carotid plexus	Thoracic Cervical cardiac neuron	Direct vascular neuron Gray rami peripheral neuron	Independent Medulla perivas-cular		Perivasc. plexus	Aortic Hypogas. plexus	Direct vascular neuron Gray rami peripheral nerves

Course of afferents	Direct vascular neuron Gray rami	Along motor cardiac neuron	Denied by some	Along splanchnics ?	Along splanchnics	Along hypogastric, sacral splanchnics	Denied by some
	Cervical Thoracic sympathetic trunk						Lower thoracic Upper lumbar
Spinal inflow	T1–T4	T1–T4	T1–T3 (T4)	T5–L2	(T10) T11–L2	T11–L2; S2–S4	

[a]The peripheral "origins" of some afferent fibers that run in sympathetic nerve trunks and the spinal levels of cord entry are also shown.

Source: Ref. 4.

others it is only 50–250 msec. Both types of hyperpolarization are associated with a decreased membrane resistance.

In central nervous system–intact and anesthetized animals, in contrast to the spinal animal (16), subthreshold synaptic potentials are present in most neurons. Action potentials are intermittently initiated from these synaptic potentials when they summate or attain sufficient amplitude (17,18).

One of the characteristics of the autonomic system is the so-called "tonus" or constant activity seen in many pre- and postganglionic neurons in the absence of external stimuli. The characteristics of this tonic activity in postganglionic fibers have been known since the pioneer work done by Bronk and his associates in the 1930s (19), when they recorded action potentials from single sympathetic fibers. Tonic activity has been recorded also from the white rami (20,21) and from neuron cell bodies directly, both extracellularly (22,23) and intracellularly (17,18). In recent years technical advances have made it possible to record such tonic firing from postganglionic sympathetic fibers in freely moving cats (24–26) and in humans (27–29).

According to Polosa et al. (23), one fourth to one fifth of all sympathetic preganglionic neurons are tonically active in central nervous system–intact anesthetized animals. This proportion seems to be uniform at all spinal cord levels. Most tonically active sympathetic preganglionic neurons fire irregularly. The mean firing rate is 1–2 imp./sec as recorded from white rami (20,21) and from spinal preganglionic neurons (22,23,30). When tonic activity is recorded as the mass discharge from the white rami at various levels the activity is relatively uniform (31).

In about half of the sympathetic preganglionic neurons the basic mode of irregular firing is rhythmically modulated at rates corresponding to that of the heart beat and that of the central respiratory activity. Respiratory modulation of sympathetic discharges has been recognized since the 1930s (32). Many papers have since appeared describing studies of the mechanism involved, but the origin and functional role of such modulations is not yet well understood (23). The activity of both sympathetic pre- and postganglionic neurons is augmented during inspiration and phrenic discharges and reduced in the absence of phrenic activity. This oscillation is considered to be due to a periodic facilitation of activity in the neurons during inspiration. Respiratory modulation is found in about one half of the active neurons in the upper thoracic cord. During these periodic bursts of discharges in spinal preganglionic neurons, rates up to 10–20 Hz may occur. Cardiac modulation is due to a depression of the neurons during part of each cardiac cycle. Afferent impulses from baroreceptors are responsible for this pulse-synchronous rhythm, since it disappears after sections of the carotid sinus and depressor nerves and the vagi.

The origin of sympathetic tone is mostly due to inputs from the central nervous system as well as from the periphery, since these neurons are connected to the sensory systems and central neuron groups. Sensory inputs come by way of various afferents originating from the skeletal muscle, skin, viscera, baro-receptors, central and peripheral chemoreceptors, vestibular and visual apparatus, and central temperature receptors (see 23 for ref.). The spinal preganglionic neurons are also connected with central nervous system structures of the brain stem reticular formation, hypothalamus, cerebellum, cerebral cortex, and others. All these inputs must play a role in tonic activity as excitatory or inhibitory influences, but the role of only a few of these afferents in tonic activity is known. Denervation of all baroreceptors increases discharge rates of spinal preganglionic neurons indicating their tonic inhibitory action; inactivation of peripheral chemoreceptors by hyperoxygenation and/or reduction of central chemoreceptor activity by low blood pCO_2 reduce sympathetic tone. The tonic discharges are reduced also be severance of the spinal cord from the medulla, though in chronic animals tonic discharges are again rather pronounced (33). Tonic activity is still present but at much reduced rates from small groups of cat cord segments even after deafferentation (30). During the last decade, much attention has been paid to a region on the ventral surface of the medulla that particularly influences tonic sympathetic activity (34-36).

During tonic activity in which the spinal preganglionic neurons fire irregularly, intracellular recording (17,18) has shown that there are many short-lasting excitatory postsynaptic potentials (EPSPs) that are not of sufficient amplitude to discharge a cell. The excitatory postsynaptic potentials have to be approximately 4-5 mV to reach threshold. It seems that generation of activity in the preganglionic neuron is not a consequence of a pacemaker potential originating locally or intrinsically or from supraspinal "oscillators," but the activity results from simple summation of synaptic events, much as occurs in a motoneurons of the lumbar spinal cord. The high sensitivity of these spinal neurons to the input and the continuation of an input may be the reason why they maintain a tonic discharge after isolation of the spinal cord. Rhythmically modulated discharges (cardiac and respiratory) can occur as a result of periodic fluctuation in synaptic action on the spinal preganglionic neurons.

Since rates of discharge in the spinal sympathetic neurons are rather low, Polosa and his associates have studied the inhibitory influences which set the limit to the firing frequency (37). Although the preganglionic neurons show high frequency discharges (10-20 Hz) during inspiration-synchronous bursts, this rate is maintained for only a short period. Even during reflex excitation the rate only slightly exceeds the normal value. Low frequency of the spinal preganglionic discharge as compared to other motoneurons can be attributed to several factors. One is the postexcitatory depression of sympathetic preganglionic neurons; the neuron's excitability decreases for nearly 300 msec after an antidromic or spontaneously occurring excitation. When the neurons are firing at a faster than average rate, the postexcitatory inhibition can add and result in a "silent period" that lasts for several seconds. Intracellular recordings show that hyperpolarization can persist for up to 200 msec subsequent to a single antidromically evoked action potential (16,17,18). In vitro studies show this after-hyperpolarization in some neurons lasts for as long as 1-7 sec following direct intracellular or focal stimulation (18a).

Another factor is the possibility of recurrent inhibition of the preganglionic neurons, although existence of such a phenomenon is still controversial. Finally, inhibition of these neurons can also spread within the cord, since in chronic spinal cats stimulation of myelinated afferent fibers in hindlimb somatic nerves can produce long-lasting inhibition of thoracic spinal preganglionic neurons; long inhibitory interspinal pathways are known to exist.

The mechanism of postexcitatory depression of sympathetic neurons is not clear but must be due to processes similar to those occurring in somatic motoneurons. The inhibitory pathways in the cord, the nature and the location of inhibitory interneurons, and so on, are not completely known. Moreover, except for inhibition originating from baroreceptors, the functional role played by inhibition of the sympathetic neurons is not clear, other than that it has a beneficial braking action. Effector organs—smooth muscles and glands—show the maximum response when efferent outflows are held between 6-8 imp./sec; the response is rather reduced at higher frequencies of discharge in sympathetic nerves.

IV. FUNCTIONAL CAPABILITIES OF THE SYMPATHETIC SYSTEM: REFLEX ACTIVITY AND DESCENDING INFLUENCES

Afferent inputs that affect these autonomic neurons, evoking reflex responses are numerous: baro- and chemoreceptors, other visceral afferents, such as those originating in receptors in the atria or ventricles of the heart, kidney, gastrointestinal tract, pelvic viscera, and other organs, and somatic afferents. Afferent fibers from viscera run in the vagus or sympathetic nerves. Somatic afferents entering the spinal cord produce sympathetic reflexes as well as somatic reflexes, affecting both sympathetic preganglionic neurons and somatic motoneurons. Afferent impulses evoke excitation or inhibition of preganglionic neurons through both supraspinal and spinal pathways (38,39).

A. Baroreceptor Reflex

The most clear-cut inhibition of the pre- and postganglionic neurons occurs with the excitation of baroreceptors (see 40,41 for reviews). The sympathetic rhythm synchronous with the pulse is due to the activity of baroreceptor afferents, though some preganglionic neurons, for example, those innervating vessels and sweat glands in the skin of humans show no cardiac rhythm except during strong sudomotor activity produced by high temperatures and are not much affected by baroreceptor input (29,42,43).

The baroreceptor-sympathetic reflex has a long latency, over 150 msec in cats (see 41 for ref.). The identification of the descending pathways conveying this inhibition from the medulla to the preganglionic neurons is still uncertain; this path can act either directly or through spinal interneurons on the preganglionic sympathetic neurons. The existence of such interneurons has been suggested (44).

B. Chemoreceptor Reflex

The most prominent effects produced by excitation of chemoreceptors are changes in respiration, but the stimulus also causes some changes in the sympathetic neuron activity through supraspinal reflex pathways (38,45). The excitation of arterial chemoreceptors by hypoxia or hypercapnia causes a mixed effect on preganglionic neurons in the cat thoracic cord (46), since reflex responses of postganglionic fibers are not uniform. For example, those innervating vasoconstrictors in muscle are strongly excited by the chemoreceptor excitation, while those innervating other tissues, for example, the heart (47,48) and various structures in the skin (49) behave differently. Central chemoreceptors, particularly those located in structures of the ventral medulla, also affect the sympathetic neurons (36,50).

C. Reflexes Originating From Receptors in Viscera

Excitation of afferents from various visceral organs evoke sympathetic reflex responses. There are receptors in atria and ventricles of the heart (51-56) sensitive to chemical and mechanical stimulation that evoke cardiovascular reflexes involving sympathetic neurons. There are receptors also in the lungs and great veins that affect the autonomic system (57). Most of these afferents enter the medulla through the vagus nerves, producing supraspinal sympathetic reflexes. Thus, these responses are altered after spinal cord transection (58). There are afferents that run in the sympathetic cardiac nerves to the spinal cord, evoking spinally mediated reflexes (59,60). These afferents are excited by distension of the aorta, chemical stimulation or occlusion of the coronary artery, and so forth, and evoke excitation or inhibition of sympathetic neurons acting on the cardiovascular system. That these afferent impulses are not produced by pain has been demonstrated by evoking similar reflex responses in unanesthetized freely moving animals without any sign of distress. Although such spinal reflexes are said to be present in central nervous system–intact animals and probably in humans, normally supraspinal structures are also involved.

Receptors in the kidney are known to cause sympathetic reflexes (61,62). There have been several reports that afferents in the splanchnic nerve produce blood pressure changes mediated by sympathetic neurons; these are activated by distension of the gallbladder, pinching of the intestine, pulling of the mesentery, and so forth (63). It is interesting to note that these responses increase after spinal transection (64); this is in contrast with the fact that somatic system reflexes in spinal preparations are generally reduced. There must be some difference in the organization of viscerosomatic and visceroautonomic reactions. In this connection, it should be noted that visceral afferents, such as those in the splanchnic nerves, have an organization within the cord that enables afferent impulses to evoke sympathetic reflexes from a greater number of segments of the cord than are involved in somatic discharges.

Afferents from pelvic organs also produce sympathetic reflexes. Distension of the bladder or stimulation of afferents from the gastrointestinal tract cause changes in activity of sympathetic neurons innervating the bladder and intestine (63,65).

D. Somatosympathetic Reflex

Practically all afferents except the largest fibers—group Ia,b fibers originating from muscle spindles and tendon organs—affect preganglionic sympathetic neurons in the cord (38,66). Figure 3 (33,67) shows sympathetic preganglionic discharges recorded from a white ramus simultaneously with somatic motoneuron discharges recorded from a ventral root. As seen in Figure 3, the supraspinal component of the sympathetic reflex is quite large and shows a similar pattern at various segmental levels, while the spinal component of the reflex response differs depending on the level of impulse entry. The advantage of supraspinal reflex responses is that afferent impulses entering the spinal cord can produce widespread and bilateral responses of similar magnitude throughout the entire thoracolumbar outflows; in contrast to this, the spinal reflex has a "local sign" and a less extensive effect. In intact animals, owing to supraspinal involvements, there are many cardiovascular reactions in which vasoconstrictor nerves have a similar effect throughout wide areas of the body. There are, of course, variations in reflex outputs depending on the stimulus; this will be discussed later.

The excitation of preganglionic neurons evoked by stimulation of somatic afferents is followed by long-lasting inhibition of background or tonic discharges ("silent period"). These biphasic responses are observed in both spinal and supraspinal sympathetic reflexes (33,38,66,68). A recent study shows that in unanesthetized spinal cats one third of all thoracic spinal preganglionic neurons responding display this dual response to somatic nerve stimulation (69).

Afferent fiber groups of types II-IV are known to evoke such biphasic reflex responses, but larger afferent fibers, particularly those of group II, may

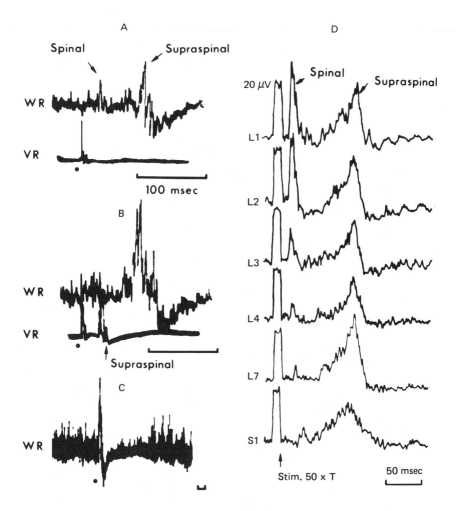

Figure 3 A, Sympathetic reflex responses recorded from cat lumbar white ramus, WR, following single-shock stimulations (marked by dots) of sciatic nerve. Tracings labeled VR are somatic reflex responses simultaneously recorded from lumbar seventh ventral root. Sympathetic reflex consists of short-latency spinal and long-latency supraspinal response. Somatic reflex shows mono- and polysynaptic components. B, Stronger stimulus is shown to evoke greater autonomic reflexes and larger somatic spinal reflex (mono- and polysynaptic reflexes fused in initial response) as well as somatic supraspinal reflex (second large deflection, VR). C, Record was taken at slow-sweep speed from white ramus and shows silent period that follows initial responses. D, Sympathetic reflex recorded from L1 white ramus (L1WR), but stimuli were applied to spinal nerves at various segmental levels, as indicated by arrow. Each record is average of 10 individual reflexes. Initial rectangular deflection is calibration pulse (20 μV). Early spinal reflex tends to be segmental and is reduced as afferent impulses enter more distant segments, whereas the supraspinal reflex remains constant. (A, B, and C from Ref. 33; D from Ref. 67.)

produce only inhibition in some cases (66). The reflex produced by excitation of unmyelinated afferents (group IV or C-fibers) has been well studied. The efferent discharge thus evoked reaches the effector organ much later than that caused by myelinated afferents. Thus, different effector organ reactions often occur when both myelinated and unmyelinated afferent fibers are excited by a stimulus (38,66,70,71).

Functional contributions of the spinal component of somatosympathetic reflexes in the central nervous system–intact animal is not yet well understood. Spinal reflexes are carried through polysynaptic pathways, judging from the central delay. In the chronic spinal animal the threshold of the spinal reflex is reduced and its magnitude is increased (38,72).

E. Differential Control of the Sympathetic Outflow

Although the sympathetic system can act in an emergency as a whole ("fight or flight reaction" of Cannon), analyses of postganglionic neuron responses have shown that there are also differential controls in the system. This suggests that differentially controlled discharge patterns must be present also in preganglionic neurons. In certain reflexes, for example, the chemoreceptor reflex and those involved in temperature regulation, differential discharges of sympathetic neurons do occur among the outflows to different effector organs (47,48,73–76). The most clearly demonstrated examples of differential control are shown by reflexes affecting vasoconstrictors in the muscle and the skin in humans. Sundlöf and Wallin (43) have found that the patterns of activity in sympathetic outflows to different skeletal muscles are remarkably uniform regardless of the region of the body, but they greatly differ from the activity shown by vasoconstrictors to the skin. Moreover, the muscle vasoconstrictors are affected by baroreceptors, but those innervating the skin are not; but they are activated by temperature changes and mental activity. Similar findings have been reported in anesthetized animals (77,78). Since there are no similarities between discharge patterns in postganglionic neurons innervating the muscle and the skin, it was suggested that sympathetic ganglia contain at least two different populations of neurons, each receiving its own characteristic preganglionic drive (43). Recently, an attempt has been made to investigate functional segregations among preganglionic neurons (79). It has been found that four groups of postganglionic fibers (skin and muscle vasoconstrictors and sudomotor and pilomotor fibers) are controlled by four corresponding groups of preganglionic neurons emanating from the lumbar cord. These groups show characteristic tonic and reflex patterns. It is still a question why a high proportion of preganglionic neurons (73%) that project to postganglionic neurons subserving the skin and muscle are silent and do not participate in reflex activity. It is also an interesting question as to how these distinct connections from pre- to postganglionic neurons and to the effecter organs are formed and maintained (80).

F. Descending Influences

Although the spinal cord isolated from central connections is capable of organizing sympathetic reflex responses, normally sympathetic neurons in the cord constantly receive impulses from "higher centers." These descending influences are both excitatory and inhibitory. A number of investigators have claimed that these two descending controls coming from the medulla, midbrain, hypothalamus, and limbic structures are conveyed by separate pathways in the spinal cord. Consensus is that the excitatory path descends in the dorsolateral funiculus, which also contains some inhibitory pathways. An exclusively inhibitory path descends in the ventral funiculus. These descending fibers can act either directly or via spinal interneurons on the preganglionic sympathetic neurons (see refs. 41 and 81 for more detailed discussion).

One thing seems clear; recently developed techniques for identifying fiber connections in the central nervous system have revealed many descending fibers making "direct" connections from the medulla and the hypothalamus (81,82). In particular, the "direct" connection between the paraventricular nucleus and intermediolateral column neurons has aroused much interest among morphologists because of the involvement of this hypothalamic structure in endocrine function (83-85). Most investigators now agree that neurons projecting to the cord are different from those projecting to the pituitary gland. The "direct" pathways from the medulla are mainly from the nucleus tractus solitarius (86) and from the ventral medulla (14,81,87). The latter contains monoaminergic fibers that probably originate in areas A1 and A5 of the catecholaminergic cell groups (87,88). These monoaminergic pathways exert a tonic inhibitory influence on sympathetic neurons in the intermediolateral column and may also be involved in supraspinal reflex responses (87,89). Iontophoretic application of norepinephrine to these sympathetic neurons also inhibits their activity (90), while iontophoretically applied 5-hydroxytryptamine excites the majority of spinal preganglionic neurons (91,92). The pharmacology of sympathetic preganglionic neurons and the transmitters that affect them and are released by them are not yet well known.

V. THE SACRAL PARASYMPATHETIC DIVISION: ITS MORPHOLOGY, PROPERTIES OF THE PREGANGLIONIC NEURONS, AND THEIR FUNCTION

A. Morphology

In the sacral outflow of the parasympathetic system preganglionic nerve fibers arise from the lateral gray matter of the spinal cord and travel by way of the midsacral ventral roots into the pelvic region. They leave the sacral spinal nerves and run independently to postganglionic cell bodies in the pelvic plexus and in the walls of the bladder, colon, rectum, and reproductive organs (4).

Recent anatomic investigations utilizing the horseradish peroxidase (HRP) technique have yielded new information about the morphology of the spinal preganglionic neurons in various animal species (93). In cats, there are two groups of neurons: a lateral and dorsal band containing 64% and 34%, respectively, of all parasympathetic neurons in the sacral cord. The cell bodies of these nuclei are spindle-shaped or elongated and triangular in shape. At least in cats, preganglionic neurons in the lateral and dorsal bands in addition to exhibiting a different morphology also innervate different effector organs. Cells in the lateral band are larger than those in the dorsal band, are oriented dorsoventrally, and innervate the urinary bladder, while cells in the dorsal band have mainly a mediolateral orientation and innervate the large intestine. This viscerotopic organization in the sacral cord was also confirmed by electrophysiologic techniques (93). Axons of preganglionic neurons of the cat innervating the bladder are B-fibers, while those innervating the large intestine are unmyelinated C-fibers (see 65 and 94 for references). Neurons seen to be situated between the lateral and dorsal bands of the sacral parasympathetic neurons are probably interneurons receiving primary afferent collaterals and are perhaps involved in intersegmental and supraspinal autonomic reflexes.

It is interesting that the somatic motoneurons related to micturition and defecation (those innervating the striated sphincter muscles and muscles of the pelvic floor) and the autonomic neurons of the sacral cord comprise an almost continuous band of cells that extends in an arc from the base of the dorsal horn to the ventral horn (Fig. 4). Moreover, as in their autonomic counterparts, the ventral group of somatic motoneurons innervate urethral sphincters, while dorsal groups innervate the anal sphinctors (95). In this connection, it should be pointed out that the pattern of activity of these somatic motoneurons is inversely related to the pattern of preganglionic parasympathetic neuron discharges; somatic motoneurons are inhibited during micturition and defecation and are excited in the period when urine and feces are stored (96).

B. Properties of Sacral Parasympathetic Preganglionic Neurons: Tonic Activity

The sacral preganglionic neurons have been studied extensively using intra- and extracellular recording techniques (97–99). Intracellularly recorded antidromic potentials have a duration of more than 5 msec with an amplitude between 20–90 mV. These potentials show a clear inflection on their rising phase that corresponds with the initial segment-somadendritic inflection. On the falling phase of the action potentials of some of these neurons another inflection is also observed. This latter phenomenon and the long duration of the action potentials resemble occurrences in sympathetic neurons described previously (16,18). An after-hyperpolarization is present that lasts approximately 60 msec. Parasympathetic neurons are inhibited by iontophoretic application of 5-hydroxytryptamine, norepinephrine, glycine and GABA(γ-aminobutyric acid) and are excited

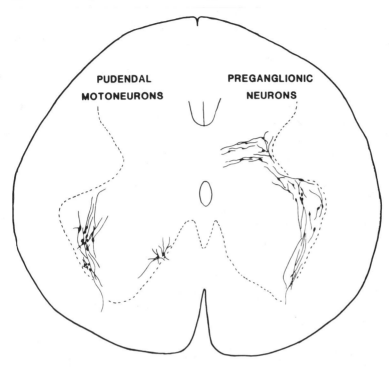

Figure 4 Anatomic location of sacral parasympathetic preganglionic neurons and pudendal motoneurons in the first sacral segment of the spinal cord. Cells were labeled by HRP applied to the central cut ends of the right pelvic nerve and the left pudendal nerve in an adult cat. Cells were drawn with camera lucida and represent the number obtained in two consecutive 70 μm sections. (From Ref. 93.)

by DL-homocysteic acid and glutamic acid, but they are not affected by acetylcholine (see 94 for reference).

Sacral preganglionic neurons behave differently depending on whether they are concerned with the bladder or large intestine, at least in cats (94). Those involved in micturition are quiescent and have no tonic activity when the bladder is empty or the intravesical pressure is lower than threshold for inducing a micturition reflex (0–5 cm H_2O). When the bladder is distended and the intravesical pressure exceeds the threshold level for micturition, preganglionic discharges occur in high-frequency bursts, reaching a level of 15–60 imp./sec. This rhythmic preganglionic neuron activity corresponds to bladder contractions, but it occurs prior to the contraction waves. The mean firing frequency of preganglionic neurons is related to intravesical pressure once it exceeds the micturition threshold. The mean frequency of discharges increases with any increase in bladder distension and ranges between 2-8 imp./sec. Unlike the preganglionic neurons, some interneurons that are situated in the region of the nuclei from which preganglionic neurons originate show tonic activity even when the bladder is empty, and their activity is very similar to that of preganglionic neurons when the bladder is distended.

Sacral parasympathetic neurons innervating the colon, on the other hand, show some spontaneous firing in the absence of intestinal distension. An enhanced discharge occurs prior to the beginning of spontaneous or evoked propulsive waves in the colon.

C. Reflex Responses of the Sacral Parasympathetic System

Recent studies have increased our knowledge of the micturition and defecation reflexes and how they are organized by the sacral parasympathetic neurons (65,93,94). Reflex pathways served by the sacral cord controlling the bladder and large intestine are quite different. Micturition is initiated by myelinated afferents receiving signals from sensors in the bladder wall ("A-fiber reflex") and is dependent mainly on supraspinal mechanisms, as F. J. F. Barrington pointed out first in the 1920s. In this reflex, firing occurs with a long latency (mean: 100 msec in cats) and the central delay is 60-75 msec following stimulation of myelinated vesical afferents in pelvic nerves. Intracellular recordings also show excitatory postsynaptic potentials with a latency of 60-100 msec. It is interesting that there is a reflex initiated by unmyelinated afferents from the bladder, but these produce only a spinal reflex. This latter spinal reflex ("C-fiber reflex") is observed in only 60% of central nervous system-intact animals and has a latency of 180-200 msec and a central delay of 45-65 msec (Fig. 5).

Stimulation of somatic afferents from the perineal region and from the hindlegs produce reflex responses in parasympathetic neurons. Intracellular records from the parasympathetic neurons show short latency (5 msec) inhibitory postsynaptic potentials (IPSPs) followed by longer latency (60-80 msec) excitatory postsynaptic potentials and firing. It should be noted that the same stimulus evokes, instead of an early inhibitory postsynaptic potential and late excitatory postsynaptic potentials seen in the autonomic circuit, both early and late excitatory postsynaptic potentials in sacral somatic motoneurons (65,99). The reflex responses of sacral preganglionic neurons innervating the bladder undergo great changes when the spinal cord is transected; this will be discussed later.

In contrast to the sacral outflow to the bladder, the sacral parasympathetic reflex pathway to the large intestine is organized within the sacral spinal cord and may subserve various functions. This pathway is responsible for coordinating large-amplitude sustained, propulsive contractions that occur during defecation.

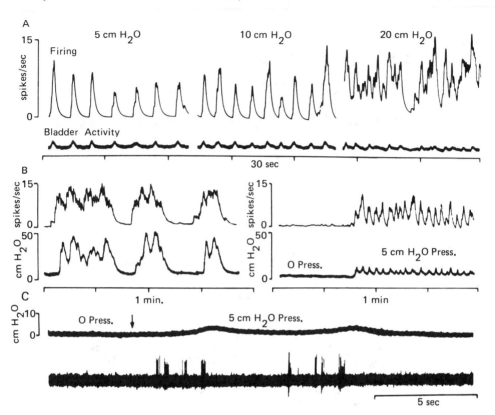

Figure 5 Discharge patterns of a bladder preganglionic neuron (B-fiber axons) in the S2 spinal segment of a cat with an intact neuraxis. A, Burst-firing with the bladder distended at 5, 10, and 20 cm H_2O constant pressure. Top tracing, ratemeter record (time constant 3 sec) of firing in spikes/sec. Bottom tracing, a recording of the fluctuations in intravesical pressure indicating rhythmic contractile activity of the detrusor. B, Left panels indicate rhythmic firing (top) and bladder contractions (bottom) with the bladder distended under constant volume conditions. Right panel shows absence of firing with bladder empty at 0 intravesical pressure and burst discharge and rhythmic bladder activity when intravesical pressure was raised to 5 cm H_2O. C, Firing pattern of the neuron when intravesical pressure was raised (arrow) from 0 to 5 cm H_2O. Top trace, bladder pressure; bottom trace, unit firing. Records show that bursts of firing seen in ratemeter tracings in A and B are subdivided into several short-duration bursts separated by intervals of 0.2–1.2 sec. (From Ref. 94.)

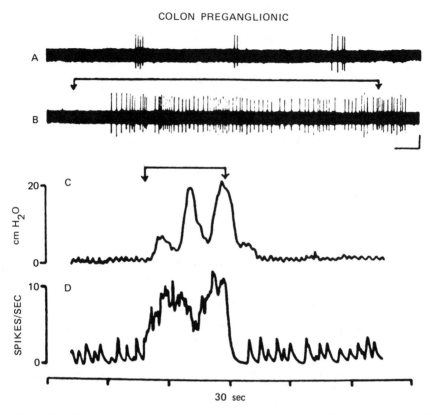

Figure 6 Discharge of a preganglionic neuron in the dorsal part of the sacral autonomic nucleus. A, Spontaneous firing. B, Firing evoked by mechanical stimulation (indicated by the arrows) of the rectum-anal canal. C and D, Simultaneous recording of intraluminal pressure (cm H_2O) in the midcolon and firing of a sacral preganglionic neuron during stimulation of rectum-anal canal (between arrows). Horizontal and vertical calibrations in A represent 1 sec and 250 μV, respectively. (From Ref. 65.)

In addition, it seems to be involved in the control of secretion and of ion transport and of the modulation of myenteric inhibitory pathways to the rectum and colon (65,93). The defecation reflex has a long latency (180–300 msec) owing to a slowly conducting spinal pathway comprised of both unmyelinated afferent and preganglionic efferent components (Fig. 6). The estimated central delay in cats is long (45–60 msec), indicative of polysynaptic pathways. In the chronic spinal preparation this is essentially unchanged, though the reflex is transiently depressed after transection. There are, of course, descending excitatory and inhibitory influences from supraspinal structures that normally function in control of defecation and micturition (96-98).

The sacral parasympathetic system also serves the reproductive organs. The behavior of preganglionic parasympathetic neurons concerned with these functions have not been much studied, although there is evidence that indicates that these neurons are responsible for various reproductive functions (100).

VI. SYMPATHETIC-PARASYMPATHETIC INTERACTIONS: CENTRAL AND PERIPHERAL

The most complex interactions of the sympathetic and parasympathetic divisions of the autonomic system are organized in the medulla and higher centers that generate either reciprocal actions or coactivations of the sympathetic and vagal fibers that converge on organs such as the heart where they are assumed to have a completely antagonistic action. Which of these associated actions occurs, reciprocal or synergistic, depends on the reflexes evoked, what hypothalamic area is stimulated, or what conditions prevail (1,101,102). If we ignore the uncoordinated interactions between spinally directed sympathetic and the brain-directed vagal actions at the periphery, we can say that in spinal animals the spinal interactions possible are between the sympathetics and sacral parasympathetics that innervate lower viscera and body parts. The two outflows, however, are not as clearly antagonistic as are, for example, the sympathetics and vagi in their actions on the heart. Unquestionably, the sacral parasympathetics are the motor nerves chiefly responsible for micturition, defecation, and erection in the male, but sympathetic nerves that are primarily inhibitory in certain circumstances can also cause weak erections and bladder contractions, possibly due to peripheral interactions. Both cooperate in the vasodilation-produced distension and ejaculation essential to the male act of reproduction. In brief, one sees not only reciprocal actions in reflex responses, but also some synergistic and supplementary or cooperative functions. When pathways for reciprocal action and coactivation are anatomically present in the cord they still operate in spinal reflexes. Presumably, in the spinal defecation reflex the inhibitory action of the sympathetic supply is turned off when the parasympathetic-promoted act of defecation is evoked (39). This assumes the presence of some intraspinal thoracolumbar/sacral cord connector pathways. These pathways must operate in the reflex activities of spinal animals.

There are other peripheral sympathetic-parasympathetic interactions that continue to operate in spinal preparations. During the last few years, the existence of peripheral or ganglionic reflexes has again been accepted (103). Such reactions are dependent upon what is occurring in ganglia and here too much new knowledge has been obtained (104). Sympathetic fibers actually converge on parasympathetic pelvic ganglia and affect transmission there (105).

Finally, in plexuses of the heart, the gut, and pelvic organs there is interaction between the terminals of parasympathetic and sympathetic efferents (106,107). It is not appropriate to our commission to discuss the details and relative significances of central, ganglionic, and peripheral interactions. The principal thought to convey is that the two divisions of the autonomic system cooperate in many ways and at many sites in promoting body functions, including those entrusted to the spinal cord.

VII. THE SPINAL CORD'S CAPABILITY AS A SENSOR AND OTHER INTRINSIC ABILITIES RELATIVE TO AUTONOMIC SYSTEM FUNCTION

The spinal cord in addition to mediating reflex action and generating tonic discharges in the sympathetic and parasympathetic efferents has some capability as a sensor. In the early 1930s, it was found that chronic spinal animals show a sympathoadrenal reaction to hypoglycemia induced by insulin and to the hypotension of reduced blood flow produced by hemorrhage even after dorsal roots are cut (108,109). Jourdan (110) claimed that asphyxia of upper thoracic regions of the cord of a spinal animal causes an increased secretion from the adrenals. The most impressive evidence, however, of this ability has been provided by studies of cord reactions to heat and cold. Those who have tried to maintain chronic spinal animals know that after a few days it is much easier to maintain a normal body temperature. In 1924, Sherrington (111) published some observations on temperature regulation after spinal transection and observations on shivering. Some authors (e.g., Thauer [112]) have long maintained that spinal animals are capable of a degree of thermoregulation, and it has been confirmed that those responses that can be generated by manipulating hypothalamic temperature can also be produced by warming and cooling the cord. Warming the cord has been shown to induce skin vasodilatation, panting, salivation, and the inhibition of shivering in dogs (113), rabbits (114), oxen (115), and guinea pigs (116). Conversely, reducing cord temperature can bring about shivering in drogs (117), pigeons (118), and other species. Toxins can also produce a low grade of fever in a chronic spinal animal. The neurons responsible for these reactions to heat and cold appear to lie in the ventrolateral region of the upper cord (119). It seems that normal cord temperature variations and gradients and cord temperatures at which reactions occur have not as yet been accurately determined. Cells sensitive to heat and cold have been located in the cord (120,121).

There is still another aspect of intraspinal function that is receiving scant attention; that is, its neuroendocrine involvement. It is very difficult to find any extensive analyses of what peptides or what neurohormones are produced within the cord relative to intra- or extra spinal cord functions. Attention has been focused primarily on the hypothalamus and ganglia with respect to these compounds. About all one finds in the literature are statements such as, "It is now clear that many peptides, including the so-called hypothalamic hormones, are distributed throughout the central nervous system including the spinal cord" (122,123).

Immunocytochemical techniques using various antisomatostatin agents have been employed for the cellular localization of somatostatin (SS). Somatostatin-like materials or activity (SLA) have been found in various parts of the brain, chiefly in the hypothalamus, but also in the spinal cord (124,125). Hökfelt et al. (126,127) identified SLA by immunocytochemistry in the substantia gelatinosa of the dorsal horn and in adjacent parts of the lateral funiculus as well as in spinal ganglion cell bodies. It is suggested that SS might function as a neuro-modulator (128). Other neuroendocrine products that can conceivably have a localized or more general action are produced in the cord, but no clear defini-tions of their functional roles can be given. It is conceivable, however, that their receptor mechanisms may be involved in "denervation sensitization" and the effects of pharmacologic agents on the cord.

VIII. THE SPINAL CORD IN THE ACUTE AND CHRONIC STATE: SPINAL SHOCK, SENSITIZATION, PLASTICITY, AND REGENERATIVE ABILITIES

Those physiologists who first tried to locate the "center" controlling cardio-vascular tone and reflex actions were the ones who initially observed the effects of cord section on autonomic system function. Those who performed studies worthy of mention were Bezold (1863) (129), Goltz (1864), Owsjannikow (1871), Dittmar (1873), Sherrington (1906), and Ranson and Billingsley (1916). Thousands of such experiments have revealed a sequence of phenomena subse-quent to transection. First, it was observed that though section reduced blood pressure drastically, there remained sufficient sympathetic tone and peripheral resistance to sustain a pressure of 40–50 mm Hg. Pithing the cord or cutting the splanchnics further reduced and practically abolished arterial pressure (see 130). Goltz, in 1864, found that after the medulla was severed from the cord vascular tone in the frog recovered quickly. He also demonstrated in the dog that if the cord was cut at the upper thoracic level, temperature became high in the lower limbs because of vasodilatation. Gradually, vessel tone was restored but dilata-tion occurred again if the cord was destroyed. Modern techniques have shown also that sympathetic fibers retain a considerable degree of tonic activity after cord section and that it is further reduced by cord destruction. Tone increases with time and normal pressures are restored if the cord, though isolated from higher centers, remains intact. Early as well as late investigations have revealed also that the cord though seemingly temporarily depressed could still mediate reflex actions of the autonomic system after transection.

The second observation that has been made consistently is that cutting the cord causes "spinal shock." The intensity and duration of this shock, or depression, depends on the degree of cord traumatization and the degree of cephalization possessed by the species used. In lower forms, inactivating shock lasts for only minutes. In cats and dogs it lasts for hours and in man for days. Although most studies of spinal shock have involved only the somatic system, the autonomic system is similarly affected and the general concept is that spinal shock is due to loss of facilitatory influences from higher centers—a sort of deprivation suppression. Studies of the effects of "shock" have produced some interesting data. Certain afferent groups cannot elicit responses during shock. For example, Sato (131) found that reflexes evoked by group IV somatic afferents disappear in the acute spinal animal but reappear some 8-12 weeks later in the chronic state. Reactions evoked by larger diameter fibers are suppressed but not blocked even temporarily.

A third consequence of cord section is loss of the inhibitory as well as facilitatory or excitatory influence of higher centers. In the sympathetic reflex evoked by stimulation of peripheral afferents under normal conditions the operation of an inhibitory component is revealed by a "silent period" in the sympathetic discharge that has a duration of 300-800 msec. In the spinal animal a silent period is perceptible but of brief duration (38,132). Loss of inhibition and the integrative power of higher centers is responsible for the "release phenomena" observed in spinal preparations in the chronic state.

A fourth phase in the sequence of phenomena revealed after cord section is restoration of responsiveness and even a hyperactivity inappropriate to the nature or intensity of a stimulus. Sherrington, in 1906, (133) noted the return of blood pressure, vascular tone, and reflexes to a rather normal state. A number of individuals actually reported a high spinal control of cardiovascular reactions and of the adrenals (110,134-136). Certainly, the cord in chronic preparations can mediate many cardiovascular reactions (11,137,138), and it has already been stated that chronic spinal animals can mount sympathoadrenal resistance to insulin-induced hypoglycemia and to hemorrhage. The system does tend to "fire as a whole," as in the normal animal under stress of asphyxia or other abnormal states and stimuli. The cord has not lost intrinsic integrative mechanisms. When a strong stimulus enters one dorsal root it evokes a major response from that segment, but there is a spread of the excitation and discharge from adjacent segments as well (139,140). In the absence of higher controls, this spread may go beyond normal bounds and result in hyperactivity.

Spinal cord section evidently results in a degree of "denervation sensitivity." Initially, it was observed that a unilateral increase in responsiveness of neurons to drugs and other stimuli develops below the level of a cord hemisection. There is now abundant pharmacologic evidence that a receptor sensitivity develops at all autonomic synapses when deprived of presynaptic nerves and transmitters. With respect to the cord, however, the most impressive display of sensitization or hyperresponsiveness and a "release phenomenon" is the "mass reflex" that occurs in spinal animals and in man. The mass reflex, according to *Blakiston's New Gould Medical Dictionary*, 1st ed. (1949), is "a complex reflex phenomenon induced by stimuli below the level of a complete transverse lesion of the spinal cord and characterized by flexor spasms of the legs, involuntary evacuation of the bladder, and sweating below the level of the lesion." Other autonomic accompaniments of this reflex are erection and even ejaculation in the male. This abnormal association of somatic, sympathetic, and parasympathetic reactions is more of a convulsive seizure than a physiologic reaction. It can be triggered by what are normally ineffective stimuli.

A final phenomenon that can be referred to as adaptive plasticity is best illustrated by reactions that involve the sacral parasympathetic as well as the sympathetic system. Studies of the micturition and defecation reflex have revealed considerable differences in their mediation and control and adaptation (93). Defecation, though normally under learned voluntary control, is primarily dependent upon a spinal reflex. Transection of the spinal cord only transiently depresses defecation, which quickly becomes automatic, though still triggered by the usual stimuli (39). Presumably, the roles of the sympathetic and parasympathetic systems must be somewhat the same because a periodicity is retained. Micturition is a more complex phenomenon and the bladder paralysis that occurs subsequent to cord section is relatively long lasting, and when a degree of automaticity does appear days or weeks later emptying is incomplete and residual urine remains.

The total complexity of the situation presented briefly is as follows. In the cat at birth and for a few weeks subsequently, micturition is evoked by a perineum-bladder reflex triggered by the mother's cleaning processes. This is a spinal "C-fiber reflex." At birth, no spinal bladder-to-bladder reflex has been detected (93). In the adult, stimulation of the perineum or sex organs inhibits micturition, so this perineal-bladder reflex disappears. It was thought for a while that the perineum-bladder reflex reappears in the chronic spinal animal (141), since a spinal bladder reflex does develop, but recent work does not confirm this. A bladder-to-bladder supraspinal reflex ("A-fiber reflex") is detectable in animals 5 to 72 days of age. It eventually becomes dominant and the perineum reflex disappears. If the cord of a kitten is cut, there is establishment of a bladder-to-bladder C-fiber reflex within a very few days. This indicates a high level of plasticity in the cord. This kitten bladder-to-bladder reflex is bilateral in action. In the adult cat there is an A-fiber supraspinal reflex and also a spinal C-fiber reflex (in 60% of animals studied). This C-reflex in the adult is bilateral in action. It is under some higher control in association with the bulbar reflex (A-reflex) because on transection of the cord the C-reflex is suppressed for quite a while. When the spinal C-reflex does recover and automatic micturition begins

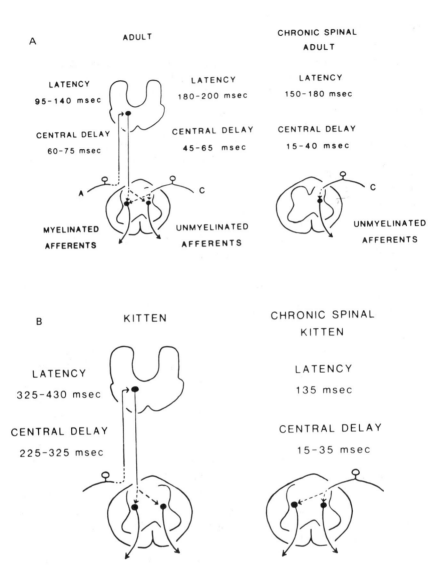

Figure 7 Diagrams of bladder reflexes in adult cats and kittens before and after transection of the cord. A, Adult cat, showing (left) supraspinal and spinal micturition reflex pathways (latency and central delay indicated). Spinal reflex path in chronic state (right); note that reflex path is unilateral. Latencies and central delays of supraspinal reflex shown on left of figure and latencies and central delays of spinal reflex to right of diagram. Note decreases in latencies and central delays of spinal reaction. B, Kitten, showing only a supraspinal reflex previous to cord section; note latencies and central delay. After section, a bilateral spinal reflex develops—and its latencies and central delay. Apparently, the adult has lost plasticity demonstrated by kitten. (From Ref. 93.)

again it has a shorter than normal latency, but it is still somewhat deficient because a unilateral stimulation produces only a unilateral response (Fig. 7). The spinal C-fiber reflex established in the more adaptive cord of the kitten is bilateral and has an even shorter latency than the spinal reflex that becomes functional after cord section in the adult (93). Evidently, the potential for adaptive plasticity within the spinal cord diminishes with age.

IX. CONCLUSIONS AND GENERALIZATIONS

The sympathetic and sacral parasympathetic components of the autonomic system originate from the neural crest as the spinal cord and the segmental components of the somatic system develop. Although higher brain centers control through facilitatory and inhibitory directives the major activities of the spinal autonomic efferent outflow, contributing tonic drives and organizing reciprocal and synergic activities of the sympathetic and parasympathetic neurons, there are rather autonomous spinally mediated responses even in intact normal animals. Although these spinal reflexes are more localized in effect than when the medulla and higher centers are involved, they still suffice to sustain the functions of the viscera required for survival after cord section. In the spinal animal there is sufficient cardiovascular sympathetic discharge to maintain an adequate pressure and blood flow and adjustments thereof. There is some compensatory reaction to heat and cold and some neuroendocrine reaction potential; release of the adrenal medulla secretions can be modulated, energy can be made available from storage, and waste products can be eliminated. Somatic deficiencies, not autonomic failures, impair reproductive abilities. On the whole, autonomic functions are of the same order of magnitude, but they are probably less impaired than the somatic functions by severance of the spinal cord.

REFERENCES

1. Brooks, C. McC., and Lange, G. (1982). Patterns of reflex action, their autonomic components and their behavioral significance. *Pavlovian J. Biol. Sci. 17*:55–61.
2. Sheehan, D. (1936). The discovery of the autonomic nervous system. *Arch. Neurol. Psychiat. 35*:1081-1115.
3. Sheehan, D. (1941). The autonomic nervous system prior to Gaskell. *N. Engl. J. Med. 224*:457-460.
4. Pick, J. (1970). *The Autonomic Nervous System: Morphology, Comparative, Clinical and Surgical Aspects*, Lippincott, Philadelphia.
5. Le Douarin, N. (1981). Plasticity in the development of the peripheral nervous system. In *Development of the Autonomic Nervous System*, G. Burnstock (Ed.), Pitman Books, London, pp. 19-50.
6. Burnstock, G. (Ed.) (1981). *Development of the Autonomic Nervous System*, Ciba Symposium 83, Pitman Books, London.

7. Garrett, J. R., and Howard, E. R. (1981). Myenteric plexus of the hindgut: Developmental abnormalities in humans and experimental studies. In *Development of the Autonomic Nervous System*, G. Burnstock (Ed.), Pitman Books, London, pp. 326–343.

8. Appenzeller, O. (1982). *The Autonomic Nervous System: An Introduction to Basic and Clinical Concepts*, 3rd ed., Elsevier, New York.

9. Bevan, J. A., Godfraind, T., Maxwell, R. A., and Vanhoutte, P. M. (1980). Development and ageing. In *Vascular Neuroeffector Mechanisms*, J. A. Bevan, T. Godfraind, R. A. Maxwell, and P. M. Vanhoutte (Eds.), Raven, New York, pp. 335–346.

10. Collins, K. J., Exton-Smith, A. N., James, M. H., and Oliver, D. J. (1980). Functional changes in autonomic nervous responses with ageing. *Age Ageing 9*:17–24.

11. Wurster, R. D. (1977). Spinal sympathetic control of the heart. In *Neural Control of the Heart*, W. C. Randal (Ed.), Oxford University Press, New York, pp. 213–246.

12. Chung, K., Lavelle, F. W., and Wurster, R. D. (1980). Ultrastructure of HRP-identified sympathetic preganglionic neurons in cats. *J. Comp. Neurol. 190*:147–155.

13. Deuschl, G., and Illert, M. (1981). Cytoarchitectonic organization of lumbar preganglionic sympathetic neurons in the cat. *J. Auton. Nerv. Syst. 3*:193–213.

14. Lowey, A. D., and McKellar, S. (1980). The neuroanatomical basis of central cardiovascular control. *Fed. Proc. 39*:2495–2503.

15. Petras, J. M., and Cummings, J. F. (1972). Autonomic neurons in the spinal cord of the Rhesus monkey: A correlation of the findings of cytoarchitectonics and sympathectomy with fiber degeneration following dorsal rhizotomy. *J. Comp. Neurol. 146*:189–218.

16. Fernandez de Molina, A., Kuno, M., and Perl, E. R. (1965). Antidromically evoked responses from sympathetic preganglionic neurons. *J. Physiol. (Lond.) 180*:321–335.

17. Coote, J. H., and Westbury, D. R. (1979). Intracellular recordings from sympathetic preganglionic neurones. *Neuroscience Lett. 15*:171–175.

18. McLachlan, E. M., and Hirst, G. D. S. (1980). Some properties of preganglionic neurons in the upper thoracic spinal cord of the cat. *J. Neurophysiol. 43*:1251–1265.

18a. Yoshimura, M., and Nishi, S. (1982). Intracellular recordings from lateral horn cells of the spinal cord in vitro. *J. Auton. Nerv. Syst. 6*:5–11.

19. Bronk, D. W. (1933-4). The nervous mechanism of cardiovascular control. *Harvey Lecture 29*:245–262.

20. Kaufman, A., and Koizumi, K. (1971). Spontaneous and reflex activity of single units in lumbar white rami. In *Research in Physiology. A Liber Memorialis in Honor of Professor Chandler McCuskey Brooks*, F. F. Kao, M. Vassalle, and K. Koizumi (Eds.), Aulo Gaggi, Bologna, pp. 469–481.

21. Sato, A. (1972). The relative involvement of different reflex pathways in somatosympathetic reflexes, analyzed in spontaneously active single preganglionic sympathetic units. *Pflugers Arch. 333*:70–81.

22. Mannard, A., and Polosa, C. (1973). Analysis of background firing of single sympathetic preganglionic neurons of cat cervical nerve. *J. Neurophysiol. 36*:398-408.

23. Polosa, C., Mannard, A., and Laskey, W. (1979). Tonic activity of the autonomic nervous system: Functions, properties, origins. In *Integrative Functions of the Autonomic Nervous System*, C. McC. Brooks, K. Koizumi, and A. Sato (Eds.), University of Tokyo Press, Tokyo, and Elsevier-North Holland, New York, pp. 342-354.

24. Kirchner, F. (1973). Spontaneous activity of the renal sympathetic nerve in the unanesthetized cat. *Acta Physiol. Pol. 24*:129-134.

25. Schad, H., and Seller, H. (1975). A method for recording autonomic nerve activity in unanesthetized, freely moving cats. *Brain Res. 100*:425-430.

26. Ninomiya, I., and Yonezawa, Y. (1979). Sympathetic nerve activity, aortic pressure and heart rate in response to behavioral stimuli. In *Integrative Functions of the Autonomic Nervous System*, C. McC. Brooks, K. Koizumi, and A. Sato (Eds.), University of Tokyo Press, Tokyo; and Elsevier-North Holland, New York, pp. 433-442.

27. Delino, W., Hagbarth, K-E., Hongell, A., and Wallin, B. G. (1972). General characteristics of sympathetic activity in human muscle nerves. *Acta Physiol. Scand. 84*:65-81.

28. Vallbo, A. B., Hagbarth, K-E., Torebjörk, H. E., and Wallin, B. G. (1979). Somatosensory, proprioceptive, and sympathetic activity in human peripheral nerves. *Physiol. Rev. 59*:919-957.

29. Bini, G., Hagbarth, K-E., and Wallin, B. G. (1981). Cardiac rhythmicity of skin sympathetic activity recorded from peripheral nerves in man. *J. Auton. Nerv. Syst. 4*:17-24.

30. Polosa, C. (1968). Spontaneous activity of sympathetic preganglionic neurons. *Can. J. Physiol. Pharmacol. 46*:887-897.

31. Koizumi, K., Seller, H., Kaufman, A., and Brooks, C. McC. (1971). Pattern of sympathetic discharges and their relation to baroreceptor and respiratory activity. *Brain Res. 27*:281-294.

32. Adrian, E. D., Bronk, D. W., and Phillips, G. (1932). Discharges in mammalian sympathetic nerves. *J. Physiol. (Lond.) 74*:115-133.

33. Koizumi, K., Sato, A., Kaufman, A., and Brooks, C. McC. (1968). Studies of sympathetic neuron discharges modified by central and peripheral excitation. *Brain Res. 11*:212-224.

34. Guertzenstein, P. G., and Silver, A. (1974). Fall in blood pressure produced from discrete regions of the ventral surface of the medulla by glycine and lesions. *J. Physiol. (Lond.) 242*:489-503.

35. Hanna, B. D., Lioy, F., and Polosa, C. (1979). The effect of cold blockade of the medullary chemoreceptors on the CO_2 modulation of vascular tone and heart rate. *Can. J. Physiol. Pharmacol. 57*:461-468.

36. Schläfke, M. E., and See, W. R. (1980). Ventral medullary surface stimulus response in relation to ventilatory and cardiovascular effects. In *Central Interaction Between Respiratory and Cardiovascular Control Systems*, H. P. Kopechen, S. M. Hilton, and A. Trzebski (Eds.), Springer-Verlag, Berlin, pp. 56-63.

37. Polosa, C., Schondorf, R., and Laskey, W. (1982). Stabilization of the discharge rate of sympathetic preganglionic neurons. *J. Auton. Nerv. Syst.* 5: 45–54.

38. Koizumi, K., and Brooks, C. McC. (1972). The integration of autonomic system reactions: A discussion of autonomic reflexes, their control and their association with somatic reactions. *Ergeb. Physiol.* 67:1–68.

39. Koizumi, K., and Brooks, C. McC. (1980). The autonomic system and its role in controlling body functions. In *Medical Physiology*, 14th ed., V. B. Mountcastle (Ed.)., Mosby, St. Louis, pp. 893–922.

40. Kirchheim, H. R. (1976). Systemic arterial baroreceptor reflexes. *Physiol. Rev.* 56:100–176.

41. Spyer, K. M. (1981). Neural organization and control of baroreceptor reflex. *Rev. Physiol. Biochem. Pharmacol.* 88:23–124.

42. Wallin, B. G., Sundlöf, G., and Delius, W. (1975). The effect of carotid sinus nerve stimulation on muscle and skin nerve sympathetic activity. *Pflugers Arch.* 358:101–110.

43. Sundlöf, G., and Wallin, B. G. (1977). The variability of muscle nerve sympathetic activity in resting recumbent man. *J. Physiol. (Lond.)* 272: 383–397.

44. McCall, R. S., Gebber, G. L., and Barman, S. M. (1977). Spinal interneurons in the baroreceptor reflex arc. *Am. J. Physiol.* 232:H657–H665.

45. Korner, P. I. (1971). Integrative neural cardiovascular control. *Physiol. Rev.* 51:312–367.

46. Preiss, G., and Polosa, C. (1977). The relation between end-tidal CO_2 and discharge patterns of sympathetic preganglionic neurons. *Brain Res.* 122:255–269.

47. Kollai, M., and Koizumi, K. (1977). Differential responses in sympathetic outflow evoked by chemoreceptor activation. *Brain Res.* 138:159–165.

48. Kollai, M., Koizumi, K., and Brooks, C. McC. (1978). Nature of differential sympathetic discharges in chemoreceptor reflex. *Proc. Natl. Acad. Sci. USA,* 75:5239–5243.

49. Blumberg, H., Jänig, W., Rieckmann, C., and Szulczyk, P. (1980). Baroreceptor and chemoreceptor reflexes in postganglionic neurones supplying skeletal muscle and hairy skin. *J. Auton. Nerv. Syst.* 2:223–240.

50. Hanna, B. D., Lioy, F., and Polosa, C. (1981). Role of carotid and central chemoreceptors in the CO_2 response of sympathetic preganglionic neurons. *J. Auton. Nerv. Syst.* 3:421–435.

51. Coleridge, H. M., Coleridge, J. C. G., and Kidd, C. (1964). Cardiac receptors in the dog, with particular reference to two types of afferent endings in the ventricular wall. *J. Physiol. (Lond.)* 174:323–339.

52. Paintal, A. S. (1973). Vagal sensory receptors and their reflex effects. *Physiol. Rev.* 53:159–227.

53. Koizumi, K., Ishikawa, T., Nishino, H., and Brooks, C. McC. (1975). Cardiac and autonomic system reactions to stretch of the atria. *Brain Res.* 87:247–261.

54. Kollai, M., Koizumi, K., Yamashita, H., and Brooks, C. McC. (1978). Study of cardiac sympathetic and vagal activity during reflex responses produced by stretch of the atria. *Brain Res. 150*:519–532.
55. Linden, R. J. (1975). Reflexes from the heart. *Prog. Cardiovasc. Dis. 18*:201–221.
56. Hainsworth, R., Kidd, C., and Linden, R. J. (Eds.) (1979). *Cardiac Receptors*, Cambridge University Press, Cambridge, England.
57. Coleridge, H. M., and Coleridge, J. C. G. (1979). Afferents of the pulmonary vascular bed and their role. In *Integrative Functions of the Autonomic Nervous System*, C. McC. Brooks, K. Koizumi, and A. Sato (Eds.), New York, University of Tokyo Press, Tokyo; and Elsevier–North Holland, New York, pp. 98–110.
58. Koizumi, K., Nishino, H., and Brooks, C. McC. (1977). Centers involved in the autonomic reflex reactions originating from stretching of the atria. *Proc. Natl. Acad. Sci. USA, 74*:2177–2181.
59. Malliani, A., Lombardi, F., and Pagani, M. (1981). Functions of afferents in cardiovascular sympathetic nerves. *J. Auton. Nerv. Syst. 3*:231–236.
60. Malliani, A. (1979). Afferent cardiovascular sympathetic nerve fibres and their function in the neural regulation of the circulation. In *Cardiac Receptors*, R. Hainsworth, C. Kidd, and P. J. Linden (Eds.), Cambridge University Press, Cambridge, England, pp. 319–338.
61. Recordati, G., Moss, N. G., Genovesi, S., and Rogenco, P. (1981). Renal chemoreceptors. *J. Auton. Nerv. Syst. 3*:237–251.
62. Rogenes, P. R. (1982). Single-unit and multiunit analyses of renorenal reflexes elicited by stimulation of renal chemoreceptors in the rat. *J. Auton. Nerv. Syst. 6*:143–156.
63. Newman, P. P. (1974). *Visceral Afferent Functions of the Nervous System*, Edward Arnold, London; and Williams & Wilkins, Baltimore.
64. Downman, C. B. B., and McSwiney, B. A. (1946). Reflexes elicited by visceral stimulation in the acute spinal animal. *J. Physiol. (Lond.) 105*:80–94.
65. de Groat, W. C., Booth, A. M., Krier, J., Milne, R. J., Morgan, C., and Nadelhaft, I. (1979). Neural control of the urinary bladder and large intestine. In *Integrative Functions of the Autonomic Nervous System*, C. McC. Brooks, K. Koizumi, and A. Sato (Eds.), University of Tokyo Press, Tokyo; and Elsevier–North Holland, New York, pp. 50–67.
66. Sato, A., and Schmidt, R. F. (1973). Somatosympathetic reflexes: Afferent fibers, central pathways, discharge characteristics. *Physiol. Rev. 53*:916–947.
67. Sato, A., and Schmidt, R. F. (1971). Spinal and supraspinal components of the reflex discharges into lumbar and thoracic white rami. *J. Physiol. (Lond.) 212*:839–850.
68. Polosa, C. (1967). Silent period of sympathetic preganglionic neurons. *Can. J. Physiol. Pharmacol. 45*:1033–1045.

69. Laskey, W., Schondorf, R., and Polosa, C. (1979). Intersegmental connections and interactions of myelinated somatic and visceral afferents with sympathetic preganglionic neurons in the unanesthetized spinal cat. *J. Auton. Nerv. Syst. 1*:69–76.

70. Koizumi, K., Collin, R., Kaufman, A., and Brooks, C. McC. (1970). Contribution of unmyelinated afferent excitation to sympathetic reflexes. *Brain Res. 20*:99–106.

71. Horeyseck, G., and Jänig, W. (1974). Reflex activity in postganglionic fibers within skin and muscle nerve elicited by somatic stimuli in chronic spinal cats. *Exp. Brain Res. 21*:155–168.

72. Sato, A., Kaufman, A., Koizumi, K., and Brooks, C. McC. (1969). Afferent nerve groups and sympathetic reflex pathways. *Brain Res. 14*:575–587.

73. Simon, E., and Riedel, W. (1975). Diversity of regional sympathetic nerve activity in integrative cardiovascular control patterns and metabolism. *Brain Res. 87*:323–333.

74. Iriki, M., and Korner, P. I. (1979). Central nervous interactions between chemoreceptor and baroreceptor mechanisms. In *Integrative Functions of the Autonomic Nervous System*, C. McC. Brooks, K. Koizumi, and A. Sato (Eds.), University of Tokyo Press, Tokyo; and Elsevier–North Holland, New York, pp. 415–426.

75. Riedel, W., and Iriki, M. (1979). Autonomic nervous control of temperature homeostasis. In *Integrative Functions of the Autonomic Nervous System*, C. McC. Brooks, K. Koizumi, and A. Sato (Eds.), University of Tokyo Press, Tokyo; and Elsevier–North Holland, New York, pp. 399–414.

76. Kollai, M., and Koizumi, K. (1980). The mechanism of differential control in the sympathetic system studied by hypothalamic stimulation. *J. Auton. Nerv. Syst. 2*:377–389.

77. Jänig, W. (1979). Reciprocal reaction patterns of sympathetic subsystem with respect to various afferent inputs. In *Integrative Functions of the Autonomic Nervous System*, C. McC. Brooks, K. Koizumi, and A. Sato (Eds.), University of Tokyo Press, Tokyo; and Elsevier–North Holland, New York, pp. 263–274.

78. Jänig, W., and Kümmel, H. (1981). Organization of the sympthetic innervation supplying the hairless skin of the cat's paw. *J. Auton. Nerv. Syst. 3*:215–230.

79. Jänig, W., and Szulczyk, P. (1981). The organization of lumbar preganglionic neurons. *J. Auton. Nerv. Syst. 3*:177–191.

80. Purves, D., and Lichtman, J. W. (1978). Formation and maintenance of synaptic connections in autonomic ganglia. *Physiol. Rev. 58*:821–862.

81. Loewy, A. D. (1981). Descending pathways to sympathetic and parasympathetic preganglionic neurons. *J. Auton. Nerv. Syst. 3*:265–275.

82. Saper, C. B. (1979). Anatomical substrates for the hypothalamic control of the autonomic nervous system. In *Integrative Functions of the Autonomic Nervous System*, C. McC. Brooks, K. Koizumi, and A. Sato (Eds.), University of Tokyo Press, Tokyo; and Elsevier–North Holland, New York, pp. 333–341.

83. Hosoya, Y., and Matsushita, M. (1979). Identification and distribution of the spinal and hypophyseal projection neurons in the paraventricular nucleus of the rat. A light and electron microscopic study with the horseradish peroxidase method. *Exp. Brain Res. 35*:315-331.

84. Armstrong, W. E., Warach, S., Hatton, G., and McNeill, T. H. (1980). Subnuclei in the rat hypothalamic paraventricular nucleus: A cytoarchitectural, horseradish peroxidase and immunocytochemical analysis. *Neuroscience 5*:1911-1958.

85. Swanson, L. W., and Kuypers, H. G. J. M. (1980). The paraventricular nucleus of the hypothalamus: Cytoarchitectonic subdivision and organization of projections to the pituitary, dorsal vagal complex, and spinal cord as demonstrated by retrograde fluorescence double-labeling methods. *J. Comp. Neurol. 194*:555-570.

86. Loewy, A. D., and Burton, H. (1978). Nuclei of the solitary tract: Efferent connections to the lower brain stem and the spinal cord of the cat. *J. Comp. Neurol. 181*:421-450.

87. Dembowsky, K., Lackner, K., Czachurski, J., and Seller, H. (1981). Tonic catecholaminergic inhibition of the spinal somato-sympathetic reflex originating in the ventrolateral medulla oblongata. *J. Auton. Nerv. Syst. 3*:277-290.

88. Loewy, A. D., McKellar, S., and Saper, C. B. (1979). Direct projections from the A5 catecholamine cell group to the intermediolateral cell column. *Brain Res. 174*:309-314.

89. Neil, J. J., and Loewy, A. D. (1982). Decrease in blood pressure in response to L-glutamate microinjections into the A5 catecholamine cell group. *Brain Res. 241*:271-278.

90. Coote, J. H., Macleod, V. H., Fleetwood-Walker, S., and Gilbey, M. P. (1981). The response of individual sympathetic preganglionic neurons to microelectrophoretically applied endogenous monoamines. *Brain Res. 215*:135-145.

91. de Groat, W. C., and Ryall, R. W. (1967). An excitatory action of 5-hydroxy-tryptamine on sympathetic preganglionic neurones. *Exp. Brain Res. 3*:299-303.

92. Coote, J. H., Macleod, V. H., and Martin, T. L. (1978). Bulbospinal tryptaminergic neurones, a search for the role of bulbospinal tryptaminergic neurones in the control of sympathetic activity. *Pflugers Arch. 377*:109-116.

93. de Groat, W. C., Nadelhaft, I., Milne, R. J., Booth, A. M., Morgan, C., and Thor, K. (1981). Organization of the sacral parasympathetic reflex pathways to the urinary bladder and large intestine. *J. Auton. Nerv. Syst. 3*: 135-160.

94. de Groat, W. C., Booth, A. M., Milne, R. J., and Roppolo, J. P. (1982). Parasympathetic preganglionic neurons in the sacral spinal cord. *J. Auton. Nerv. Syst. 5*:23-43.

95. Kuzuhara, S., Kanazawa, I., and Nakanishi, T. (1980). Topographical localization of the Onuf's nuclear neurons innervating the rectal and vesical striated sphincter muscles: A retrograde fluorescent double labeling in cat and dog. *Neurosci. Lett. 16*:125-130.

96. Mackel, R. (1979). Segmental and descending control of the external urethral and anal sphincters in the cat. *J. Physiol. (Lond.) 294*:105-122.
97. de Groat, W. C., and Ryall, R. W. (1968). The identification and characteristics of sacral parasympathetic preganglionic neurones. *J. Physiol. (Lond.) 196*:563-578.
98. de Groat, W. C., and Ryall, R. W. (1968). Recurrent inhibition in sacral parasympathetic pathways to the bladder. *J. Physiol. (Lond.) 196*:579-592.
99. de Groat, W. C., and Ryall, R. W. (1969). Reflexes to sacral parasympathetic neurones concerned with micturition in the cat. *J. Physiol. (Lond.) 200*:87-108.
100. Bell, C. (1972). Autonomic nervous control of reproduction: Circulatory and other factors. *Pharmacol. Rev. 24*:657-736.
101. Koizumi, K., and Kollai, M. (1981). Control of reciprocal and nonreciprocal action of vagal and sympathetic efferents: Study of centrally induced reactions. *J. Auton. Nerv. Syst. 3*:483-502.
102. Koizumi, K., Terui, N., Kollai, M., and Brooks, C. McC. (1982). Functional significance of co-activation of vagal and sympathetic cardiac nerves. *Proc. Natl. Acad. Sci. USA* (in press).
103. Archakova, L. I., Bulygin, I. A., and Netukova, N. I. (1982). The ultrastructure organization of sympathetic ganglia of the cat. *J. Auton. Nerv. Syst. 6*:83-93.
104. Libet, B. (1979). Slow postsynaptic actions in ganglionic functions. In *Integrative Functions of the Autonomic Nervous System*, C. McC. Brooks, K. Koizumi, and A. Sato (Eds.), University of Tokyo Press, Tokyo; and Elsevier-North Holland, New York, pp. 197-222.
105. de Groat, W. C., Booth, A. M., and Krier, J. (1979). Interaction between sacral parasympathetic and lumbar sympathetic inputs to pelvic ganglia. In *Integrative Function of the Autonomic Nervous System*, C. McC. Brooks, K. Koizumi, and A. Sato (Eds.), University of Tokyo Press, Tokyo; and Elsevier-North Holland, New York, pp. 234-247.
106. Burnstock, G. (1979). Interactions of cholinergic, adrenergic, purinergic and peptidergic neurons in the gut. In *Integrative Functions of the Autonomic Nervous System*, C. McC. Brooks, K. Koizumi, and A. Sato (Eds.), University of Tokyo Press, Tokyo; and Elsevier-North Holland, New York, pp. 145-158.
107. Wood, J. D. (1979). Neurophysiology of the enteric nervous system. In *Integrative Functions of the Autonomic Nervous System*, C. McC. Brooks, K. Koizumi, and A. Sato (Eds.), University of Tokyo Press, Tokyo; and Elsevier-North Holland, New York, pp. 177-193.
108. Brooks, C. McC. (1934). The resistance of long surviving spinal animals to hypoglycemia induced by insulin. *Am. J. Physiol. 107*:577-583.
109. Brooks, C. McC. (1935). The reaction of chronic spinal animals to hemorrhage. *Am. J. Physiol. 114*:30-39.
110. Jourdan, F. (1936). Prisence de centres adrénalino-sécreteurs dans le moelle cervicale haute chez le Chien. Contribution a la topographie du Systeme nerveaux adrénalino-sécreteur. *Arch. Int. Pharmacodyn. 53*:71-79.

111. Sherrington, C. S. (1924). Notes on temperature after spinal transection with some observations on shivering. *J. Physial. (Lond.) 58*:405–424.

112. Thauer, R. (1935). Wärmeregulation und Fieberfähigkeit nach operativen Eingriffen am Nervensystem homoiothermer Sängetiere. *Pflugers Arch. ges. Physiol. 236*:102–147.

113. Jessen, C. (1967). Auslösung von Hecheln durch isolierte Wärmung des Rückenmarks am wachen Hund. *Pflugers Arch. ges Physiol. 297*:53–70.

114. Iriki, M. (1968). Änderung der Hautdurchblutung bei unnarkotisierten Kaninchen durch isolierte Wärmung des Rückenmarkes. *Pflugers Arch. ges. Physiol. 299*:295–310.

115. Hales, J. R. S., and Jessen, C. (1969). Increase of cutaneous moisture loss caused by local heating of the spinal cord of the ox. *J. Physiol. (Lond.) 204*:40–42P.

116. Brück, K., and Wunnenberg, W. (1966). Beziehung zwischen Thermogenese im "braunen" Fettgewebe Temperatur im cervicalen Anteil des Vertebralkanals im Kältezittern. *Pflugers Arch. ges. Physiol. 290*:167–183.

117. Jessen, C., Simon, E., and Kullmann, R. (1968). Interaction of spinal and hypothalamic thermodetectors in body temperature regulation of the conscious dog. *Experientia 24*:694–695.

118. Rautenberg, W. (1969). Die Bedeutung der zentralnervösen Thermosensitivität für die Temperaturregulation der Taube. *Z. vergl. Physiol. 62*:235–266.

119. Simon, E. (1974). Temperature regulation: The spinal cord as a site of extrahypothalamic thermoregulatory functions. *Rev. Physiol. Biochem. Pharmacol. 71*:1–76.

120. Hardy, J. D., Gagge, A. P., and Stolwijk, J. A. J. (1970). *Physiological and Behavioral Temperature Regulation*, Charles C Thomas, Springfield, Illinois.

121. Hellon, R. F. (1972). Central thermoreceptors and thermoregulation. In *Handbook of Sensory Physiology–Enteroceptors*, vol. III/1, E. Neil (Ed.), Springer-Verlag, Berlin, pp. 161–186.

122. Jeffcoate, S. L., White, N., Bennett, G. W., Edwardson, J. A., Griffiths, E. C., Forbes, R., and Kelly, J. A. (1979). Studies of the release and degradation of hypothalamic releasing hormones by the hypothalamus and other CNS areas *in vitro*. In *Central Regulation of the Endocrine System*, K. Fuxe, T. Hökfelt, and R. Luft, (Eds.), Plenum, New York, pp. 61–70.

123. Fuxe, K., Hökfelt, T., and Luft, R. (Eds.) (1979). *Central Regulation of the Endocrine System*, Plenum, New York.

124. Vale, W., Brazeau, P., Rivier, C., Brown, M., Boss, B., Rivier, J., Burgus, R., Ling, N., and Guillemin, R. (1975). Somatostatin. *Recent Prog. Horm. Res. 31*:365–397.

125. Kobayashi, R. M., Brown, M., and Vale, W. (1977). Regional distribution of neurotensin and somatostatin in rat brain. *Brain Res. 126*:584–588.

126. Hökfelt, T., Elde, R., Johansson, O., Ljungdahl, A., Schultzberg, M., Fuxe, K., Goldstein, M., Nilsson, G., Pernow, B., Terenius, L., Ganten, D., Jeffcoate, S. L., Rehfeld, J., and Said, S. (1978). The distribution of peptide containing neurons in the nervous system. In *Psychopharmacology:*

A Generation of Progress, M. Lipton, A. Di Moscio, and K. Killam (Eds.), Raven, New York, pp. 39–66.

127. Hökfelt, T., Efendic, S., Hellerström, S., Johansson, O., Luft, R., and Arimura, A. (1975). Cellular localization of somatostatin in endocrine-like cells and neurons of the rat with special reference to the A cells of the pancreas islets and to the hypothalamus. *Acta Endocrinol. 80*(Suppl. 200): 5–41.

128. Vale, W., Rivier, C., and Brown, M. (1980). Physiology and pharmacology of hypothalamic regulatory peptides. In *Physiology of the Hypothalamus*, P. J. Morgane and J. Panksepp (Eds.), Marcel Dekker, New York, pp. 165–252.

129. Bezold, A. (1863). *Untersuchungen über die innervation des Harzen*, vol. I, W. Engelmann, Leipzig, pp. 165–328.

130. Tigerstedt, R. (1923). *Die Physiologie des Kreislaufes*, W. de Gruyter, Berlin.

131. Sato, A. (1973). Spinal and medullary reflex components of the somato-sympathetic reflex discharges evoked by stimulation of group IV somatic afferents. *Brain Res. 51*:307–318.

132. Wyszogrodski, I., and Polosa, C. (1973). The inhibition of sympathetic preganglionic neurons by somatic afferents. *Can. J. Physiol. Pharmacol. 51*:29–38.

133. Sherrington, C. (1906). *The Integrative Action of the Nervous System*, Yale University Press, New Haven, Connecticut.

134. Stewart, G. N., and Rogoff, J. M. (1917). The relation of the spinal cord to the spontaneous liberation of epinephrine from adrenals. *J. Exp. Med. 26*:613–637.

135. Takahashi, W. (1931). Zur Lokalizationsfrage der Zentren für die Epinephrinsekretion. *Tohoku J. Exp. Med. 18*:339–381.

136. Brooks, C. McC. (1931). A delimitation of the central nervous mechanisms involved in reflex hyperglycemia. *Proc. Soc. Exp. Biol. Med. 28*:524–526.

137. Brooks, C. McC. (1933). Reflex action of the sympathetic system in the spinal cat. *Am. J. Physiol. 106*:251–266.

138. McDowall, R. J. S. (1956). *The Control of the Circulation of the Blood*, 2nd ed., W. M. Dawson, London, p. 619.

139. Beacham, W. S. (1964). Characteristics of a spinal reflex. *J. Physiol. (Lond.) 173*:431–448.

140. Beacham, W. S., and Perl, E. R. (1964). Background and reflex discharge of sympathetic preganglionic neurons in the spinal cat. *J. Physiol. (Lond.) 172*:400–416.

141. de Groat, W. C., Douglas, J. W., Glass, J., Simons, W., Weimer, B., and Werner, P. (1975). Changes in somato-vesical reflexes during postnatal development in the kitten. *Brain Res. 94*:150–154.

18
LOCAL SPINAL CORD BLOOD FLOW AND OXYGEN METABOLISM

Nariyuki Hayashi* and Barth A. Green   *University of Miami School of Medicine, Miami, Florida*

Richard P. Veraa   *National Spinal Cord Injury Association, Lauderhill, Florida*

The author has been impressed throughout the work by the close structural similarity of the rat to man and by the fact that only the texts on human anatomy were useful when it came to the identification of details of structure (1).

I. INTRODUCTION

The spinal cord of the rat provides an excellent model for the study of blood flow and metabolism, both from the standpoints of similarity of vascular structure to that of the human and the relative availability of experimental animals in large enough numbers to establish statistically significant norms. A traditional difficulty with such studies has been the small size of the rat cord, but recently developed high-resolution microelectrode techniques for hydrogen clearance and oxygen analysis have permitted experimental measurements of local spinal cord blood flow (lSCBF), and local tissue oxygen tension (lTO$_2$), and local tissue oxygen consumption (lTO$_2$C) in very small volumes of tissue as small as specific tracts of rat spinal cord (2–4).

II. HIGH-RESOLUTION HYDROGEN CLEARANCE MEASUREMENTS

The principles of the hydrogen clearance technique were described in 1964 by Auklund et al. (5), and applied to the spinal cord by Kobrine et al. (6). The

---

**Present affiliation*: Nihon University Medical School, Tokyo, Japan

The method is based on the ability to determine the concentration of H_2 by the oxidation of molecular H_2 at the surface of a positively referenced platinum electrode (+400 mV in the studies described here). The measured current is directly proportional to H_2 concentration and permits blood flow measurement by determining the clearance according to the Fick principle. Simultaneous measurement of local spinal cord blood flow and local tissue oxygen tension are derived from the following formula (7):

$$i = 2\,FA\,(K_1 CsO_2 + K_2 CsH_2 O_2)$$

where

    i = electrode current
    F = Faraday's constant
    A = Surface area of electrode tip
    CsO_2 and $CsH_2 O_2$ = surface concentrations of O_2 and $H_2 O_2$, respectively.
    K_1 and K_2 = reaction rate coefficient of O_2 and $H_2 O_2$.

From this, it may be seen that the greater the length of the electrode tip (e.g., > 250 μm), the more stable the measurement. However, by the same token, the less specific and less consistent will be the flow values using the hydrogen washout technique. In the high-resolution results reported by Hayashi et al. (2-4), the electrical current generated at the microelectrode tip (35 μm) is small, so that an increase in amplification of the current was needed to reliably sense 16 pA. In addition, this technique required standardization of the current for each local spinal cord blood flow and local tissue oxygen tension recording site as shown in Figure 1. The high sensitivity of these microelectrodes was made feasible by taking into consideration the standardization of the microelectrode resistance. The resistance is affected by the length and diameter of the insulated shank of the electrode as well as by the shape of the electrode tip in proportion to its length. The exposed length of the electrode tip was, therefore, a critical factor in these studies. It was found that a clean, smooth, and tapered microelectrode tip performed most consistently.

Microelectrode techniques for the measurement of local tissue oxygen tension and blood flows in brain have been reported by Lubbers (8) and Baumgartl et al. (9). However, these techniques cannot consistently measure local spinal cord blood flow because of artifacts associated with respiratory excursions and the corresponding difficulty in establishing blood flow values. In addition, movements of the electrode tip caused by the incompatibility between fixed microelectrode holders and spinal cord physiologic movements created tissue damage around the electrode implantation sites. To minimize these problems, a microelectrode placement technique has been developed that uses a floating clamp technique similar in principle to the adjustable electrode

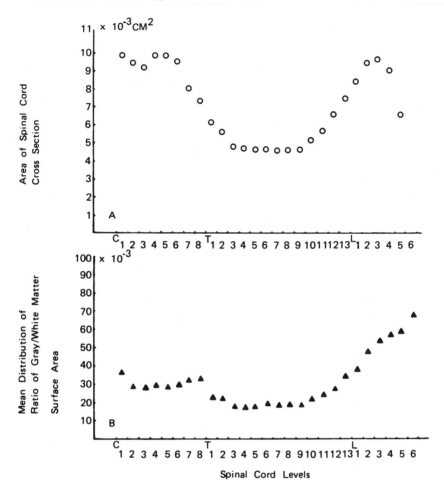

Figure 1 A, Anatomic cross-sectional variations in size of spinal cord at each cord level. B, Mean ratio of gray to white matter cross-sectional area at each cord level.

suspension technique reported by Kobrine et al. (6). The floating clamp is capable of inserting the microelectrode into the tissue and then releasing it. Because of its microsize and weight, the electrode produces little or no distortions of the cord tissue even when the latter moves rhythmically with respirations. Results using the floating clamp approach are illustrated by the data shown in Tables 1 and 2. (See Ref. 2 for a detailed description of these methods.)

Table 1   Spinal Cord Blood Flow (SCBF) and Blood Gases in Rats

Specimen and parameter	Rexed's laminae	lSCBF (ml/100 g/min)	SD[a]	No. of experiments
Gray matter				
	I	39.6	5.44	6
	II	49.4	6.97	12
Dorsal horn	III	53.8	4.12	10
	IV	50.1	7.90	10
	V	52.3	6.18	14
Intermediate gray	VII,X	79.4	4.29	18
	VIII	69.8	2.82	10
Ventral horn	IX	56.2	5.76	8
White matter				
Dorsal funiculus		21.0	3.44	10
Lateral funiculus		18.6	2.80	11
Ventral funiculus		23.3	3.13	5
Mean SCBF				
Gray matter		64.5	5.36	88
White matter		20.4	3.12	26
Interface zone		36.8	3.12	35
Blood gases (mmHg)				
$PaCO_2$		40.7	4.17	46
PaO_2		95.6	9.27	46
pH		7.38	0.052	46
MABP[b] (mmHg)		109.3	13.74	46
Body temperature (°C)		36.5	0.61	46

[a]SD = standard deviation.
[b]MABP = mean arterial blood pressure.

Mean values for gray and white matter local spinal cord blood flow of 64.5 and 20.4 ml/100 g/min are consistent with values of 61.4 and 15.2 reported using [^{14}C]-antipyrine (10) for the measurement of spinal cord blood flow in the rat. Previous spinal cord blood flow measurements obtained by means of hydrogen clearance have reported white matter flows ranging from 10 to 14 ml/100 g/min and gray matter flows slightly higher, ranging from 10.8 to 17.5 ml/10 g/min (6,11,12). These gray matter spinal cord blood flow values are inconsistent with flow values of 48.4–57.6 ml/100 g/min obtained by the use of autoradiographic techniques (10,13,14). It has been suggested that the low values of gray matter blood flow measured by the hydrogen washout method may have been caused by the rapid diffusion of hydrogen gas between gray and

Table 2 Summarized Results of lSCBF, lTO$_2$, and lTO$_2$C in Rat Spinal Cord[a]

	lSCBF (ml/100g/min ± SD)	lTO$_2$ (torr ± SD)	lTO$_2$C (ml/100g/min ± SD)
Cervical spinal cord			
Gray matter	63 ± 5.7	17 ± 4.3	3.5 ± 0.34
White matter	20 ± 3.5	15 ± 5.4	1.1 ± 0.37
Thoracic spinal cord			
Gray matter	62 ± 4.8	19 ± 3.9	3.4 ± 0.59
White matter	19 ± 2.8	16 ± 4.6	1.0 ± 0.01
Lumbar spinal cord			
Gray matter	64 ± 5.1	16 ± 4.7	3.6 ± 0.09
White matter	20 ± 3.3	15 ± 5.2	1.1 ± 0.31
Gray matter ($\bar{X}$)	63 ± 5.2	17 ± 4.2	3.4 ± 0.34
White matter ($\bar{X}$)	20 ± 3.2	15 ± 5.0	1.0 ± 0.23
Number	21	18	18

[a]Local spinal cord blood flow (lSCBF), local tissue oxygen tension (lTO$_2$) and tissue oxygen consumption (lTO$_2$C) in cervical, thoracic, and lumbar spinal cord in the rat.

white matter (15). However, other factors are more significant, such as trauma induced by the size of the electrode during insertion into the spinal cord, the sensitivity of the recording apparatus, the physical configuration of the electrode, including its tip size in relation to the length and diameter of the shaft, its insulation, and the caliber of its connecting wire. It was found, for example, that if the microelectrode bare tip diameter is >35 μm and measures >200 μm in length, gray and white matter flow values may be recorded simultaneously, resulting in falsely lower gray matter flow values. A possible example may be seen from previously reported hydrogen clearance blood flow values for central nervous system gray matter using relatively large bare electrode tips (8,11,16). De la Torre and Boggen (17) used 300-μm electrode tips and reported spinal cord blood flow values in gray matter of 49, while Tamura et al. (18), using 500–1000-μm tips, reported 38 ml/100 g/min. Other studies reported even lower gray matter flow values ranging from 10.8 to 17.5 with electrode tips measuring 1000 μm (6,11).

Spinal cord tissue oxygen tension is considered to be directly proportional to the oxygen supply of the tissue and depends upon the cord's oxygen affinity and the diffusion coefficient for oxygen in the blood and spinal cord. Local tissue oxygen tension also decreases in proportion to spinal cord tissue oxygen consumption in a fashion similar to that reported in brain (19). Consequently, spinal cord tissue oxygen is altered by the balance between oxygen supply and oxygen consumption in the spinal cord. It has been found that local tissue oxygen tension in gray and white matter (14 and 11 torr, respectively) is very similar to reported brain tissue oxygen values of 5-30 torr (20-22).

III. EXTRINSIC BLOOD SUPPLY

The extrinsic blood supply of the rat spinal cord is primarily derived from the spinal radicular arteries (23-25), which arise from extraspinal arteries (C1-C6), the ascending cervical branch of the subclavian (C7-C8), the superior intercostal branch of the subclavian (T1-T2), the intercostal vessels (T3-T2), the intercostal vessels (T3-T12), the lumbar vessels (L1-L4), the low lumbar vessels (L5), and the medial and lateral sacral arteries (S1-S3) (26).

The distribution of the radicular system is variable (2,5,27-29). At the cervical level there are usually two or three vessels of equal size, the most consistently present being at the C6 level (26). In the upper thoracic levels, only one or two small vessels are present. The lower thoracic and lumbar spinal cord levels are supplied by one to three vessels. The most prominent usually lies on the left between L1 and L3 (the artery of Adamkiewicz) (26). The most significant vessels for distal supply accompany the L3-L5 roots.

IV. CONTROL OF LOCAL BLOOD FLOW

Transverse blood flow is in continuity with the bidirectional flow between adjacent radicular arteries via longitudinally directed blood flow on the spinal cord surface. It has been suggested that intrinsic capillary anastomoses provide a protective mechanism for maintenance of local spinal cord blood flow in the face of ischemia caused by obstruction of a singular radicular artery (26).

Reports indicate that central nervous system local blood flow values are dependent upon local blood supply at the capillary level and local tissue metabolic activity (28,29). Therefore, to maintain consistency of mean intrinsic local spinal cord blood flow and metabolism between various cord levels, blood supply must be maintained at the capillary level.

The spinal cord has been categorized as "a long tube of tissue with least susceptibility to anoxia, gram for gram, of any central nervous system tissue" (23), and thus, it must be able to control its intrinsic blood supply in spite of decreased extrinsic vascular supply. This effect is best illustrated at thoracic levels. The decreased size of the thoracic spinal cord allows the maintenance of mean local spinal cord blood flow values similar to those at cervical and lumbar levels in spite of its decreased total spinal cord blood flow. A decrease in the gray to white matter area ratio and the smaller area of the thoracic cord produces a decreased total spinal cord blood flow demand. In addition, the

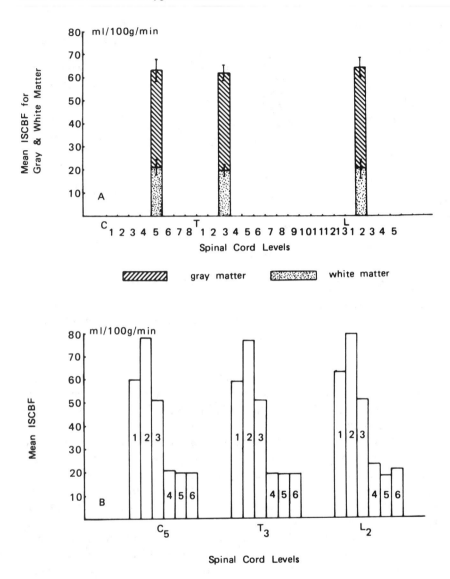

Figure 2 Variations of lSCBF at cervical, thoracic, and lumbar spinal cord levels in the rat. (N = 21). A, Mean lSCBF for gray and white matter at C5, T3, and L2 levels. B, Mean lSCBF at different sites in the gray and white matter at C5, T3, and L2: 1, ventral horn; 2, intermediate gray; 3, dorsal horn; 4, ventral funiculus; 5, lateral funiculus; 6, dorsal funiculus.

Mean Local Spinal Cord
Tissue O_2 Consumption
(ml/100g/min)

Gray Matter [*]
3.41 ± 0.341
(n = 18)

White Matter [**]
1.14 ± 0.061
(n = 15)

Mean Local Spinal Cord
Blood Flow (ml/100g/min)

Gray Matter [*]
63.0 ± 4.29
(n = 18)

White Matter [**]
18.6 ± 2.80
(n = 11)

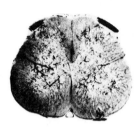

Mean Local Spinal Cord
Tissue O_2 Tension (torr)

Gray Matter [*]   15 ± 4.2   (n = 21)

White Matter [**]   12 ± 5.1   (n = 19)

[*] = Gray Matter (Ventral Horn) ,   [**] = White Matter (Lateral Funiculus)

Figure 3 Microangiogram of the rat spinal cord cross section summarizes normal mean lSCBF, lTO$_2$, and lTO$_2$C values in the gray and white matter (N = 52).

thoracic spinal cord has a unique hemodynamic blood flow pattern that varies from that of cervical and lumbar levels. Variations in spinal cord parenchymal architecture at various levels are shown in Figure 2A. The ratio of gray to white matter area within each spinal cord level is shown in Figure 2B.

White matter area in the thoracic spinal cord is three times greater than gray matter. In the cervical spinal cord it is 1.8 times greater and in the lumbar spinal cord white and gray matter are almost equal. Thus, we can see that demands upon total spinal cord blood flow at the thoracic levels are maintained at lower values than at cervical or lumbar levels because of its specific anatomic architecture.

Variations in intrinsic vasculature among the various human spinal cord levels have been described by Crock and Yoshizawa (30). In the cervical and lumbar regions of the spinal cord dorsal and ventral penetrating arteries lie in a straight line along the horizontal plane. At thoracic levels the central arteries are more widely spaced at the origins along the anterior spinal arteries; they course backward obliquely and branch out. On sagittal section, the main stems of the central thoracic arteries form wedgelike patterns with arteries penetrating the posterior surface of the cord (30). This specific configuration of intrinsic thoracic vessels seems to be very effective in hydrodynamically perfusing a large area with a decreased number of small-caliber vessels.

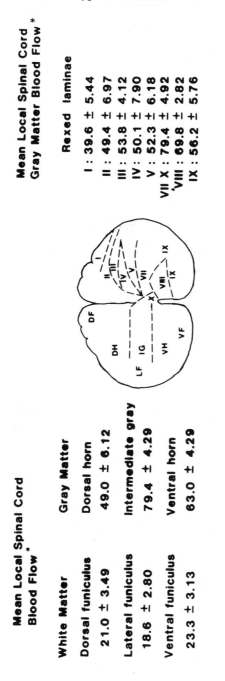

Mean Local Spinal Cord Blood Flow*

White Matter

Dorsal funiculus
21.0 ± 3.49

Lateral funiculus
18.6 ± 2.80

Ventral funiculus
23.3 ± 3.13

Gray Matter

Dorsal horn
49.0 ± 6.12

Intermediate gray
79.4 ± 4.29

Ventral horn
63.0 ± 4.29

Mean Local Spinal Cord Gray Matter Blood Flow*

Rexed laminae

I : 39.6 ± 5.44

II : 49.4 ± 6.97

III : 53.8 ± 4.12

IV : 50.1 ± 7.90

V : 52.3 ± 6.18

VII X : 79.4 ± 4.92

VIII : 69.8 ± 2.82

IX : 56.2 ± 5.76

*: (n = 114)' (blood flow : ml/ 100g/min)

Figure 4 Summary of mean SCBF values in gray and white matter regions are shown on the left side. Right side shows Rexed's laminae blood flow values in the gray matter.

Observed data suggest the existence of specific anatomicophysiologic mechanisms responsible for the maintenance of consistent values for blood flow and oxygen metabolism at all spinal cord levels. There are no differences in mean local spinal cord blood flow and oxygen metabolism values between white and gray matter areas within the cervical, thoracic, and lumbar spinal cord (Figures 3 and 4).

V. INTRINSIC VASCULARIZATION

The intrinsic perfusion arises from the anterior and posterior spinal cord arteries at each segmental level (23). This blood flow pattern is arranged in a two-dimensional system; longitudinally directed flow on the surface of the cord and transversely directed flow within the cord tissue. The intramedullary or transversely directed blood flow is in two different directions: proceeding inwardly from the surface (centripetal system) and outwardly from the spinal cord center (centrifugal system) (31). In the white matter and in the dorsal half of the gray matter, local spinal cord blood flow is provided primarily by the centripetal system. In contrast, the ventral region of the spinal cord gray matter derives its flow from the centrifugal system. The directional pattern of gray matter blood flow may correspond to the direction of neuronal transmission.

Normal spinal cord blood flow is maintained by autoregulation with average values of 63 ml/100 g/min in the gray matter and 18.6 ml/100 g/min in the white matter, whereas local spinal O_2 consumption maintains the same 3:1 ratio with values of 3.41 and 1.14 ml/100 g/min, respectively (3). The difference in these flow values may be dependent upon the metabolic demands and morphologic arrangement of specific neuronal groups. Regionally, vascular density is higher in the gray than in the white matter and in the ventral half of the gray matter (centrifugal arterial system) than in the dorsal half (centripetal system) (27). These bidirectional arterial systems allow the formation of a rich vascular bed in the gray matter. On the other hand, the gray matter venous outflow is by means of five intraparenchymal venous roots in the dorsal funiculus, dorsal horn, lateral funiculus, ventral horn, and ventral spinal fissure (30,32). The gray matter, therefore, is hydrodynamically perfused in a heterogeneous flow pattern.

Studies by Hayashi et al. (3) show that local spinal cord blood flow in the intermediate gray (Rexed's laminae VII and X) and in the ventral horn (lamina VIII) was 69-79 ml/100 g/min. These values are higher than those found in the motoneuron pool (lamina IX) (56 ml/100 g/min) and higher than those in the more dorsal regions of the cord (laminae III-V) (52 ml/100 g/min). The high blood flow area is concentrated around the internuncial cell region of the gray matter. The dorsal horn of the gray matter has been designated laminae I-IV. It has been found that local spinal cord blood flow in the marginal zone and substantia gelatinosa (laminae I and II) is lower than that seen in more ventral areas (laminae III–V). Lamina I, in particular, is about 10 ml lower than other dorsal horn areas. It is possible that this difference results from the fact that local spinal cord blood flow in lamina I is measured in so small an area that H_2 escaped into the subarachnoid space and produced errors in studies using the H_2 clearance method.

In white matter, blood flow is also supplied by two systems composed of peripheral arteries (centripetal system) and central arteries (centrifugal system) (24). Most of the blood flow to the white matter is supplied by the centripetal system. The peripheral arteries in the white matter form a rich anastomotic network on the surface of the spinal cord and send central penetrating branches to all levels of spinal cord tissue (25,26). It would seem, therefore, that the hydrodynamic distribution of local blood flow in the white matter depends mainly on the surface vascularization of the cord, unlike the hydrodynamic vascular distribution in the gray. Hayashi et al. (3) found that the white matter hydrogen washout curves were all monoexponential except in the area interfacing with the gray matter, where 68% of washout curves were found to be biexponential and 32% monoexponential. This may reflect the bidirectional nature of the system in this "watershed" zone of spinal cord white matter (23). The mean values of white matter blood flow in the centripetal arterial feeding areas and in the interface zone were 20 and 38 ml/100 g/min, respectively. However, the interface zone is such a small area that the possibility of simultaneous recording of gray and white matter may have occurred. Thus, the observed local spinal cord blood flow values for the interface zone may not reflect a true measurement of that region.

In addition to the higher vascular density and metabolic activity of the intermediate gray and lamina VIII in the ventral horn area, these regions are also highest in catecholaminergic nerve terminals as evaluated by fluorescence microscopy (32). The relationship of high blood flow to high concentrations of transmitter is similar to that reported for areas in the hypothalamus where regions of high vascular density such as the supraoptic and paraventricular nuclei also contain the highest catecholamine terminal concentrations. However, the precise relationship between density of vascular networks and concentration of transmitters is a matter of speculation.

VI. CONCLUSION

In summary, we may view the spinal cord, both of rats and humans, as an exquisite example of autoregulation of blood flow to meet metabolic requirements. A better understanding of the regulatory mechanisms involved will bring us a great deal closer to comprehending the function of the spinal cord.

REFERENCES

1. Greene, E. C. (1963). *Anatomy of the Rat*. Hafner, New York.
2. Hayashi, N., Green, B. A., Mora, J., Gonzales-Carvajal, M., and Veraa, R. P. (1983). Simultaneous measurement of local blood flow and tissue oxygen in rat spinal cord. *Neurol. Res. 5*:49–57.
3. Hayashi, N., Green, B. A., Gonzales-Carvajal, M., Mora, J., and Veraa, R. P. (1983). Local blood flow, oxygen tension and oxygen consumption in the rat spinal cord. I: Oxygen metabolism and neuronal function. *J. Neurosurg. 58*:516–525.
4. Hayashi, N., Green, B. A., Gonzales-Carvajal, M., Mora, J., and Veraa, R. P. (1983). Local blood flow, oxygen tension and oxygen consumption in the rat spinal cord. II: Relation to segmental level. *J. Neurosurg. 58*:526–530.
5. Auklund, K., Bower, B. F., and Berliner, R. W. (1964). Measurement of local blood flow with hydrogen gas. *Circ. Res. 14*:164–187.
6. Kobrine, A. I., Doyle, T. F., and Martins, A. N. (1976). Spinal cord blood flow in the rhesus monkey by the hydrogen clearance method. *Surg. Neurol. 2*:197–200.
7. Tang, T. W., Barr, R. E., Murphy, V. G., and Hahn, N. W. (1977). A working equation for oxygen sensing disk electrodes. In *Oxygen Transport to Tissue* vol. III, I. A. Silver (Ed.), Plenum, New York, pp. 9–15.
8. Lubbers, D. W. (1967). Regional cerebral blood flow and micro-circulation. In *Blood Flow Through Organs and Tissues: Proceedings of an International Conference*. W. H. Bain, and A. M. Harper (Eds.), Williams & Wilkins, Baltimore, pp. 162–168.
9. Baumgartl, H., Grunewald, W., and Lubbers, D. W. (1974). Polarographic determination of the oxygen partial pressure field by Pt microelectrodes using the O_2 field in front of a Pt microelectrode as a model. *Pflugers Arch. 347*:49–61.
10. Rivlin, A. S., and Tator, C. H. (1978). Regional spinal cord blood flow in rats after severe cord trauma. *J. Neurosurg. 49*:844–853.
11. Griffiths, I. R., Rowan, J. O., and Crawford, R. A. (1975). Flow in the gray and white matter of the spinal cord measured by a hydrogen clearance technique. In *Blood Flow and Metabolism in the Brain: Proceedings of the 7th International Symposium on Cerebral Blood Flow and Metabolism*. A. M. Harper, W. B. Jennet, J. D. Miller, and J. O. Rowen (Eds.), Churchill Livingston, Edinburgh, pp. 4.20–4.21.
12. Senter, H. J., Burgess, D. L., and Metzler, J. (1978). An improved technique for measurement of spinal cord blood flow. *Brain Res. 149*:197–203.
13. Bingham, W. G., Goldman, H., Friedman, S. J., Murphy, S., Yashon, D., and Hunt, W. E. (1975). Blood flow in normal and injured monkey spinal cord. *J. Neurosurg. 43*:162–171.
14. Sandler, A. N., and Tator, C. H. (1975). The effect of spinal cord trauma on spinal cord blood flow in primates. In *Blood Flow and Metabolism in the Brain: Proceedings of the 7th International Symposium on Cerebral Blood*

Flow and Metabolism. A. M. Harper, W. B. Jennet, J. D. Miller, and J. O. Rowen (Eds.), Churchill Livingston, Edinburgh, pp. 4.22–4.26.

15. Halsey, J. H., Capra, N. F., and McFarland, R. S. (1977). Use of hydrogen for measurement of regional cerebral blood flow. *Stroke 8*:351–357.

16. Morawetz, R. B., DiGirolami, V., Ojeman, R. G., and Marcous, F. W. (1978). Cerebral blood flow determined by hydrogen clearance during middle cerebral artery occlusion in unanesthetized monkeys. *Stroke 9*: 143–149.

17. de la Torre, J. C., and Boggan, J. E. (1980). Neurophysiological recording in rat spinal cord trauma. *Exp. Neurol. 70*:356–370.

18. Tamura, A., Asano, T., and Sano, K. (1978). Measurement of spinal cord blood flow in rabbits: Central gray matter flow and CO_2 reactivity. *Brain and Nerve 30*:383–386.

19. Hayashi, N., de la Torre, J. C., and Green, B. A. (1980). Regional spinal cord blood flow and tissue oxygen content after spinal cord trauma. *Surg. Forum 31*:461–463.

20. Kessler, M. (1974). Oxygen supply to tissue in normoxia and in oxygen deficiency. *Microvas. Res. 8*:283–290.

21. Leninger-Follert, E., and Hossman, K. A. (1977). Microflow and cortical oxygen pressure during and after prolonged cerebral flow. *Stroke 8*:351–357.

22. Lubbers, D. W. (1967). Regional cerebral blood flow and microcirculation. In *Blood Flow Through Organs and Tissues: Proceedings of an International Conference*. W. H. Bain, and A. M. Harper (Eds.), Williams & Wilkins, Baltimore, pp. 162–168.

23. Schlossberger, P. (1974). Vasculature of the spinal cord: A review. I. Anatomy and physiology. *Bull. L.A. Neurol. Soc. 39*:71–84.

24. Turnbull, I. M., Brieg, A., and Nassler, O. (1966). Blood supply of the cervical spinal cord in man. *J. Neurosurg. 24*:951–965.

25. Wollen, D. H. M., and Millen, J. W. (1955). The arterial supply of the spinal cord and its significance. *J. Neurol. Neurosurg. Psychiat. 18*:97–102.

26. Tveten, L. (1976). Spinal cord vasculature. *Acta Radiol. (Diagn.) 17*:385–398.

27. Jellinger, K. (1974). Comparative studies on spinal cord vasculature. In *Pathology of Cerebral Microcirculation*. J. Cervos-Navarro (Ed.), Walter de Gruytor, Berlin, pp. 45–58.

28. Espagno, J., and Lazorthes, Y. (1970). Blood flow of the cerebral cortex related to anatomical electroencephalography and angiographic data. In *Recent Advances in the Study of Cerebral Circulation*. J. M. Taveras, H. Fishgold, and D. Dilengo (Eds.), Charles C Thomas, Springfield, Illinois, pp. 112–118.

29. Sokoloff, L. (1961). Local cerebral circulation at rest and during altered activity induced by anesthesia or visual stimulation. In *The Regional Chemistry, Physiology, and Pharmacology of the Nervous System*. Pergamon Press, Oxford, pp. 107–117.

30. Crock, H. V., and Yoshizawa, H. (1977). *The Blood Supply of the Vertebral Column and Spinal Cord in Man*, Springer-Verlag, New York, pp. 114–117.
31. Hukuda, S., and Wilson, C. B. (1972). Experimental cervical myelopathy; effects of compression and ischemia on the canine cervical cord. *J. Neurosurg. 37*:631–652.
32. Gillilan, L. A. (1970). Vein of the spinal cord. *Neurology 20*:860–867.

AUTHOR INDEX

Numbers in parentheses are reference numbers and indicate that an author's work is referred to although the name is not cited in text. Italic numbers give page on which the complete reference is listed.

A

Abdelmoumene, M., 140(22), 152 (86), 155(86), 158(86), 165 (22,86), *170*, *174*, 424(329), *455*, 768(54–56), 770(54,55), 771(54,55), 772(54,55), *776*, *777*

Acuna, C., 711(195), *745*

Adair, R., 410(199), *447*

Adam, D., 525(469, 470), *557*, 640 (87), *646*

Adam, J. E. R., 627(63), *645*

Adams, D. J., 221(92), 224(92), *241*

Adams, P. R., 214(77), 221(90, 91), *240*, *241*

Adams, R. J., 142(33), 143(33), *170*, 183(60), *196*

Adrian, E. D., 91(175), 94(190), *125*, *126*, 305(107), *314*, 788 (32), *809*

Aitken, J. T., 200(5), *236*, 245(15), *262*, 317(33), *373*

Ake, N., 412(216), *448*

Akert, K., 386(26–28), *437*

Albe-Fessard, D., 687(85a), *738*

Albert, A., 90(168), *124*, 190(78), *197*

Aldskogius, H., 34(33), *45*, 82(86), *120*

Aléonard, P., 424(329), *455*

Alger, B. E., 258(77), *266*, 385(8), *436*

Allum, J. H. J., 595(144), *607*

Alnaes, E., 107(321), *133*, 488(252), *543*

Altman, J., 659(150, 151), *671*

Alvarez-Feefmans, F. J., 359(181), *382*

Alvord, E. C., 619(27), *643*

Anastasijevic, R., 473(132, 133), 481 (132, 133, 193), 489(132, 193), 506(193), *536*, *540*

Anden, N. E., 401(121), 417(257), 421(257), *443*, *451*, 491(276), *545*

Andersen, P., 702(168), 720(247), *743*, *748*

Anderson, E. G., 415(246), 417(267), *450*, *451*

Anderson, F. D., 83(91), *120*

Anderson, J. H., 589(128), 593(128), *606*

Anderson, M. E., 369(204), *384*

Anderson, P., 424(324, 325), *455*

Anderson, S. A., 702(164, 168), *743*

Anderson, S. D., 167(119), *176*

Andersson, O., 659(125, 126, 138), 660(125, 126, 130), *669*, *670*

Andreassen, S., 629(72), 631(76), *645*

831

Homma, S., 473(146, 147), 481(194, 196-199), *537, 540*
Hong, T., 90(171), 91(181), 94(181), 102(171), 109(171), *124, 125*
Hongell, A., 788(27), *809*
Hongo, T., 105(297), 109(327), *132, 134,* 157(94), *174,* 182 (34), 192(86), *194, 197,* 316 (23, 26), 317(23, 26), 318(26), 320(23, 26), 324(26), 326(23, 26), 328(23, 26), 345(26), 328 (23, 26), 345(26), 370(207, 208), *372, 373, 384,* 397(91), 398(88, 89, 91), 399(91), 400 (109, 112), 401(91, 109, 112), 417(268), 424(331), *441, 442, 451, 456* 485(217, 223), 495 (308), 496(308), 509(373), 514 (407), *541, 547, 551, 553*
Horch, K. W., 84(125), 91(125), 96 (125), 98(125), 100(125), *122,* 681(42), 682(42), 726(42), *735*
Horcholle-Bossauit, G., 258(70), *265*
Hore, J., 720(249), 721(249), *748*
Horeyseck, G., 794(71), *812*
Horridge, G. A., 48(2), 50(2), 51(2), 52(2), *73*
Horsley, V., 406(164), *445*
Hösli, E., 412(221), *449*
Hösli, L., 412(221), 429(342), *449, 456*
Hosoya, Y., 142(32), *170,* 183(59), *196,* 759(28), *775,* 795(83), *813*
Hossman, K. A., 822(21), *829*
Hostetter, G., 698(148), 729(148), *742*
Hotson, J. R., 212(71), *240*
Houk, J., 107(322), 109(322), *133*
Houk, J. C., 360(189), 361(189), *383,* 401(121a), *443,* 561(14), 570(14), 571(64, 67, 68), 573 (64, 67, 68, 70), 574(68), 576 (64, 68), 579(68, 70), 585(108, 111, 112), 586(111, 112, 117), 587(111), 588(111), 589(111),

[Houk, J. C.] 590(131), 592(131), 593(137), 595(142), 597(14), *599, 602, 604-607,* 610(1), 613(14), 614 (14) 615(14), 618(19, 20), 620 (39), 625(14), 626(14), 628(14, 68), 629(14, 68-70), 630(73), 631(73), 633(78), 635(4), 636 (39), 637(39), *641, 642, 643, 646*
House, C. R., 142(36), *170*
Howard, E. R., 783(7), *808*
Howe, J. F., 681(47), 687(47), *736*
Howland, B., 351(154), *380,* 407 (191), 431(191), *447*
Hu, J. W., 752(6), 753(6), 754(6), 755(6), 757(6), 759(29), 760 (29), 761(6, 29), 764(6), 768 (6), *773, 775*
Huang, S. P., 167(124), *176*
Hubbard, J. I., 105(302), *132,* 352 (164), *381*
Hubbard, J. L., 56(26), *74,* 517(422, 425), 518(422), 519(422), *554*
Huber, G. C., 48(1), 50(1), 51(1), 52 (1), *73*
Hughes, J., 403(137, 138), *444*
Hulliger, M., 566(41), 573(72), 574 (72), 575(41, 72, 75), 579(95), *600, 602, 604,* 617(18), *642*
Hultborn, H., 101(272-274), 106 (272-274), *130,* 181(23), 192 (93), *193, 198,* 388(46), 397 (74-76, 79, 80, 83-85), 398(46, 74, 79, 80, 83-87, 90), 399(75, 76, 83), 402(76), 419(76), *438, 440-442,* 461(23), 464(58, 69), 466(58), 472(124), 473(148, 149), 473(165), 476(165), 479 (124), 485(58, 226), 499(165, 323), 500(69, 323), 501(23, 69, 226), 502(330), 504(330), 505 (23), 511(58, 226, 388, 389), 512(58, 69, 226, 386, 388, 389, 391, 391a, 392, 394-396), 513 (58, 69, 226, 388, 399, 403,

SUBJECT INDEX

A

Accessory cuneate nucleus, 25, 50
Accessory olivary nucleus, 35
Accommodation, 205, 206
Acetylcholine, 463, 471, 797
Action potential, 201–203, 211, 212,
    214, 215, 218, 225–228, 233,
    255, 477, 685
autonomic nervous system, 788
dendrite, 260
initial segment spike, 201–203,
    206, 214–215, 225–228, 233,
    785
motoneuron, 328, 500
muscle spindle, 566
soma-dendritic spike (SD spike),
    201–203, 214–215, 225–228,
    233, 785
spike threshold, 205, 231–233, 235
Achilles tendon, 561
Actomyosin, 613, 634
Acupuncture, 763
Adaptation, 204
Adenosine triphosphatase (ATPase),
    285–287, 292, 294, 295, 563
Adiadokokinesis, 716
Adrenal medulla, 782, 783
A-fiber reflex, 798, 805
Afterhyperpolarization (AHP)
  alpha motoneurons, 499, 500, 504

[Afterhyperpolarization (AHP)]
  gamma motoneurons, 507, 508
  motoneuron, 203, 212, 217, 219–
    231, 255, 260, 306
  sympathetic preganglionic neurons,
    785, 788, 790, 796
  Renshaw cell, 471
Aganglionosis, 783
Alar plate, 48
Alpha-gamma coactivation, 399
Alpha-response, 492, 493, 497
4-Aminopyridine, 219, 350
Ammonium ion, 390, 391, 393, 396
Amphicytes, 17
Amygdaloid nucleus, 42
Amyotrophic lateral sclerosis, 783
Analgesia, 765
Anastomoses, 822
Anesthetics, 342, 343
Angiotensin, 434
Anomalous rectification, 212, 214,
    219
Antenna neurons, 142
Anterior funiculus, 21, 22, 37, 40,
    41 (see also Ventral funiculus)
Anterior horn, 22, 52, 59, 65, 67,
    70, 71, 200 (see also Ventral
    horn)
Anterior horn cells (see Motoneurons)
Anterior horn nuclear group, 213
Anterior median fissure, 7, 8